MW00452733

# Handbook of
# MIND-BODY
# MEDICINE
## for Primary Care

# Handbook of
# MIND - BODY
# MEDICINE
# for Primary Care

## Editors

### Donald Moss
Western Michigan Behavioral Health Services,
Grand Haven and Muskegon, Michigan

### Angele McGrady
Medical College of Ohio

### Terence C. Davies
Eastern Virginia Medical School

### Ian Wickramasekera

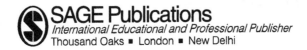
**SAGE Publications**
*International Educational and Professional Publisher*
Thousand Oaks ▪ London ▪ New Delhi

*For information:*

Sage Publications, Inc.
2455 Teller Road
Thousand Oaks, California 91320
E-mail: order@sagepub.com

Sage Publications Ltd.
6 Bonhill Street
London EC2A 4PU
United Kingdom

Sage Publications India Pvt. Ltd.
M-32 Market
Greater Kailash I
New Delhi 110 048 India


**Library of Congress Cataloging-in-Publication Data**


Handbook of mind-body medicine for primary care / edited by  Donald Moss ... [et. al.].
    p. cm.
Includes bibliographical references and index.
ISBN 0-7619-2323-3 (c : alk. paper)
   1. Medicine, Psychosomatic—Handbooks, manuals, etc. 2. Mind and body therapies—Handbooks, manuals, etc. 3.  Biofeedback training—Handbooks, manuals, etc. I. Moss, Donald, Ph. D.
RC49 .H327 2002
616.08—dc21
2002008957


This book is printed on acid-free paper.

03  04  05  06  10  9  8  7  6  5  4  3  2  1

| | |
|---|---|
| *Acquisitions Editor:* | Jim Brace-Thompson |
| *Editorial Assistant:* | Karen Ehrmann |
| *Production Editor:* | Sanford Robinson |
| *Copy Editor:* | Barbara McGowran |
| *Typesetter:* | C&M Digitals (P) Ltd. |
| *Indexer:* | Teri Greenberg |
| *Cover Designer:* | Michelle Lee |

# Contents

Foreword: Common Problems in Primary Care: The Need
for a New Biopsychosocial and Psychophysiological Model   ix

TERENCE C. DAVIES AND FRANK V. DEGRUY, III

## Part I. Models and Concepts for Mind-Body Medicine   1

1   Mind-Body Medicine, Evidence-Based Medicine, Clinical
    Psychophysiology, and Integrative Medicine   3
    DONALD MOSS

2   The High Risk Model of Threat Perception and
    the Trojan Horse Role Induction: Somatization
    and Psychophysiological Disease   19
    IAN WICKRAMASEKERA

3   Psychophysiological Foundations of the Mind-Body
    Therapies   43
    ANGELE MCGRADY

4   Complementary, Alternative, and Integrative Medicine   57
    JAMES LAKE

5   The Placebo Effect and Its Use in Biofeedback Therapy   69
    IAN WICKRAMASEKERA

6   A Comprehensive Approach to Primary Care Medicine:
    Mind and Body in the Clinic   83
    TERENCE C. DAVIES

7   Professional Ethics and Practice Standards
    in Mind-Body Medicine   93
    SEBASTIAN STRIEFEL

# Part II. Basic Clinical Tools    107

8    **Biofeedback and Biological Monitoring**    109
CHRISTOPHER GILBERT AND DONALD MOSS

9    **Neurofeedback, Neurotherapy, and Quantitative EEG**    123
THEODORE J. LA VAQUE

10    **Progressive Relaxation, Autogenic Training, and Meditation**    137
PAUL LEHRER AND PATRICIA CARRINGTON

11    **Hypnotherapy**    151
IAN WICKRAMASEKERA

12    **Cognitive-Behavioral Therapies for the Medical Clinic**    167
MARK A. LAU, ZINDEL V. SEGAL, AND ARI E. ZARETSKY

13    **Acupuncture**    181
EMANUEL STEIN

14    **Spirituality and Healing**    191
STANLEY KRIPPNER

# Part III. Applications to Common Disorders    203

15    **The Biobehavioral Treatment of Headache**    205
STEVEN M. BASKIN AND RANDALL E. WEEKS

16    **Temporomandibular Disorders and Facial Pain**    223
ALAN G. GLAROS AND LEONARD LAUSTEN

17    **Asthma**    235
PAUL LEHRER, MAHMOOD SIDDIQUE, JONATHAN FELDMAN,
AND NICHOLAS GIARDINO

18    **Coronary Disease and Congestive Heart Disorder**    249
NARAS BHAT AND KUSUM BHAT

19    **Back Pain: Musculoskeletal Pain Syndrome**    259
GABRIEL E. SELLA

20    **The Metabolic Syndrome: Obesity, Type 2 Diabetes,
Hypertension, and Hyperlipidemia**    275
ANGELE McGRADY, RAYMOND BOUREY, AND BARBARA BAILEY

21  Functional Bowel and Anorectal Disorders  299
    OLAFUR S. PALSSON AND ROBERT W. COLLINS

22  Urinary Incontinence  313
    OLAFUR S. PALSSON

23  Fibromyalgia  323
    C. C. STUART DONALDSON AND GABRIEL E. SELLA

24  Chronic Fatigue Syndrome  333
    CHARLES W. LAPP

25  Attention Deficit Hyperactivity Disorder  347
    JOEL F. LUBAR

26  Anxiety Disorders  359
    DONALD MOSS

27  Mood Disorders  377
    ELSA BAEHR AND J. PETER ROSENFELD

28  Sleep and Sleep Disorders  393
    SUZANNE WOODWARD

29  Rheumatoid Arthritis  407
    CHERYL BOURGUIGNON AND DIANA TAIBI

30  Premenstrual Syndrome and Premenstrual
    Dysphoric Disorder  419
    ANNABAKER GARBER

31  Caring for the Person With a Chronic Condition  429
    SHARON WILLIAMS UTZ

Part IV. Education for Mind-Body Medicine  441

32  Medical Education for Mind-Body Medicine  443
    MARGARET DAVIES AND OLAFUR S. PALSSON

33  Nursing Education for Mind-Body Nursing  449
    DEBRA E. LYON AND ANN GILL TAYLOR

34  The Professional Role and Education of Physician
    Assistants in Mind-Body Medicine  457
    ROBERT W. JARSKI

35  The Behavioral Health Provider in Mind-Body Medicine  467
    RICHARD GEVIRTZ

36  Existential and Spiritual Dimensions of Primary Care: Healing the
    Wounded Soul  477
    DONALD MOSS

    Author Index  489

    Subject Index  517

    About the Editors  535

    About the Contributors  537

# Foreword: Common Problems in Primary Care

*The Need for a New Biopsychosocial and Psychophysiological Model*

**Abstract:** The foreword introduces the importance of primary care in health care and the central place of mind-body problems within primary care. The authors, both educators in primary care medicine, define primary care and review its scientific and intellectual paradigm. They describe the role of managed care organizations in increasing the importance of primary care within American health care, enlarging the function of the primary care physician, and creating incentives that redirect the priorities and resources of primary care. Mental health is indivisible from physical health, and the authors see mental health problems as a major challenge for primary care. Finally, the authors project their vision for primary care and the need for a practical, integrated mind-body approach to health care within the one undivided house of primary care.

## INTRODUCTION

The case for primary care as an obligation of society is derived from the special vulnerability and the universal fact of illness. This vulnerability generates a need that takes on the substance of a relative right because of the promises inherent in our social and political structures.

We have, in a sense, all made a set of mutual promises to guarantee to each other a certain kind of society, one which is sensitive to and secures those things closest to our needs as humans. We would break our communal promise, tell a communal lie, and live an inauthentic social life if we neglected to exert every effort to assure the minimum security of access to primary care whenever it is needed. (Pellegrino & Thomasma, 1981, p. 243)

The necessity for sick people to have access to healers is such a fundamental reality that we might wonder why it was not included within the founding fathers' Bill of Rights. In the ongoing dispute regarding government-provided universal health care, many people support the viewpoint of Pellegrino and Thomasma (1981), who maintain that primary health care services, at least, should be "the minimum security of access . . . whenever it is needed" (p. 243). However, this belief leaves unstated a definition of the scope and responsibility of primary health care, and in view of the currently inadequate level of support for mental health services at a primary care level (by both practicing clinicians and third-party payors), one is left to question the potential sufficiency of a future response to societal needs for mind-body treatments, even within a universally insured, primary care–oriented government health care system.

The centrality of primary care within a well-functioning health care system is by this time indisputable. Most of the world's countries have established their health care systems around a solid core of primary care, and in a comparison of 12 different Western industrialized nations, Starfield (1994) demonstrated that countries with a stronger orientation to primary care were indeed more likely to have better health levels and lower costs. Sadly, the United States spends more money on its health care system than any other country, and yet because of the inadequacy of its primary care services, it is ranked behind many countries whose overall health care expenditures are far less (Starfield, 1994). Even within the British National Health Service, which has suffered such extremities of financial shortcoming that rationing of some specialized services became a necessity, the ready availability of general practice care has been held sacrosanct. If primary health care is destined to become a universal "right," it is imperative that the human health problems encompassed by primary care be researched and managed to the highest degree possible so that maximum benefit can result—for optimal cost, to the greatest number. An ever increasing body of research now reveals that a majority of these health problems can be defined in terms of mind-body illness, and therefore the publication of this work, at this point in time, becomes a matter of considerable significance.

This is an ambitious volume. It would be enough to pull together a coherent inventory of the common problems that arise at the interface between mind and body. It would be more than enough to then create a compendium of the tools that are useful against these problems. The authors have done all that and more; they have gone on to describe the use of these methods in primary care settings, where indeed they are most needed. They imply that our system of primary care should be able to accommodate these methods but that we may need to develop a new model of health care to do so. In our opinion, this is a correct interpretation, although it will not be easy. This foreword will describe a few elements of primary care—what it is, where it came from, how it fits into the larger house of medicine, what can be accomplished there—so we can understand how the principles of psychophysiological medicine can be incorporated into the primary health care of patients.

Before proceeding further, we want to state that we will make no apology for the fact that much of this volume will be construed by many to be contentious. If the place and relevance of primary care services in the scheme of things is a matter of continued debate, then the proper role and significance of many mind-body and complementary and alternative medicine (CAM) therapies is even more controversial. Equally controversial will be many of the interpretations and philosophies associated with the practice of the clinical methods that are discussed in this volume. As commentators, we have even suggested that a more appropriate title for this book might have been *A Handbook of Controversies in Mind-Body Medicine and Primary Care Practice*, but this is not to detract from the timeliness and importance of this body of work. As discussed later, primary care and mental health go hand in hand; therefore, an assessment of mind-body practices within the field of primary care medicine is long overdue. But this is "cutting-edge" knowledge that often defies rigorous definition. Hence, controversy is inevitable—and in the best spirit of intellectual advancement, it should be welcomed!

## A DEFINITION OF PRIMARY CARE

In 1996, the Institute of Medicine published the findings of its Committee on the Future of Primary Care in a volume entitled *Primary Care: America's Health in a New Era* (Donaldson et al., 1996). The committee recommended adoption of the following definition of primary care:

> Primary care is the provision of integrated, accessible health care services by clinicians who are accountable for addressing a large majority of personal health care needs, developing a sustained partnership with patients, and practicing in the context of family and community. (p. 1)

The committee elaborated on this definition by describing six core attributes that characterize primary care:

1. Excellent primary care is grounded in both the biomedical and the social sciences.

2. Clinical decision making in primary care differs from that in specialty care.

3. Primary care has at its core a sustained personal relationship between patient and clinician.

4. Primary care does not consider mental health separately from physical health.

5. Important opportunities to promote health and prevent disease are intrinsic to primary care practice.

6. Primary care is information intensive.

These six characteristics of primary care provide a frame of reference that will assist the reader in understanding this book's topic material.

## SCIENTIFIC AND INTELLECTUAL BASIS OF PRIMARY CARE

Medical specialties have arisen because they were necessary, because they were possible, because it made sense to divide medicine's work along certain lines. Therefore, we should not demand of any medical specialty too high a standard of conceptual coherence. Primary care, which emerged just over 30 years ago as a medical specialty in the form of family practice, turns out to be extraordinarily useful to any health care system, and its shape has as much to do with what needs to be done and who is around to do it as with intellectual consistency. Since primary care has become defined as a specialty of breadth, of personal relationship, and of continuity, then it follows that certain approaches to understanding the problems and getting the work done are better suited than others. Although the reductionistic approach to scientific inquiry has catapulted medicine into an era of unprecedented progress, many clinical problems are resistant to reductionistic methods, and primary care is a clinical domain where much of this resistant material is found. Dubos (1971) has called reductionism "the doctrine of specific etiology," but it is well recognized that chronic diseases (which now constitute over half of all illnesses) are inevitably multifactorial in origin. In addition, much of human morbidity is associated with personal and social behaviors that directly damage health; and behavior-related illness cannot be understood or managed within a reductionistic paradigm. Consequently, medicine is still only capable of curing, in a specific and permanent fashion, less than one-fifth of the total burden of human disease. Nowhere is this statistic more evident than in primary care.

George Engel (1977) introduced a concept that expanded or augmented the biomedical approach, naming it the biopsychosocial model. The biopsychosocial paradigm represents an extrapolation of the work of Ludwig von Bertalanffy, the father of general system theory. Von Bertalanffy may be one of the least appreciated intellectuals of the 20th century; although he was nominated for a Nobel Prize in 1972, he died before his nomination could be considered (Davidson, 1983). Briefly, Engel elaborated a model that conceptualized a hierarchy of factors or variables that influenced health and disease. In addition to the biomedical, with its impetus to look for explanations at progressively "lower," or "simpler" levels of analysis—organ to tissue to cell to gene, and so on—he elaborated a set of "upward" levels—the psychological and social—that held equal sway over the course of human illness and disease. Moreover, these different levels of interaction themselves interact with one another such that psychological distress, for example, can be expected to affect endocrine function, or social isolation can be expected to affect the course of tuberculosis. This reformulation has huge implications for what becomes the legitimate business of clinicians, and nowhere has this new paradigm affected the fundamental assumptions of a clinical discipline more than in family medicine.

Applying this contextual orientation of general systems theory to family medicine, some early advocates drew attention to the potential clinical application of Bowen's family system theory (Bowen, 1966; Christie-Seely, 1981). Use of the "relational genogram" to analyze and understand family group morbidity was promoted (Crouch & Roberts, 1987), and at least one attempt was made to link intrafamilial system developments on a time-measured scale (Rainford & Schuman, 1981). While this perspective has withstood the challenges of the past two decades, it has only gained an uneven purchase as an organizing conceptual model for medicine at large, and even the primary care disciplines have not yet evolved a particularly coherent clinical posture that follows from the biopsychosocial model. Nevertheless, it is legitimate to claim that in primary care, complex problems are not routinely dismembered to help clinicians understand them, simple technical solutions are not assumed for complex clinical problems, and clinicians generally appreciate that in many cases there is no single right answer or single cause for a problem. The reader would do well to bear this in mind while reading through the material in this volume, which is deeply concerned with associations across different levels of analysis.

In summary, it could be said that primary care is engaged in the process of formulating an original scientific paradigm that integrates at least two existing perspectives: the ontological (or causally focused) and the holistic (which prioritizes a systems perspective). This integration is difficult and far from complete. The recent enthusiasm for "evidence-based" knowledge should guarantee that however eclectic the vision becomes, it will be grounded in validated fact.

## MANAGED CARE

The hand of managed care has been shaping American medicine for well over a decade now, perhaps most conspicuously in primary care. Three changes are most notable: the change in the importance of primary care, the change in function expected of primary care, and the change in incentives and resources with which to work.

Managed care has certainly changed the centrality of primary care within the health care system. In many cases, rendering a service in a primary care setting is less expensive than rendering that same service in a specialty setting. In some cases, rendering a service in primary care is the only option, as patients will not go elsewhere for certain kinds of care. This phenomenon has been most fully characterized for certain mental health services, described in some detail later in this foreword. Early on, managed care companies figured all this out and began hiring and contracting with more primary care clinicians. This created a demand for primary care clinicians and accelerated the growth and prestige of the constituent specialties. Managed care organizations also began using contracting and other means to "push" new functions and higher levels of "productivity" into this setting. This has made it difficult to honor several of the core attributes of primary care as enumerated at the beginning of this foreword, such as establishing a personal relationship and offering comprehensive care. More recently, certain health plans have also used financial incentives, provision of additional resources, and plan-level disease management programs to add even more responsibilities. Some of this is for good reasons; for example, prevention, screening, and case finding are best done in the primary care setting and can lead to better health and less expensive health care. Sometimes the reasons have not been good and have injured primary care clinicians' ability to function therapeutically. For example, the gatekeeper role assigned to primary care clinicians was seen as a way to limit access to more expensive specialist care, thereby saving managed care companies money and sparing them the unpleasant task of denying expensive care themselves.

As the field of clinical medicine progresses, new means of improving or protecting health are discovered. As previously noted, it often becomes evident that the best place to accomplish this work is in the primary care setting. One of the ubiquitous pressures in primary care comes from the hope and expectation from the larger house of medicine that primary care clinicians will take on these new tasks, such as screening for an ever expanding list of conditions and risk factors, managing and monitoring an ever growing list of diseases, and practicing preventive medicine. This expectation creates a set of competing demands whereby the primary care clinician must choose, from an impossibly long list of things that "should" be done, the few things that she or he will actually do on a visit. Those things rise to the top that the patient deems most important, that the clinician deems most important, that can be accomplished most easily, that the clinician is most comfortable managing, that the clinician is rewarded for doing, that resources are readily available to manage, and that the clinician is evaluated on. Many innovators in the house of medicine have been disappointed by the unwillingness or inability of the primary care system to adopt this new screening tool or that clinical intervention simply because it has been shown to be efficacious. A whole set of barriers stand between the demonstration of an efficacious intervention and its successful, enduring implementation into ordinary primary care. The concept of competing demands must be understood by anyone who hopes to introduce into primary care any new technology, pattern of care, or any other new clinical demand.

## MENTAL HEALTH PROBLEMS

Earlier we offered a definition and a list of six core attributes of primary care tendered by the Institute of Medicine in 1996 in a volume entitled *Primary Care: America's Health in a New Era* (Donaldson et al., 1996). The fourth attribute, "Primary care does not consider mental health separately from physical health," was described in some detail in that monograph by one of us (deGruy, 1996) and is particularly relevant to the business of this book. Therefore, we revisit a few highlights from that argument and update them with developments that have transpired since 1996. We organize this material under three points.

   *1. The Indivisibility of Mental from Physical Health.* This point deserves the strongest emphasis, foremost to counteract the fundamental misconception that leads to such language as "mental health" or "physical problem." These very notions are erroneous and incomplete and are belied by simple clinical phenomena. One can hardly find in a primary care patient evidence of psychological distress or mental symptomatology without accompanying physical symptomatology (Bridges & Goldberg, 1985; Kroenke et al., 1994). Conversely, physical—so-called medical—problems are always accompanied by psychological symptoms. It is impossible to render adequate primary care without attending to both. DeGruy (1996) has commented on the disadvantages of splitting mind and body in health care:

> Systems of care that force the separation of "mental" from "physical" problems consign the clinicians in each arm of this dichotomy to a misconceived and incomplete clinical reality that produces duplication of effort, undermines comprehensiveness of care, hamstrings clinicians with incomplete data, and ensures that the patient cannot be completely understood. (p. 286)

   Patients understand this concept better than clinicians, and all clinical psychophysiologists who aspire to render any care to primary care patients must fully grasp it. Primary care patients have repeatedly shown their resistance to leaving the primary care setting for special care, particularly care of a psychological nature, no matter how efficient or effective such care may in fact be (Olfson, 1991; Orleans, George, Haupt, & Brodie, 1985). Thus efforts to introduce new therapies to primary care patients are in general more likely to succeed if they can be offered within the context of ordinary primary care.

   It may be worth pointing out that mental diagnoses are themselves extremely common in primary care settings, affecting over a third of the patients seen, and that their presentation is heavily tilted toward somatic rather than psychological symptomatology. Thus somatization—the presentation of physical symptoms without a physical explanation—is an extremely prevalent and difficult problem in such settings. Moreover, many patients, somatizing patients included, may manifest insufficient psychological symptoms to meet the diagnostic criteria for a DSM mental diagnosis yet show profound functional impairment and distress. These so-called subthreshold patients clearly need help, but we have much to learn about how to help them and when our help will actually be beneficial.

*2. The Inadequacy of Mental Health Care in Primary Care Settings and the Reasons for This.* We seem to have settled on the understanding that under conditions of usual care, about half the primary care patients with mental disorders are recognized as such, and less than half of those patients are treated adequately. The data supporting this assertion are largely derived from depression studies, and the generalization is subject to wide variation. After a decade of miscellaneous efforts to improve the treatment of depression in primary care, the general level of recognition and management of this particular condition is probably higher, but it is probably lower for other mental conditions. Interestingly, the finding prevails even among clinicians who believe that mental disorders are important problems for their patients. Why are common, disabling conditions apparently so neglected? The reasons are more compelling and intractable than they might appear on first flush. The barriers occur at the level of the patient, the clinician, the office or clinic, and the larger health care system.

At the level of the patient, mental disorders are perceived as stigmatizing, and a patient will sometimes avoid reporting psychological symptoms or acknowledging mental distress out of shame or a desire to keep a mental diagnosis out of his or her medical record. The fact that mental syndromes frequently manifest with physical symptomatology often leads the patient to believe that the problem itself is of a physical nature; in other words, primary care patients tend to *somatize*. Finally, a patient who might meet criteria for a mental diagnosis is usually not seeing a primary care clinician for that reason but for some other medical problem, and the mental symptoms are thought of as incidental or irrelevant.

At the level of the clinician, most are not sufficiently familiar with the formal diagnostic criteria for specific mental disorders to confidently make diagnoses. Moreover, many clinicians believe that the criteria are inappropriate and result in the inclusion of patients who are not sufficiently distressed or impaired by their diagnoses to justify treatment. Just as patients somatize, so do clinicians. Our medical education has tilted us in the biomedical direction, and we tend to look for physical explanations for physical symptomatology. Many clinicians shy away from mental diagnoses, even if they suspect them, because of the amount of time it takes to deal with such problems and the havoc they wreak on tight patient care schedules. But even when the clinician is confident of the diagnosis and is ready to deal with it, she or he may avoid making and recording such a diagnosis out of consideration of the negative consequences to the patient. A mental diagnosis can sometimes find its way back to an employer, where it can adversely affect job evaluation and promotability, or to the insurer, where it can adversely affect insurability.

At the level of the practice, mental diagnoses do not generally fare well in the competition for a clinician's precious time with a patient, particularly if a mental problem is not the reason the patient has appeared for care. Primary care practices are rarely equipped to make the case-finding efforts necessary to identify patients with mental disorders, and they rarely have the resources to treat and monitor these patients appropriately.

At the level of the larger health care system, primary care clinicians are often not reimbursed to identify and manage mental disorders. Even in managed care plans that expect such management from the primary care clinician, rarely are the clinicians provided the proper incentive to render adequate mental health care.

*3. Recent Efforts to Create a Sustainable System of Mental Health Care That Is Part of the Fabric of Primary Care.* Several recent efforts are particularly relevant for the care of depressed primary care patients. Important too are the implications for those who might wish to incorporate psychophysiological interventions into primary care settings. A decade ago, we understood that most patients with mental diagnoses were appearing in primary care settings, that they were severely impaired and thus in need of help, that excellent treatments were available, and that the clinicians still were not dealing with the problems. Excellent case-finding tools, such as PRIME-MD (Primary Care-Mental Diagnoses) and its subsequent refinement, the PHQ (Primary Care Health Questionnaire), had been developed and validated. Clinicians could be persuaded to use these tools but tended to stop when the studies stopped. Even when they persisted in using them, this alone did not result in better outcomes for patients afflicted with mental disorders. Outstanding patient education and physician education programs have been developed, and these have been shown to increase both patients' and clinicians' knowledge about recognizing and treating mental disorders. Unfortunately, the programs alone have produced no corresponding improvement in patient outcomes. Improved access to mental health resources causes almost no improvements in mental health outcomes because primary care patients will not leave their primary care clinicians to access them.

A set of progressively sophisticated care management protocols have also been developed for primary care settings, involving access to care managers, cognitive-behavioral therapists, and psychiatrists. These have resulted in definite improvements in the care process and in some instances have resulted in better health outcomes for patients, but these practice-level structural changes tend to disappear when the research support that creates them disappears. We have reached the point of realizing that a chain of conditions, each necessary but not alone sufficient, must be met to introduce into the primary care setting effective, sustainable mental health care. As of this writing, it appears that the most effective mental health care conforms to the principles of chronic disease management, such as the model developed by Wagner (Wagner, Austin, & Von Korff, 1996). Wagner's model of care generally contains elements of patient education and motivation for self-care; clinician education; easy-to-use office tools for case finding, diagnosis, tracking and monitoring, and outcomes measurement; care management; and simple guidelines or algorithms. These elements must be supported by an incentive structure that actually rewards the primary care clinician for implementing multidimensional changes in their practices.

## FUTURE PROSPECTS

Many authors in this book describe innovations in clinical care that are supported by compelling evidence of their benefits. The trick will be to figure out how to get them in use and maintain their use long enough to convince everyone of their benefits. Time and progress are on our side. Increasingly sophisticated information systems make the difficult practice-level innovations, such as case-finding and tracking systems, more available and useful. The concepts of collaborative care and clinical teamwork are replacing the earlier cultural norm of the primary care clinicians as solely responsible for the health and health care of their patients. Most important, evidence is accumulating of the importance of the psychophysiological connections and the value of reaching across these connections with new therapies. This evidence will have more researchers and innovators searching for ways to bring new developments to the patients who need them, and those patients are found in primary care settings.

## REFERENCES

Bowen, M. (1966). The use of family theory in clinical practice. *Comprehensive Psychiatry,* 7, 345–374.

Bridges, K. W., & Goldberg, D. P. (1985). Somatic presentation of DSM-III psychiatric disorders in primary care. *Journal of Psychosomatic Research, 29,* 563–569.

Christie-Seely, J. (1981). Teaching the family system concept in family medicine. *Journal of Family Practice, 13*(3), 391–401.

Crouch, M., & Roberts, L. (1987). *The family in medical practice: A family systems primer.* New York: Springer-Verlag.

Davidson, M. (1983). *Uncommon sense. The life and thought of Ludwig von Bertalanffy, father of general systems theory.* Los Angeles: Tarcher.

deGruy, F. V., III (1996). Mental health care in the primary care setting. In M. S. Donaldson, K. D. Yordy, N. Lohr, & N. A. Vanselow (Eds.), *Primary care: America's health in a new era* (pp. 285–311). Washington, DC: National Academy Press.

Donaldson, M. S., Yordy, K. D., Lohr, N., & Vanselow, N. A. (1996). *Primary care: America's health in a new era.* Washington, DC: National Academy Press.

Dubos, R. (1971). *Mirage of health.* New York: Harper & Row.

Engel, G. L. (1977). The need for a new medical model: A challenge for biomedicine. *Science, 196,* 129–136.

Kroenke, K., Spitzer, L. R., Williams, J. B., Linzer, M., Hahn, S. R., deGruy, F. V., III, & Brody, D. (1994). Physical symptoms in primary care: Predictors of psychiatric disorders and functional impairment. *Archives of Family Medicine, 3*(9), 774–779.

Olfson, M. (1991). Primary care patients who refuse specialized mental health services. *Archives of Internal Medicine, 151,* 129–132.

Orleans, C., George, L., Haupt, J., & Brodie, H. (1985). How primary care physicians treat psychiatric disorders: A national survey of family practitioners. *American Journal of Psychiatry, 142,* 52–57.

Pellegrino, E. D., & Thomasma, D. C. (1981). *A philosophical basis of medical practice.* New York: Oxford University Press.

Rainford, G. L., & Schuman, S. H. (1981). The family in crisis. A case study of overwhelming illness and stress. *Journal of the American Medical Association, 1,* 246.

Starfield, B. (1994). Primary care: Is it essential? *Lancet, 344,* 1129–1133.

Wagner, E. H., Austin, B. J., & Von Korff, M. (1996). Organizing care for patients with chronic illness. *Milbank Quarterly, 74*(4), 511–544.

Terence C. Davies, MD
*Professor and Chair of Family and Community Medicine, Eastern Virginia Medical School*

Frank V. deGruy, III, MD
*Woodward-Chisholm Professor and Chair of Family Medicine, University of Colorado School of Medicine*

# Part I

# MODELS AND CONCEPTS FOR MIND-BODY MEDICINE

# Mind-Body Medicine, Evidence-Based Medicine, Clinical Psychophysiology, and Integrative Medicine

## DONALD MOSS

**Abstract:** The author introduces the concepts of mind-body medicine, evidence-based medicine, clinical psychophysiology and biofeedback, integrated care, and integrative medicine. The chapter emphasizes a mind-body approach that recognizes the unitary psychophysiological nature of both illness and healing. Many common medical problems are functional or chronic disorders exacerbated by lifestyle, situational stress, and psychosocial factors. Managing or reducing the symptoms of such disorders requires patients to make behavioral changes. Mind-body medicine offers patients an active role in recovery and health maintenance. Scientific research offers a guiding "evidence-based" light in designing the optimal mind-body treatment plan. Together, biofeedback and clinical psychophysiology offer powerful tools for mind-body medicine. The mastery of self-regulation skills is a primary tool for health. Today's health problems require an integrated care model, involving a partnership of physician, nurse, psychologist, and other behavioral health professionals. This partnership delivers behavioral interventions directly into primary care settings, integrates complementary and conventional therapies, and modifies treatment paradigms to benefit larger numbers of patients in primary care settings.

## MIND-BODY MEDICINE

> Mind/body medicine . . . should be an integral part of evidence-based, cost-effective, quality health care. (Sobel, 2000, p. 1705)

Mind-body medicine is a revolutionary 21st-century approach to health care that includes a wide range of behavioral and lifestyle interventions on an equal basis with traditional medical interventions. The patient in mind-body medicine is understood as a totality of body, mind, and spirit. Interventions are directed at each of these aspects of the person. The medical conditions linked with human suffering today, in the affluent societies of the developed world, are caused as much by lifestyle, dietary habits, activity level, and life stress as they are by such traditional causes of disease as infection, virus, bacteria, and physical trauma. The mind-body medicine approach creates a partnership among practitioners of the medical and mental specialties, including physicians, nurse practitioners, and psychologists, as well as mind-body specialists, such as biofeedback practitioners, chiropractors, nutritionists, spiritual counselors, and yoga teachers. The result is an integrated team of caregivers who address mind, body, and spirit with each patient.

The acute care medical model has provided tremendous advances in the health of human beings. Based on a dualistic dichotomy of body and mind, the acute care model is a mechanistic approach to disease and treatment. The model emphasizes the use of a diagnostic symptom-oriented interview, extensive laboratory work, and sophisticated imaging studies to identify a specific disease or condition causing the patient's complaints (Cassell, 1997). The corresponding treatment model places a heavy reliance on pharmacology and a lesser emphasis on surgical intervention. Although most physicians acknowledge the importance of life stress, diet, and exercise, these factors are largely addressed only after conventional therapeutic strategies have failed. Psychological specialists are regarded as secondary and tertiary caregivers to be consulted when the primary care physician has been unable to provide relief or when no physical cause can be identified for a disorder. In many cases, a referral takes place only after the patient's condition has become more severe and chronic and thus less amenable to behavioral intervention.

The education that physicians receive in medical schools often does not prepare them well for the typical patient in primary care (see Chapters 6, 32, and 33). Patients are more likely to present with symptoms that fall into several overlapping categories: somatization disorder, "undifferentiated complaints," psychophysiological disorders related to psychosocial stress, posttraumatic conditions, somatic symptoms of psychiatric disorders, and symptoms of chronic disease. The mismatch between the health needs of the typical patient and the standard medical response produces a waste of medical resources, frustration for patient and physician, and the danger that acute conditions become chronic.

Mind-body medicine includes behavioral and psychosocial interventions among the first line of interventions. The patient is given an active role from the beginning in developing a treatment plan and takes more responsibility for directing the psychosocial and lifestyle aspects of that plan. Mind-body medicine emphasizes patient education and patient self-management as integral parts of clinical practice, from the first day of well care (Blonshine, 1998; Kotses et al., 1995; Nakagawa-Kogan, 1994). Smoking cessation is one example of a critical area for patient education, addressing the number one risk factor that is currently manageable, with dramatic consequences for morbidity and mortality. One in five Americans dies as a result of complications related to smoking (U.S. Department of Health and Human Services, 1994). For many patient groups, research has shown that relatively brief and inexpensive mind-body interventions can improve the patient's recovery process, speed healing, shorten inpatient stays, and reduce the cost of treatment (Blanchard et al., 1985; Sobel, 2000).

## CHALLENGING PROBLEMS IN PRIMARY CARE

This section highlights some of the most challenging patient groups in primary care.[1] Patients in these groups require a shift in paradigms. Treating their problems can be frustrating for medical professionals unless managed within an integrated mind-body approach from the beginning.

## Somatization Disorder

Somatization disorder involves the translation of emotional distress into physical symptoms, when no significant organic bases have been identified for the complaints. A patient's tendency to develop physical symptoms often begins at an early age and continues for many years, even decades (Quill, 1985). Physicians may contribute to the genesis of somatization disorder by failing to detect signs of the somatization process and aggressively pursuing diagnostic testing (e.g., X rays, CT scans, blood tests), which confirms the patient's preconception that some serious disease is lurking undetected (Groth-Marnat & Edkins, 1996).

## Undifferentiated Complaints

Michael Balint (1964) pointed out that many patients in primary care present "undifferentiated complaints" (see also, E. Balint & Norell, 1973). Undifferentiated complaints are vague presentations of symptoms that have not yet developed into clear-cut physical or medical illnesses. Kroenke and Mangelsdorff (1989) observed that only 20 percent of visits to primary care physicians involve discoverable organic causes, and only 10 percent are clearly psychological disorders without confounding physical symptoms. The complaints most commonly presented in the family practitioner's office today include chest pain, fatigue, dizziness, headache, edema, back pain, dyspnea, insomnia, abdominal pain, numbness, impotence, weight loss, cough, and constipation (Blount, 1998, p. 6). The first 10 complaints in this list account for 40 percent of all visits. For patients with these complaints, only

10 percent to 15 percent were determined, after one year, to have clear organic diagnoses (Blount, 1998, pp. 6–7).

According to Balint (1964), the majority of primary care patients' complaints lie in a twilight zone between body and mind, marked by overlapping psychosocial stress, physical discomfort, relationship conflicts, life-stage dissatisfaction, and unfulfilled aspirations. The response of the physician is critical because unless the patient is assisted to identify psychosocial aspects of his or her distress, the patient will continue to shape his or her complaints in the direction of an established somatic disorder. There is a significant risk with such patients of a harmful "over-medicalisation" (Smith, 1995). Balint suggested using the doctor-patient relationship as a tool to enable patients to become aware of the nonmedical aspects of their distress and thus avoid the somatization process. (Chapter 2 describes the high risk model of threat perception, which provides guidance for steering in this twilight zone by identifying specific psychosocial factors that increase the risk for somatic symptoms, serve as triggers for symptoms, or create a buffer against symptoms.)

## Psychophysiological Disorders

Many of the undifferentiated complaints just mentioned also qualify as psychophysiological disorders. They involve measurable modifications in physiology but worsen under the influence of situational stress or internal cognitive distress (Gatchel & Blanchard, 1993). Sternbach's (1966) stress-diathesis model states that each human being shows a certain response stereotypy, responding physiologically to situations in a particular way. Some individuals are cardiovascular responders, some musculoskeletal, some gastrointestinal, and some cognitive. Then, if the individual's coping resources do not keep his or her physiology within bounds, new life stressors will produce new somatic symptoms (Sternbach, 1966). If one adopts a broadened focus, identifying complaints that are not clear-cut psychiatric disorders but are "psychological in some way," one discovers that 75 percent to 80 percent of primary care patients present evidence of at least some psychosocial or psychophysiological component in their symptom presentation. Many of these patients benefit greatly from education in stress management and self-regulation skills.

### Posttraumatic Conditions

Many patients who present in primary care settings suffer delayed consequences of physical and sexual abuse, traumatic experiences, and losses. A prospective study of 1,007 members of a Michigan HMO reported that a history of posttraumatic stress disorder (PTSD) was associated with significantly more somatic symptoms in general and with an increased incidence of somatization symptoms (Andreski, Chilcoat, & Breslau, 1998). In many cases, neither the patient nor the physician recognizes the connection between current symptoms and earlier emotional trauma. Research by van der Kolk et al. (1996) showed that PTSD, dissociation, and somatization are highly interrelated. Individuals with childhood trauma show the greatest vulnerability to somatization, although individuals with adult trauma or loss also show heightened incidence of somatization. Lingering "unconscious trauma" involves measurable physiological arousal patterns. As Wickramasekera (1988, 1998) observed, individuals can push trauma out of their minds but not out of their bodies. Biofeedback and clinical psychophysiology provide useful tools in this context, monitoring autonomic nervous arousal through such modalities as heart rate, skin conductance, and peripheral temperature and detecting traumatic memories in the course of assessment (see Chapters 2 and 8).

### Somatic Symptoms of Psychiatric Disorders

Unrecognized psychiatric disorders account for a large portion of the complaints in primary care. Patients with anxiety and depressive disorders present physical symptoms in both primary care and specialty clinics. An estimated 65 percent of individuals with anxiety-related disorders seek treatment from primary care physicians (Danton, Altrocchi, Antonuccio, & Basta, 1994). A study of patients with acute chest pain showed that 17.5 percent had panic disorder and 23.1 percent had depression (Yingling, Wulsin, Arnold, & Rouan, 1993). Patients with panic disorder or depression were much more likely to have made an emergency room visit in the preceding 12 months than were the patients without psychiatric conditions.

In a study of 1,000 primary care patients, deGruy (1994) examined the relationship between the occurrence of 15 common physical symptoms and the presence of psychiatric disorders. The more physical symptoms were present, the higher the likelihood of a psychiatric disorder. The relationship between physical symptoms and mood problems is reciprocal. Anxious and depressed individuals are more vulnerable to developing functional symptoms, and persons who suffer a variety of medical complaints are more vulnerable to the onset of depression and anxiety (deGruy, 1996). Kroenke (2000) argues for an equal emphasis on the identification of anxiety, depression, and somatization disorders and highlights the commonalities of the three disorders.

Depressed individuals seek help most often in primary care settings; yet they are often neither well diagnosed nor well managed in primary care. Rost et al. (1998) identified 98 adults with current major depression. Thirty-two percent of these primary care patients remained undetected for up to one year. Simply identifying patients with anxiety and depression already comprises a breakthrough service in any primary care clinic.

## Chronic Conditions

Patients with chronic illness account for between 46 percent and 75 percent of costs in health care. This includes such diverse conditions as diabetes mellitus, arthritis, hypertension, and chronic heart disease. Lifestyle, diet, exercise, habits such as smoking, and situational stress play a major part in both the etiology and course of such conditions. Medical management via medication is a losing battle unless the behavioral factors are addressed. Once a chronic condition progresses to a more advanced stage, treatment is palliative and not curative, and both patient and physician are forced to modify expectations. On the other hand, targeted behavioral services can reduce needless suffering and successfully reduce medical costs by 18 percent to 31 percent for individuals with such chronic conditions as diabetes and hypertension (Lechnyr, 1992).

When the patient's condition is chronic or complex and involves chronic irreversible changes in anatomy and physiology, the acute care model clearly reaches its limits. In frustration, physicians typically add medication after medication to manage the ever multiplying list of complaints. The use of polypharmacy then produces an array of interactive adverse effects, typically including fatigue, lethargy, weight gain, inactivity, and loss of any sense of internal control over body and health. The individual with a chronic condition eventually comes to see him- or herself in a passive patient role, submitting to tests and procedures, and awaiting the physician's next decision or intervention. The patient's lifestyle frequently becomes organized around a never ending series of medical visits, lab tests, and medications. The secondary effects of the more sedentary

lifestyle are interactive with the original disease or condition, producing a loss of muscle tone, aerobic conditioning, and general vitality. Treatment compliance becomes a major issue for the physician because the patient often shows little "ownership" in the medical care plan. The individual often struggles with whether to accept a diagnosis and cooperate with prescribed medication or resist the diagnosis and the prescribed treatment.

In many chronic conditions, personal choices and lifestyle play a role in initiating and maintaining the illness (McLellan, Lewis, O'Brien, & Kleber, 2000). These psychological factors interact with genetics and familial/cultural factors in the onset of the disorder. The decision to drink the first drink and the habit of regular excessive drinking interact with the genetic vulnerability to alcohol dependence to create the chronic illness of alcoholism and the eventual end-state condition of liver disease. Similarly, salt sensitivity is an inherited risk factor for hypertension, yet individual dietary choices and familial salt use patterns influence which individuals end up with hypertension. Voluntary, lifestyle, and familial variables also contribute to creating some of the strongest health risk factors, including obesity, stress level, and inactivity, which exacerbate many chronic conditions (McLellan et al., 2000).

## EVIDENCE-BASED MEDICINE

Evidence-based medicine is a systematic effort to bring science and research-based knowledge into the heart of clinical practice. (Sackett, Straus, Richardson, Rosenberg, & Haynes, 2000)

The clinical judgment of health care providers is easily distorted by coincidental improvements in a handful of patients (Jonas, Linde, & Walach, 1999). Research tests the efficacy of treatments for a specific condition in a systematic fashion, with methodological safeguards to produce reliable conclusions (Geyman, Deyo, & Ramsey, 2000). Evidence-based medicine at its best rates a new intervention or therapy on both the *direction* and the *level* of the evidence—in other words, on whether a therapy is empirically supported and on how strong the evidence for or against the therapy is (Ernst, Pittler, Stevinson, & White, 2001). Research can weigh the relative benefits, costs, and risks of interventions, providing practical information relevant in treatment planning. One of the relatively common objections in mainstream medicine to complementary and alternative therapies is the lack of extensive outcomes research on these interventions (Grollman, 2001).

Jonas, Linde, and Walach (1999, p. 73) asserted that six kinds of knowledge should ideally be considered in the course of reaching evidence-based treatment decisions:

1. Patient preferences and meaning.

2. Mechanisms of action.

3. Safety and efficacy.

4. Treatment effect probabilities in the open clinical setting from observational and outcomes research.

5. Precise estimations of effects through systematic summaries and calculation of confidence intervals when possible.

6. Demonstration of utility and benefit under normal health service conditions examining the impact of access, feasibility, and costs.

Under typical conditions, fortunately, the same authors concede that it is sufficient to weigh "clinical expertise, patient relevance, and research evidence," providing a three-legged foundation for evidence-based practice (p. 74).

Under evidence-based medicine, assessing a patient's condition and selecting treatment are collaborative processes in which physician and patient make decisions together based on up-to-date knowledge about the relative efficacy and risks of available treatment options. Following evidence-based medicine means that not all new patients will be given the same treatment interventions regardless of their complaints. The provider's preference for a specific modality does not justify the use of that modality if current outcome research shows that another modality has a clear advantage in effectiveness, cost, or reduced risk to the patient (Dams, 1997).

If the patient presents with a panic disorder, for example, there is strong outcome data showing the efficacy of cognitive-behavioral therapy, alone or combined with medication (Barlow, Gorman, Shear, & Woods, 2000). There is also an increasingly strong body of literature showing the presence of hyperventilation and other dysfunctional breathing patterns in panic disorder (Wilhelm & Roth, 1998) and the effectiveness of biofeedback training in diaphragmatic breathing to moderate both abnormal breathing and panic. No such research supports the use of intensive psychoanalytic therapy for panic disorder. Therefore, the provider would violate the patient's right to an effective, inexpensive, and nonharmful treatment were he or she to follow personal preference and deliver psychoanalytic therapy.

On the physical medicine side, it is clear that a patient should not be steered into cardiac bypass surgery, risking life, inflicting pain, and requiring weeks of healing and rehabilitation, if outcome data show that patients with similar angiograms do equally well on medication. In mind-body medicine, the evidence-based principle means that providers should consider which modalities and treatment strategies hold up best in research, which are available in the locale, and which are available given the patient's means and health insurance coverage. Then the patient's response to each intervention reopens the decision-making process.

Another challenge in evidence-based medicine is paradigm shifting. When a condition is medical, the most effective intervention may nevertheless be behavioral. The federal Health Care Finance Administration recently recognized that biofeedback should be the first line of treatment for urinary incontinence (Perry, 2000). Biofeedback uses electromyographic sensors to monitor pelvic floor muscle activity, and the patient learns better muscular control (see Chapter 22). Yet medical caregivers still frequently think in terms of medication or corrective surgery for this disorder.

Similarly, the outcome research on irritable bowel syndrome shows that cognitive behavioral therapy, hypnosis, and biofeedback are all effective, noninvasive, and cost-effective (Blanchard, 2001); medication remains more widely used yet is less effective (see Chapter 21). Choosing within behavioral approaches should be guided by research and access. The outcome research is strongest on hypnosis and cognitive-behavioral therapy, so one would lean toward choosing these modalities. However, the unavailability of a qualified hypnotherapist or cognitive-behavioral therapist and the availability of a qualified biofeedback practitioner might steer the decision differently. Similarly, cultural factors play a role in the selection of a treatment—for example, if the patient has a religious bias against hypnotism that cannot be dispelled by a brief education about medical hypnotism.

Evidence-based practice recognizes the powerful role of faith and placebo in the healing process. Nonspecific factors play a major role in the patient's response to treatment. The use of interventions widely regarded as efficacious increases the patient's faith (Ader & Cohen, 1993; Wickramasekera, 1999). Similarly, complementary and alternative therapies that have the cachet of something new and powerful are useful in eliciting this nonspecific healing effect. Trousseau's old comment is apt, that one "should treat as many patients as possible with the new drugs while they still have the power to heal" (Trousseau, 1854, cited by Wickramasekera, 1999, p. 1a). Current research on the placebo as a form of conditioning improves one's ability to use this nonspecific effect while continuing to practice within the framework of evidence-based practice (Ader, 1988).

Finally, evidence-based medicine has to adapt the relatively black-and-white guidelines of outcome research to the realities of a given individual. Outcome research is largely based on homogeneous samples of patients with a given disorder, and many individuals are excluded from such studies due to comorbid conditions, the use of confounding medications, or the chronicity of their conditions. In the world of clinical practice, one is faced with individuals who have complex, chronic conditions and multiple comorbid problems and are already using a variety of medications and other therapies. The science of evidence-based medicine must serve the art of clinical practice. The health care provider weighs each of the individual's medical and psychological conditions when selecting and delivering a new treatment intervention.

## BIOFEEDBACK AND CLINICAL PSYCHOPHYSIOLOGY

Biofeedback is an evidence-based treatment paradigm that opens up a broad avenue for the mind-body approach (Moss, 1998; Schwartz & Associates, 1995). The biofeedback instrument measures a biological process such as muscle tension by means of a sensor and provides an immediate visual or auditory display of this signal to the subject (Lawlis, 2001). The feedback of the biological signal increases the individual's awareness of his or her own body and enables the individual to establish control over the physiological system (see Figure 1.1).

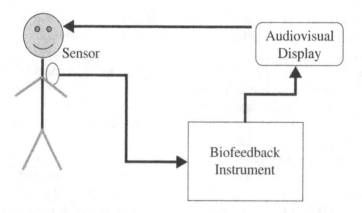

**Figure 1.1**    Basic Biofeedback System

SOURCE: Moss (2001). Reprinted with the permission of Academic Press.

The modality of biofeedback supports a philosophy of self-regulation and the acquisition of voluntary controls over one's own body and life. The individual gains self-efficacy by learning control over a muscle, brain wave, or other physiological process, by reducing the severity of symptoms, and by increasing a sense of participation in personal wellness. Self-efficacy, the inner conviction that one can do something that will make a positive difference, often generalizes into a more active personal mastery over psychosocial and relationship problems.

Chapter 8 by Gilbert and Moss summarizes the procedures and applications of biofeedback, and several chapters in this book highlight the applications of biofeedback to common medical and emotional disorders. Biofeedback has proven effective in controlling many physiological processes—including muscle tension, skin temperature, respiration, autonomic nervous tension, heart rate, electrical wave activity in the brain, and brain blood flow—and has applications in health care, mental health, rehabilitation, education, sports psychology, and the performing arts. Within primary care, a broad range of biofeedback applications have been documented, from headache to asthma, hypertension, and chronic pain (see Chapter 8). There

are also well-documented applications to mental health problems, including anxiety, depression, attention deficit disorders, alcoholism and addictions, and general psychotherapy (Moss, 2001, 2002).

Biofeedback is a useful tool for helping individuals understand the mind-body link. The biofeedback display shows the patient vividly how memories or thoughts induce an immediate physiological change. Biofeedback practice rests on the psychophysiological principle that mind and body are so delicately interwoven that any change in the bodily state will evoke a psychological change and any change in the mind will evoke a physiological change (Green, Green, & Walters, 1970, p. 3). Biofeedback quickly teaches heightened body awareness, as the instrument detects the individual's subtle physiological reactions and the individual learns to consciously feel what had been automatic and below awareness. Biofeedback speeds the acquisition of relaxation skills. It also serves as a Trojan horse, accepting the patient's somatic orientation, gaining the patient's trust for a seemingly medical and physiological approach, and leading the patient to an understanding of mind-body linkages (see Chapter 2; Wickramasekera, 1988; Wickramasekera, Davies, & Davies, 1996).

Finally, biofeedback enables the individual to strategically modify key physiological variables relevant in his or her disease or suffering, with measurable health consequences. Chapter 3 explores the role of physiological mechanisms and behavioral change in healing and recovery.

Biofeedback is not practiced in isolation but is part of a comprehensive mind-body approach called clinical psychophysiology. Clinical psychophysiology uses current knowledge of behavior-change skills and an understanding of physiologic functioning to produce simultaneous changes in mind and body. Practitioners typically design a customized behavioral treatment package for each patient, which may include any or all of the following:

- Education about physiology relevant to the presenting symptoms
- Relaxation skills training, including progressive muscle relaxation, autogenic training, and diaphragmatic breathing
- Stress management to buffer the family or job problems exacerbating physical symptoms
- Cognitive restructuring to modify thought patterns that maintain physical tensions
- Behavior therapy to reduce maladaptive or self-defeating behavior
- Physiological monitoring during psychotherapy, utilizing autonomic nervous system arousal to identify implicit emotional issues (Wickramasekera, 1988, 1998).

Biofeedback and clinical psychophysiology provide a model for mind-body medicine because they form a three-decade-old mind-body approach founded on scientific research and dedicated to enlarging the individual's control over body and mind.

## INTEGRATED CARE

The patient of the future will encounter an integrated system of behavioral and medical care, involving a partnership of behavioral practitioners, physicians and nurses, in "one house" and "one system." (Cummings & Cummings, 2000)

The ideal of integrated care requires that the full range of mind-body interventions be included from the first day of any patient's health care and remain a part of each successive episode of treatment (Nadeau & Moss, 1999). This means that simple and inexpensive counseling on lifestyle changes and the use of nutritional and habit-changing procedures are made available to each patient at each visit, wherever they may serve to prevent the onset of illness or alleviate current symptoms. Similarly, every patient entering surgery should receive at least a brief educational session with an office nurse, a written handout depicting the surgical procedure and its impact on the body, and an audiotape on relaxation skills, including visualization and hypnotic-type suggestions of rapid healing. Research has shown that such presurgical education can reduce blood loss, speed wound healing, and reduce days admitted (Dreher, 1998; Kiecolt-Glaser, Page, Marucha, MacCallum, & Glaser, 1998).

For over four decades, authors in behavioral medicine and psychosomatic medicine have criticized the Cartesian mind-body split in medical thinking. In 1977, George Engel proposed a unitary biopsychosocial model for all of medicine. Most medical researchers today agree that clinical disorders are better understood from a unitary and integrative mind-body perspective. However, the physical organization of medical practice, including the sharp division between physical medicine and the mental health specialties, has continued the mind-body split in an equally destructive fashion. Physical medicine specialists throw up their hands and declare, "This problem belongs in psychiatry." The patient arrives in the psychiatric specialty clinic hurt, bitter, and discouraged, declaring that "My doctor thinks my problem isn't real" or "My doctor says the symptoms are in my head, but I know they are not."

When physicians and behavioral specialists attempt to create truly integrated care, many obstacles intervene. There are significant differences in education and professional culture between physicians and behavioral specialists (Haley et al., 1998). Practitioners in each group think, behave, and approach problems differently in their daily clinical practice. As a result, medical institutions frequently exclude or limit the scope of practice of psychologists and other behavioral professionals. Sample differences in professional culture include (1) physicians are more authoritarian in interpersonal style, operate on a faster pace, and arrive at decisions rapidly by objective criteria; and (2) psychologists tend to be more egalitarian and team oriented in interpersonal style, gather information over a longer period, and often rely on intuition and global impressions as much as objective criteria (Haley et al., 1998).

The organization of reimbursement also creates numerous barriers to integrated care. Behavioral practitioners are frequently informed that they cannot be reimbursed for the treatment of physical disorders, such as gastric ulcers, diabetes, or even pain disorders. They must identify psychiatric diagnoses if they wish to be reimbursed. Similarly, many insurance companies only reimburse bills for certain diagnoses, such as chronic pain, when the services are billed on a hospital billing form that outpatient mental health providers cannot use.

Finally, many managed care companies use a "mental health carve-out." The treatment of all psychiatric diagnoses falls under a separately managed and capitated budget. The effectiveness of the gatekeeper is judged solely on the funds within this mental health carve-out. Thus authorizing psychotherapeutic or behavioral services for a patient with multiple somatic complaints may save money by reduced use of medical services, but the mental health gatekeeper receives no recognition for these cost savings because they are not credited to his or her budget.

One positive step addresses some of these reimbursement barriers: Foxhall (2000) reports that the American Medical Association committee on Current Procedural Terminology (CPT) codes has approved six new codes covering psychosocial and behavioral services for patients with physical health diagnoses. This includes two codes for health and behavior assessment and four codes for health and behavior intervention services.

## INTEGRATIVE MEDICINE: THE USE OF COMPLEMENTARY AND ALTERNATIVE THERAPIES

In a primary care setting, *integrated care* means that behavioral health providers are present to offer psychosocial, educational, and psychophysiological interventions as part of the primary treatment of patient distress. Inclusion of behavioral health providers is an implementation of what research has long supported. Many typical patient complaints have more to do with the patient's psychosocial problems than with diagnosable diseases, infections, injuries, or pathophysiological processes.

Integrative medicine takes this model one step farther, making the entire range of complementary and alternative medicine (CAM) interventions available within the primary care clinic. Today CAM interventions range from acupuncture to nutritional therapies to Eastern disciplines such as yoga, prayer, and spiritual healing (see Box 1.1). Biofeedback, herbal supplements, acupuncture, and chiropractic therapies lie at the more widely accepted end of the spectrum for health care providers, because a significant number of research studies and case reports show their efficacy. Research today is accumulating showing the effectiveness of many other CAM interventions (Ernst et al., 2001; Jonas & Levin, 1999). The general public in the United States already shows a readiness to accept and

---

**Box 1.1** Complementary and Alternative Medicine Therapies

| | |
|---|---|
| Acupuncture | Hypnotherapy |
| Aromatherapy | Manual therapies |
| Biofeedback | Massage therapy |
| Bioenergetics | Nutritional counseling |
| Chiropractic | Prayer |
| Exercise therapies | Spiritual healing |
| Feldenkrais technique | Tai chi, qigong |
| Herbal therapies | Yoga |

---

spend large amounts of personal funds on CAM therapies, regardless of documented efficacy (Eisenberg et al., 1998). Similar trends are evident in the use of alternative therapies by individuals with disabilities (Krauss, Godfrey, Kirk, & Eisenberg, 1998). *The Handbook of Mind-Body Medicine for Primary Care* emphasizes the elements within mind-body medicine and CAM that have the best empirical documentation.

Freeman and Lawlis (2001), Jonas (2001), Jonas and Levin (1999), and Whorton (1999) have overviewed current trends in complementary and alternative medicine. A distinctive CAM paradigm comprises the following:

1. Emphasis on a holistic and unitary view of mind, body, and spirit.

2. Treating the patient as a unique human being and person.

3. Emphasis on a more personal, supportive relationship between the CAM healer and the patient.

4. Attribution of an active role to the patient in the healing process.

5. Belief in the inherent healing power of the living organism.

6. Prescription of lifestyle and habit changes to optimize health.

7. Emphasis on interventions that elicit the body's healing powers.

8. Distrust of invasive treatments that crush disease but harm the patient as a whole.

9. Belief in eclecticism and empiricism.

10. Readiness to accept unconventional interventions and unorthodox theoretical models that appear to work.

11. Openness to prayer, meditation, and spiritual practices as supportive for healing and health.

12. Integration of physical, psychological, and spiritual practices.

The majority of patients today want health care that has some or all of these elements. Patients want their health care provider to know them as human beings, not just as cases, and they resent a lack of such personalism in medicine. They want holism as well. They don't want to be referred to a psychiatrist with the implication that their problem is "in their heads," yet they want their physician to pay attention to and care about their life problems. Harold Koenig has remarked, "Patients want to be seen and treated as a whole person, not as diseases. A whole person is someone whose being has physical, emotional, and spiritual dimensions. Ignoring any of these aspects of humanity leaves the person incomplete and may even interfere with healing" (Koenig, 2000, p. 1708).

The public is sometimes drawn to CAM therapies for the same reasons that arouse the objections of health care professionals (Beyerstein, 2001, p. 230). The origin of many CAM procedures in premodern religious and medical systems lends them a mystique with the public and stirs skepticism in the professional community. Qigong is a branch of Traditional Chinese Medicine, as is acupuncture, and Ayurvedic medicine originated in India's ancient Vedic religious traditions (Jonas & Levin, 1999; Xiangcai, 2000). Research continues to accumulate showing that regardless of origins, many traditional interventions have efficacy for specific disorders (Jonas & Levin, 1999). Integrative medicine involves a systematic effort to cull the active and effective elements within traditional medicine, demonstrate their efficacy through modern scientific research, and educate the professional community and public about discriminate use of CAM therapies.

The integration of CAM therapies in mainline medical clinics may seem to strain the bounds of clinical medicine too far. Yet outcome research is accumulating showing positive efficacy for a number of CAM therapies for specific disorders (Jonas, 2001; Jonas & Levin, 1999). If a tai chi class will reduce the number of falls and hip fractures in elderly individuals, for example, then why shouldn't that class be offered within the internal medicine clinic (Wolf et al., 1996)? The physician-patient relationship is a powerful motivational tool to increase patient compliance with such CAM practices.

Current research tells us that patients are already using CAM therapies in enormous numbers and that 60 percent of these patients are not telling their primary care physicians about their use of CAM (Eisenberg et al., 1998). Consequently, the patient's health care is fragmented, and the possibility for adverse interactions among CAM therapies and conventional therapies is increased. Wayne Jonas, who headed the federal Office of Alternative Medicine, advocates that health care providers become cognizant of CAM and use the available online databases to identify CAM therapies for which clinical efficacy has been documented.[2] He emphasizes a four-step process, the "Four Ps," in which the physician (1) *protects* the patient from potentially harmful CAM remedies; (2) *permits* the patient to use any harmless and inexpensive remedy, even when efficacy has not been established, in hopes that nonspecific placebo effects will be mobilized; (3) *promotes* proven CAM practices—that is, encourages any safe and proven CAM therapies; and (4) *partners* with any outside CAM therapists that patients are using (Jonas, 2001). These guidelines open the door to a medicine that is once again whole.

## NOTES

1. Portions of this section are adapted with permission from an article published in *Biofeedback* (Moss, 1999).
2. Jonas cites the National Center for Complementary and Alternative Medicine database, with over 100,000 citations, available at http://www.nccam.nih.gov/databases.html, and the *British Medical Journal*'s book *Clinical Evidence*, available at http://www.clinicalevidence.com.

## REFERENCES

Ader, R. (1988). The placebo effect as a conditioned response. In R. Ader, H. Weiner, & A. Baum (Eds.), *Experimental foundations of behavioral medicine: Conditioning approaches* (pp. 47–66). Hillsdale, NJ: Lawrence Erlbaum.

Ader, R., & Cohen, N. (1993). Psychoneuroimmunology: Conditioning and stress. *Annual Review of Psychology, 44,* 53–85.

Andreski, P., Chilcoat, H., & Breslau, N. (1998). Post-traumatic stress disorder and somatization symptoms: A prospective study. *Psychiatric Research, 79*(2), 131–138.

Balint, E., & Norell, J. S. (Eds.). (1973). *Six minutes for the patient: Interactions in general practice consultation.* London: Tavistock.

Balint, M. (1964). *The doctor, his patient, and the illness.* New York: International Universities Press.

Barlow, D. H., Gorman, J. M., Shear, M. K., & Woods, S. W. (2000). Cognitive-behavioral therapy, imipramine, or their combination for panic disorder: A randomized controlled trial. *Journal of the American Medical Association, 283*(19), 2529–2536.

Beyerstein, B. L. (2001). Alternative medicine and common errors of reasoning. *Academic Medicine, 76*(3), 230–237.

Blanchard, E. B. (2001). *Irritable bowel syndrome: Psychosocial assessment and treatment.* Washington, DC: American Psychological Association.

Blanchard, E. B., Andrasik, F., Appelbaum, K. A., Evans, D. D., Jurish, S. E., Teders, S. J., et al. (1985). The efficacy and cost-effectiveness of minimal-therapist-contact, non-drug treatments of chronic migraine and tension headache. *Headache, 25*(4), 214–220.

Blonshine, S. (1998). Patient education: The key to asthma management. *Home Care Providers, 3*(3), 153–159.

Blount, A. (Ed.). (1998). *Integrated primary care: The future of medical and mental health collaboration.* New York: Norton.

Cassell, E. J. (1997). *Doctoring: The nature of primary care medicine.* New York: Oxford University Press.

Cummings, N., & Cummings, J. (2000). *The essence of psychotherapy: Reinventing the art in the age of data.* San Diego, CA: Academic Press.

Dams, P.-C. (1997). Providing effective interventions may not be enough: The importance of cost analysis in the behavioral health system. *Behavior and Social Issues, 7*(2), 141–152.

Danton, W. G., Altrocchi, J., Antonuccio, D., & Basta, R. (1994). Nondrug treatment of anxiety. *American Family Physician, 49*(1), 161–166.

deGruy, F. V., III. (1994). Physical symptoms in primary care: Predictors of psychiatric disorders and functional impairment. *Archives of Family Medicine, 3*(9), 774–779.

deGruy, F. V., III. (1996). *Mental health care in the primary care setting.* Washington, DC: Institute of Medicine, National Academy Press.

Dreher, H. (1998). Mind-body interventions for surgery: Evidence and exigency. *Advances in Mind-Body Medicine, 14,* 207–222.

Eisenberg, D. M, Davis, R. B., Ettner, S., Appel, S., Wilkey, S., Van Rompay, M., et al. (1998). Trends in alternative medicine use in the United States, 1990–1997: Results of a follow-up national survey. *Journal of the American Medical Association, 280,* 1569–1575.

Engel, G. L. (1977). The need for a new medical model: A challenge for biomedicine. *Science, 196,* 129–136.

Ernst, E., Pittler, M. H., Stevinson, C., & White, A. (2001). *The desktop guide to complementary and alternative medicine: An evidence-based approach.* St. Louis, MO: Mosby.

Foxhall, K. (2000). New CPT codes will recognize psychologists' work with physical health problems. *Monitor on Psychology, 31*(10), 46–47.

Freeman, L. W., & Lawlis, G. F. (2001). Mosby's complementary and alternative medicine: A research-based approach. St. Louis, MO: Mosby.

Gatchel, R. J., & Blanchard, E. B. (1993). *Psychophysiological disorders: Research and clinical applications*. Washington, DC: American Psychological Association.

Geyman, J. P., Deyo, R. A., & Ramsey, S. D. (Eds.). (2000). *Evidence-based clinical practice: Concepts and approach*. Boston: Butterworth-Heinemann.

Green, E., Green, A. M., & Walters, E. D. (1970). Voluntary control of internal states: Psychological and physiological. *Journal of Transpersonal Psychology, 2*, 1–26.

Grollman, A. P. (2001). Alternative medicine: The importance of evidence in medicine and medical education. *Academic Medicine, 76*(3), 221–223.

Groth-Marnat, G., & Edkins, G. (1996). Professional psychologists in general health care settings: A review of the financial efficacy of direct treatment interventions. *Professional Psychology: Research and Practice, 27*(2), 161–174.

Haley, W. E., McDaniel, S. H., Bray, J. H., Frank, R. G., Heldring, M., Johnson, S. B., et al. (1998). Psychological practice in primary care settings: Practical tips for a clinician. *Professional Psychology: Research and Practice, 29*(3), 237–244.

Jonas, W. B. (2001). Advising patients on the use of complementary and alternative medicine. *Applied Psychophysiology and Biofeedback, 26*(3), 205–214.

Jonas, W. B., & Levin, J. S. (Eds.). (1999). *Essentials of complementary and alternative medicine*. Philadelphia: Lippincott, Williams, & Wilkins.

Jonas, W. B., Linde, K., & Walach, H. (1999). How to practice evidence-based complementary and alternative medicine. In W. B. Jonas & J. S. Levin (Eds.), *Essentials of complementary and alternative medicine* (pp. 72–87). Philadelphia: Lippincott, Williams, & Wilkins.

Kiecolt-Glaser, J. K., Page, G. G., Marucha, P. T., MacCallum, R. C., & Glaser, R. (1998). Psychological influences on surgical recovery: Perspectives from psychoneuroimmunology. *American Psychologist, 53*(11), 1209–1218.

Koenig, H. (2000). Religion, spirituality, and medicine: Application to clinical practice. *Journal of the American Medical Association, 284*(13), 1708.

Kotses, H., Bernstein, I. L., Bernstein, D. I., Reynolds, R. V., Korbee, L., Wigal, J. K., et al. (1995). A self-management program for adult asthma. Part I: Development and evaluation. *Journal of Allergy and Clinical Immunology, 95*(2), 529–540.

Krauss, H. H., Godfrey, C., Kirk, J., & Eisenberg, D. M. (1998). Alternative health care: Its use by individuals with physical disabilities. *Archives of Physical Medicine and Rehabilitation, 79*(11), 1440–1447.

Kroenke, K. (2000). Somatization in primary care: It's time for parity. *General Hospital Psychiatry, 22*(3), 141–143.

Kroenke, K., & Mangelsdorff, A. D. (1989). Common symptoms in ambulatory care: Incidence, evaluation, therapy, and outcome. *American Journal of Medicine, 86*(3), 262–266.

Lawlis, G. F. (2001). Biofeedback. In L. W. Freeman & G. F. Lawlis (Eds.), *Mosby's complementary and alternative medicine: A research based approach* (pp. 196–224). St. Louis, MO: Mosby.

Lechnyr, R. (1992). Cost savings and effectiveness of mental health services. *Journal of the Oregon Psychological Association, 38*, 8–12.

McLellan, A. T., Lewis, D. C., O'Brien, C. P., & Kleber, H. D. (2000). Drug dependence, a chronic medical illness. *Journal of the American Medical Association, 284*(13), 1689–1695.

Moss, D. (1998). Biofeedback, mind-body medicine, and the higher limits of human nature. In D. Moss (Ed.), *Humanistic and transpersonal psychology: A historical and biographical sourcebook* (pp. 145–161). Westport, CT: Greenwood.

Moss, D. (1999). Biofeedback, mind-body medicine, and primary care. *Biofeedback, 27*(1), 4–11.

Moss, D. (2001). Biofeedback. In S. Shannon (Ed.), *Handbook of complementary and alternative therapies in mental health* (pp. 135–158). San Diego, CA: Academic Press.

Moss, D. (2002). The anxiety disorders: Identification and management. In B. Horwitz (Ed.), *Communication apprehension: Origins and management* (pp. 74–113). San Diego, CA: Singular/Thompson Learning.

Nadeau, M., & Moss, D. (1999). Integrated health care: A provider's primer. *Biofeedback, 27*(2), 15–25.

Nakagawa-Kogan, H. (1994). Self-management training: Potential for primary care. *Nurse Practitioners Forum, 5*(2), 77–84.

Perry, J. (2000). HCFA decision sooner than expected. *Biofeedback, 28*(3), 6A.

Quill, T. E. (1985). Somatization disorder: One of medicine's blind spots. *Journal of the American Medical Association, 254,* 3075–3079.

Rost, K., Zhang, M., Fortney, J., Smith, J., Coyne, J., & Smith, G. R., Jr. (1998). Persistently poor outcomes of undetected major depression in primary care. *General Hospital Psychiatry, 20*(1), 12–20.

Sackett, D. L., Straus, S. E., Richardson, W. S., Rosenberg, W., & Haynes, R. B. (Eds.). (2000). *Evidence-based medicine: How to practice and teach EBM.* Edinburgh, Scotland: Churchill Livingstone.

Schwartz, M., & Associates. (Eds.). (1995). *Biofeedback: A practitioner's guide* (2nd ed.). New York: Guilford.

Smith, S. (1995). Dealing with the difficult patient. *Postgraduate Medicine Journal, 71*(841), 653–657.

Sobel, D. S. (2000). Mind matters, money matters: The cost-effectiveness of mind/body medicine. *Journal of the American Medical Association, 284*(13), 1705.

Sternbach, R. (1966). *Principles of psychophysiology: An introductory text and readings.* San Diego, CA: Academic Press.

U.S. Department of Health and Human Services. (1994). *Healthy people 2000: National health promotion and disease prevention objectives.* Washington, DC: Government Printing Office.

van der Kolk, B. A., Pelcovitz, D., Roth, S., Mandel, F. S., McFarlane, A., & Herman, J. L. (1996). Dissociation, somatization, and affect dysregulation: The complexity of adaptation to trauma. *American Journal of Psychiatry, 153*(Suppl. 7), 83–93.

Whorton, J. C. (1999). The history of complementary and alternative medicine. In W. B. Jonas & J. S. Levin (Eds.), *Essentials of complementary and alternative medicine* (pp. 16–30). Philadelphia: Lippincott, Williams, & Wilkins.

Wickramasekera, I. (1988). *Clinical behavioral medicine: Some concepts and procedures.* New York: Plenum.

Wickramasekera, I. (1998). Secrets kept from the body but not the body or behavior: The unsolved problems of identifying and treating somatization and psychophysiological disease. *Advances in Mind-Body Medicine, 14,* 81–98.

Wickramasekera, I. (1999). The faith factor, the placebo, and AAPB. *Biofeedback, 27*(1), 1A–3A.

Wickramasekera, I., Davies, T., & Davies, M. (1996). Applied psychophysiology: A bridge between the biomedical model and the biopsychosocial model in family medicine. *Professional Psychology: Research and Practice, 27,* 221–233.

Wilhelm, F. H., & Roth, W. T. (1998). Taking the laboratory to the skies: Ambulatory assessment of self-report, autonomic and respiratory responses in flying phobia. *Psychophysiology, 35*(5), 596–606.

Wolf, S. L., Barnhart, H. X., Kutner, N. G., McNeely, E., Coogler, C., & Xu, T. (1996). Reducing frailty and falls in older persons: An investigation of tai chi and computerized balance training. Atlanta FICSIT group. Frailty and injuries:

Cooperative studies of intervention techniques. *Journal of American Geriatric Society, 44*(5), 489–497.

Xiangcai, X. (2000). *Qigong for treating common ailments: The essential guide to self-healing.* Boston: YMAA Publication Center.

Yingling, K. W., Wulsin, L. R., Arnold, L. M., & Rouan, G. W. (1993). Estimated prevalence of panic disorder and depression among consecutive patients seen in an emergency department with acute chest pain. *Journal of General Internal Medicine, 8,* 2315.

# CHAPTER 2

# The High Risk Model of Threat Perception and the Trojan Horse Role Induction: Somatization and Psychophysiological Disease

IAN WICKRAMASEKERA

**Abstract:** The identification and therapy of somatoform and psychophysiological disorders are major problems for medicine. This paper identifies three measurable risk factors (Wickramasekera, 1979, 1988, 1993a, 1993b, 1995) that are empirically associated with somatoform and psychophysiological disorders: high hypnotic ability, low hypnotic ability, and high repressive coping. Patients who are positive on one or more of these risk factors (all of which can constrict consciousness) have a high likelihood of having somatoform and psychophysiological disorders and should be assessed for the additional risk factors proposed in the high risk model of threat perception (HRMTP). Treatment of patients should begin with the Trojan horse role induction procedure (Wickramasekera, 1988), which enables patients, who might otherwise resist psychological interpretations of their physical problems, to recognize that unconscious threat perceptions could be driving their somatic symptoms. Understanding this relationship reduces their resistance to psychotherapy. A case study is presented of a patient without identifiable pathophysiology or psychopathology to account for somatic symptoms that were largely resistant to standard medical therapy. The patient was positive for several of the psychosocial and psychophysiological risk factors of the HRMTP and after experiencing the Trojan horse role induction showed improvement in somatic symptoms.

## THE CHALLENGE OF TREATING SOMATIZING PATIENTS

Somatization is the name medicine gives to the process by which an individual, "hiding" from threatening psychological information, expresses (or in more technical terms, transduces) his or her emotional distress into physical symptoms or maladaptive behavior. A partial list of physical symptoms that could be emotionally derived includes chronic fatigue, chronic allergic reactions, chronic pain, muscular and vascular headache, irritable bowel syndrome, temporomandibular joint pain, primary insomnia, low-back pain, and primary hypertension. Somatization may sound exotic, a phenomenon to be found in only a small number of patients. Nothing could be further from the truth. Estimates have determined that somatizing patients probably represent as many as half of the people seen by primary care doctors (Brown, Robertson, Kosa, & Alpert, 1971; deGruy, 1996; Roberts, 1994).

Numbers do not tell the whole story. Three facts make somatizing patients—who recently came to be labeled somatoform patients—perhaps the largest single challenge facing primary care medicine, a challenge that is both intellectual and economic. First, somatizing patients are difficult to identify. Second, they are difficult to successfully manage. Third, problems in diagnosis and management make these patients extremely costly to the medical system. The problem in a nutshell is this: Though somatizing patients represent the largest group of primary care patients, doctors are basically at a loss to know who they are and what to do about them.

Why are somatizing patients so difficult for primary care physicians to identify?

In theory, the identification process seems simple enough: Simply sort out patients who have no serious identifiable organic disease that accounts for their symptoms but who do have significant psychopathology. In reality, the problem is far more complex. The disturbing and puzzling fact is that at least 50 percent of the patients who bring somatic complaints to doctors display neither any serious organic identifiable disease (Brown et al., 1971; Roberts, 1994), which would suggest that they are somatoform patients, nor any significant psychopathology, the very criteria by which the *Diagnostic and Statistical Manual of Mental Disorders IV* says a somatizing patient is to be identified (deGruy, 1996). In other words, with our current methodological tools, there is no easy way to determine whether 50 percent of the patients who bring somatic complaints to primary care physicians are

somatizers or are suffering from (hard-to-identify) physical disorders.

Of course, in a certain percentage of cases, patients are quite capable of describing events in their lives that alert physicians would likely view as traumatic. For example, McCauley et al. (1997) reported that 22 percent of a large sample of nearly 2,000 internal medicine primary care patients were capable of verbally reporting childhood physical and sexual abuse associated with physical symptoms, psychological symptoms, and substance abuse. The problem of identifying somatizing patients involves the patients who do not recall or are unwilling to report traumatic or distressing events, because these events frequently remain inaccessible to our prevalent methodologies. There is little doubt, as my argument will help make clear, that the 22 percent figure in the McCauley study is only a portion of the somatizing patients in this sample of approximately 2,000 patients.

For medicine, the hard-to-identify somatizing patients represent the worst sort of lose-lose situation: The patients continue to suffer, and doctors experience a sense of failure. What the physicians see are individuals with chronic somatic complaints but, so far as the doctors can tell, no significant organic findings and no significant psychopathology. To help the patients find some relief and partly out of fear of malpractice lawsuits, doctors often refer these patients to medical specialists or subspecialists, who in turn proceed with their investigations by means of usually costly and invasive techniques that can have iatrogenic consequences. It is such tests that drive up the cost of managing somatoform patients, which on the average is nine times higher than the national norm (Smith, 1994). Further, if a patient is identified as (or thought to be) a somatizer, the situation is complicated even more by the fact that one third to one half of primary care patients refuse their doctors' referrals to mental health professionals (deGruy, 1996), presumably the very people who might help. A substantial portion of patients who have ills in their bodies do not want to be told that somehow the ills come from their psyches.

All this explains why somatization has been called medicine's "blind spot" (Quill, 1985) and medicine's "unsolved problem" (Lipowski, 1987). My aim here is to bring some light to this blind spot. My approach is twofold. First, I offer one solution to the problem of identifying somatoform patients that puts in the hands of primary care physicians the tools they need to determine whether a patient is likely to be a somatizer. The need for specialists and their tests is then reduced, and the costs of somatoform patients decline accordingly. Second, I offer an approach to treating somatoform patients that makes patients willing partners in the search within themselves for the source of their difficulties. In my conclusion, I set out six testable predictions that follow from the model that underlies my analysis. As I note there, proof that any of the predictions is false would cast doubt on the model.[1]

## SOMATOFORM PATIENTS

For reasons that I will explain, I have hypothesized that most patients who present somatic complaints without organic findings and who deny or are unaware of emotional distress or refuse a referral to the mental health sector are likely to have one or more of three predisposing psychometric risk factors (Wickramasekera, 1979, 1988, 1993a, 1993b; Wickramasekera & Atkinson, 1993; Wickramasekera, Davies, & Davies, 1996a; Wickramasekera & Kenkel, 1996a, 1996b). Briefly, these risk factors are *high hypnotic ability* (a score of 12 to 9 on the Harvard Group Scale of Hypnotic Susceptibility; Shor & Orne, 1962); *low hypnotic ability*

(a score of 3 to 0 on the Harvard scale); and a *high score on the Marlowe-Crowne scale* (17 or greater). The Marlowe-Crowne scale measures the capacity for blocking aversive perceptions, memories, and moods from consciousness; this process appears to operate by promoting inattention to aversive situations and by amplifying positive situations (Crowne & Marlowe, 1960).

The common feature of the three risk factors is that they reduce or block from consciousness negative emotions (as expressed in verbal reports by patients) but do not block their behavioral effects (which include violence, avoidance of certain situations, and reliance on self-soothing substance abuse) or their physiological effects (which I hypothesize include dysregulation of the autonomic nervous system and the immune system). In practice, the result is an incongruence (Wickramasekera, 1988, 1993a, 1993b, 1994a, 1994b) between what people are consciously aware of, as measured by their insistence that nothing is troubling them, and what their behavior or bodily responses reveal. For example, somatizers may be angry, fearful, or ashamed, as indicated by high measures of autonomic sympathetic activation (skin conductance, muscle tension, heart rate, blood pressure, hand temperature), but they will have minimal or no conscious perception of their anger, fear, or shame—or, more broadly, the negative affect they feel (Watson & Tellegen, 1985).

Put simply, the patient is being disturbed or made sick by a distressing, secret perception, memory, or mood that the patient blocks from consciousness. The character of the secrets can vary. They may pertain to a recent painful perception or to old traumatic memories of "unfinished" business that color and distort current perceptions. The critical point—the point that makes the person a somatoform patient—is that the secret is hidden from the self.

## THREE RISK FACTORS AND THEIR CORRELATION WITH SOMATIC DISORDERS

This perspective, a bit like a jigsaw puzzle, clearly consists of several major pieces. The first piece, without which there would be little reason to explore anything else, is whether or not empirical research has shown any association between the three elements that I label predisposing risk factors and the disorders that are common among somatoform and psychophysiological patients. More precisely, are there data to show a connection between high or low hypnotic ability and/or high Marlowe-Crowne scores and the kinds of medical problems that are typically regarded as expressions of somatization and psychophysiological disease?

The answer is a qualified yes. The three risk factors have been associated with a large variety of disorders often seen in somatoform and psychophysiological patients. Qualifying the association is the fact that the frequency of the risk factors is not yet known in people without such disorders. Yet the sheer variety of the disorders that have been empirically associated with the three risk factors is itself suggestive, strengthening the likelihood that this is a legitimate association. The disorders include primary insomnia (Perlstrom, Morin, Wickramasekera, Strong, & Ware, 1995; Perlstrom, Morin, Wickramasekera, & Ware, 1996; Wickramasekera, Ware, & Saxon, 1992); chronic somatoform complaints, such as functional muscular and vascular headache, temporomandibular joint pain, vasovagal syncope, low-back pain, primary dysmenorrhea, primary hypertension, idiopathic flushing, and hyperhydrosis (Wickramasekera, 1988, 1994b, 1995); irritable bowel syndrome (Toner, Koyama, Garfinkel, & Jeejeebhoy, 1992); morbid obesity (Wickramasekera & Price, 1997); moderate obesity (Wickramasekera & Atkinson, 1993); nonorganic chest pain (Saxon &

Wickramasekera, 1994); chronic pain (Remler, 1990; Stam, McGrath, Brooke, & Cosire, 1986); chronic urticaria (Shertzer & Lookingbill, 1987); posttraumatic stress disorder symptom intensity (Spiegel, Hunt, & Dondershine, 1988; Stutman & Bliss, 1985); nightmares (Belicki & Belicki, 1986); and bulimia and substance abuse (Pettinati, Horne, & Staats, 1985; Pettinati et al., 1990).

In some studies, too, a risk factor characterizes a higher than expected number of patients with a typical somatic disorder. For example, in a sample of patients with moderate to severe asthma, Wagaman (1996) found significantly more high hypnotizables ($p<.001$) and more high Marlowe-Crowne scores ($p<.001$). A study of cardiac surgery patients by Greenleaf, Fisher, Miaskowski, and DuHamel (1992) revealed significantly more low hypnotizables (though the researchers did not remark on the finding), and found that the lows took longer than others to recover from cardiac surgery and that cardiopulmonary function took longer to stabilize in patients who were low or high in hypnotic ability ($p<.05$).

## THE THREE RISK FACTORS BLOCK CONSCIOUSNESS

The next question, the second piece of the puzzle, is how the three risk factors—both high and low hypnotic ability and high scores on the Marlowe-Crowne scale—serve to block an individual's awareness of his or her negative feelings or experiences. In particular, how can high and low hypnotic ability have a comparable blocking effect on consciousness? As I have indicated, the basic general point with all three risk factors is that they seem to be associated with peculiarities in the processing of cognitive and emotional information, producing an incongruence between conscious and unconscious perceptions, memories, and moods.[2] In short, high hypnotizables, low hypnotizables, and people with high Marlowe-Crowne scores represent three different cognitive styles that have important repercussions for health.

## Cognitive Style
## of High Hypnotizables

I begin with the features of the people who are high in hypnotic ability. It is empirically well established that these people can block or significantly reduce from consciousness (as manifested by their verbal reports) even surgical and experimental laboratory pain (Hilgard & Hilgard, 1975) and can also block memories from consciousness, as in post-hypnotic amnesia (Hilgard, 1977). I maintain that it is the chronic (unconscious) use of such cognitive and perceptual inhibitory mechanisms to block negative emotions that places people with high hypnotic ability at risk at first for somatization and later perhaps even organic disease (Wickramasekera, 1993a, 1993b, 1998). Many features of these "highs" add to their problems with healthy living.

A paradoxical feature is that despite their lack of awareness of their negative emotions, highs can also be *hypersensitive* to events, as the fairy-tale princess was hypersensitive to the pea at the bottom of the stack of mattresses on which she was trying to sleep. Being acutely alert, hypersensitive highs often develop insomnia (Perlstrom et al., 1995; Wickramasekera, Ware, & Saxon, 1992), particularly if they cannot mobilize their analgesic and amnesiac abilities to block out painful sensations and aversive memories. This hypersensitivity is likely related to the tendency of such highs to see meaning and pattern in events that appear randomly distributed to people with moderate or low hypnotic ability, a propensity I call surplus pattern recognition. The upside of this propensity is that it puts these people "at risk" for creativity in art and science if they

can discipline their talents to see meaning and pattern. But if the meaning they perceive is threatening, they can cognitively elaborate or amplify the presumed threat to the point that they become agitated and episodically dysfunctional. In this context, their cognitive amnesia and analgesia abilities (Hilgard, 1982, 1987), when effectively mobilized, are probably adaptive sensitivity-reducing mechanisms of compensation that support survival (Wickramasekera, 1988, 1994a). Nonetheless, when the feature of surplus pattern recognition interacts with negative affect, the likely consequence is a downward spiral of fear, panic, and depression (Wickramasekera, 1994a, 1994b, 1994c; Wickramasekera, Pope, & Kolm, 1996).

Some highs are also prone to surplus empathy, to the point that they become so absorbed in the problems of others that they may develop empathic somatic symptoms (including pains, wounds, stigmata, and cardiovascular responses), unless they carefully monitor their own boundaries. These highs are at major risk for transference and countertransference problems in close personal relationships, in psychotherapy as well as in life in general.

Another important feature of highs is that they tend to leap cognitively from specific instances to general expectations very rapidly and are therefore at risk for excessive credulity if they do not concurrently practice critical logical thinking. This trait of highs, the quick leap to general expectations, is seen in the relative ease with which they are conditioned, which occurs more rapidly with highs than it does with lows (Das, 1958a, 1958b; King & McDonald, 1976; Webb, 1962; Wickramasekera, 1970). Studies have shown that the speed of Pavlovian conditioning is based on how quickly expectations about rewards or punishments are acquired (Rescorla, 1988).

The rapid acquisition of expectations can be maladaptive. Consider a finding that deals with a phenomenon called absorption, which is a correlate of hypnotic ability. Being high on absorption means that the individual's cognitive styles are marked by a profound capacity for involvement in internal or external events that alter perception, memory, mood, and physiology in a "top-down" fashion (Sperry, 1980). High absorbers are at greater risk for developing anticipatory nausea and vomiting during cancer chemotherapy than are people low on absorption (Challis & Stam, 1992; Wickramasekera & Saxon, 1988). Importantly, studies show that absorption is a cognitive style that seems stable across time and situations and has a 50 percent heritability index in monozygotic versus dizygotic twins, even when they are reared apart (Tellegen, Lykken, Bouchard, Wilcox, & Rich, 1988). The maladaptiveness can be intellectual and behavioral. Highs are prone to leap to surplus inferences, forming and dissolving belief systems rapidly, which puts them at risk for "conversions" to cults.

Studies have also found that during (stressful) verbal information processing, those high in hypnotic ability are prone to perceive psychological events (perceptions, memories, moods) as occurring involuntarily or outside their control, both during and outside hypnosis (Bowers, 1982; Dixon, Brunet, & Laurence, 1990; Dixon & Laurence, 1992). This perception of intrusive, uncontrollable, and unpredictable events can amplify fear and pain (Mineka & Kihlstrom, 1978). Highs' perception of sensory and motor events (for example, "automatic" movements) or memories as intrusively "occurring" by themselves or automatically can make life seem out of control—as in the comic example of the ex-Nazi plagued by an automatic hand salute in Stanley Kubrick's movie *Dr. Strangelove*. Not surprisingly, then, a recent study of chronic pain patients found that in highs, negative, stressful events are physiologically amplified more than in moderates or lows (Wickramasekera, Pope, & Kolm, 1996)—a

very important finding theoretically because it shows that two unrelated (orthogonal) variables (hypnotic ability and stress) can interact, amplifying sympathetic reactivity (expressed in the fight-or-flight response). It is likely that highs also perceive positive events as occurring involuntarily or effortlessly (Grove & Lewis, 1996; Wickramasekera, 1988), as in creative inspiration from the "muse" or as an expression of what has been called flow (Csikszentmihalyi & Massimini, 1975; Grove & Lewis, 1996). There are no detrimental health effects from seeing positive events as involuntary unless the euphoria becomes exaggerated to the point of delusions of grandeur. It is the perceived involuntariness of emotional events that places highs at risk for mood oscillations (Crowson, Conroy, & Chester, 1991; Velten, 1968).

In sum, because highs are prone to hypersensitivity, surplus pattern recognition, and surplus empathy, because they acquire expectations (conditioned responses) so rapidly, and because many perceive psychological events as occurring automatically, their cognitive style appears to put them at risk for excessive credulity and mood fluctuations—yet all the while they may remain unaware of the source of their own negative feelings. Clinically, extreme forms of this credulity and empathy can manifest themselves as the psychophysiological plasticity caricatured by Woody Allen in his movie *Zelig*.

### Cognitive Style of Low Hypnotizables

People who are low on hypnotic ability, on the other hand, are likely to be *hyposensitive*, to have a diminished sensitivity to the emotional somatic component of psychosocial threats. Clinically, lows are observed to be mainly skeptical, rational, and analytic about most events. They are reluctant to go from specific instances to general expectations, particularly regarding the etiology of unpleasant emotional somatic information emanating from their own bodies. Rather, they are prone to look for mechanical, chemical, or physical explanations of their distress and tend to prefer chemical, surgical, or physical solutions (Wickramasekera & Price, 1997).

In contrast to highs, little is known about the features of lows, except of course for their lack of words to acknowledge and describe their feelings (Frankel, Apfel-Savitz, Nemiah, & Sifneos, 1977). The reason for the relative lack of information is partly because lows skeptically avoid psychological studies like the plague.

Clinically, I have observed lows to have a "bottom-up" (Sperry, 1980) cognitive style that searches for and needs to be shown (not just told about) external mechanical or physical explanations of natural phenomena. Consider a study in Virginia of the absorption scores of two different samples of medical students totaling 200 people (Wickramasekera, Davies, & Davies, 1996b). Remember that absorption is a correlate of hypnotic ability and that absorption is the cognitive capacity to be profoundly involved in imagination and fantasy in ways that may alter perception, memory, mood, and physiology. The study found that the mean absorption scores of both samples of medical students were significantly below the national norm. These students, in other words, needed to be shown, not told, about the mind-body connection. If the finding of a lower mean absorption score is replicated at other medical schools and is found, as predicted, to be even *lower* at schools that train medical educators (e.g., Harvard and Stanford), it is not surprising that our health care services and system are limited to, and controlled by, a belief in "bottom-up" biomedical reductionism.

Empirically, it has been found that the sympathetic reaction of low hypnotizable chronic pain patients (as manifested in, for example, their electrodermal reactivity) is lower than the reactivity of highs during cognitive stress (Wickramasekera, Pope, & Kolm, 1996), indicating a diminished fight-or-flight response. But, of course, this diminished sympathetic response, about which much is known, may tell us nothing *directly* about reactivity or dysregulation in the parasympathetic division of the autonomic nervous system, about which much less is known. A recent study of 70 morbidly obese patients seeking gastric exclusion surgery—most patients weighed more than 400 pounds (182 kg) and had a body mass index of 40 or more (normal is 25)—may offer some insight into the hypothesis of parasympathetic dysregulation (Wisen, Rossner, & Johansson, 1987) under conditions of chronic stress (Wickramasekera & Price, 1997).

The study found that low absorption scores occurred more frequently in the morbidly obese patients ($p<.001$) and that these patients had very high measures of negative affectivity ($p<.001$), which means, in a word, that they were notably fearful or depressed. Surgeons would likely argue that the weight of the patients was the source of their depression. No doubt there is some truth to this, but the question is, Why did these patients become morbidly obese in the first place? Wickramasekera and Price (1997) maintain that it is partly related to both their high negative affectivity (their marked fear or depression) and the cognitive style associated with their low absorption measures. Thus, both traits probably existed before the morbid obesity. Further, people with low absorption would tend not to acknowledge depression or anxiety but instead would use a behavioral coping style like overeating or drinking to soothe their emotional pain or sadness. Hence, in the presence of depression and anxiety, the skeptical and rational cognitive style of these people contributed to their overeating, and this coping style eventually contributed to the dysregulation of the parasympathetic division of their autonomic nervous systems and to their morbid obesity. Given their cognitive style, moreover, it is no surprise that these patients fail in behavioral weight control programs, which probably have low credibility for them in the first place, and eventually seek surgery.

Several additional studies support the contention that low hypnotic ability is a personality feature that contributes to increased risk of organic disease (Wickramasekera, 1979, 1988, 1993a, 1993b). For example, in a primary medical care setting, the bulk of patients complaining of chest pain were found to be low on absorption ($p<.005$), and a subset of them had significant organic findings (Saxon & Wickramasekera, 1994). The previously mentioned study of cardiac surgery patients (Greenleaf et al., 1992), which found that low hypnotizable patients took longer to recover from cardiac surgery than did moderates or highs, also reported, but did not otherwise comment on, the fact that this sample of patients contained significantly more lows ($n = 19$) than moderates ($n = 8$) or highs ($n = 5$).

Further, Harris, Porges, Carpenter, and Vincenz (1993) found that low hypnotizable "normals"—people without symptoms or pathophysiology—have higher baseline heart rates and lower cardiac vagal tones than do highs. The importance of the higher baseline heart rate is clear: It may increase the risk for heart disease. The lower cardiac vagal tone also has negative implications for health, because high cardiac vagal tone has been associated with positive health, greater alertness, and, as a likely consequence of this increased alertness, greater reactivity to the environment (Donchin, Feld, & Porges, 1985; Donchin, Constantini, Szold, Byrne, & Porges, 1992; Porges, 1991, 1992). In line with this finding of low cardiac vagal tone among low hypnotizables, DeBenedittis, Cigada, and Bianchi (1994) found that during hypnosis, low hypnotizables were less able to reduce their fight-or-flight response—that is, increase their vagal tone—than were highs. The study by Harris

et al. (1993) also found that during experimental mood induction (for example, happy and sad moods), lows showed less cardiovascular reactivity than highs, a sign, it would seem, of the low sensitivity of lows to psychosocial stimulation and the environment. Consistent with DeBenedittis's observation, we had found that during high cognitive stress, normal low hypnotizable college students had lower subjective perceptions of the stressor ($p<.001$) than did highs (Pomerantz & Wickramasekera, 1988). In a later study on chronic-pain patients who were low hypnotizables, Wickramasekera, Pope, and Kolm (1996) similarly found that during cognitive stress, they had less stress-related reactivity (such as electrodermal reactivity) than highs had.

The important question then is, Do lows who are more reactive during resting baseline conditions (higher heart rates, lower vagal tones; Harris et al., 1993) make an extra conscious or unconscious effort (parasympathetically) during threatening stimulation (stress)? And do they endeavor to block psychosocial cognitive stress from both consciousness and physiology? If so, what, if any, are the long-term biological consequences of such a stress-blocking cognitive style for the dysregulation of the autonomic nervous system and specifically for the parasympathetic nervous system and the immune system (Wickramasekera, 1988, 1993a, 1993b, 1994a)? Some suggestive evidence is the finding that among patients who had clear pathophysiology and who complained of chest pain, a larger than expected number were low on absorption (Saxon & Wickramasekera, 1994) and were morbidly obese (Wickramasekera & Price, 1997). Arguably, the cognitive style of low absorption and the behavioral response of overeating enabled these people to reduce from their awareness any conscious recognition of negative emotional signs that they might be becoming ill. Relevant here is the finding that changes in mood and feelings, like an early warning system, can precede the onset of even infections and organic diseases (Canter, 1972; Canter, Cluff, & Imboden, 1972; Canter, Imboden, & Cluff, 1966; Hall, Popkin, Devaul, Faillace, & Stickney, 1978).

In my clinical practice, I have observed that most people who are low on hypnotic ability or absorption tend to be rigidly skeptical, critical, and analytical in their cognitive styles and often minimize subjective sources of information (particularly negative emotions) in favor of evidence that is objective and ocular ("Show me!") rather than instructional. Is emotional stoicism and skepticism of symbolic and subjective sources of information associated with delays in seeking medical investigation of distress? Do these delays contribute to the establishment of organic disease in lows?

People with low hypnotic ability may also be more vulnerable to psychosocial stress because they are less able to recognize it and tend to deny psychological causation of physical dysfunction or distress. In addition, the retarded rate of Pavlovian conditioning in low hypnotizables (Das, 1958a, 1958b; Wickramasekera, 1970, 1988) may mean that these people generally discount or minimize the role of conditioned or symbolic stimuli and delay responding until the onset of the physical stimulus (an unconditioned stimulus). Metaphorically, it is not the sound of rustling leaves, a conditioned stimulus, that is lethal to the deer but the wolf's unconditioned stimulus of teeth and claws. The same process may be at work in low hypnotizables. Given their cognitive style, they may discount the conditioned signals of an early warning system and see no reason to flee until they observe the unconditioned stimulus of canines in their jugular.

I am proposing, then, that lows have a diminished sensitivity to subtle psychosocial threats, partly because of their rigidly rational-skeptical cognitive style, and therefore are less able to recognize and cope with subtle cognitive emotional threats than are people who approach their experience with a wider emotional range.

In sum, both excessive credulity, as in the highs, and excessive skepticism, as in the lows, appear to be risk factors for somatoform disorders.

## Cognitive Style of People With High Marlowe-Crowne Scores

Finally, and briefly, people who score high on the Marlowe-Crowne test avert their inner eyes from the unpleasant. They appear to operate in ways that block threatening perspectives and memories from consciousness (Wickramasekera, 1993a, 1994a, 1994b, 1995), or in a more complex system, to practice self-deception or repression (Schwartz, 1990; Weinberger, 1990). While these people may be verbally and subjectively unaware of threatening perceptions, memories, or moods, their negative emotions—such as fear and anger—nonetheless leak through into avoidance behavior (phobias, insomnia) or induce chronic sympathetic activation (leading to a disorder like primary hypertension). The incongruence between the verbal report that fails to include any perceived threat on the one hand and the behavioral and physiological measures of threat on the other hand may further lead to the dysregulation of the autonomic nervous system and place such people at risk for neuroendocrine and immune disorders (Wickramasekera, 1988, 1993a). The findings of several studies that associate high Marlowe-Crowne scores with excessive sympathetic activation, high endorphin levels, and possible immunosuppression (Jamner, Schwartz, & Leigh, 1988; Jensen, 1987) help lay the groundwork for such possibilities.

Other studies add to the picture. We found that among patients with organic findings who complained of chest pain, significantly more ($p<.0001$) had high Marlowe-Crowne scores (Saxon & Wickramasekera, 1994).

Another study (Palsson, Wickramasekera, Rutledge, Davies, & Downing, 1997) found that among 54 normal medical students, the average baseline finger temperature of high Marlowe-Crowne scorers was 5.3 °F (3 °C) lower than in those with low scores (83 °F versus 88.3 °F; 28.3 °C versus 31.3 °C), signifying a considerably higher baseline fight-or-flight response in the high Marlowe-Crowne scorers. Wagaman (1996) found elevated Marlowe-Crowne scores in patients with moderate to severe asthma, and Toner et al. (1992) found elevated Marlowe-Crowne scores in irritable bowel syndrome patients.

I hypothesize that rigidly limiting oneself to one of three cognitive styles that can reduce access to threatening negative emotional information can be maladaptive and even lethal in the long run. Hence, therapy for high and low hypnotizables should consist of learning to extend their range of cognitive operations to the cognitive style of moderately hypnotizable people, even episodically; and therapy for high Marlowe-Crowne scorers should consist of extending their cognitive style to the style of low scorers, again, even episodically.

## PREVALENCE AND PSYCHOPHYSIOLOGY OF THE HIDDEN

The last pieces of the puzzle concern the impact of negative emotions, disturbing secrets, or hidden, troubling information on the psyche and the body. How prevalent is an effect and how, biochemically, does it occur? For decades, clinicians have been aware that unperceived, disturbing emotions can make one physically sick and contribute to maladaptive or even self-destructive behavior (Freud, 1948; Jung, 1969; Vaughan, 1997). Research studies are now adding to our understanding of how this can happen in many people.

Today strong and growing empirical evidence exists that cognitive and emotional factors can constrict consciousness, not just in patients but also in normal people (Shedler, Mayman, & Manis, 1993; Shevrin, 1991; Shevrin, Bond, Brakel, Hertel, & Williams, 1996; Weinberger, 1990; Wickramasekera, 1976, 1988, 1993a, 1994a, 1994b, 1994c; Wickramasekera, Pope, & Kolm, 1996). These studies lay the groundwork for understanding the everyday beginnings by which common cognitive coping styles can sometimes lead to somatization and even to serious psychophysiological disease.

Research in cognitive neuroscience, neuropsychology, and experimental hypnosis is also showing that complex and simple unconscious factors can influence behavior and biology in everyday life. This work empirically supports the reality of many previously contested and controversial phenomena, including unintended and unattended thought in daily life, subliminal or implicit perception, nonconscious social information processing, sleep learning, and learning under anesthesia (Bentin & Moscovitch, 1990; Greenwald, 1992; Kihlstrom, 1987; Lewicki, 1986; Shedler, Mayman, & Manis, 1993; Shevrin et al., 1996; Uleman & Bargh, 1989). Again, these studies, by documenting such phenomena, testify to the plenitude and commonness of the processes that can lead to somatization and, more broadly, explain the psyche's contribution to disease.

At the same time, the nexus between feeling and thinking is receiving new, clarifying attention. Extremely valuable here is the work of the neurologist and neuroscientist Damasio (1994), who argues that feeling is an "integral component of the machinery of reason" (p. xii). This perspective helps provide a framework for understanding how blocking from consciousness threatening or aversive emotions can be associated with poor judgment and can be maladaptive both behaviorally and biologically. Put simply, such blocking deprives reason of what it needs to make sense of complex events and is hypothesized to impair autonomic, neuroendocrine, and immune responses mediated by the brain. As Damasio says, "Consciousness buys an enlarged protection policy" (p. 133).

Both Damasio (1994) and Dennett (1991) point out additionally that the strong intuitive perception of the so-called Cartesian theater of an integrated mind from "parcellated activities" for vision, sound, taste, smell, shape, and so on is an illusion. There is, in fact, no single region in the human brain equipped to process simultaneous input from all the sensory modalities we experience simultaneously. Damasio proposes that our strong illusory sense of an integrated mind is created from "synchronizing sets of neural activity in separate brain systems, in effect a trick of timing" (p. 93).

I have hypothesized that the three risk factors can selectively *disable* negative emotional input to this "binding system" (Wickramasekera 1993a, 1993b) and that the chronic failure to detect potent information from reflexive emotional states can have important negative behavioral and health consequences, mostly by blocking negative emotions *based on and associated with neuroendocrine and immune responses* (National Academy of Sciences, 1989). This loss of information to consciousness appears to dysregulate the adaptive functions of the autonomic nervous system and the immune system. At the same time, it constricts the range of cognitive perspectives and the range of behavioral coping responses to threatening but inevitable human predicaments (including failures, births, deaths, divorce, loss of support systems, disappointments).

It is becoming clear that our automatic, unconscious emotional responses to the inevitable "risk taking" involved in human development are, in fact, composed of powerful neuroendocrine and immune responses mediated by neuropeptides that constitute a natural "emotional pharmacy" (Dafter, 1996), which can be toxic or healing. Unconscious emotions may contain important information (as in the case study described later in this chapter) that should rationally be factored into conscious judgments and conscious decisions in living. In the famous statement by Pascal, who perhaps is not sufficiently appreciated for his understanding of the link between emotion and thought, "The heart has reasons that reason does not know."

To all the previous observations, I would add one further note by way of emphasis: Under conditions of psychosocial threat or trauma, the blocking operation of the three risk factors increases in probability.

## THE PROCEDURE IN BRIEF

I have gone far from the office of the primary doctor to explain my proposition that testing for high or low hypnotizability and high Marlowe-Crowne scores can be used to help identify somatoform and psychophysiological patients. To close this part of the discussion, let me return to that office and to the procedure that I believe will give primary care physicians a new grip on one of medicine's most recalcitrant, discouraging, and costly problems.

In sum, then, I propose that all patients in primary care medicine who present chronic somatoform symptoms without obvious organic disease and without the diagnosable psychopathology listed in *Diagnostic and Statistical Manual of Mental Disorders IV* be routinely tested for the three risk factors of high or low hypnotic ability and a high Marlowe-Crowne score while their medical investigations for pathophysiology continue.[3] People with one or more of these three factors may well have blocked or reduced negative emotional information from their consciousness, the lack of which, as I have tried to explain, can impair judgment and adaptive behavior.

When one or more of the three risk factors is identified, further testing may be useful. I have developed what I call a high risk model of threat perception, or somatization, which includes measures that are specialized for identifying additional triggering and buffering factors (Wickramasekera, 1979, 1988, 1995). The model contains tests for catastrophizing (Zocco, 1984), negative affectivity (Watson & Clark, 1984), major life changes (Holmes, 1981), hassles (Zarski, 1984), support systems (House, Landis, & Umberson, 1988; Sarason, Levine, Basham, & Sarason, 1983), and coping skills (Moos, 1993). For the interested reader, I include a blank patient profile worksheet (Figure 2.1), on which I score the various components that compose the model (Wickramasekera, 1988, 1993a, 1995).

Similarly, the verbal report by a patient showing that he or she is consciously unaware of any threatening feelings or experiences, in conjunction with a psychophysiological stress profile (Wickramasekera, 1976, 1988, 1993a, 1994b, 1994c; Wickramasekera, Davies, & Davies, 1996a) showing that the patient does in fact react to such feelings or experiences, would increase the index of suspicion.

In any case, these procedures—especially testing for the three predisposing risk factors—should allow primary care physicians to determine with a fair degree of confidence whether a person, like some estimated 50 percent of the people seen by primary care physicians, is a somatoform patient or may have a significant psychophysiological component to his or her disease.

## TREATING THE SOMATOFORM PATIENT

The question of how to treat a somatoform patient is almost as vexing as how to identify one. As I noted earlier, many people who go to their doctors with physical problems do not, as a rule, like to be told that the problems are "in their heads." How can one make this clear without antagonizing a patient and, more important, gain the patient's collaboration in resolving the problem?

To reveal and assess the "secrets" that somatoform patients are keeping from themselves, I have developed a treatment that I call the Trojan horse role induction (Wickramasekera, 1988, 1989a, 1989b, 1996b). It begins by first putting out the "fire" of chronic distressing somatic symptoms (e.g., headaches, irritable bowel syndrome, vasovagal syncope, insomnia) with a variety of empirically effective techniques like biofeedback, hypnosis, and cognitive behavior therapy (National Institutes of Health Technology Assessment Panel, 1996; Olness, 1996, Wickramasekera, 1970, 1976, 1977, 1988, 1994c; Wickramasekera & Kenkel, 1996a, 1996b). Concurrently, it uses psychophysiological monitoring techniques to identify, track, and explore the physiological changes associated with the "matches" that have started the patient's "fire" —the secrets blocked from consciousness that drive the somatic symptoms. This is not lie detection but truth detection.

When the primary focus of the therapist's attention is first on the effective reduction of the patient's chronic distressing symptoms, a powerful positive transference relationship can be developed that enables the bypassing of typical psychological security operations and allows the patient to talk about threatening secrets "kept from the self." The Trojan horse role induction, along with psychophysiological monitoring (Wickramasekera 1988, 1994a, 1994b, 1994c; Wickramasekera, Davies, & Davies, 1996a) appears to disable, at least temporarily, the risk factors maintaining mind-body incongruence or self-deception and improves psychophysiological self-regulation. This combined approach converts somatizers into curious psychotherapy patients engaged in a therapeutic alliance whose aim is

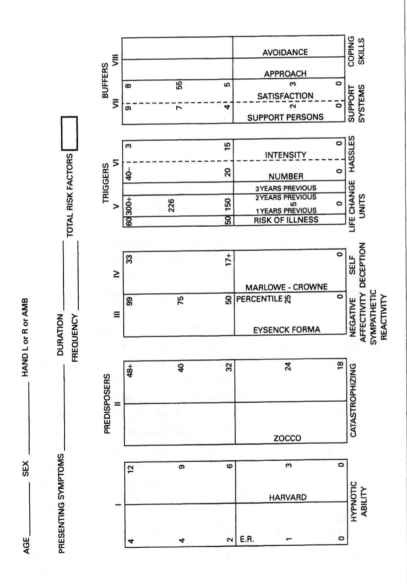

**Figure 2.1  High Risk Model of Threat Perception**

SOURCE: Wickramasekera (1988, figure 26, p. 218).

not simply to put out the fire but to find the matches blocked from consciousness.

## CASE STUDY: THE TWO-MILLION-DOLLAR MAN

The following abbreviated case study illustrates the combination of Trojan horse role induction with psychophysiological therapy.

K.C. is a 35-year-old white, married father of two children. In the five years before seeking help, K.C. had developed several somatic symptoms, including uncontrolled hypertension, severe idiopathic flushing, severe headaches, and mild depression. He was studied more than 20 times for extensive periods (on both in- and outpatient bases) at three famous medical school centers, two in the Midwest and one in the South. His health insurance company had spent more than $2 million over three years on highly technical biomedical studies. But only his headaches were moderately improved by a combination of several drugs. The other somatic symptoms were unaltered or had worsened during the three years of expensive and invasive tests. Psychiatric interviews and conventional psychological testing at the three major academic medical centers found no evidence of any significant psychopathology. Because of K.C.'s failure to respond to any type of blood pressure medication and his unpredictable episodic surges of blood pressure, his Midwestern internist considered his situation life threatening and referred him for a series of rare and highly specialized neuroendocrine tests. When this series of tests was also negative, the medical neuroendocrinologist, who knew of my work with the psychophysiology of somatization, referred the patient to me for evaluation.

K.C.'s history revealed that because of his uncontrolled somatic symptoms, he had quit work three years earlier and progressively had become, in his words, "an invalid." He felt that he was barely able to perform simple

housekeeping and child care activities. He also gained weight and increased his alcohol intake. Prior to his assorted symptoms, he had been an excellent student, a leader in college, and a very successful salesman on the fast track to a top executive position with a major national corporation. K.C.'s chronic somatic symptoms, doctor shopping, and self-declared invalid status enabled his wife to resuscitate her own promising professional career that had been interrupted by the birth of the children. He reported some mild marital stress accompanying his lack of employment, weight gain, and increased alcohol intake, but he denied any recent or remote significant distress or trauma at home, at work, or in any social relationships. He reported he missed seeing his parents, who lived several hundred miles away. He explained that he frequently saw his in-laws, who lived close to him. He stated that if his somatic symptoms were controlled, he could return to work, and his depression would resolve.

Psychological testing indicated that K.C. was high on both hypnotic ability (Harvard scale = 9; Stanford Hypnotic Susceptibility Scale Form C = 9; absorption = 70 percent) and the Marlowe-Crowne test (20). Because he had two psychometric risk factors for somatization, I suspected that his verbal report data and conventional psychological testing (Symptom Check List–90 [SCL-90]) would be relatively uninformative. Previous psychiatric interviews at major medical school centers had identified no diagnosable psychopathology (as indicated in the *Diagnostic and Statistical Manual of Mental Disorders IV*), and psychological testing on standard personality tests (e.g., the Beck Depression Inventory and the Minnesota Multiphasic Personality Inventory) were all within the normal range. In fact, his SCL-90 scales were nearly all in the normal range except for depression, which was an elevated $T = 74$ ($T = 50$ is normal), and hostility, which at $T = 41$ was his lowest score ($T = 50$ is normal).

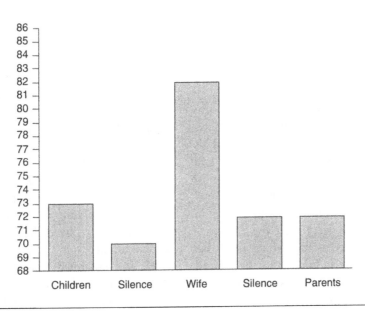

**Figure 2.2**    Blood Pressure and Conversational Topic

In spite of the adversities of the last several years, K.C. appeared cheerful, humorous, and socially outgoing. Nonetheless, he had a cold and wet handshake. His psychophysiological stress profile (Wickramasekera, 1976, 1988, 1993a; Wickramasekera, Davies, & Davies, 1996a) confirmed the source of his cold and wet hands. Even resting baseline measures indicated a sympathetically activated body. His most reactive systems were cardiovascular: a low resting baseline hand temperature of 73.6 °F, or 23.1 °C (normal is 88 °F, or 31.1 °C), a resting heart rate of 86.08 beats per minute (normal is from 70 to 80 beats per minute), low blood volume pulse (no absolute normal values, only relative values) indicating peripheral vasoconstriction, a high skin conductance of 17.74 μ mhos (a measure of sweat gland activity in which normal is 5.0 μ mhos), and a high frontal electromyogram of 11.78 microvolts (normal is approximately 7.0 microvolts). Hence, even under resting baseline conditions, K.C.'s body was on a "red alert" status. But this apparently was a "secret" to him. During the measurements, he reported feeling calm (on a visual analogue of the Subjective Units of Distress Scale).

The incongruence between, on the one hand, his low level of verbally reported subjective distress and his cheerful manner and, on the other, the strong physiological baseline indicators of chronic sympathetic activation suggested that most of his stress was outside consciousness. Hence, any productive clinical-verbal investigation would require concurrent physiological monitoring to reveal to K.C. the "secrets" he was keeping from himself. Because of his stress profile data, I chose to monitor his blood pressure continuously, first under baseline conditions (eyes open 3 minutes, eyes closed 3 minutes) and later while he was talking about several topics that included his parents, children, wife, job, and friends. (Since some question surrounds such measurements, I note that I used equipment manufactured by Critikon-Dinamap Johnson & Johnson). Figure 2.2 illustrates his blood pressure response under three conditions.

As the figure makes clear, his strongest response occurred when he talked about his wife. In the course of the monitoring, I changed to a neutral topic, then returned to his wife and replicated the same blood pressure response three times before I showed

K.C. the data. He acknowledged the reliability of his blood pressure response to the topic of his wife, but he denied any conscious perception of blood pressure increase or any associated emotion.

Because he was visiting our medical center, he spoke to his wife daily from his motel room. I asked him to measure and record his blood pressure twice before, during, and after speaking to his wife. His records indicated the same strong blood pressure elevation while talking to his wife and a delay in blood pressure recovery after the conversation. He also experienced flushing across his face, chest, and back. In addition, he noticed a feeling of sadness and irritation during this "in vivo" conversational stimulation.

In the course of three weeks of intensive psychophysiological psychotherapy (three times a week), K.C. became aware of intense rage toward his wife, whom he perceived as "jealous" both of his prior professional success, because it left her "trapped" as a housewife, and of his relationship to his parents. He perceived her as very domineering and seeking to separate him from his children and his parents. He felt she blamed him for the pregnancies that had interrupted her promising professional career, which was now slowly prospering during his illness.

At the conclusion of the three weeks of therapy, K.C.'s physician had withdrawn him from all blood pressure medications, and his systolic and diastolic levels were within the normal range. His blood pressure surges were infrequent, and the flushing had stopped. He recognized that he had very frustrated and angry feelings toward his wife. He also realized that he had always had ambivalent sexual feelings toward other men, about which he felt shame, and that he now felt profoundly ashamed of what had become of his promising career and of his present life. When he left Virginia, I referred him to a skilled psychotherapist back in the Midwest to continue to work on his personal and marital problems and specifically his sexual conflicts.

When he returned for a three-month medical and psychological follow-up, all his somatic symptoms had declined in frequency and intensity by more than 80 percent. He reported that his headaches had dropped to zero and that he was off all pain medications. His flushing had improved more than 95 percent, and his episodic blood pressure surges had become even less frequent, even without any blood pressure medication. However, he had not reduced his weight or his alcohol intake.

He had separated from his wife, built a closer relationship with his children, and was contemplating divorce and another adult relationship. For the first time in his marriage, he had twice visited his parents just with his children, and he felt supported by his family. He reported that he used the self-hypnosis skills he had learned in Virginia to soothe his negative emotions only on an erratic basis. He also reported, however, that the self-hypnosis enabled him to see old situations freshly.

This case study illustrates how the identification of two psychometric risk factors for blocking threatening emotions from consciousness influenced the selection of techniques of therapy and led to the surprising short-term psychosocial and somatic outcomes. Remember that K.C. had his symptoms for more than three years and that his health insurance company had paid out more than $2 million in an effort to learn how to resolve them.

K.C.'s unconscious emotional reactions of rage (driving hypertension and headaches) and shame (driving idiopathic flushing or blushing) were associated with autonomic and neuroendocrine responses that, I maintain, drove his somatic symptoms, at least in part. As I have proposed, the chronic occlusion or blocking from consciousness of salient cognitive-emotional/neuroendocrine information can have seriously deleterious consequences for behavior and biology. In this case, the lack of conscious information about his important emotions clearly seems to have impaired his judgment and behavioral choices in everyday life. I would further hypothesize that the occlusion of conscious information about his emotions *amplified* the pharmacological component of emotion that drove his somatic symptoms. I maintain that the delivery of such emotional information to *consciousness* (feelings of rage, shame, etc.) reduces the intensity of the *pharmacological* component of the response (rage, shame, etc.) and provides the patient with more behavioral options in living, as it did for K.C.

## EMPIRICAL TESTS OF THE MODEL

In conclusion, I want to summarize the high risk model of threat perception that underlies this discussion by proposing six predictions that follow from the model. If any of these predictions proves false, it would cast doubt on the model. The model, in short, is amenable to scientific validation and, like any such proposition, is vulnerable to being disproved. To date, research continues to accumulate to support these six predictions.

1. The probability of stress-related symptoms is *always* a function of multifactorial psychosocial, predisposing, triggering, and buffering risk factors interacting with genetic predispositions.

2. Negative affect (state) or negative affectivity (trait) is an *essential* but not a *sufficient* condition for the development of stress-related psychological, somatic, or organic symptoms.

3. High hypnotizables who block threatening secrets from consciousness will develop both psychological and somatic symptoms, whereas low hypnotizables and people with high Marlowe-Crowne scores will develop mainly somatic symptoms.

4. Few high hypnotizables with somatoform or psychophysiological disease will remain in primary care or in the medical-surgical sector because they more readily recognize negative affect and accept referral for mental health services.

5. The bulk of somatoform and psychophysiological disease patients in primary care or in the medical-surgical sector will have low hypnotic ability (as in the Greenleaf et al. 1992 study discussed previously) and/or score high on the Marlowe-Crowne test. These patients are most likely to require both psychophysiological monitoring of the autonomic nervous system to detect high negative affect and a Trojan horse role induction to reduce their resistance to referral for mental health services, the induction preferably to be provided within primary care or the medical-surgical sector.

6. Somatoform patients who are low on hypnotic ability or high on the Marlowe-Crowne test and who are referred for mental health service *outside* primary care or the medical-surgical service are very likely to become "dropouts" and will not follow through on the referral.

## NOTES

1. My thanks to Harris Dienstfrey for his editorial assistance, which aided me in articulating my theoretical concepts and empirical observations and, at times, made me more conscious of my own ideas; and to my wife, Judy Wickramasekera, for her help with this paper.

2. It is important to note that hypnotic ability and Marlowe-Crowne scores are statistically independent. They are orthogonal and probably interacting pathways into mind-body incongruence and autonomic nervous system dysregulation (Wickramasekera 1993a, 1993b, 1994a, 1994b; Wickramasekera & Atkinson, 1993).

3. The measurement of hypnotic ability with the Harvard or Stanford scales requires specialized training and skills. For this reason, I recommend during at least the initial screening the use of the 34-item absorption scale (Tellegen & Atkinson, 1974), which correlates modestly with hypnotic ability independent of context effects (Nadon, Hoyt, Register, & Kihlstrom, 1991), along with the 33-item Marlowe-Crowne scale. This testing should take approximately 20 minutes.

## REFERENCES

Belicki, K., & Belicki, D. (1986). Predisposition for nightmares: A study of hypnotic ability, vividness of imagery, and absorption. *Journal of Clinical Psychology, 42*, 714–718.

Bentin, S., & Moscovitch, M. (1990). Psychophysiological indices of implicit memory performance. *Bulletin of the Psychonomic Society, 23*, 346–352.

Bowers, P. E. (1982). The classic suggestion effect: Relationships with scales of hypnotizability, effortless experiencing and imagery vividness. *International Journal of Clinical and Experimental Hypnosis, 3*, 270–279.

Brown, J. W., Robertson, L. S., Kosa, J., & Alpert, J. J. (1971). A study of general practice in Massachusetts. *Journal of the American Medical Association, 216*, 301–306.

Canter, A. (1972). Changes in mood during incubation of acute febrile disease and the effects of pre-exposure psychologic states. *Psychosomatic Medicine, 34*, 424–430.

Canter, A., Cluff, L. E., & Imboden, J. B. (1972). Hypersensitive reactions to immunization innoculations and antecedent psychological vulnerability. *Journal of Psychosomatic Research, 16*, 99-101.

Canter, A., Imboden, J. B., & Cluff, L. E. (1966). The frequency of physical illness as a function of prior psychological vulnerability and contemporary stress. *Psychosomatic Medicine, 28*, 344–350.

Challis, G. B., & Stam, H. J. (1992). A longitudinal study of the development of anticipatory nausea and vomiting in cancer chemotherapy patients: The role of absorption and autonomic perception. *Health Psychology, 11*, 181–189.

Crowne, D. P., & Marlowe, D. (1960). A new scale of social desirability independent of psychopathology. *Journal of Consulting Psychology, 24*, 349–354.

Crowson, J. J., Conroy, A. M., & Chester, T. D. (1991). Hypnotizability as related to visually induced affective reactivity. *International Journal of Clinical and Experimental Hypnosis, 39*, 140–144.

Csikszentmihalyi, M., & Massimini, F. (1975). *Beyond boredom and anxiety*. San Francisco: Jossey-Bass.

Dafter, R. E. (1996). Why "negative" emotions can sometimes be positive: The spectrum model of emotions and their role in mind-body healing. *Advances: The Journal of Mind-Body Health, 12,* 6–19.

Damasio, A. R. (1994). *Descartes' error: Emotion, reason, and the human brain.* New York: Avon Books.

Das, J. P. (1958a). The Pavlovian theory of hypnosis: An evaluation. *Journal of Mental Sciences, 104,* 82–90.

Das, J. P. (1958b). Conditioning and hypnosis. *Journal of Experimental Psychology, 56,* 110–113.

DeBenedittis, G., Cigada, M., & Bianchi, A. (1994). Autonomic changes during hypnosis: A heart rate variability power spectrum analysis as a marker of sympatho-vagal balance. *International Journal of Clinical and Experimental Hypnosis, 42,* 140–152.

deGruy, F., III (1996). Mental health care in the primary care setting. In M. S. Donaldson, K. D. Yordy, N. Lohr, & N. A. Vanselow (Eds.), *Primary care: America's health in a new era* (pp. 285–311). Washington, DC: National Academy Press.

Dennett, D. (1991). *Consciousness explained.* Boston: Little Brown.

Dixon, M., Brunet, A., & Laurence, J. R. (1990). Hypnotizability and automaticity: Toward a parallel distributed processing model of hypnotic responding. *Journal of Abnormal Psychology, 99,* 336–343.

Dixon, M., & Laurence, J. R. (1992). Hypnotic susceptibility and verbal automaticity: Automatic and strategic processing differences in the Stroop color-naming task. *Journal of Abnormal Psychology, 101,* 344–347.

Donchin, Y., Constantini, S., Szold, A., Byrne, E. A., & Porges, S. W. (1992). Cardiac vagal tone predicts outcome in neurosurgical patients. *Critical Care Medicine, 20,* 942–949.

Donchin, Y., Feld, J. M., & Porges, S. W. (1985). Respiratory sinus arrhythmia during recovery from isoflurane-nitrous oxide anesthesia. *Anesthesia and Analgesia, 64,* 811–815.

Frankel, F. H., Apfel-Savitz, R., Nemiah, J. C., & Sifneos, P. E. (1977). The relationship between hypnotizability and alexithymia. *Psychotherapy and Psychosomatics, 8,* 172–178.

Freud, S. (1948). *The ego and the mechanism of defense.* New York: International Universities Press. (Original work published 1926).

Greenleaf, M., Fisher, S., Miaskowski, C., & DuHamel, K. (1992). Hypnotizability and recovery from cardiac surgery. *American Journal of Clinical Hypnosis, 35,* 119–128.

Greenwald, A. G. (1992). New look 3: Unconscious cognition reclaimed. *American Psychologist, 47,* 766–779.

Grove, J. R., & Lewis, M. A. E. (1996). Hypnotic susceptibility and the attainment of flowlike states during exercise. *Journal of Sport and Exercise Psychology, 18,* 380–391.

Hall, R. C. W., Popkin, M. K., Devaul, R. A., Faillace, L. A., & Stickney, S. K. (1978). Physical illness presenting as psychiatric disease. *Archives of General Psychiatry, 35,* 1315–1320.

Harris, R. M., Porges, S. W., Carpenter, M. E., & Vincenz, L. M. (1993). Hypnotic susceptibility, mood state, and cardiovascular reactivity. *American Journal of Clinical Hypnosis, 36*(1), 15–25.

Hilgard, E. R. (1977). *Divided consciousness: Multiple controls in human thought and action.* New York: Wiley.

Hilgard, E. R. (1982). Hypnotic susceptibility and implications for measurement. *International Journal of Clinical and Experimental Hypnosis, 30,* 394–403.

Hilgard, E. R. (1987). Research advances in hypnosis: Issues and methods. *International Journal of Clinical and Experimental Hypnosis, 35*, 248–264.

Hilgard, E. R., & Hilgard, J. R. (1975). *Hypnosis in the relief of pain.* Los Altos, CA: William Kaufmann.

Holmes, R. H. (1981). *Schedule of recent events.* Seattle, WA: University of Washington Press.

House, J. S., Landis, K. R., & Umberson, D. (1988). Social relationships and health. *Science, 241*, 540–545.

Jamner, L. D., Schwartz, G. E., & Leigh, H. (1988). The relationship between repressive and defensive coping styles and monocyte, eosinophil, and serum glucose levels: Support for the opioid peptide hypothesis of repression. *Psychosomatic Medicine, 50*, 567–575.

Jensen, M. R. (1987). Psychobiological factors predicting the course of breast cancer. *Journal of Personality, 55*, 315–342.

Jung, C. G. (1969). *Man and his symbols.* New York: Doubleday.

Kihlstrom, J. F. (1987). The cognitive unconscious. *Science, 237*, 1445–1452.

King, D. R., & McDonald, R. D. (1976). Hypnotic susceptibility and verbal conditioning. *International Journal of Clinical and Experimental Hypnosis, 24*, 29–37.

Lewicki, P. (1986). Nonconscious social information processing. Orlando, FL: Academic Press.

Lipowski, Z. J. (1987). Somatization: Medicine's unsolved problem [Editorial]. *Psychosomatics 28*, 294–297.

McCauley, J., Kern, D. E., Kolodner, K., Dill, L., Schroeder, A. F., DeChant, H. K., Ryden, J., Derogatis, L. R., & Bass, E. B. (1997). Clinical characteristics of women with a history of childhood abuse. *Journal of the American Medical Association, 227*, 1362–1368.

Mineka, S. L., & Kihlstrom, J. F. (1978). Unpredictable and uncontrollable events: A new perspective on experimental neurosis. *Journal of Abnormal Psychology, 87*, 256–271.

Moos, R. H. (1993). *Coping responses inventory. CRI–Adult Form professional manual.* Odessa, FL: Psychological Assessment Resources Inc.

Nadon, R., Hoyt, I. P., Register, P. A., & Kihlstrom, J. F. (1991). Absorption and hypnotizability: Context effects reexamined. *Journal of Personality and Social Psychology, 60*, 144–153.

National Academy of Sciences, Institute of Medicine. (1989). *Behavioral influences on the endocrine and immune systems.* Washington, DC: Author.

National Institutes of Health Technology Assessment Panel. (1996). The integration of behavioral and relaxation approaches into the treatment of chronic pain and insomnia. *Journal of the American Medical Association, 276*(4), 313–318.

Olness, K. (1996). Introduction: Hypnosis and biofeedback with children and adolescents: Clinical, research, and educational aspects. *Journal of Developmental and Behavioural Pediatrics, 17*, 299.

Palsson, O. S., Wickramasekera, I. E., Rutledge, C., Davies, M., & Downing, B. (1997). Social desirability, repression, and finger temperature. *Applied Psychophysiology and Biofeedback, 22*, 143.

Perlstrom, J. R., Morin, C. M., Wickramasekera, I. E., Strong, S. R., & Ware, J. C. (1995). The high risk model of threat perception: Clinical and theoretical implications for sleep disorders. *Sleep Research, 24*, 177.

Perlstrom, J. R., Morin, C. M., Wickramasekera, I. E., & Ware, J. C. (1996). Hypnotizability in insomnia and apnea patients. *Sleep Research, 25*, 172.

Pettinati, H., Horne, R. L., & Staats, J. M. (1985). Hypnotizability in patients with anorexia nervosa and bulimia. *Archives of General Psychiatry, 42,* 1014–1016.

Pettinati, H. M., Kogan, L. G., Evans, F. J., Wade, J. H., Home, L., & Staats, J. M. (1990). Hypnotizability of psychiatric inpatients according to two different scales. *American Journal of Psychiatry, 147, 69–75.*

Pomerantz, B., & Wickramasekera, I. (1988). Hypnotizability and subjective distress. Paper presented at the meeting of the Society for Experimental & Clinical Hypnosis, Asheville, NC.

Porges, S. W. (1991). Vagal tone: An autonomic mediator of affect. In J. A. Gaber & K. A. Dodge (Eds.), *The development of affect regulation and dysregulation* (pp. 111–128). New York: Cambridge University Press.

Porges, S. W. (1992). Vagal tone: A physiological marker of stress vulnerability. *Pediatrics, 90,* 498–503.

Quill, T. E. (1985). Somatization disorder: One of medicine's blind spots. *Journal of the American Medical Association, 254,* 3075–3079.

Remler, H. (1990). *Hypnotic susceptibility, suggestion and compliance with treatment in patients with chronic pain.* Unpublished doctoral dissertation, Virginia Consortium for Professional Psychology, Norfolk, VA.

Rescorla, R. A. (1988). Pavlovian conditioning: It's not what you think it is. *American Psychologist, 43,* 151–160.

Roberts, S. J. (1994). Somatization in primary care: The common presentation of psychosocial problems through physical complaints. *Nurse-Practitioner, 19,* 47, 50–56.

Sarason, I. G., Levine, H. M., Basham, R. B., & Sarason, B. R. (1983). Assessing social support: The social support questionnaire. *Journal of Personal and Social Psychology, 44,* 127–139.

Saxon, J., & Wickramasekera, I. (1994, October). Discriminating patients with organic disease from somatizers among patients with chest pain using factors from the high risk model of threat perception. Paper presented at the meeting of the Society for Experimental and Clinical Hypnosis, San Francisco, CA.

Schwartz, G. E. (1990). Psychobiology of regression and health: A systems approach. In J. L. Singer (Ed.), *Repression and dissociation* (pp. 405–434). Chicago: University of Chicago Press.

Shedler, J., Mayman, M., & Manis, M. (1993). The illusion of mental health. *American Psychologist, 48,* 1117–1131.

Shertzer, C. I., & Lookingbill, D. P. (1987). Effects of relaxation therapy and hypnotizability in chronic urticaria. *Archives of Dermatology, 123,* 913–916.

Shevrin, H. (1991, May). Discovering how event-related potentials reveal unconscious processes. *Biofeedback Newsmagazine, 19*(1), 12–15.

Shevrin, H., Bond, J. A., Brakel, L. A., Hertel, R. K., & Williams, W. J. (1996). *Conscious and unconscious processes: Psychodynamic, cognitive, and neurophysiological convergences.* New York: Guilford Press.

Shor, R. E., & Orne, E. C. (1962). *Manual of Harvard Group Scale of Hypnotic Susceptibility.* Palo Alto, CA: Consulting Psychologies Press.

Smith, G. R. (1994). The course of somatization and its effects on utilization of health care resources. *Psychosomatics, 35,* 263–267.

Sperry, R. (1980). Mind-brain inferaction. *Neuroscience, 5,* 195–206.

Spiegel, D., Hunt, T., & Dondershine, H. (1988). Dissociation and hypnotizability in post-traumatic stress disorder. *American Journal of Psychiatry, 145,* 301–305.

Stam, H., McGrath, P., Brooke, R., & Cosire, F. (1986). Hypnotizability and the treatment of chronic facial pain. *International Journal of Clinical and Experimental Hypnosis, 34,* 182–191.

Stutman, R. K., & Bliss, E. L. (1985). Post-traumatic stress disorder, hypnotizability, and imagery. *American Journal of Psychiatry, 142*, 741–743.

Tellegen, A., & Atkinson, G. (1974). Openness to absorbing and self-altering experiences ("absorption"), a trait related to hypnotic susceptibility. *Journal of Abnormal Psychology, 83*, 268–277.

Tellegen, A., Lykken, D. T., Bouchard, T. J., Jr., Wilcox, K. J., & Rich, S. (1988). Personality similarity in twins reared apart and together. *Journal of Personality and Social Psychology, 54*, 1031–1039.

Toner, B. B., Koyama, E., Garfinkel, P. E., & Jeejeebhoy, K. N. (1992). Social desirability and irritable bowel syndrome. *International Journal of Psychiatry in Medicine, 22*, 99–103.

Uleman, J. S., & Bargh, J. A. (1989). *Unintended thought.* New York: Guilford Press.

Vaughan, S. C. (1997). *The talking cure: The science behind psychotherapy.* New York: Grosset/Putnam.

Velten, E. (1968). A laboratory task for induction of mood states. *Behavioral Research Therapy, 18*, 79–86.

Wagaman, M. J. (1996, August). Hypnotic susceptibility and repressive coping in asthma patients. Paper presented at the annual meeting of the American Psychological Association, Toronto, Canada.

Watson, D., & Clark, L. A. (1984). Negative affectivity. The disposition to experience aversive emotional states. *Psychological Bulletin, 96*, 465–490.

Watson, D., & Tellegen, A. (1985). Toward a consensual structure of mood. *Psychological Bulletin, 98*, 219–235.

Webb, R. A. (1962). Suggestibility and verbal conditioning. *International Journal of Clinical and Experimental Hypnosis, 10*, 275–279.

Weinberger, D. A. (1990). The construct validity of the repressive coping style. In J. L. Singer (Ed.), *Repression and dissociation: Implications for personality theory, psychopathology, and health* (pp. 337–386). Chicago: University of Chicago Press.

Wickramasekera, I. (1970, August). The effects of hypnosis and a control procedure on verbal conditioning. Paper presented at the annual meeting of the American Psychological Association, Miami, FL.

Wickramasekera, I. (1976). *Biofeedback, behavior therapy and hypnosis: Potentiating the verbal control of behavior for clinicians.* Chicago: Nelson Hall.

Wickramasekera, I. (1977). On attempts to modify hypnotic susceptibility. *Annals of New York Academy of Science, 296*, 143–153.

Wickramasekera, I. (1979). A model of the patient at high risk for chronic stress related disorders: Do beliefs have biological consequences? *Proceedings of the Annual Convention of the Biofeedback Society of America*, San Diego, CA.

Wickramasekera, I. (1988). *Clinical behavioral medicine: Some concepts and procedures.* New York: Plenum.

Wickramasekera, I. (1989a). Enabling the somatizing patient to exit the somatic closet: A high risk model. *Psychotherapy, 26*, 530–544.

Wickramasekera, I. (1989b). Somatizers, the health care system, and collapsing the psychological distance that the somatizer has to travel for help. *Professional Psychology: Research and Practice, 20*, 105–111.

Wickramasekera, I. (1993a). Assessment and treatment of somatization disorders: The high risk model of threat perception. In J. W. Rhue, S. J. Lynn, & I. Kirsch (Eds.), *Handbook of clinical hypnosis* (pp. 587–621). Washington, DC: American Psychological Association.

Wickramasekera, I. (1993b, August). High hypnotic ability and high neuroticism as risk factors for psychopathology and pathophysiology. Paper presented at the annual meeting of the American Psychological Association, Toronto, Canada.

Wickramasekera, I. (1994a). On the interaction of two orthogonal risk factors, 1) hypnotic ability and 2) negative affectivity (threat perception) for psychophysiological dysregulation in somatization, II. In V. De Pascalis (Chair), *Suggestion and suggestibility.* Symposium conducted at the University of Rome, Italy.

Wickramasekera, I. (1994b). Psychophysiological and clinical implications of the coincidence of high hypnotic ability and high neuroticism during threat perception in somatization disorders. *American Journal of Clinical Hypnosis, 37,* 22–33.

Wickramasekera, I. (1994c). Somatic to psychological symptoms and information transfer from implicit to explicit memory: A controlled case study with predictions from the high risk model of threat perception. *Dissociation, 7,* 153–166.

Wickramasekera, I. (1995). Somatization: Concepts, data and predictions from the high risk model of threat perception. *Journal of Nervous and Mental Disease, 183,* 15–23.

Wickramasekera, I. (1998). Secrets kept from the mind but not the body or behavior: The unsolved problems of identifying and treating somatization and psychophysiological disease. *Advances: The Journal of Mind-Body Medicine, 14,* 81–132.

Wickramasekera, I., & Atkinson, R. (1993, August). High hypnotic ability and high neuroticism as risk factors for moderate obesity. Paper presented at the annual meeting of the American Psychological Association, Toronto, Canada.

Wickramasekera, I., Davies, T., & Davies, M. (1996a). Applied psychophysiology: A bridge between the biomedical model and the biopsychosocial model in family medicine. *Professional Psychology: Research and Practice, 27,* 221–233.

Wickramasekera, I., Davies, M., & Davies, T. (1996b, March). Applied psychophysiology and primary care. Paper presented at the 27th annual meeting of the Association of Applied Psychophysiology, Albuquerque, New Mexico.

Wickramasekera, I., & Kenkel, M. B. (Eds.). (1996a). Somatization, applied psychophysiology, and effective mind-body therapies [Special section]. *Professional Psychology: Research and Practice, 27,* 217.

Wickramasekera, I., & Kenkel, M. B. (Eds.). (1996b). Somatization, primary care, and applied psychophysiology II [Special section]. *Professional Psychology: Research and Practice, 27,* 537.

Wickramasekera, I., Pope, A. T., & Kolm, P. (1996). On the interaction of hypnotizability and negative affect in chronic pain: Implications for the somatization of trauma. *Journal of Nervous and Mental Disease, 184,* 628–635.

Wickramasekera, I., & Price, D. (1997). Morbid obesity, absorption, neuroticism and the high risk model of threat perception. *American Journal of Clinical Hypnosis, 34,* 291–302.

Wickramasekera, I., & Saxon, J. (1988). Absorption, neuroticism, and anticipatory nausea and vomiting in chemotherapy. Paper presented at the 19th annual meeting of the Biofeedback Society of America, Colorado Springs, CO.

Wickramasekera, I., Ware, C., & Saxon, J. (1992, August). EEG defined insomnia and hypnotic ability with pathophysiology excluded. In I. Wickramasekera (Chair), *Hypnotic ability as a risk factor for psychopathology and pathophysiology.* Symposium conducted at the annual meeting of the American Psychological Association, Washington, DC.

Wisen, O., Rossner, S., & Johansson, C. (1987). Gastric secretion in massive obesity: Evidence for abnormal response to vagal stimulation. *Digestive Diseases and Sciences, 32,* 968–972.

Zarski, J. J. (1984). Hassles and health: A replication. *Health Psychology, 3,* 243–251.

Zocco, L. (1984). *The development of a self-report inventory to assess dysfunctional cognitions in phobics.* Unpublished doctoral dissertation, Virginia Consortium for Professional Psychology, Norfolk, VA.

# CHAPTER 3

# Psychophysiological Foundations of the Mind-Body Therapies

ANGELE MCGRADY

**Abstract:** The health care provider in a primary care setting frequently encounters patients with comorbid emotional and physical problems. The presence of chronic stress, mood or anxiety disorders, and personality characteristics complicates diagnosis and interferes with management and compliance. Models have been proposed to explain the mediation of the effects of stress via the nervous, endocrine, and immune systems. Intervention by primary care providers can be office based or by referral and may vary from short-term to complex, ongoing therapy. Effects of mind-body therapies are based on solid psychophysiological data and are well suited to the problems seen in patients in primary care practice.

## COMORBIDITY OF EMOTIONAL AND PHYSICAL ILLNESS

Mental and emotional illnesses are very common in the primary care sector and affect every aspect of physical illnesses. The presence of mood and anxiety disorders as well as subclinical anxiety and depression prevent patients from reaching optimal quality of life (Spitzer et al., 1995). Chronic pain is also a frequent complaint of people seeking services in primary care. The transformation of an acute, time-limited, curable illness into a chronic problem depends more on psychosocial factors than it does on physical variables. Frequency, severity, and chronicity of illness influence patients' needs for services and the time spent in managing them when they are ill (Sullivan, Turner, & Romano, 1991).

Patients suffering with mood or anxiety disorders and functional impairments are more likely to be considered difficult by primary care physicians than are patients with the same degree of severity of physical illness but no emotional problems (Hahn et al., 1996). Difficult relationships in the primary care setting lead to unmet expectations and affect utilization of services (Kroenke, Jackson, & Chamberlin, 1997). For example, the number of physical problems reported on the PRIME-MD questionnaire was correlated with the number of phone calls to the office and the perceived difficulty of the encounter from the physician's perspective (Wahl, McGrady, Lynch, & Nagel, 2000). Patients who demonstrated a tendency to somatize psychological distress had higher negative affect, were more focused on physical symptoms, and used services more than patients without this tendency. Patients with somatoform pain disorder demonstrated similar characteristics (McGrady, Lynch, Nagel, & Zsembik, 1999). Frequently treated patients at a gastroenterology clinic who did not demonstrate organic disease were more likely to have psychiatric diagnoses and histories of sexual abuse. However, they attributed their symptoms more frequently to organic causes and less frequently to psychological factors (Bass, Bond, Gill, & Sharpe, 1999).

The diagnosis of chronic illness, even when the prognosis is good, is associated with an emotional reaction. During acuity or when complications from a chronic illness develop, the patient grieves about actual or perceived loss of physical abilities and faces increased difficulty in maintaining his or her usual roles. The patient's emotional response to illness affects family members and interpersonal relationships (Brenner, 1997). Yet too often the physician focuses predominantly on treating the physical aspects of the illness to the detriment of assessing and managing the emotional accompaniments.

Despite the high prevalence of emotional disorders in patients seeking primary care services, symptoms of anxiety or depression are often not reported, and when verbalized, not recognized or adequately treated. On the other hand, the presence of medically unexplained symptoms or hypochondriasis increases the rate of recognition of emotional illness by physicians (Kirmayer, Robbins, Dworkind, & Yaffe, 1993). Histories of traumatic life events are not uncommon in primary care patients but are often poorly assessed. In a recent study, the 10 percent of primary care patients who had experienced traumatic events during the past year were more likely to have psychiatric disorders and also used more medical services than patients without these experiences (Holman, Silver, & Waitzkin, 2000).

What are the factors that influence the inadequate reporting and identification of emotional illness in primary care? For a chronic-pain patient, disclosure is affected by perceived stigma, the effect of pain on memory, and the physician's ability to elicit the information. Pain interferes with the ability to focus and learn, so instructions may not be remembered or understood (Kuhajda, Thorn, & Klinger, 1998). The patient's willingness to exhibit illness behavior resulting from pain as well as emotional distress is affected by his or her prediction of the physician's reaction to this display.

Primary care practitioners are accustomed to observing the behaviors that accompany physical illness, such as the person with back pain moving more slowly and stiffly. Similarly, the appearance and actions of a person with depression or anxiety can provide clues to a diagnosis (Lewis & Lubkin, 1998). Behavioral indicators of morbidity resulting from disturbances of mood, such as days of work missed, less frequent church attendance, and fewer social events attended, also provide important indicators of emotional distress.

To illustrate further, emotional and social factors are very important in the management of obese persons, who are criticized by society, their peers, and health care providers. An obese patient's disclosure of depressive symptoms may be thwarted by the provider's exclusive focus on the obesity. Subsequently, poor compliance is attributed solely to unwillingness to change, whereas depression is actually preventing such healthy behaviors. Certainly, the obese person with depression is unlikely to fulfill behavior requirements for weight loss (Clark, Niaura, King, & Para, 1996). On the other hand, the person who loses weight successfully usually demonstrates a decrease in depressive symptoms and improvement in self-esteem (Devlin, Yanovski, & Wilson, 2000).

## THE ROLE OF EMOTIONAL STRESS IN THE DEVELOPMENT AND MAINTENANCE OF PHYSICAL DISORDERS

Stress increases the intensity of physical symptoms and lowers the threshold for seeking medical help. Repeated stress makes people more likely to conclude that ill-defined or vague bodily sensations are due to physical disease. Interpretation of symptoms such as fatigue, difficulty sleeping, or mild gastrointestinal disruptions as "sickness" facilitates the identification of oneself as "sick." The sick role with its attendant behaviors is more easily accepted over time (Barsky & Borus, 1999). Individuals appraise potentially stress-inducing situations and assess their ability to manage or control the stress. If demand exceeds perceived capability, the stress response ensues (Lazarus & Folkman, 1984). Successful adaptation means that each stressor is countered in a timely manner and without long-term damage.

Individuals are equipped with complex, overlapping, yet distinct behavioral and physiological stress response systems. As Dantzer (1991) summarizes, a pathogen, a predator, and a poison have nothing in common except that they disrupt normal psychophysiological functioning, so the responses to those three stressors will involve different systems. In contrast, Barsky and Borus (1999) maintain that persons with functional somatic syndromes (which may result from chronic stress) share many symptoms, such as unexplained physical distress, fatigue, sleeplessness, and elevated rates of psychiatric disorders.

The ability to respond and to achieve stability through change is referred to as allostasis. Instead of the narrow normal range limits of homeostatic systems, allostatic systems function under more varied conditions, allowing individuals to cope and readjust without long-term harm. Load on the system results from chronic overactivity or underactivity of the hypothalamic-pituitary-adrenal axis that normally protects the body from the effects of stressful events. Individual differences in response are due to genetic predisposition, past experience, and the person's perception of the event (McEwen, 1998). Cacioppo et al. (2000) studied the physiological and psychological characteristics of persons who care for their spouses with dementia to elucidate the effects of high allostatic load on function. (*Allostatic load* here means the total burden on the individual for adaptation and coping.) Higher levels of baseline sympathetic tone and plasma adrenocorticotrophic hormone, as well as more depressive symptoms and poorer immune function, were observed.

The physiological effects of stress are mediated by the central, autonomic, endocrine, and immune systems. Hyperactivity of the sympathoadrenal system is associated with increased heart rate and blood pressure, decreased heart rate variability, and impaired digestion. Stress also predisposes susceptible individuals to obesity. When the body's fight-or-flight response is triggered, hunger and appetite for carbohydrates ensues because the hypothalamus anticipates an expenditure of calories following the stress stimulus. Ingestion of carbohydrates triggers the release of serotonin, which is associated with decreased negative affect. Overeating in stressful circumstances is reinforced by positive sensations such as fullness and a more positive mood (Goodnick, Henry, & Buki, 1995).

Common central nervous system pathways mediate stress-induced disruptions of behavioral and emotional homeostasis. The cells of the nervous, endocrine, and immune systems communicate via neurotransmitters and neuropeptides (nervous), hormones (endocrine), and cytokines (immune). Communication is bidirectional between the nervous and immune systems. Sympathetic fibers innervate both primary and secondary lymphoid tissues (Ader, Cohen, & Felten, 1995), and both T and B lymphocyte cells have receptors for stress hormones. Glucocorticoids exert a counter-regulatory effect on inflammation. Disruptions in communication among the major biological systems during and after serious stress or the accumulation of multiple, minor, difficult events increase the risk for physical and emotional illness (Sternberg, Chrousos, Wilder, & Gold, 1992).

One of the by-products of negative mood is observed in the ability of the immune system to respond to stress (Kemeny & Miller, 1999). The immune system is capable of a relatively rapid response, but most effects take hours or days. Depending on the individual's perception of the severity of the threat and past success at coping with the same stressor, the hypothalamic-pituitary-adrenal axis and the sympathetic nervous system will be activated to a lesser or greater degree, with resulting immunological sequelae (Maier, Watkins, & Fleshner, 1994). For example, the person who undergoes chronic stress shows inhibition of the delayed hypersensitivity response. One of the many consequences of this is an increased sensitivity to the common cold. In contrast, more frequent social contacts lessen the impact of the stress response on the immune system and decrease the frequency of colds in an otherwise healthy population (Cohen, Doyle, Skoner, Rabin, & Gwaltney, 1997).

Interrelationships among the immune and cardiovascular systems under stressful conditions are common (Cacioppo, 1994; Skinner, 1991). Normal levels of cortisol can raise blood pressure, and stress-induced higher levels of cortisol can produce sustained elevations of blood pressure (Walker, Unützer, & Katon, 1998). Adrenergic receptors are sensitized by cortisol so that low levels of catecholamines can produce a hyperarousal response (Nelesen & Dimsdale, 1994). Constantly reliving a traumatic event is similar to the effects of such an event being prolonged and represents a chronic stress to the nervous, cardiovascular, and immune systems. Besides the resulting increased blood pressure and heart rate, the fibrinogen system is more reactive during stress, and this reactivity is associated with increased risk of myocardial infarction.

Low blood pressure that occurs during stressful situations is as maladaptive a response as continued high blood pressure after the stress is removed. In susceptible individuals, emotional distress initially produces a strong sympathetic response followed by paradoxical withdrawal of adrenergic activity. Blood pressure decreases abruptly, and the person faints. Patients with autonomic dysfunction usually present with complaints of fatigue, dizziness, and negative mood, similar to many other illnesses. In fact, there is a high degree of comorbidity between syncope and depression. Therefore, selective serotonin reuptake inhibitors are frequent choices for treatment of these patients (Kosinski & Grubb, 1994). In the animal world, hyporesponsiveness in the face of stress is sometimes the best adaptive choice. Bradycardia in the hog-nosed snake that feigns death and in the iguana immobilized by fear permits these animals to be protected from predators. In mammals, reflex bradycardia reduces oxygen resources and metabolic output; the traditional fight-or-flight response is reduced in favor of the freeze response (Porges, 1995). Nonetheless, syncope as an adaptive response to stress in humans is difficult to understand.

Psychiatric disorders are commonly associated with cortisol dysregulation. In particular, failure of inhibition of the normal feedback system for cortisol is a hallmark of depressive disorders. On the contrary, patients with post-traumatic stress disorder have reduced cortisol levels, perhaps due to neuroanatomical changes resulting from extreme psychological stress (Yehuda et al., 1990). Cortisol inhibits serotonin, norepinephrine, and dopamine, neurotransmittors that normally maintain

---

**Box 3.1**      Format of Assessment for Well Patients

1. Use PRIME-MD.
2. Use Life Events Scale.
3. Assess changes in physical and emotional health from last year.
4. Ask about social support.
5. Remain alert about possible changes in normal self-satisfying activities.
6. Promote the maintenance of healthy behaviors.
7. Suggest an increase in wellness activities.
8. Emphasize self-care.
9. Predict upcoming stress.
10. Explain mind-body-spirit influences on continued health.

---

normal mood. For the short term, high levels of cortisol allow the brain to modify the memory of emotional events. But a high concentration of cortisol in the hippocampus for prolonged periods can destroy hippocampal neurons (Corcoran, Gallitano, Leitman, & Malaspina, 2001). If cortisol secretion does not increase in response to stress, secretion of inflammatory cytokines increases, putting the individual at risk for autoimmune diseases. Humans who underrespond biochemically are more likely to develop fibromyalgia, chronic fatigue syndrome, and later posttraumatic stress disorder. Depressive reactions comprise the emotional accompaniment to physiological hypoarousal.

## MIND-BODY MODELS APPLICABLE TO PRIMARY CARE

The diagnosis and management of emotional disorders in primary care must be improved. Physicians and other primary care practitioners can increase their efficiency of handling stress-related emotional disorders through training, education, and on-site consultation with behavioral health consultants. Several interventions to improve physician awareness of mood and anxiety disorders have been tested in a primary care setting. These include

providing screening tools to identify depression and anxiety, giving feedback of symptom scores, and videotaping encounters between depressed patients and physicians and providing feedback. The use of more intensive training for providers than a single continuing medical education (CME) lecture format has been supported (Kroenke, Taylor-Vaisey, Dietrich, & Oxman, 2000). In addition, patients who are currently well but want to decrease their risk and request methods to do so must be taken seriously. Often patients who ask for risk-reduction interventions are dismissed with vague recommendations to "exercise and watch what you eat."

### Wellness Checkups

Box 3.1 presents the format for an assessment of well patients that can help physicians identify potential or developing problems. Short questionnaires such as the PRIME-MD and the Life Events Scale (LES) can be used while patients wait to be seen for wellness checkups. The LES in particular tells the physician what major events the patient has experienced in the past year; this information facilitates the encounter (Miller & Rahe, 1997). With these simple tools, the physician is prepared to ask the appropriate questions during the visit and can allot time to relevant

---

**Box 3.2     Format for Assessment of Chronically Ill Patients**

1. Use PRIME-MD and Life Events Scale every six months.
2. Follow with depression and anxiety inventories if necessary.
3. Observe illness behaviors.
4. Assess adherence to treatment; explore reasons for nonadherence if appropriate.
5. Check on behavioral indicators of morbidity.
6. Ask about emotional adjustment to illness.
7. Assess degree of social support and number of social roles.
8. Ask about history of physical abuse, sexual abuse, and neglect.
9. Assume that there is an emotional reaction, even though it may not be stated.
10. Explain the effects of stress on exacerbation of illness.
11. Agree on and set goals for the next visit.
12. Foster adherence from an empowerment perspective.
13. Emphasize patient strengths and abilities to manage illness.

---

issues. Emphasis is placed on maintaining or improving wellness and decreasing risk. The patient's healthy self-management routines are encouraged and praised. Additional wellness activities are recommended, followed by discussion of the wellness plan. Goals are set, community resources are mentioned, and the appointment for the following year is made.

### Visits for Chronic Illness

Box 3.2 provides the format for a more detailed investigation of emotional factors that may be increasing the severity of the illness or impeding compliance in a patient with chronic illness. Again, short questionnaires may be used to inform the physician about changes in activities. Any indication of incipient mood or anxiety disorders can be investigated with self-report paper-and-pencil inventories and followed up with longer assessment tools or referral if necessary.

Illness conviction (the person's belief that there is something wrong and what is wrong must be fixed by medical intervention) must be considered and acknowledged in a person with persistent illness. The person's explanatory model of illness, including the treatments

that they think will be beneficial, should be elicited (Sullivan et al., 1991). When a person is chronically ill, prior roles must be modified to accommodate the disability resulting from the illness. Persons' views of themselves—as handicapped or disabled and their personality characteristics—will influence their behaviors and how they interact with their physicians. So, although behaviors of individuals with mental and emotional illnesses may be subtle, health care providers must be able to assess them.

### Models for Mind-Body Therapies

Once emotional issues are identified, several models can facilitate the physician's understanding of the appropriate mind-body therapies. The high risk model of threat perception, developed by Wickramasekera (1995), was discussed in detail in Chapter 2. Cohen and Rodriguez (1995) proposed a model in which negative affect and affective disorders are linked to physical disorders and illness behavior through biological, behavioral, cognitive, and social pathways. Repeated activation of the hypothalamic-pituitary-adrenal axis can directly initiate flare-ups as well as increase severity of illness. Mood disorders also influence behavior so that self-care is compromised and normal family and occupational roles are disrupted. The model is bidirectional, so physical illness and sick role behaviors link to negative mood and eventual mood and anxiety disorders through the same pathways. A study by McCauley et al. (1997) found that women with histories of abuse report more physical symptoms and are more likely to have a comorbid substance abuse problem than women without such histories. This research supports the need for an assessment of emotional state and abuse history in every patient with chronic illness.

Allostatic load can be lessened if patients modify their behavior by eating a healthy diet and reducing tobacco and alcohol use. The patient who is encouraged to extend social networks and reduce inactivity, perhaps in a social context, benefits by improved ability to manage stress (McEwen, 1998). Current support systems should be assessed and extended if found lacking.

A stress model designed for both prevention and intervention in primary care has been proposed. The person's appraisal of the potential threat due to a stressful situation and the success of stress-mitigating behaviors are superimposed on a genetic and cultural backdrop (Boone & Christensen, 1997). Some individuals use health-enhancing behaviors such as exercise or relaxation to decrease the impact of stress, while others rely on health degrading activities, such as smoking and alcohol use. The primary care provider needs to elicit information from patients about their perception of stressful situations and their use of stress-mitigating behaviors. Predisposition to cardiovascular, gastrointestinal, neurological, or psychiatric illnesses due to family history, personality, or environmental factors is important. Type D personality (high negative affect and social inhibition) increases risk for cardiac events.

The convergence of multiple risk factors (Type D personality, younger age, and decreased left ventricular ejection fraction) predicts poorer treatment response in patients with coronary heart disease (Denollet, Vaes, & Brutsaert, 2000). To illustrate further, stressful life events are associated with the onset of major depressive disorders. Approximately one third of the association is noncausal, because individuals predisposed to depressive disorders self-select themselves into high-risk environments (Kendler, Karkowski, & Prescott, 1999). General questions about socioeconomic status, living conditions, health habits, and leisure activities can yield important data on the patient's risk for illness and attitude toward self-care.

The physician may find an analysis of predisposing, precipitating, and perpetuating factors in regard to physical and emotional illness helpful. Patients may be at risk for stress-related illness because of genetic factors, history of abuse, low social support, or chronic stress. Precipitating factors such as the breakup of a marriage are the initiating events associated with the onset of illness. Finally, certain aspects of the patient's life maintain or exacerbate the illness. For example, weight gain resulting from inactivity, boredom, and social isolation increases the probability of obesity. The overweight patient or the person steadily gaining a few pounds a year creates fertile territory for subsequent diabetes, hypertension, and depressive illness (Walker et al., 1998). Recognizing the predisposing and precipitating factors for onset of illness prior to a well or illness visit increases the probability of a mutually satisfying, efficient encounter and successful intervention if needed.

The physician dealing with a patient with chronic illness is well advised to consider the persistent impact of psychological and emotional factors on the patient's day-to-day disease management, particularly in crisis. The physician should recognize that the person's attempts to regulate his or her emotions to deal with highly charged events may have cognitive consequences. The interpretation of a traumatic event is influenced by perception, past experience, and the emotion related to the event. Trying to suppress a strong emotion resulting from observing or being the victim of trauma is associated with poor memory, so less vivid recall protects the person from distressing images (Richards & Gross, 2000). Coping by disengagement is often observed in a patient with a past history of serious abuse (Coffey, Leitenberg, Henning, Turner, & Bennett, 1996). Anticipation of a stressful situation and its potential upsetting effects can lessen its emotional impact and the potential for later trauma (Holman et al., 2000). However, the physician may interpret the patient's reticence as intentional withholding of information. Patients' attempts to manage their stressful lives should be respected, even if poorer reporting of events is the result.

### Spiritual Factors

Some individuals use prayer and meditation to help them deal with stressful situations. Research has shown that frequency of church attendance was positively related to physical health and negatively related to depression. Watching religious television shows did not confer the same benefits (Harmon & Myers, 1999). To some people, prayer and church attendance are important aspects of life, so a physician's general questioning about how a patient is coping with illness should include spiritual factors. Recent research supports a relationship between religious involvement and lower mortality (McCullough, Hoyt, Larson, Koenig, & Thoresen, 2000).

### Motivation for Change

Motivation for change varies among individuals and is affected by a person's perception of the severity of the illness and his or her capability for self-care. The physician should estimate the patient's readiness for change and explain the stages involved in making a permanent change in behavior. A patient's current level of stress can predict a relapse to former maladaptive behaviors; for example, a patient may overeat during forced overtime at work or turn to alcohol after long periods of abstinence when faced with a personal crisis (Prochaska, Norcross, & Diclemente, 1994). A person who becomes sleep deprived during stressful times should be informed that regular and sufficient sleep maintains, in part, glucose balance and normal growth hormone regulation. It follows, therefore, that families of low socioeconomic status who are awakened by noise at night have a higher allostatic load and are thereby at greater risk for diabetes, hypertension, and obesity (Van Cauter & Spiegel, 1999).

### Treating Stress and Mood Disorders

Treatment of stress-related illness and mood disorders has been shown to improve physical health, add to quality of life, and decrease demand for services. Two behavioral medicine interventions decreased reported distress and service use in comparison to an information session about stress and health. The intervention group was given actual practice in relaxation, education about mind-body relationships, and cognitive behavioral therapy (Hellman, Budd, Borysenko, McClelland, & Benson, 1990). In patients with cardiovascular disease, results of treatment of depression on morbidity and mortality are variable, but quality of life improves as depressive symptoms are resolved. Further, depressed patients are at increased risk for death after myocardial infarction and are less likely to adhere to medical treatment recommendations (Musselman, Evans, & Nemeroff, 1998). Treatment of depressive illness has been shown to improve clinical outcome and quality of life, but overall, costs of treatment in a group of high users increased (Simon et al., 2001). Patients most likely to accept referrals for psychological or psychophysiological therapy and to respond positively should be identified (Kroenke & Swindle, 2000).

## Managing Functional Syndromes

Barsky and Borus (1999) recommend a multistep process for management of patients with functional syndromes. Vague, poorly defined symptoms should be evaluated, though not with exhaustive testing. Assessment of major depressive disorder and panic disorder is important. The patient should be engaged in a collaborative effort to improve quality of life. Education about the role of psychosocial factors in disease and cautious reassurance about the absence of life-threatening disease can be made part of each office visit. The physician should be aware of community resources for cognitive behavioral therapists, psychophysiological therapists, support groups, and appropriate complementary services. By demonstrating their knowledge about the appropriate uses of yoga, meditation, relaxation, and biofeedback for well and ill people, physicians place value on these therapies. Patients are thereby encouraged to invest the time and money needed to learn the techniques (Barnes, Treiber, Turner, Davis, & Strong, 1999).

## Brief Interventions

The potential benefits of short-term or brief interventions should not be ignored. A four-session self-care intervention for patients with back pain changed attitudes about use of services (Saunders, Von Kroff, Pruitt, & Moore, 1999). Physician recommendations to patients that they should stop smoking, and reduce substance abuse can be as effective as more costly therapist-intensive approaches

(Heather, 1995). Patients who have problems with alcohol were shown to benefit from a few minutes of advice followed by booster phone calls (Pinto, Goldstein, & Marcus, 1998). Calfas, Salis, Oldenburg, and French (1997) showed that primary care physicians who talk with patients about increasing physical activity were effective in improving awareness of the necessity for exercise. These patients also increased activity compared to those who had no such discussion. Some minimal therapist interventions for chronic headache that comprise 3 to 5 sessions instead of the usual 10 to 12 have similar success rates (Rowan & Andrasik, 1996). Positive outcomes of less pain, better sleep, and lower severity of depression and anxiety resulted from a short-term, mind-body wellness intervention. Participants with depression, sleep disturbances, and pain were provided with relaxation training, cognitive restructuring, and learned simple behaviors. Both the home study course and classroom instruction were better than the no-intervention control (Rybarczyk, DeMarco, DeLaCruz, & Lapidos, 1999).

## Therapist-Intensive Interventions

Review and meta-analysis of studies dealing with psychological or stress management interventions in people who have chronic stressors demonstrated improvements in immune function. These effects included increased natural killer cell cytotoxicity and lymphocyte proliferation in response to an antigen (Miller & Cohen, 2001). Turner, Linden, van der Wal, and Schamberg (1995) compared a treatment program that combined stress management and exercise with a program of exercise alone in patients with heart disease. Blood pressure reactivity to psychological challenge, which is an important risk factor for cardiovascular disease, was reduced after the combined treatment. A recent Canadian consensus report summarizes the use of stress management as an effective intervention in essential hypertension. Multicomponent therapy results were comparable to other nonpharmacological interventions and to some drug therapies (Spence, Barnett, Linden, Ramsden, & Taenzer, 1999).

whom emotional factors or mood disorders are influencing physical illness. Once the impact of psychological factors is known, the physician has multiple resources available, ranging from brief in-office recommendations to short-term behavioral interventions to long-term psychological and complementary therapies.

## SUMMARY

This chapter has provided several strategies for eliciting information from patients in

---

## REFERENCES

Ader, R., Cohen, N., & Felten, D. (1995). Psychoneuroimmunology: Interactions between the nervous system and the immune system. *Lancet, 345,* 99–103.

Barnes, V. A., Treiber, F. A., Turner, R., Davis, H., & Strong, W. B. (1999). Acute effects of transcendental meditation on hemodynamic functioning in middle-aged adults. *Psychosomatic Medicine, 61,* 525–531.

Barsky, A. J., & Borus, J. F. (1999). Functional somatic syndromes. *Annals of Internal Medicine, 130,* 910–921.

Bass, C., Bond, A., Gill, D., & Sharpe, M. (1999). Frequent attenders without organic disease in a gastroenterology clinic. Patient characteristics and health care use. *General Hospital Psychiatry, 21,* 30–38.

Boone, J. L., & Christensen, J. F. (1997). Stress & disease. In M. D. Feldman & J. F. Christensen (Eds.), *Behavioral medicine in primary care: A practical guide* (pp. 265–276). Stamford, CT: Appleton & Lange.

Brenner, G. F. (1997). Chronic illness. In M. D. Feldman & J. F. Christensen (Eds.), *Behavioral medicine in primary care: A practical guide* (pp. 313–320). Stamford, CT: Appleton & Lange.

Cacioppo, J. T. (1994). Social neuroscience: Autonomic, neuroendocrine, and immune responses to stress. *Psychophysiology, 31,* 113–128.

Cacioppo, J. T., Burleson, M. H., Poehlmann, K. M., Malarkey, W. B., Kiecolt-Glaser, J. K., Berntson, G. G., et al. (2000). Autonomic and neuroendocrine responses to mild psychological stressors: Effects of chronic stress on older women. *Annals of Behavioral Medicine, 22*(2), 140–148.

Calfas, K. J., Salis, J. F., Oldenburg, B., & French, M. (1997). Mediators of change in physical activity following an intervention in primary care: PACE. *Preventive Medicine, 26*(3), 297–304.

Clark, M. M., Niaura, R., King, T. K., & Para, V. (1996). Depression, smoking, activity level, and health status: Pretreatment predictors of attrition in obesity treatment. *Addictive Behavior, 21*(4), 509–513.

Coffey, P., Leitenberg, H., Henning, K., Turner, T., & Bennett, R. T. (1996). The relation between methods of coping during adulthood with a history of childhood sexual abuse and current psychological adjustment. *Journal of Consulting and Clinical Psychology, 64,* 1090–1093.

Cohen, S., Doyle, W. J., Skoner, D. P., Rabin, B. S., & Gwaltney, J. M., Jr. (1997). Social ties and susceptibility to the common cold. *Journal of the American Medical Association, 277*(24), 1940–1944.

Cohen, S., & Rodriguez, M. S. (1995). Pathways linking affective disturbances and physical disorders. *Health Psychology, 14*(5), 374–380.

Corcoran, C., Gallitano, A., Leitman, D., & Malaspina, D. (2001). The neurobiology of the stress cascade and its potential relevance for schizophrenia. *Journal of Psychiatric Practice, 7*(1), 3–14.

Dantzer, R. (1991). Stress and disease: A psychobiological perspective. *Annals of Behavioral Medicine, 13*(4), 205–210.

Denollet, J., Vaes, J., & Brutsaert, D. L. (2000). Inadequate response to treatment in coronary heart disease: Adverse effects of type D personality and younger age on 5-year prognosis and quality of life. *Circulation, 102*(6), 630–635.

Devlin, M. J., Yanovski, S. Z., & Wilson, G. T. (2000). Obesity: What mental health professionals need to know. *American Journal of Psychiatry, 157*(6), 854–865.

Goodnick, P. J., Henry, J. H., & Buki, V. M. (1995). Treatment of depression in patients with diabetes mellitus. *Journal of Clinical Psychiatry, 56,* 128–136.

Hahn, S. R., Kroenke, K., Spitzer, R. L., Brody, D., Williams, J. B. W., Linzer, M., & deGruy, F. V., III (1996). The difficult patient: Prevalence, psychopathology and functional impairment. *Journal of General Internal Medicine, 11,* 1–8.

Harmon, R. L., & Myers, M. A. (1999). Prayer and meditation as medical therapies. *Physical Medicine and Rehabilitation Clinics of North America, 10*(3), 651–662.

Heather, N. (1995). Brief intervention strategies. In R. K. Hester & W. R. Miller (Eds.), *Handbook of alcoholism treatment approaches: Effective alternatives* (2nd ed., pp. 105–122). Boston: Allyn & Bacon.

Hellman, C. J. C., Budd, M., Borysenko, J., McClelland, D. C., & Benson, H. (1990). A study of the effectiveness of two group behavioral medicine interventions for patients with psychosomatic complaints. *Behavioral Medicine, 16*(4), 165–173.

Holman, E. A., Silver, R. C., & Waitzkin, H. (2000). Traumatic life events in primary care patients. *Archives of Family Medicine, 9,* 802–810.

Kaplan, N. M. (1986). Therapeutic implications from clinical trials for the treatment of hypertension. *Journal of Clinical Hypertension, 2*(Suppl. 3), 22S–27S.

Kemeny, M. E., & Miller, G. E. (1999). Effects of psychosocial interventions on immune functions. In M. Schedlowski & U. Tewes (Eds.), *Psychoneuroimmunology: A textbook* (pp. 373–415). New York: Plenum.

Kendler, K. S., Karkowski, L. M., & Prescott, C. A. (1999). Causal relationship between stressful life events and the onset of major depression. *American Journal of Psychiatry, 156,* 837–841.

Kirmayer, L. J., Robbins, J. M., Dworkind, M., & Yaffe, M. J. (1993). Somatization and the recognition of depression and anxiety in primary care. *American Journal of Psychiatry, 150,* 734–741.

Kosinski, D. J., & Grubb, B. P. (1994). Neurally mediated syncope with an update on indications and usefulness of head-upright tilt table testing and pharmacologic therapy. *Current Opinion of Cardiology, 9,* 53–64.

Kroenke, K., Jackson, J. L., & Chamberlin, J. (1997). Depressive and anxiety disorders in patients presenting with physical complaints: Clinical predictors and outcome. *American Journal of Medicine, 103*(5), 339–347.

Kroenke, K., & Swindle, R. (2000). Cognitive-behavioral therapy for somatization and symptom syndromes: A critical review of controlled clinical trials. *Psychotherapy and Psychosomatics, 69*(4), 205–215.

Kroenke, K., Taylor-Vaisey, A., Dietrich, A. J., & Oxman, T. E. (2000). Interventions to improve provider diagnosis and treatment of mental disorders in primary care. A critical review of the literature. *Psychosomatics, 41*(1), 39–52.

Kuhajda, M. C., Thorn, B. E., & Klinger, M. R. (1998). The effect of pain on memory for affective words. *Annals of Behavioral Medicine, 20*(1), 31–35.

Lazarus, R. S., & Folkman, S. (1984). *Stress, appraisal, and coping.* New York: Springer.

Lewis, P., & Lubkin, I. M. (1998). Illness roles. In I. M. Lubkin & P. D. Larsen (Eds.), *Chronic illness: Impact and interventions* (4th ed., pp. 77–102). Boston: Jones & Bartlett.

Maier, S. F., Watkins, L. R., & Fleshner, M. (1994). Psychoneuroimmunology. The interface between behavior, brain, and immunity. *American Psychologist, 49*(12), 1004–1017.

McCauley, J., Kern, D. E., Kolodner, K., Dill, L., Schroeder, A. F., De Chant, H., et al. (1997). Clinical characteristics of women with a history of childhood abuse: Unhealed wounds. *Journal of the American Medical Association 277*(17), 1362–1368.

McCullough, M. E., Hoyt, W. T., Larson, D. B., Koenig, H. G., & Thoresen, C. (2000). Religious involvement and mortality: A meta-analytic review. *Health Psychology, 19*(3), 211–222.

McEwen, B. S. (1998). Protective and damaging effects of stress mediators. *Seminars in Medicine of the Beth Israel Deaconess Medical Center, 338*(3), 171–179.

McGrady, A., Lynch, D., Nagel, R., & Zsembik, C. (1999). Application of the high risk model of threat perception to a primary care patient population. *Journal of Nervous and Mental Disease, 187,* 369–375.

Miller, G. E., & Cohen, S. (2001). Psychological interventions and the immune system: A meta-analytic review and critique. *Health Psychology, 20*(1), 47–63.

Miller, M. A., & Rahe, R. H. (1997). Life changes scaling for the 1990s. *Journal of Psychosomatic Research, 43*(3), 279–292.

Musselman, D. L., Evans, D. L., & Nemeroff, C. (1998). The relationship of depression to cardiovascular diseases. *Archives of General Psychiatry, 55,* 580–592.

Nelesen, R. A., & Dimsdale, J. E. (1994). Hypertension and adrenergic functioning in adrenergic dysfunction and psychobiology. In O. G. Cameron (Ed.), *Adrenergic dysfunction and psychobiology* (pp. 257–274). Washington, DC: American Psychiatric Press.

Pinto, B. M., Goldstein, M. G., & Marcus, B. H. (1998). Activity counseling by primary care physicians. *Preventive Medicine, 27*(4), 506–513.

Porges, S. W. (1995). Orienting in a defensive world: Mammalian modifications of our evolutionary heritage. A polyvagal theory. *Psychophysiology, 32,* 301–318.

Prochaska, J. E., Norcross, J. C., & Diclemente, C. C. (1994). *Changing for good: The revolutionary program that explains the six stages of change and teaches you how to free yourself from bad habits.* New York: Morrow.

Richards, J. M., & Gross, J. J. (2000). Emotion regulation and memory: The cognitive costs of keeping one's cool. *Journal of Personality and Social Psychology, 79*(3), 410–424.

Rowan, A. B., & Andrasik, F. (1996). Efficacy and cost-effectiveness of minimal therapist contact treatments of chronic headaches: A review. *Behavior Therapy, 27,* 207–234.

Rybarczyk, B., DeMarco, G., DeLaCruz, M., & Lapidos, S. (1999). Comparing mind-body wellness interventions for older adults with chronic illness: Classroom versus home instruction. *Behavioral Medicine, 24*(4), 181–190.

Saunders, K. W., Von Kroff, M., Pruitt, S. D., & Moore, J. E. (1999). Prediction of physician visits and prescription medicine use for back pain. *Pain, 83,* 369–477.

Simon, G. E., Manning, W. G., Katzelnick, D. J., Pearson, S. D., Henk, H. J., & Helstad, C. P. (2001). Cost-effectiveness of systematic depression treatment for high utilizers of general medical care. *Archives of General Psychiatry, 58*(2), 181–187.

Skinner, J. E. (1991). Interrupting neural pathways that transduce stressful information into physiological responses. *Integrative Physiological and Behavioral Science, 26,* 330–334.

Spence, J. D., Barnett, P. A., Linden, W., Ramsden, V., & Taenzer, P. (1999). Recommendations on stress management. *Canadian Medical Association Journal, 160*(Suppl. 9), S46–S50.

Spitzer, R. L., Kroenke, K., Linzer, M., Haha, S. R., Williams, J. B., deGruy, F. V., III, et al. (1995). Health-related quality of life in primary care patients with mental disorders. Results from the PRIME-MD 1000 study. *Journal of the American Medical Association, 274*(19), 1511–1517.

Sternberg, E. M., Chrousos, G. P., Wilder, R. L., & Gold, P. W. (1992). The stress response and the regulation of inflammatory disease. *Annals of Internal Medicine, 117*(10), 854–866.

Sullivan, M. D., Turner, J. A., & Romano, J. (1991). Chronic pain in primary care. Identification and management of psychosocial factors. *Journal of Family Practice, 32*(2), 193–199.

Turner, L., Linden, W., van der Wal, R., & Schamberg, W. (1995). Stress management for patients with heart disease: A pilot study. *Heart & Lung, 24,* 145–153.

Van Cauter, E., & Spiegel, K. (1999). Sleep as a mediator of the relationship between socioeconomic status and health: A hypothesis. *Annals of the New York Academy of Sciences, 896,* 254–261.

Wahl, E., McGrady, A., Lynch, D., & Nagel, R. (2000, August). Patient characteristics: Prediction of service utilization. Presented at Ohio Academy of Family Physicians Foundation Annual Research Day, Columbus, OH.

Walker, E. A., Unützer, J., & Katon, W. J. (1998). Understanding and caring for the distressed patient with multiple medically unexplained symptoms. *Journal of the American Board of Family Practice, 11,* 347–356.

Wickramasekera, I. (1995). Somatization: Concepts, data, and predictions from the high risk model of threat perception. *Journal of Nervous and Mental Disease, 183,* 15–23.

Yehuda, R., Southwick, S. M., Nussbaum, G., Wahlby, V., Giller, E. L., Jr., & Mason, J. W. (1990). Low urinary cortisol excretion in patients with posttraumatic stress disorder. *Journal of Nervous and Mental Disease, 178,* 366–369.

# CHAPTER 4

# Complementary, Alternative, and Integrative Medicine

JAMES LAKE

**Abstract:** The author reviews the recent history of complementary and alternative medicine (CAM) in the United States as it pertains to mind-body medicine, including prospects and obstacles that will affect its continued growth. Central concepts of integrative medicine are explained. The evolution of Western medicine toward a truly integrative paradigm will likely incorporate the values and scientific principles of Dossey's Era III medicine. Premodern and emerging therapies based on presumed Era III mechanisms compose *energy medicine*. The issue of managed care impeding progress toward widespread acceptance of CAM or integrative medicine is discussed. The absence of a unifying body of theory and practice in contemporary Western psychiatry is identified as an important factor promoting openness to CAM and integrative therapies in the treatment of psychiatric and neurological disorders. Conceptual approaches to reasonable, safe integration of CAM and biomedicine are presented. Traditional Chinese Medicine, therapeutic touch, and EEG biofeedback are given as examples of emerging therapies in the United States that will play an increasing role in future mind-body medicine.

## BASIC CONCEPTS

Much of the confusion and debate surrounding mind-body medicine can be traced to ambiguous definitions of terms such as *complementary, alternative,* and *integrative.* To date, a consensus over definitions of basic concepts distinguishing conventional Western biomedicine from unconventional therapies has not been achieved. This problem of language reflects broad philosophical, scientific, and institutional issues that underlie the practice of medicine in contemporary Western societies.

## The Chantilly Report—First Steps Toward Legitimacy of Alternative Medicine

In 1991, the U.S. Senate established the Office of Alternative Medicine (OAM) within the National Institutes of Health (NIH) and gave it a mandate to "more adequately explore unconventional medical practices" (National Institutes of Health, 1995, p. iv). The federal initiative to establish the OAM was an acknowledgment of the widening gap between available conventional medical therapies and patients' unmet health care needs.

Many compelling reasons were cited for renewed interest in alternative medicine, including evidence of widespread use of alternative therapies (Eisenberg, Kessler, et al., 1993). Another reason was the growing percentage of medically uninsured people and increasing health costs generally attributed to the demographic shift toward more elderly people with debilitating chronic diseases.

Because of these concerns, the OAM convened a workshop in Chantilly, Virginia, in 1992. Leading researchers and educators in all areas of alternative medicine presented different views on the current status of alternative medical practices in the United States, summarized ongoing research, and recommended future research priorities aimed at promoting basic scientific understanding and clinical applications of the range of unconventional medical therapies. The government-issued report that contains those findings and recommendations has become known as the Chantilly report (National Institutes of Health, 1995). It remains perhaps the single most important overview of the state of affairs of alternative medical paradigms and practices in the United States and can be regarded as a manifesto of scientific principles and compelling research issues that will probably guide the evolution of medicine in this country for years to come. In 1998, in response to continued growth in the use of unconventional medicine (Eisenberg, Davis, et al., 1998), the OAM became the National Center for Complementary and Alternative Medicine (NCCAM), elevating its status and reflecting the continuing national priority on developing evidence-based practices of alternative and complementary medicine.

Participants in the Chantilly workshop proposed a systematic way of defining and categorizing the numerous fields of medical practice that are outside conventional Western biomedicine. *Mind-body medicine* was defined as a set of interventions originating in both Western and non-Western paradigms directed at treating disease or preserving health based on an assumed interconnection or *integration* of mind and body. According to the Chantilly report, mind-body interventions include psychotherapy, meditation, guided imagery, hypnosis, biofeedback, yoga, dance therapy, music therapy, art therapy, prayer, and intentional healing at a distance. Since those early efforts, a coherent taxonomy of alternative medicine has been the object of continuing discussion and debate among both conventionally trained Western physicians and many alternative practitioners. To date, there is no clear consensus about whether or how the diverse unconventional systems of medicine should be hierarchically organized with respect to one another.

## Congruency With the Western Medical Paradigm

Numerous medical treatments that are becoming popular in the United States and other Western countries were introduced in the context of highly evolved professional systems of medicine. These include, principally, Traditional Chinese Medicine (TCM), Ayurveda, homeopathic medicine, and naturopathic medicine. An estimated 70 percent to 90 percent of the world's population receives medical care from practitioners trained in these unconventional systems of medicine. Each major alternative system of medicine provides rigorous professional training to its practitioners, is accepted as legitimate by major world cultures, and is typically an important and sometimes the sole source of medical care for millions of people. It is important to note that each major alternative system of medicine embodies clinical techniques based on a coherent body of theory about mechanisms of disease causation and healing. Further, specific therapies within each system of traditional medicine are judged to be valid and "scientific," in accord with the concepts of health and disease respected by the particular paradigm and based on standards of proof embedded in the particular system of medicine. In fact, the sophisticated theories and practices that compose the major alternative systems of medicine are regarded as substantial and valid and are as strongly endorsed in their parent cultures as Western biomedicine is in the United States and Europe. An impartial observer would feel obliged to conclude that the other major systems of medicine are "alternative" only in the context of Western cultures and that it is equally wrongheaded or misguided to regard Western biomedicine as de facto "alternative" in non-Western cultures.

In attempting to understand the differences between alternative and complementary therapies, it is useful to distinguish these approaches with respect to the dominant Western paradigm of biomedicine. *Complementary treatments* are presently outside orthodox Western biomedicine but are based on theories congruent with models of disease causation and healing embedded in the conventional Western medical system. Nevertheless, practitioners of Western biomedicine do not endorse many complementary therapies, including herbal medicine, massage therapy, and EEG biofeedback. In contrast, *alternative treatments* rest on nonorthodox theories regarded by Western biomedicine practitioners as violating basic laws of science. Therefore, contemporary biomedicine rejects most alternative therapies, including acupuncture, Reiki, and homeopathy. An adequate approach to organizing the numerous CAM therapies into a hierarchy of systems of medicine awaits clarification of basic differences and similarities between emerging therapies and biomedicine. Several authors have attempted to systematically characterize all nonbiomedical therapies (Spencer & Jacobs, 1999). Some authors have focused on CAM therapies relevant to mind-body medicine (Bassman, 1998).

Finally, *integrative medicine* represents the attempt to integrate or combine various complementary, alternative, and mind-body therapies with mainstream biomedicine, in one seamless treatment process. For example, Cohen et al. (2000) used Chinese herbal medicine to treat pathogen-negative diarrhea associated with HIV within the larger context of conventional medical care for the HIV patient. Similarly, Moore and Spiegel (2000) used guided imagery for pain relief within the context of mainstream cancer care for women with metastatic breast cancer.

## Historical Roots

Most theories and treatments that are collectively described as biomedicine or modern medicine have common scientific and historical roots that can be traced to the empiricism of ancient Greek medicine and, subsequently, Descartes' philosophical arguments toward mind-body dualism and the first explicit formulation of a scientific method of experimentation requiring quantitative observation (1637, 1641/1999). For the most part, the ancient healing traditions of Ayurveda, Chinese medicine, and other major non-Western systems of medicine evolved independently of early Greek influences (Kuriyama, 1999). In contrast to Greek medicine, early non-Western paradigms were influenced by the metaphysical concepts of existence and causality inherent in major Eastern philosophical or religious systems of thought, such as the Hindu Vedas (Ayurveda) and Buddhism (Chinese medicine). Therefore, systems of medicine that evolved in the context of the major Oriental philosophical-religious traditions did not regard "diseases" as empirically measurable cause-effect patterns of pathology but as manifestations of subtle or gross imbalances in presumed fundamental energies at the core of their metaphysical worldviews. Indeed, the wide conceptual gap in understandings of the attributes and processes of the human body in time and space reflects unresolved basic differences in the philosophical origins of Western and non-Western medicine.

## FACTORS FAVORING AND LIMITING CAM

Many factors favor continuing acceptance of complementary and alternative therapies by physicians, medical societies, and the population at large. Demographic trends favoring growth of CAM in the United States have been confirmed by two studies conducted by Eisenberg at the Center for Alternative Medicine Research and Education, Beth Israel Deaconess Medical Center (Eisenberg, Davis, et al., 1998; Eisenberg, Kessler, et al., 1993). These studies demonstrated gradually increasing use of CAM therapies for a range of medical and psychiatric disorders. An important finding was widespread use of unconventional medicine despite major insurance providers not reimbursing for most CAM treatments. Reasons for this are complex (Astin, 1998) and include a common belief that conventional Western biomedical therapies often do not result in cures or substantial relief; concerns about safety issues inherent in many biomedical therapies; and increasing openness to unconventional treatments including acupuncture, homeopathy, and "energy medicine." In addition, many CAM therapies are increasingly congruent with the values of educated people, and emerging scientific evidence supporting the use of many CAM therapies continues to accumulate.

Barriers to continued growth and acceptance of CAM in the United States include (1) the absence of adequate legal and regulatory mechanisms that define allowable, appropriate, and safe uses of unconventional therapies in the context of Western biomedicine (Cohen, 1998, 2000); (2) unclear issues of liability and scope of practice relevant to

physicians who incorporate CAM therapies into their practices; (3) limited availability or limited qualifications of specialists in many CAM areas, such as Reiki and Ayurvedic healing; (4) absent or insufficient scientific evidence of the efficacy or safety of CAM therapies; (5) negative biases against CAM therapies by Western medical practitioners and their societies; and (6) the paucity of coverage for most CAM therapies by most insurance carriers.

As increasing numbers of U.S. medical schools include courses on CAM in their preclinical curricula, physicians in the future will presumably be better informed and more aware about potential benefits and risks of various CAM therapies. Further, as Western medicine becomes increasingly open to CAM, patients will expect physicians to know how to competently refer them to CAM practitioners. At the same time, physicians are increasingly motivated to learn about CAM to better serve patients' needs, while state and local medical societies carefully monitor the legal environment to assess the risks and benefits associated with specific CAM therapies.

## THE LACK OF A UNIFYING THEORY FOR WESTERN PSYCHIATRY

When placed in the evolutionary context of medicine in general, psychiatry and psychology lack a unifying body of theory or universally accepted standards of clinical practice. The issues contributing to this ambiguous state of affairs have been described in two important recent works: Grof (1985) and Wilber (2000). To summarize these arguments, the theoretical perspectives and clinical practices of Western-trained psychiatrists or psychologists largely depend on personal intellectual or other (e.g., spiritual, cultural, etc.) kinds of preferences regarding the nature and meanings of psychopathology.

Among psychiatrists, the dominant view is an extension of contemporary biomedicine, which equates psychopathology with functional abnormalities in neurochemistry. According to this model, successful "treatment" entails "correcting" a presumed neurochemical abnormality that corresponds to a specific abnormal cognitive, emotional, or behavioral state.

While psychiatrists often use cognitive-behavioral approaches or therapies directed at interpreting interpersonal dynamics, depth psychological approaches examining existential or spiritual themes are typically regarded as incidental to "more serious" pharmacological treatments. Among psychologists, numerous and often contradictory theories have yielded disparate conceptions of psychopathology, fundamentally different models of psychotherapy based on structured verbal interactions, and a range of nonverbal experiential techniques. Because of the prevailing multiplicity of theories that compose Western psychiatry, there is no consensus over a single "best" model of psychotherapy. Therefore, with few exceptions, there is no consensus over a "most appropriate" psychotherapeutic intervention for a given symptom or disorder. The result is an eclecticism that has facilitated an openness to complementary and alternative therapies in the mental health arena (Shannon, 2001). In an effort to address the fragmentation of psychiatry and psychology, Wilber (2000) has systematically reviewed divergent psychological theories of mind-body and proposed initial guidelines for the creation of an "integral psychology" that attempts to take into account the core psychological and spiritual features of many dominant theories of mind-body. An important goal of this work is the elaboration of a series of integrative psychotherapeutic strategies that are ideally suited for specific symptom patterns of mind-body, psychological, or spiritual distress.

## REDEFINING THE EVOLUTION OF MEDICINE

Many authors have examined the evolutionary progress of medicine. Perhaps the most creative and notable of these is Larry Dossey (1982, 1999), who has characterized conceptual and practical progress in medicine according to his three-era model. Dossey argues that medicine has evolved along the lines of three separate but overlapping historical and conceptual epochs, or eras. Each era is characterized by a different metaphysical or scientific view of reality that informs and limits the theory and practice of medicine.

Era I medicine, still the dominant Western medical perspective, largely rests on the mechanistic concepts of classical Newtonian physics that are internalized in contemporary biomedicine as a priori "laws" operating in disease causation and healing. Dossey (1982, 1999) defines Era II medicine as mind-body medicine. This evolutionary phase of medical understanding posits a primary healing role of mind, which functions to promote healing according to the same classical laws of causality assumed in the Era I model. Era III medicine subsumes emerging paradigms that rest on suppositions of healing and disease that cannot be adequately explained with reference to concepts of classical Newtonian physics. Invoking quantum mechanics to explain the role of directed intention, or consciousness, mind has primacy in disease causation and healing. Causal mechanisms underlying disease and healing in therapies within the domains of Eras I and II operate in the "local" space-time environment according to the laws of classical physics. In contrast, the capacity of human consciousness to invoke "nonlocal" healing effects across space and time is viewed as a fundamental characteristic of Era III therapies.

## ENERGY MEDICINE: UNITING ANCIENT HEALING METHODS WITH MODERN PHYSICS

It is significant that many core tenets of Era III medicine are also central elements of emerging or pre-modern concepts of energy medicine. According to this evolving paradigm, the proper balancing of fundamental life energies, or forces, is required for health, and disease is caused by deranged energetic balance. Historically, these vital forces have been described in different cultural contexts as qi, prana, and other presumed energetic essences. Both ancient and modern healing techniques have been grouped under energy medicine. These include qigong, acupuncture, many forms of therapeutic touch therapies, polarity therapy, the use of devices that generate magnetic fields or low-frequency sound, homeopathy, and others.

In a groundbreaking book, James Oschman (2000) provides a concise review of theories and research supporting various energetic healing methods. According to Oschman, all forms of energetic healing rely on the apparently inherent capacity of humans to generate or direct biomagnetic fields, infrared energy, very low frequency (VLF) sound, quantum fields, and possibly other heretofore undescribed kinds of energy or "information" in ways that result in symptom amelioration or healing. Oschman argues that humans are able to generate various forms of energy that can be directed as healing intention. According to this view, the human capacity to generate healing energy is the adaptive outcome of the exquisitely complex primate central nervous system, which has evolved to possess fundamental functional characteristics permitting humans to generate and direct highly organized biomagnetic fields, low-frequency sound, and perhaps also coherent quantum fields. Numerous studies have established that certain unconventional energetic healing practices including qigong

and various methods of healing touch are associated with measurable changes in infrared energy, magnetic field strength, and very low frequency sound. Further, predictable changes in energetic signals reportedly generated by healers appear to correspond to their intentions in directing this healing energy to patients. The NCCAM has recently funded several studies investigating the mechanisms and efficacy of different energetic healing practices. Definitive scientific validation or falsification of energy medicine will likely require many more years because reported effects of energetic healing practices are extremely subtle. Further, purported effects of energy medicine often elude the capacity of contemporary science to distinguish them from other subtle factors that affect healing.

In spite of the ambiguous evidence for energetic healing methods, alternative practitioners will probably continue to employ many of these subtle approaches, whose roots are embedded in the major unconventional systems of medicine.

## INTEGRATIVE MEDICINE

Integrative medicine combines complementary, alternative, and Western biomedical therapies. This approach is therefore broader and more encompassing than any single practical approach or theoretical perspective. Discussion of scientific, economic, or other justifications for integrating therapies from divergent paradigms is in an early phase. The two paramount issues in this discussion are efficacy and safety. Opponents of integration argue that from a rational perspective, combining (or excluding combinations of) different therapies is justified only when doing so yields improved outcomes compared with single-therapy treatments and only after the safety of combining specific treatments under consideration has been demonstrated.

Western science is only now beginning to formulate methods to meet the goals of efficacy and safety, but the process requires many decades. The proponents of moving toward integration before Western scientific "gold standards" of efficacy and safety are met argue that combining therapies from divergent systems of medicine is reasonable and probably safe because most complementary or alternative therapies do not "work" through biological mechanisms that can potentially result in undesirable or life-threatening interactions with conventional biomedical therapies. They might argue further that the safe and efficacious combination of many specific therapies has been demonstrated through the widespread, though still unapproved, use of numerous common alternative or complementary therapies in combination with biomedical therapies.

Although Wilber (2000) has advanced a broad theoretical framework for integral psychology, there has been little empirical basis for combining specific CAM or biomedical therapies into truly integrative treatments. Major unresolved questions of mechanisms of action, efficacy, and safety continue to obscure efforts to establish a rigorous and truly integrative medicine incorporating the diverse unconventional systems of medicine and their associated therapies.

## LIMITATIONS PRESENTED BY MANAGED CARE

Standard treatment approaches to psychiatric outpatients have become increasingly abbreviated and simplified as the practice of psychiatry in the United States becomes has been progressively limited by the dictates of time efficiency and cost constraints inherent in managed care. The currently accepted standard for outpatient psychiatric services consists of an initial interview to establish a

diagnosis and initiate psychopharmacological treatment, followed by brief monthly (or less frequent) appointments conducted strictly for the purpose of "medication management." Typically, outpatients receive only brief examinations of their mental status, cursory reviews of medication dosage and side effects, and no discussion of psychotherapeutic issues. A motivated patient can seek psychotherapy where, under most managed care contracts, he or she may be eligible to work with a psychotherapist for a total of 10 to 20 annual sessions, depending on insurance benefits, documented medical necessity, and acuity. The present economic organization of outpatient mental health care ensures that such "split therapy" will continue for the near future, with little opportunity or incentive for meaningful contact between medication-dispensing psychiatrists and "talk therapists." In the managed care model, where biological and psychotherapeutic treatments are kept separate and other kinds of treatments, including CAM, are seldom available, there is no supportive context for development or delivery of integrative treatment approaches.

## EMERGING CAM THERAPIES

In recent decades, practitioners of all major unconventional medical therapies have established a clear presence in the United States. To date, few CAM therapies have received FDA approval, acceptance by professional medical societies, or state medical boards, or through state licensure requirements of practitioners (Cohen, 1998). Major U.S. medical journals continue to publish skeptical or hostile editorials that call into question the legitimacy of major alternative medicine paradigms. To further confuse the situation, a complex, often contradictory body of legal and regulatory issues germane to the practice of CAM, or to the integration of CAM and biomedicine in conventional medical practice settings, is rapidly accumulating (Cohen, 1998, 2000). At this time, it is not clear how ongoing debates in the state and federal courts and in federal regulatory agencies will ultimately shape the practice of CAM or integrative medicine in the United States.

The NIH (1997) has formally recognized only Traditional Chinese Medicine as comprising a legitimate body of therapies but, significantly, has not recognized the validity of its theoretical basis. Though not officially endorsed by FDA or the NIH, massage and other somatic therapies, including Rolfing and applied kinesiology, are widely used in hospitals and clinics to treat a range of pain disorders, other functional impairments, and stress-related complaints. Biofeedback has commanded a strong following among psychologists for decades. EEG biofeedback is an emerging approach to diagnosing and treating mind-body problems that has created renewed controversy between conventionally trained Western physicians and many CAM practitioners. Homeopathy has also attracted rapidly growing interest among conventionally trained physicians and allied health care professionals. Numerous other CAM therapies are being explored by researchers at NIH-sponsored Centers of Alternative Medicine at universities and private institutions, under the auspices of the NCCAM. These include energy medicine techniques such as qigong (a branch of Chinese medicine), Reiki, polarity therapy and other forms of healing touch, as well as herbal medicines and other natural products. Ayurvedic medicine is also gaining popularity in the United States, and NCCAM is beginning to sponsor studies of its numerous applications in both medicine and psychiatry.

The following sections describe three areas of CAM that are coming to the forefront of integrative medical care in the United States.

## Traditional Chinese Medicine for Depression

Numerous acupuncture treatments and herbal formulas have resulted from a long history of practical experimentation by TCM doctors addressing a range of symptom patterns that Western physicians view as psychiatric disorders. Chinese medicine is one of the world's oldest systems of medicine. Its theoretical basis, *materia medica,* and techniques have evolved over at least five millennia. It shares ancient roots with Ayurvedic medicine of the Indian subcontinent, and there is no clear line of demarcation between its fundamental metaphysical tenets and Buddhism. Empirical approaches underlying the historical development of complicated herbal formulas and acupuncture treatment protocols, combined with metaphysical assumptions about esoteric "fundamental" energetic principles, are embodied in the theory and practice of Chinese medicine, which is a truly integrative system of medicine that strives to treat both spirit and body.

It is important to clarify that *depression* in Western psychiatry is not necessarily equivalent to symptom pattern discriminations in Chinese medicine that are also labeled as depressed mood (Flaws & Lake, 2001, pp. 323–344). As Chinese medicine does not distinguish between mind and body, symptoms that would be regarded by Westerners as somatic complaints are typically grouped with so-called mood or cognitive symptoms into one coherent pattern discrimination. Chinese medical practitioners use a combination of acupuncture and compound herbal formulas to treat numerous symptom patterns that manifest as depressed mood. The practitioner selects from defined combinations of acupuncture points, or prescribes an herbal formula with the goal of correcting the energetic imbalance underlying a specific symptom pattern. The mechanism of action remains unclear to Western biomedicine.

However, numerous case reports and controlled studies support the efficacy of TCM treatments of depression (in particular, see Flaws & Lake, 2001). Numerous Chinese studies and some Western studies have demonstrated the efficacy of both acupuncture and certain compound herbal formulas in treating depression, and several other independent or NIH-sponsored investigations of TCM treatments of depression are ongoing (Flaws & Lake, 2001; National Institutes of Health, 1997; Schnyer, 2001).

## Therapeutic Touch for Stress-Related Diseases

As practiced in the United States, therapeutic touch is a composite of various ancient forms of healing based on the belief that the intention of one person can correct energetic imbalances in another person, resulting in healing. Therapeutic touch is therefore included under the broad heading of energy medicine. Contrary to what the term implies, direct physical contact does not take place during a therapeutic touch session. Initially, the therapist positions his or her hands close to certain areas of the patient's body while attempting to sense energetic imbalances. This is sometimes described as scanning. After determining the characteristics of a sensed energetic imbalance, the therapist typically uses his or her hands to emit healing energy into the patient, correcting the imbalance. The central premises of therapeutic touch are therefore roughly equivalent to those of qigong, Reiki, and other specific practices whose validity and effectiveness presumes the existence of fundamental energetic essences that can result in healing when directed by conscious intention. To date, most evidence supporting an effect in therapeutic touch comes from case reports or small nonblinded trials. These studies (Bassman, 1998) purport to show the positive effects of therapeutic touch in relieving stress and

anxiety in hospitalized medically ill adults and children and in victims of natural disasters.

Therapeutic touch is not potentially harmful to hospitalized medically ill patients. That is, whether this technique operates through suggestion only (as skeptics would argue) or on the basis of subtle manipulations of a patient's energy fields, many studies support its continued use in hospitalized patients receiving concurrent pharmacological or other biomedical treatments. Therefore, therapeutic touch is arguably a safe and reasonable kind of general intervention that can be safely combined with other conventional or alternative therapies.

## Biofeedback for Anxiety Disorders and ADHD

Quantitative electroencephalography (QEEG) was developed in the 1970s. Soon afterwards, databases of normative EEG activity and various abnormal populations, including major psychiatric or neurological disorders, were developed (Evans & Arbanel, 1999). The use of electroencephalography (EEG) in biofeedback to treat psychiatric disorders dates to the mid-1960s (Budzynski, 1999). Initially, QEEG did not gain acceptance as a clinical tool because of the absence of standard EEG recording approaches, and repeated attempts to replicate findings of specific EEG abnormalities in individuals with established diagnoses failed. These issues have resulted in the reluctance of many physicians and psychologists to adopt QEEG or EEG biofeedback (also called neurofeedback or neurotherapy) as a clinical tool. In spite of these early problems, normative databases of EEG data for several psychiatric or neurological disorders have recently been developed and validated (Evans & Arbanel, 1999; John, Prichep, Fridman, & Easton, 1988; Thatcher, 1998, 1999). This progress has led, in turn, to the development of specific therapeutic EEG biofeedback protocols for many psychiatric and neurological disorders (Moss, 2001; "The State of EEG Biofeedback Therapy," 2000).

The Association for Applied Psychophysiology and Biofeedback (AAPB), founded in 1969, is a professional organization that promotes both general biofeedback and EEG biofeedback and includes a neurofeedback division devoted to research and practice on EEG biofeedback and QEEG assessment. The Society for Neuronal Regulation (SNR) was established more recently to further neurofeedback research, promote standardized recording techniques, refine databases, and suggest protocols for clinical applications using EEG biofeedback for a range of neuropsychiatric and medical disorders. Both organizations have scientific journals that publish empirical investigations on neurofeedback and biofeedback (the AAPB journal is *Applied Psychophysiology and Biofeedback*, and the SNR publication is *Journal of Neurotherapy*). Practitioners of neurofeedback argue that the de facto scientific validity of this method has been established through numerous studies demonstrating its efficacy in the treatment of attention deficit disorder, cognitive deficits following stroke, relapse prevention in alcoholism, improved functioning in chronic fatigue syndrome, and other disorders. However, the uses and efficacy of neurofeedback continue to be disputed by most physicians. Today in the United States and Western Europe, many psychologists but few MDs use EEG biofeedback to treat the wide range of neurological and psychiatric disorders. More details are provided on the use of QEEG and neurofeedback in Chapter 9.

## THE EMERGENCE OF A TRULY INTEGRATIVE MEDICINE

Currently, the chief goal of NCCAM is the validation of diverse CAM therapies through well-designed, rigorously conducted research. Considerable information has accumulated regarding a few major CAM paradigms—for example, TCM and herbal medicine. However, an understanding of other unconventional therapies and their root sources remains largely anecdotal, including healing touch and other energy therapies. Research programs have recently been initiated to systematically examine safe and appropriate strategies for combining specific CAM therapies and biomedical interventions (Riley & Heger, 1999). However, adequate information is seldom available to permit clinicians to rationally determine whether it is safe or appropriate to integrate specific CAM and biomedical therapies. In spite of this dilemma, many believe that the selective integration of CAM and conventional therapies is the next phase in the continuing evolution of Western medicine.

Historically, Western medicine has followed a course of embracing therapies from divergent paradigms only after sufficient evidence accumulates to permit an alternative therapy to be regarded as legitimate within orthodox Western medicine. A major obstacle affecting the evolution of medicine at this time is the dispute over what constitutes sufficient or good evidence of a mechanism of action or efficacy, especially when it is difficult or impossible to characterize the nature of the healing effects of numerous unconventional therapies, much less to quantify those effects using Western scientific standards (Walach, 2001).

At present, there is a paucity of reliable data supporting the efficacy of numerous CAM therapies, and the safety risks inherent in combining specific CAM therapies with other CAM or biomedical therapies are poorly understood. Because of these unresolved issues, it is reasonable to consider only broad conservative strategies for combining diverse therapies into integrative treatment approaches. Conservative guidelines for integrating CAM and biomedical treatments might include a continuum from well-supported applications through applications to be avoided, as outlined here:

• Clear evidence from randomized controlled research trials supports the efficacy and safety of integrating two or more specific therapies.

• Compelling anecdotal evidence demonstrates the absence of safety issues and probable efficacy when two or more CAM or biomedical therapies are combined.

• In spite of limited research or anecdotal evidence, an established tradition among professional CAM practitioners of integrating two or more therapies has led to informal consensus about combined use.

• Clear evidence from controlled trials combining specific CAM or biomedical therapies has demonstrated absence of efficacy, clear safety problems, or both.

• Compelling anecdotal evidence demonstrates lack of efficacy or probable safety issues when combining two or more specific CAM or biomedical therapies.

• In spite of limited research or anecdotal evidence, an established tradition among professional CAM practitioners proscribes against combining two or more specific CAM or biomedical therapies, and professional consensus supports this view. In this case, the prohibition against combining the specific treatments should be followed until research evidence eventually contradicts this view.

## REFERENCES

Astin, J. (1998). Why patients use alternative medicine: Results of a national study. *Journal of the American Medical Association, 279*(19), 1548–1555.

Bassman, L. (Ed.). (1998). *The whole mind: The definitive guide to complementary treatments for mind, mood, and emotion.* Novato, CA: New World Library.

Budzynski, T. H. (1999). From EEG to neurofeedback. In J. Evans & A. Arbanel (Eds.), *Introduction to quantitative EEG and neurofeedback* (pp. 65–79). San Diego, CA: Academic Press.

Cohen, M. (1998). *Complementary and alternative medicine: Legal boundaries and regulatory perspectives.* Baltimore: Johns Hopkins University Press.

Cohen, M. (2000). *Beyond complementary medicine: Legal and ethical perspectives on health care and human evolution.* Ann Arbor: University of Michigan Press.

Cohen, M., Mitchell, T. F., Bacchetti, P., Child, C., Crawford, S., Gaeddert, A., et al. (2000). Use of a Chinese herbal medicine for treatment of HIV-associated pathogen-negative diarrhea. *Integrative Medicine, 2*(2), 79–84.

Descartes, R. (1999). *Discourse on method* and *Meditations on first philosophy* (4th ed.; D. Cress, Trans.). Indianapolis, IN: Hackett. (Original works published in 1637, 1641)

Dossey, L. (1982). *Space, time and medicine.* Boulder, CO: Shambhala.

Dossey, L. (1999). *Reinventing medicine: Beyond mind-body to a new era of healing.* San Francisco: Harper.

Eisenberg, D. M., Davis, R. B., Ettner, S., Appel, S., Wilkey, S., Van Rompay, M., & Kessler, R. C. (1998). Trends in alternative medicine use in the United States, 1990–1997: Results of a follow-up national survey. *Journal of the American Medical Association, 280*(18), 1569–1575.

Eisenberg, D. M., Kessler, R. C., Foster, C., Norlock, F. E., Calkins, D. R., & Delbanco, T. L. (1993). Unconventional medicine in the United States: Prevalence, costs and patterns of use. *New England Journal of Medicine, 328*, 246–252.

Evans, J. R., & Arbanel, A. (Eds.). (1999). *Introduction to quantitative EEG and neurofeedback*. San Diego, CA: Academic Press.

Flaws, B., & Lake, J. (2001). *Chinese medical psychiatry: A textbook and clinical manual*. Boulder, CO: Blue Poppy Press.

Grof, S. (1985). *Beyond the brain: Birth, death, and transcendence in psychotherapy*. Albany: State University of New York Press.

John, E. R., Prichep, L. S., Fridman, J., & Easton, P. (1988). Neurometrics: Computer assisted differential diagnosis of brain dysfunction. *Science, 293,* 162–169.

Kuriyama, S. (1999). *The expressiveness of the body and the divergence of Greek and Chinese medicine*. New York: Zone Books.

Moore, R. J., & Spiegel, D. (2000). Uses of guided imagery for pain control by African-American and white women with metastatic breast cancer. *Integrative Medicine, 2*(2), 115–126.

Moss, D. (2001). Biofeedback. In S. Shannon (Ed.), *Handbook of complementary and alternative therapies in mental health* (pp. 135–158). San Diego, CA: Academic Press.

National Institutes of Health. (1995). *Alternative medicine: Expanding medical horizons*. Washington, DC: Government Printing Office.

National Institutes of Health. (1997). Acupuncture. *NIH Consensus Statements Online, 15*(5), 1–34. Retrieved March 26, 2002, from http://odp.od.nih.gov/consensus/cons/107/107_statement.htm

Oschman, J. L. (2000). *Energy medicine: The scientific basis*. Edinburgh: Churchill Livingstone.

Riley, D., & Heger, M. (1999, March). Integrative medicine data collection network (IMDCN). Presentation to the Fourth Annual Alternative Therapies Symposium, New York.

Schnyer, R. (2001). *Acupuncture in the treatment of depression: A manual for practice and research*. Edinburgh, Scotland: Churchill Livingstone.

Shannon, S. (Ed.) (2001). *Handbook of complementary and alternative therapies in mental health*. San Diego, CA: Academic Press.

Spencer, J. W., & Jacobs, J. J. (1999). *Complementary/alternative medicine: An evidence-based approach*. St. Louis, MO: Mosby.

The state of EEG biofeedback therapy (EEG operant conditioning) in 2000 [Special issue]. (2000). *Clinical Electroencephalography, 31*(1), v–viii, 1–55.

Thatcher, R. W. (1998). Normative EEG databases and EEG biofeedback. *Journal of Neurotherapy, 2* (4), 8–39.

Thatcher, R. W. (1999). EEG database guided neurotherapy. In J. R. Evans & A. Arbanel (1999). *Introduction to quantitative EEG and neurofeedback* (pp. 29–64). San Diego, CA: Academic Press.

Walach, H. (2001). The efficacy paradox in randomized controlled trials of CAM and elsewhere: Beware of the placebo trap. *The Journal of Alternative and Complementary Medicine: Research on Paradigm, Practice, and Policy, 7*(3), 213–218.

Wilber, K. (2000). *Integral psychology: Consciousness, spirit, psychology, therapy,* Boston: Shambhala.

# CHAPTER 5

# The Placebo Effect and
# Its Use in Biofeedback Therapy

IAN WICKRAMASEKERA

**Abstract:** The placebo effect is a powerful phenomenon in primary care medicine under non-double-blind conditions and can be used with positive results in biofeedback therapy. This chapter examines the scientific evidence for the placebo effect, reviews current theories of the placebo, and presents a conditioned response model to clarify the mechanism of the placebo. This conditioned response model has previously been strongly supported by psychoneuroimmunology data and recently by positron emission tomography in Parkinson's disease patients. There is evidence that biofeedback instruments operate as conditioned stimuli and that instrumentation may be a powerful tool to elicit a placebo effect. The chapter presents strategies to optimize the placebo effect in biofeedback and in health care generally.

## DEFINING THE PLACEBO EFFECT

One definition of *placebo effect* is a therapeutic response that cannot be explained by the known properties of the applied substance or procedure or the simple passage of time. This definition implies that *neutral* or inert substances or procedures can have empirically documented therapeutic efficacy that current medical theory in medicine or the simple passage of time (spontaneous remission) cannot explain. Many inert chemical substances and surgical and psychological procedures have therapeutic efficacy for conditions ranging from the common cold to cancer, but the mechanisms of the effects are unknown. The double-blind experimental design with randomized assignment of patients to either the placebo or active therapy group was designed to keep patients and therapists "blind" as to who was getting the placebo therapy and who was getting the active therapy. It was designed to control or eliminate psychosocial factors in drug or surgical studies. But it has now been shown that unless active placebos or placebos that produce side effects similar to the active drug are used, patients can discern if they are on an active drug or a placebo (Greenberg & Fisher, 1997). Hence the psychological and social effects of therapy are not controlled or held constant in double-blind studies unless active placebos are used (Greenberg & Fisher, 1997). In fact, a recent meta-analysis of fluoxetine (Prozac) found a very high correlation ($r = .85$) between the therapeutic efficacy of Prozac and the percentage of patients reporting drug side effects (Greenberg, Bornstein, Zborowski, Fisher, & Greenberg, 1994).

## EMPIRICAL EFFICACY OF THE PLACEBO

Recently, de la Fuente-Fernandez et al. (2001) reported that a neutral or conditioned stimulus released substantial endogenous dopamine in the striatum of Parkinson's disease patients, as evidenced on position emission tomography (PET) scan. This finding is supportive of the conditioned response theory of the placebo proposed by Wickramasekera (1977a, 1980) and documented by Ader (1988) and others. Reviews of 26 double-blind studies of 1,991 patients found that the severity of clinical (postsurgical) pain experienced by 35 percent of patients was reduced by at least half of its original intensity by an inert substance or placebo drug. The mean placebo rate for experimentally induced laboratory pain, however, is considerably lower (3 percent to 16 percent; Evans, 1974). The discrepancy between the placebo rate in experimental and clinical pain strongly suggests that the psychological *meaning* of the therapy situation is a major determinant of the magnitude of the placebo effect. Experimental pain is a brief, known transient event, but clinical pain is disruptive to life, and its source may be uncertain. The meaning and life consequences of pain and symptoms matter greatly in placebo studies (Evans, 1974; Wickramasekera, 1977a, 1980; Wickramasekera & Truong, 1974).

Placebo effects are not limited to chemical treatments but may include surgical and psychological therapies. In a classic paper, "Surgery as Placebo," Beecher (1961) compared the results of enthusiastic and skeptical surgeons performing the once popular internal mammary artery ligation for angina pectoris. Two independent skeptical teams (Cobb, Thomas, Dillard, Merendino, & Bruce, 1959; Dimond, Kittle, & Crockett, 1958), using a single-blind procedure, performed a bilateral skin incision on all patients under local anesthesia, and in randomly selected patients, the internal mammary artery was ligated. Dimond et al. found that 100 percent of the nonligated and 76 percent of the ligated patients reported decreased need for nitroglycerin and increased exercise tolerance. All nonligated patients showed improvement for more than six weeks, and followed patients remained improved six to eight months later. Cobb et al. stated that six months after surgery, five ligated and five nonligated patients reported more than 40 percent subjective improvement. Two nonligated patients showed dramatic improvement in exercise tolerance, and one nonligated patient even showed improved electrocardiographic results after exercise. These studies demonstrated that ligation of the internal mammary artery was no better than a skin incision and that skin incision could generate a dramatic and sustained therapeutic placebo effect. The surgery was quietly abandoned.

The mean rate of pain reduction with a placebo drug is 33 percent, plus or minus 2 percent. But actual rates in studies vary from 10 percent to 90 percent (Turner, Deyo, Loeser, Von Korff, & Fordyce, 1994). Placebo effects are not limited to the relief of acute pain. Placebos may be useful in the therapy of coughs, angina, low blood cell counts, high blood pressure, fever, insomnia, cough reflex, headaches, asthma, multiple sclerosis, the common cold, diabetes, ulcers, warts, arthritis, emesis, sea sickness, gastric secretion and motility, pupil dilation and constriction, cancer, Parkinson's disease, and other ailments (Beecher, 1955; Bergin & Garfield, 1971; Shapiro, 1971; Spanos, Stenstrom, & Johnston, 1988). Placebo effects are not limited to chemical and surgical treatments. In fact, a review of controlled studies of systematic desensitization (Kazdin & Wilcoxon, 1976) and a pioneering major double-blind study of clinical biofeedback (Cohen, Graham, Fotopoulos, & Cook, 1977) have also found equally high mean rates of placebo response for these psychological treatments.

The first controlled study of electroencephalograph (EEG) and electromyograph (EMG) clinical biofeedback found that the placebo effect was 67 percent under nonblind conditions even in the reduction of severe chronic detoxification symptoms in opiate addicts. Under double-blind conditions, the placebo rate for EEG/EMG biofeedback with the same type of patients was reduced to 34 percent, and it was found that physiological changes in EEG and EMG were unrelated to clinical outcome. The mean placebo effect in double-blind drug studies is reported to be 33 percent, plus or minus 2 percent. Hence the mean magnitude of the placebo effect in double-blind drug and EEG/EMG biofeedback studies is almost identical (34 percent vs. 33 percent; Cohen et al., 1977; Turner et al., 1994). A recent review of nonblind drug and surgical studies encompassing 6,931 patients found that the mean placebo rate was 70 percent (Roberts, Kewman, Mercier, & Hovell, 1993). This is similar to the Cohen et al. finding of a stronger placebo rate (67 percent) obtained under nonblind conditions compared with blinded studies in biofeedback training. In actual clinical work (nonblind conditions), treatments are seldom used unless both the patient and therapist have some reason to believe they work. Roberts et al. reviewed two medical therapies (glomectomy for bronchial asthma and gastric freezing for duodenal ulcer) and three drug therapies (levamisole for herpes simplex virus, or HSV; photodynamic inactivation for HSV infection; and organic solvents for HSV). However, under nonblind conditions (which are routine in actual clinical practice) or when both the patient and the doctor believed in the treatment, the mean clinical efficacy rate was a high 70 percent. Forty percent of patients received excellent clinical results, 30 percent received good results, and 30 percent received poor clinical results. Hence under real clinical conditions or ecologically valid conditions (nonblind) when both patient and therapist expectations are high, the placebo effect leaves only 30 percent of the variance in clinical outcome to be accounted for by germs and genes. These five therapies are now abandoned by the medical profession as ineffective.

The foregoing review suggests that a therapeutic phenomenon like the placebo effect, which occurs across such a wide range of clinical treatment modalities (drugs, surgery, psychotherapies, biofeedback) and across such a wide range of physical and mental symptoms (colds to cancer to depression) to people who are physically or psychologically immobilized by symptoms or in a state of health deprivation, must be a true general ingredient in all therapeutic situations. It may be a mechanism of self-healing common to a variety of symptoms and treatments that must be better understood to be applied in specific and predictable ways.

It has been found that a placebo can *potentiate*, *attenuate*, or *negate* the active ingredients in a drug. Placebos can have powerful effects on organic illness and malignancies, and can even mimic the side effects of active drugs (Shapiro, 1971). Studies have found that dose response and time effect curves for an active drug and a placebo can be similar and that the side effects of an active drug and a placebo can be similar (Evans, 1974).

A review of the literature on the placebo effect leads to several conclusions: (1) A subset of patients shows a significant (10 percent to 90 percent) therapeutic response to neutral or placebo substances, procedures, and objects in *any* clinical study; (2) no reliable procedure exists to date to identify in advance this subset of patients; (3) the same subset may not reliably respond to placebos; (4) any neutral object or procedure offered with therapeutic intent can, under the "right" conditions, generate placebo effects; and (5) the mechanism of the effect is unknown, and all the "right" conditions are unclear.

## THEORIES OF THE PLACEBO

When both patient and therapist believe in the efficacy of a therapy, what is the mechanism of this powerful placebo effect? Evans (1974) proposed that the placebo works by reducing anxiety, Barber (1959) proposed that the placebo works by mobilizing the suggestibility of the patient, and Kirsch (1997) proposed expectancy mechanisms.

Wickramasekera (1977a, 1980), Ader (1988, 1997), and Siegel (1999) proposed a memory or conditioned response (CR) mechanism of the placebo effect. Active treatments (e.g., morphine, insulin, penicillin, accurate and valid medical information) and active diagnostic procedures are unconditioned stimuli (UCS), and the vehicles in which they are delivered (e.g., pills, capsules, syringes, biomedical instruments) are neutral or conditioned stimuli (CS). The medical treatments and diagnostic procedures that people experience during their lives constitute conditioning or learning trials during which neutral vehicles are paired with active treatments. These pairings endow the neutral vehicles with the capacity to elicit the memories of therapeutic, clinical effects as conditioned responses (Ader, 1988, 1997; Wickramasekera, 1977a, 1980). The CR model of placebo responding involves the elicitation of implicit (unconscious) and explicit (conscious) psychophysiological memories of actual prior healing experiences in childhood or adolescence and the credible expectation of future healing.

The CR model states that the placebo is a complex learned mind-body response. It predicts that placebo learning, for example, based on partial reinforcement (UCS present in 50 percent of trials), will produce greater resistance to extinction than placebo learning acquired on a schedule of continuous reinforcement (UCS present in 100 percent of trials). Is there any data to support the CR model of placebo learning and more specifically the partial versus continuous reinforcement prediction of resistance to extinction of placebo learning or faith? Ader and Cohen (1982) paired saccharin (CS) and cyclophosphamide (UCS) on a 100 percent and 50 percent reinforcement schedule and showed that saccharin could delay the onset of proteinuria and death in New Zealand mice genetically prone to lupus. Several other controlled animal studies (Ader, 1997; Hernstein, 1962) and carefully controlled human studies that tested the expectancy versus the conditioning models of the placebo effect have favored the conditioning or memory model (Voudouris, Peck, & Coleman, 1989, 1990). In fact, a clinical case study (Olness & Ader, 1992) of a child with lupus showed that pairing a CS (rose perfume and cod liver oil) with a UCS (cytoxan) during chemotherapy sessions provided a clinically successful outcome with 50 percent less drug. Hence there is considerable animal and some human data to support the conditioned response model of the placebo effect (Wickramasekera, 1977a, 1980).

## PERSONALITY FACTORS THAT AMPLIFY CONDITIONED RESPONSES

The Pavlovian (Das, 1958a, 1958b) and operant conditioning data (King & McDonald, 1976; Webb, 1962; Wickramasekera, 1970a, 1976, 1988) reveal individual differences in trait hypnotic ability related to the acquisition of conditioned responses. Hypnotic ability represents the individual's readiness to respond to hypnotic induction or suggestive intervention (see Chapters 2 and 11 for further discussion of hypnotic ability). Trait hypnotic ability (Barber, 1969; Hilgard, 1965) appears to be an important determinant of the rate of acquisition ($r = .5$) and extinction ($r = .4$) of Pavlovian eyelid conditioning (Das, 1958a, 1958b). High trait negative affectivity (or anxiety) has also been shown to amplify the acquisition of conditioned responses; hence it may also amplify placebo responding, and empirical data already support this prediction (Siegel, 2000).

This analysis points out that intrinsic to all unconditioned stimuli or reliably effective interventions or events (physiochemical, behavioral/psychological, or surgical) is the potential for Pavlovian conditioning (Wickramasekera, 1977a, 1980) and therefore placebo learning, and that trait hypnotic ability and high negative affect will facilitate placebo learning. In fact, it has been found (Challis & Stam, 1992; Wickramasekera & Saxon, 1988) that anticipatory nausea and vomiting (ANV) during chemotherapy is positively correlated with high absorption, which is a correlate of hypnotic ability. ANV is also known to be amplified by high state anxiety (Challis & Stam, 1992) and high neuroticism (Wickramasekera & Saxon, 1988).

This analysis suggests that any reliable mechanisms of pathophysiology that have clearly and sharply defined onsets and offsets can operate as unconditioned responses (UCRs). To cite the previous example, nausea and vomiting can serve as UCRs. Chemicals and procedures that reliably and clearly turn on or off such pathophysiology can operate as (UCS). Hence mechanisms of both disease and healing may be responsive to conditioning effects. The UCR is a function not only of the UCS but also of any associated CS. Counterintuitively, the CR model predicts that therapists who use active ingredients (UCS) will get stronger placebo effects than those who use neutral ingredients (CS). The CR model also paradoxically predicts that progress in isolating active ingredients will inevitably lead to more and stronger placebo effects.

It is also known that conditioning can occur rapidly or with a single trial and in association especially with flavors and chemicals (Siegel, 2000; Siegel, Baptista, Kim, McDonald, & Weise-Kelly, 2000). It is known that conditioning can generalize to similar stimuli, and it is well established that once conditioned responses are acquired, they can be retained over many years. Studies have shown that multiple chemical sensitivity (headaches, nausea, pain in limbs) to odiferous stimuli can be explained in terms of conditioning (Siegel, 1999). Recently, it has been shown that the behavioral and physiological effects of caffeine, nicotine, and alcohol can also be explained in terms of conditioning. For example, caffeine and decaffeinated (placebo) coffee altered standardized tests of daytime sleepiness and auditory vigilance (Siegel, 2000; Siegel et al., 2000). Siegel et al. report that both nonalcoholic beer and a frosted mug of beer that could be handled and smelled but not drunk increased heart rate, verbally reported intoxication, plasma testosterone, and luteinizing hormone. Tolerance and withdrawal symptoms from cocaine and morphine have been explained by conditioning (Siegel, 2000; Siegel et al., 2000). Also cardiac responses to nitroglycerin and placebo nitroglycerin have been shown in dogs and humans (Siegel, 2000).

## ORIGINS OF THE CONDITIONED RESPONSE MODEL

Early in the 1970s, in the course of EMG biofeedback headache work (Wickramasekera, 1972, 1973a; Wickramasekera & Truong, 1974), I made some puzzling observations. Some patients reported relief of headache pain with startling rapidity. Often this occurred after no more than one or two sessions of EMG biofeedback therapy and several sessions *before* they demonstrated any measurable ability to reduce EMG levels of their head and neck. Changes in the verbal report of the intensity and frequency of headache pain should correlate with or follow, not precede, a drop in frontal EMG levels.

I wondered if this very short latency therapeutic response was not a learned or placebo response to the impressive and highly credible biofeedback instruments in anticipation of actual healing. It is well known that a CR mediated by the central nervous system can have a shorter latency than a UCR, or, in this case, the actual reduction in muscle tension levels in the head and neck. The rapidity of this response reminded me of the well-known clinical observation that ingestion of aspirin often relieves a headache long before its pharmacological effect (UCR) can occur.

In the late 1970s and early 1980s, a series of well-controlled clinical studies and a major double-blind clinical study (Cohen, Graham, Fotopoulos, & Cook, 1977) verified my clinical observation that physiological (EMG) change was not related to the clinical efficacy of EMG biofeedback. These studies showed that neither the magnitude nor the direction of physiological change in EMG biofeedback training was strongly related to the magnitude of the reduction of clinical symptoms. The reduction of clinical symptoms was, of course, the major reason most clinicians and the public had flocked to biofeedback. Even today, however, the empirical demonstration nearly 20 years ago that the magnitude of physiological change during biofeedback is not strongly related to clinical outcome is the best-kept secret in clinical biofeedback. For example, Cohen et al., in a carefully done double-blind EEG/EMG biofeedback study, showed that the reduction of clinical symptoms during detoxification from methadone, verified by urinalysis, was unrelated to the magnitude of specific changes in an EEG/EMG biofeedback training procedure. Patients on contingent biological feedback demonstrated more control over EMG activity, but this control was unrelated to clinical outcome under double-blind conditions. Later studies by Andrasik and Holroyd (1980) and Holroyd et al. (1984) showed that the reduction of headache pain (clinical outcome) was unrelated to changes in EMG levels. A recent review of the literature of chronic pain by Arena and Blanchard (1996) also concluded that there is no strong relationship between the magnitude and direction of physiological change and chronic pain reduction. A study of EMG biofeedback for low-back pain found that contingent EMG biofeedback was not essential for a positive clinical outcome and that high trait hypnotic ability was a significant predictor of positive clinical outcome in the placebo control group (Bush, Ditto, & Feuerstein, 1985). It appears that physiological change alone accounts for only about 20 percent of the variance in clinical biofeedback.

Many of us (30 years ago in biofeedback) believed that given sufficient specific and accurate biological feedback, people would walk on water. Fortunately, my earliest interest in biofeedback was not related to the reduction of clinical symptoms. I was searching for a reliable and clinically acceptable procedure to induce the two known conditions (mental relaxation and sensory restriction) that have been shown, at least temporarily, to increase a person's trait hypnotic ability (Wickramasekera, 1970b, 1973b, 1977b).

## WHY DOES BIOFEEDBACK WORK?

I have stated that the well-established empirical efficacy of biofeedback (Hatch, Fisher, & Rugh, 1987; Wickramasekera & Kenkel, 1996a, 1996b) in clinical symptom reduction is due to at least three mechanisms that deserve more empirical study. First, EMG and EEG biofeedback temporarily increase state and probably trait hypnotic ability (Engstrom, London, & Hart, 1970; Wickramasekera, 1973b, 1977b). This increased hypnotic responsivity is theorized to be associated with the patient's greater openness to altered perceptions, moods, and memories of the factors triggering and maintaining clinical symptoms (Costa & McCrae, 1986). Second, biomedical instruments used in biofeedback can automatically elicit a therapeutic mind-body conditioned placebo response based on the memory of prior healing associated with biomedical instruments (Wickramasekera, 1977a, 1980). Third, biofeedback recruits one of the primary mechanisms underlying risk—the interaction between trait hypnotic ability (high or low) and negative affect—and positively reverses its direction of action (Wickramasekera, 1979, 1986, 1988, 1993, 1994, 1995, 1998).

### Does Biofeedback Increase Trait Hypnotic Ability and Increase Openness to Change?

Several studies have shown that biofeedback works better for low rather than high trait absorption people (Qualls & Sheehan, 1981) and that absorption is a modest correlate of trait hypnotic ability (Tellegen & Atkinson, 1974). The first mechanism through which EEG and EMG biofeedback reduce clinical symptoms is by temporarily increasing trait hypnotic ability (Engstrom, 1976; Engstrom et al., 1970; Wickramasekera, 1973b, 1976, 1977b, 1999). Biofeedback probably increases the patient's openness to alternative cognitive explanations and perceptions of clinical symptoms (Costa & McCrae, 1986). For example, insomnia or pain may now be seen as temporary reactions to some prior stress that have no current utility. Reframed in this way, insomnia and pain are viewed as habits that can be unlearned. In the face of trauma or threat, deficits in cognitive flexibility or openness can be more immobilizing than the absence of an arm or leg.

### Do Biomedical Instruments Used in Biofeedback Elicit an Automatic Conditioned Placebo Hope Response?

The second hypothesized mechanism through which biofeedback reduces clinical symptoms is by eliciting a conditioned placebo *hope response*. Biomedical instruments used in biofeedback training are hypothesized to elicit a therapeutic placebo conditioned response (CR) based on memories of prior healings that can stimulate current hope and reduce current fear of symptoms (Wickramasekera, 1977a, 1977b, 1980, 1988, 2000). The CR is based on a prior reinforcement history of healing with biomedical instruments associated with vivid memories of previous healings. Mobilizing this placebo effect of biomedical instruments can boost the credibility and efficacy of cognitive reconstructions of the causes of present clinical symptoms.

Several empirical studies show that biomedical instruments per se can have placebo effects. For example, Hashish, Feinman, and Harvey (1988) found that an ultrasound instrument was effective at reducing both pain and swelling (a local response to tissue damage) whether it was turned on or not, if *both* the patient and therapist *believed* it was emitting sound. In the above study, pain and edema were an acute response to wisdom tooth extraction. Placebo responses to medical and surgical tools are well documented (Long, Uematsu, & Kouba, 1989; Schwitzgebel & Traugott, 1968). The affective component of low-back pain reduction with transcutaneous electrical nerve stimulation (TENS) may be a placebo response (Marchand, Charest, Li, Chenard, Lavignolle, & Laurencelle, 1993). Sox, Margulies, and Hill (1981) showed that medical diagnostic tests alone were independent predictors of clinical recovery from non-specific chest pain. Hence there is empirical evidence that some part of the initial reduction in clinical symptoms in biofeedback training may be a conditioned placebo response to biomedical instruments (Wickramasekera, 1977a, 1977b, 1980, 1988, 2000).

## MAXIMIZING THE PLACEBO EFFECT

The conditioned response model of placebo responding that I propose involves the elicitation with biofeedback instruments of implicit (unconscious) and explicit (conscious) memories of actual prior healing experiences in childhood or adolescence and the credible expectation of future healing. Beliefs constructed from memories seem central to the placebo response. Theoretically, alterations in cognitions, emotions, and beliefs induced by a placebo drug that is believed to have healing properties can directly alter physiology (Ader, 1988, 1997; Siegel, 2000; Siegel et al., 2000). Beliefs may also indirectly alter physiology through behavioral mechanisms (e.g., exercise, diet). Roberts et al. (1993) found that the degree of belief or faith in the potency of a therapy can be a powerful factor in placebo efficacy. In the study ($N = 6,931$), the mean magnitude of the placebo effect was 70 percent when both the patient and doctor believed in the efficacy of the therapy.

It appears that a learning or CR model of the placebo effect is the most effective method of installing reliable response expectancies in the general population (Ader, 1997; Voudouris et al., 1989, 1990; Wickramasekera, 1977a, 1980, 1999, 2000). Because alterations in physiology and clinical symptoms induced with placebos are notoriously unreliable, it is crucial in the initial investigation of this CR model to select

subjects in whom mind-body effects occur powerfully and reliably. People high in hypnotic ability rapidly acquire conditioned responses both respondently, through the autonomic nervous system, and operantly, through the central nervous system (Barber, 1969; Hilgard, 1965), and they overlearn or automate conditioned responses more quickly than do people of low to moderate hypnotic ability (Das, 1958a, 1958b; King & McDonald, 1976; Webb, 1962; Wickramasekera, 1970a, 1976, 1980, 1988, 2000). The CR model of the placebo predicts that people of high hypnotic ability trained on a partial reinforcement schedule will produce the most rapidly acting and reliable placebo responding with the greatest resistance to extinction (Wickramasekera, 1977a, 1980, 1999, 2000) — for example, when the patient is eventually switched to a strictly placebo schedule of delivery (e.g., a beta blocker is totally withdrawn).

The power of placebo or "top-down" healing is most likely to be manifested under conditions of strong anxiety or emotional arousal (Frank, 1965) in skillfully managed life-threatening clinical situations. Consider the example of the Greek drama of the surgical operating theater, where surgeons, the robed and masked high priests of the medical establishment, perform life-threatening surgical rituals (Cobb et al., 1959; Dimond et al., 1958). In the surgical placebo studies previously mentioned, the mean placebo rates were as high as 90 percent. Evans (1974) and Beecher (1961) have reported that the patients' state anxiety level is positively related to placebo efficacy.

The CR model also predicts that progress in isolating physiochemically active ingredients (such as morphine, nitroglycerin, or antibiotics) and psychologically active ingredients (such as high hypnotic ability, accurate empathy, and warmth) or unconditioned stimuli for healing will be associated with more powerful placebo effects because of the inevitable learned or conditioned response component in all active therapies (Wickramasekera, 1980, 1988, 1999, 2000).

Living organisms, human or animal, can learn and use any psychophysiologically active ingredient (e.g., nitroglycerin, insulin, morphine, warmth, accurate empathy, high hypnotic ability) or UCS for healing or disease in their environments. Microbiologists are starting to realize this, and it was recently bluntly stated by Bull and Levin (2000) that even mice are not "simply furry petri dishes." There are major differences between drug experiments done in test tubes and those done in animals that can learn and use learned interactions with drugs. Important here too is the "vulnerability" of the animal or the patient to learning. The symptomatically immobilized and dependent patient in a state of health deprivation (in an aversive state not unlike food deprivation) is an ideal candidate for conditioning and learning.

Counterintuitively, then, this conditioned response model of the placebo effect predicts that therapists who use active ingredients (UCS, such as morphine, empathy, high hypnotic ability, etc.) will get stronger placebo effects than those who use neutral or inert ingredients (CS, such as saline or professional detachment). The CR model also paradoxically predicts that biomedical progress in isolating active ingredients will inevitably lead to both more and stronger placebo effects (Wickramasekera, 1980, 1988, 1999, 2000). Put another way, the more effective the therapy, the stronger the placebo effect of anything associated with the delivery of the therapy. This paradox of healing is predicted by the CR model of the placebo (Wickramasekera, 1977a, 1980).

The practical implication of this learned or memory-based CR model of the placebo effect is that people currently on high and lifetime doses of hypertensive medications, nitroglycerin, insulin, or Ritalin may be able to control their hypertension, diabetes, angina, or attention deficit disorder with only half their current dose if trained on a partial reinforcement schedule. This reduction in medication use may enable patients to control their symptoms while avoiding the toxic side effects of active drugs. In short, the theoretical analysis (Wickramasekera, 1977a, 1980), which remains to be empirically tested in humans (Olness & Ader, 1992) with drugs and surgery, strongly suggests that the mind, through learning mechanisms (CR), can alter the body both physiochemically and behaviorally.

**REFERENCES**

Ader, R. (1988). The placebo effect as a conditioned response. In R. Ader, H. Weiner, & A. Baum (Eds.), *Experimental foundations of behavioral medicine: Conditioning approaches* (pp. 47–66). Hillsdale, NJ: Lawrence Erlbaum.

Ader, R. (1997). The role of conditioning in pharmacotherapy. In A. Harrington (Ed.), *Placebo* (pp. 138–165). Cambridge: Harvard University Press.

Ader, R., & Cohen, N. (1982). Behaviorally conditioned immunosuppression and murine systemic lupus erythematous. *Science, 215,* 1534–1536.

Andrasik, F., & Holroyd, K. A. (1980). A test of specific and nonspecific effects in the biofeedback treatment of tension headache. *Journal of Consulting and Clinical Psychology, 48,* 575–586.

Arena, J. G., & Blanchard, E. B. (1996). Biofeedback and relaxation therapy for chronic pain disorders. In R. J. Gatchel and D. C. Turk (Eds.), *Chronic pain: Psychological perspectives on treatment* (pp. 179–230). New York: Guilford.

Barber, T. X. (1959). Toward a theory of pain: Relief of chronic pain by prefrontal leucotomy, opiates, placebos, and hypnosis. *Psychological Bulletin, 56,* 430.

Barber, T. X. (1969). *Hypnosis: A scientific approach.* New York: Litton Educational Publishing.

Beecher, H. K. (1955). The powerful placebo. *Journal of the American Medical Association, 159,* 1602–1606.

Beecher, H. K. (1961). Surgery as placebo. *Journal of the American Medical Association, 176,* 1102–1107.

Bergin, A., & Garfield, S. (Eds.). (1971). *Handbook of psychotherapy and behavior change.* New York: Wiley.

Bull, J., & Levin, B. (2000). Mice are not furry petri dishes. *Science, 287,* 1409–1410.

Bush, C., Ditto, B., & Feuerstein, M. (1985). A controlled evaluation of paraspinal EMG biofeedback in the treatment of chronic low back pain. *Health Psychology, 4*(4), 307–321.

Challis, G. B., & Stam, H. J. (1992). A longitudinal study of the development of anticipatory nausea and vomiting in cancer chemotherapy patients: The role of absorption and autonomic perception. *Health Psychology, 11*(3), 181–189.

Cobb, I. A., Thomas, G. I., Dillard, D. H., Merendino, R. A., & Bruce, R. A. (1959). An evaluation of internal-mammary-artery ligation by a double blind technique. *New England Journal of Medicine, 260,* 1115–1118.

Cohen, H. D., Graham, C., Fotopoulos, S. S., & Cook, M. R. (1977). A double-blind methodology for biofeedback research. *Psychophysiology, 14*(6), 603–608.

Costa, P. T., Jr., & McCrae, R. R. (1986). Personality stability and its implications for clinical psychology. *Clinical Psychology Review, 6,* 407–423.

Das, J. P. (1958a). Conditioning and hypnosis. *Journal of Experimental Psychology, 56,* 110–113.

Das, J. P. (1958b). The Pavlovian theory of hypnosis: An evaluation. *Journal of Mental Sciences, 104,* 82–90.

de la Fuente-Fernandez, R., Ruth, T. J., Sossi, V., Schulzer, M., Calne, D. B., & Stoessl, A. J. (2001). Expectation and dopamine release: Mechanism of the placebo effect in Parkinson's disease. *Science, 293,* 1164–1166.

Dimond, E. G., Kittle, C. F., & Crockett, J. E. (1958). Evaluation of internal mammary artery ligation and sham procedure in angina pectoris. *Circulation, 18,* 712–713.

Engstrom, D. R. (1976). Hypnotic susceptibility, EEG-alpha, and self-regulation. In G. E. Schwartz & D. Shapiro (Eds.), *Consciousness and self-regulation: Advances in research* (vol. 1, pp. 173–222). New York: Plenum.

Engstrom, D. R., London, P., & Hart, J. T. (1970). Hypnotic susceptibility increased by EEG alpha training. *Nature, 227,* 1261–1262.

Evans, F. J. (1974). The power of a sugar pill. *Psychology Today, 7*(4), 32.

Frank, J. D. (1965). *Persuasion and healing.* Baltimore, MD: Johns Hopkins University Press.

Greenberg, R. P., Bornstein, R. F., Zborowski, M. J., Fisher, S., & Greenberg, M. D. (1994). A meta-analysis of fluoxetine outcome in the treatment of depression. *Journal of Nervous and Mental Disease, 182,* 547–551.

Greenberg, R. P., & Fisher, S. (1997). Mood-mending medicines: Probing drug, psychotherapy, and placebo solutions. In S. Fisher & R. P. Greenberg (Eds.), *From placebo to panacea: Putting psychiatric drugs to the test* (pp. 115–172). New York: Wiley.

Hashish, L., Feinman, C., & Harvey, W. (1988). Reduction of postoperative pain and swelling by ultrasound: A placebo effect. *Pain, 83,* 303–311.

Hatch, J. P., Fisher, J. G., & Rugh, J. D. (1987). *Biofeedback studies in clinical efficacy.* New York: Plenum.

Hernstein, R. J. (1962). Placebo effect in the rat. *Science, 138,* 677–678.

Hilgard, E. R. (1965). *Hypnotic susceptibility.* New York: Harcourt, Brace and World.

Holroyd, K. A., Penzien, D. B., Hursey, K. G., Tobin, L. R., Holm, J. E., Marcille, P. J., Hall, J. R., & Chila, A. G. (1984). Change mechanisms in EMG biofeedback training: Cognitive changes underlying improvements in tension headache. *Journal of Consulting and Clinical Psychology, 52,* 1039–1053.

Kazdin, A. E., & Wilcoxon, L. A. (1976). Systematic desensitization and nonspecific treatment effects: A methodological evaluation. *Psychological Bulletin, 83*(5), 729–758.

King, D. R., & McDonald, R. D. (1976). Hypnotic susceptibility and verbal conditioning. *International Journal of Clinical and Experimental Hypnosis, 24,* 29–37.

Kirsch, I. (1997). Specifying nonspecifics: Psychological mechanisms. In A. Harrington (Ed.), *The placebo effect* (pp. 166–186). Cambridge, MA: Harvard University Press.

Long, D. W., Uematsu, S., & Kouba, R. B. (1989). Placebo responses to medical device therapy for pain. *Stereotactic and Functional Neurosurgery, 53,* 149–156.

Marchand, S., Charest, J., Li, J., Chenard, J. R., Lavignolle, G., & Laurencelle, L. (1993). Is TENS purely a placebo effect? A controlled study on chronic low back pain. *Pain, 54,* 99–106.

Olness, K., & Ader, R. (1992). Conditioning as an adjunct in the pharmacotherapy of lupus erythematosus. *Developmental and Behavioral Pediatrics, 13*(2), 124–125.

Qualls, P. J., & Sheehan, P. W. (1981). Electromyograph biofeedback as a relaxation technique. A critical appraisal and reassessment. *Psychological Bulletin, 90*(1), 21–42.

Roberts, A. H., Kewman, D. G., Mercier, L., & Hovell, M. (1993). The power of nonspecific effects in healing: Implications for psychosocial and biological treatments. *Clinical Psychology Review, 13,* 375–391.

Schwitzgebel, R., & Traugott, M. (1968). Initial note on the placebo effect of machines. *Behavioral Science, 13,* 267–273.

Shapiro, A. (1971). Placebo effects in medicine, psychotherapy and psychoanalysis. In A. Bergin & S. Garfield (Eds.), *Handbook of psychotherapy and behavior change* (pp. 439–474). New York: Wiley.

Siegel, S. (1999). Multiple chemical sensitivity as a conditional response. *Toxicology and Industrial Health, 15,* 323–330.

Siegel, S. (2000). Explanatory mechanisms of the placebo effect: Pavlovian conditioning. Paper presented at *The science of the placebo: Toward an interdisciplinary research agenda.* Symposium conducted at a meeting of the National Institutes of Health, Washington, DC.

Siegel, S., Baptista, M. A., Kim, J. A., McDonald, R. V., & Weise-Kelly, L. (2000). Pavlovian psychopharmacology: The associative basis of tolerance. *Experimental and Clinical Psychopharmacology, 8*(3), 276–293.

Sox, H. C., Jr., Margulies, I., & Hill, C. (1981). Psychologically mediated effects of diagnostic tests. *Annals of Internal Medicine, 95,* 680–685.

Spanos, N. P., Stenstrom, R. J., & Johnston, J. C. (1988). Hypnosis, placebo, and suggestion in the treatment of warts. *Psychosomatic Medicine, 50,* 245–260.

Tellegen, A., & Atkinson, G. (1974). Openness to absorbing and self-altering experiences ("absorption"), a trait related to hypnotic susceptibility. *Journal of Abnormal Psychology, 83,* 268–277.

Turner, J. A., Deyo, R. A., Loeser, J. D., Von Korff, M., & Fordyce, W. E. (1994). The importance of placebo effects in pain treatment and research. *Journal of the American Medical Association, 271*(20), 1609–1614.

Voudouris, N. J., Peck, C. L., & Coleman, G. (1989). Conditioned response models of placebo phenomena: Further support. *Pain, 38,* 109–116.

Voudouris, N. J., Peck, C. L., & Coleman, G. (1990). The role of conditioning and verbal expectancy in the placebo response. *Pain, 43,* 121–128.

Webb, R. A. (1962). Suggestibility and verbal conditioning. *International Journal of Clinical and Experimental Hypnosis, 10,* 275–279.

Wickramasekera, I. (1970a, August). *The effects of hypnosis and a control procedure on verbal conditioning.* Paper presented at the annual meeting of the American Psychological Association, Miami, FL.

Wickramasekera, I. (1970b). Effects of sensory restriction on susceptibility to hypnosis. *Journal of Abnormal Psychology, 76,* 69–75.

Wickramasekera, I. (1972). Electromyographic feedback training and tension headache: Preliminary observations. *The American Journal of Clinical Hypnosis, 15*(2), 83–84.

Wickramasekera, I. (1973a). The application of verbal instructions and EMG feedback training to the management of tension headache preliminary observations. *Headache, 13*(2), 73–76.

Wickramasekera, I. (1973b). Effects of electromyographic feedback on hypnotic susceptibility: More preliminary data. *Journal of Abnormal Psychology, 82*(1), 74–77.

Wickramasekera, I. (1976). *Biofeedback, behavior therapy and hypnosis: Potentiating the verbal control of behavior for clinicians.* Chicago: Nelson-Hall.

Wickramasekera, I. (1977a). The placebo effect and medical instruments in biofeedback. *Journal of Clinical Engineering, 2*(3), 227–230.

Wickramasekera, I. (1977b). On attempts to modify hypnotic susceptibility: Some psychophysiological procedures and promising directions. *Annals of the New York Academy of Sciences, 296,* 143–153.

Wickramasekera, I. (1979). A model of the patient at high risk for chronic stress related disorders: Do beliefs have biological consequences? In *Proceedings of the annual convention of the Biofeedback Society of America,* San Diego, CA.

Wickramasekera, I. (1980). A conditioned response model of the placebo effect predictions from the model. *Biofeedback & Self-Regulation, 5*(1), 5–18.

Wickramasekera, I. (1986). A model of people at high risk to develop chronic stress-related somatic symptoms: Some predictions. *Professional Psychology: Research and Practice, 17*(5), 437–447.

Wickramasekera, I. (1988*). Clinical behavioral medicine: Some concepts and procedures.* New York: Plenum.

Wickramasekera, I. (1993). Assessment and treatment of somatization disorders: The high risk model of threat perception. In J. W. Rhue, S. J. Lynn, & I. Kirsch (Eds.), *Handbook of clinical hypnosis* (pp. 587–621). Washington, DC: American Psychological Association.

Wickramasekera, I. (1994). On the interaction of two orthogonal risk factors, 1) hypnotic ability and 2) negative affectivity (threat perception) for psychophysiological dysregulation in somatization. In V. De Pascalis (Chair), *II. Symposium on suggestion and suggestibility,* University of Rome, Italy.

Wickramasekera, I. (1995). Somatization: Concepts, data and prediction from the high risk model of threat perception. *The Journal of Nervous and Mental Disease, 183*(1), 15–23.

Wickramasekera, I. (1998). Secrets kept from the mind but not the body or behavior: The unsolved problems of identifying and treating somatization and psychophysiological disease. *Advances: The Journal of Mind-Body Medicine, 14*, 81–132.

Wickramasekera, I. (1999). How does biofeedback reduce clinical symptoms and do memories and beliefs have biological consequences? Toward a model of mind-body healing. *Applied Psychophysiology and Biofeedback, 24*(2), 91–105.

Wickramasekera, I. (2000). How to produce not only powerful but, more importantly, reliable placebo healing and analgesia. *Advances in Mind-Body Medicine, 16*, 211–216.

Wickramasekera, I., & Kenkel, M. B. (1996a). Special section: Somatization, applied psychophysiology, and effective mind-body therapies. *Professional Psychology: Research and Practice, 27*(3), 217.

Wickramasekera, I., & Kenkel, M. B. (1996b). Special section: Somatization, primary care, and applied psychophysiology II. *Professional Psychology: Research and Practice, 27*(6), 537.

Wickramasekera, I., & Saxon, J. (1988, March). *Absorption, neuroticism, and anticipatory nausea and vomiting in chemotherapy*. Paper presented at the 19th annual meeting of the Biofeedback Society of America, Colorado Springs, CO.

Wickramasekera, I., & Truong, X. T. (1974). Biofeedback. *Archives of Physical Medicine and Rehabilitation, 55*, 483–484.

# CHAPTER 6

# A Comprehensive Approach to Primary Care Medicine: Mind and Body in the Clinic

TERENCE C. DAVIES

**Abstract:** The philosophy of Cartesian dualism has resulted in a separation of mind from body in the diagnosis and treatment of disease states, and this intellectual attitude has crippled the progress of holistic medical treatment for the past three and a half centuries. It has led to a reductionistic, mechanistic view of biological function that has only recently been challenged by the advent of system theory. Engel's biopsychosocial model provides a more appropriate paradigm for the symptom presentations encountered in primary care practice. Primary care practitioners spend an estimated 75 percent of their time and effort dealing with somatization and mental health diagnoses for which they currently have no clearly defined management methods. Globally, the majority of mental health care occurs in the primary health care sector. Every effective resource that can be used to improve the management of this massive burden of disease worldwide must be identified, mobilized, and integrated into the primary health care delivery systems. Inevitably, this has to include complementary and alternative (CAM) health care providers whose methods are so clearly associated with mind-body interaction and who are known to have a high level of public recognition and support. Ultimately, this process has to be conducted with the same degree of intellectual rigor and outcome analysis that has characterized the course of 20th-century, "scientific" medicine. The goal can be nothing less than to define and establish a new, integrated mind-body, health and disease management, whole-person paradigm. Primary health care practitioners and mental health clinicians of all disciplined backgrounds need to unify in pursuing this task.

## THE DEATH OF CARTESIAN MIND-BODY DUALISM?

In a book titled *Descartes' Error*, the neurologist Antonio Damasio (1994) made a compelling case for emotion and feelings as being preeminent in influencing humankind's thinking and behavior. He stated his argument as follows:

Long before the dawn of humanity, beings were beings. At some point in evolution, an elementary consciousness began. With that elementary consciousness came a simple mind; with greater complexity of mind came the possibility of thinking and, even later, of using language to communicate and organize thinking better. For us then, in the beginning it was being, and only later was it thinking. And for us now, as we come into the world and develop, we still begin with being, and only later do we think. We are, and then we think, and we think only inasmuch as we are, since thinking is indeed caused by the structures and operations of being. (p. 248)

The concept of a "point in evolution [when] an elementary consciousness began" was explored some time previously in a widely discussed book by the Princeton psychologist Julian Jaynes (1976). In their theories of the emergence of the human mind, both Damasio and Jaynes illustrated the principle of ontogeny recapitulating phylogeny (the history of the individual's development reflecting the evolutionary history of the race). As the newborn child first feels and reacts emotionally to its environment and later becomes self-aware and develops cognition, so we can imagine early man and his successors following a similar sequence of mental development over the course of eons.

Damasio (1994) directly challenged the long-standing influence of Cartesian mind-body dualism. His ideas are stated at the beginning of this chapter because if medicine is ever to recover from the profound impact of Descartes' mind-body separation philosophy, a radical reorientation of approach is necessary. Damasio regarded the brain and the rest of the body as an indissoluble organism that is integrated via mutually interactive biochemical and neural regulatory circuits (including endocrine, immune, and autonomic neural components). As such, the organism interacts with the environment as an ensemble, and the physiological operations that we call mind are derived from the structural and functional ensemble rather than from the brain alone. Accordingly, mental phenomena can be fully understood only in the context of the organism's interactions within an environment (pp. xvi–xvii). This description is exactly consistent with the principles and practice of applied psychophysiology and represents a core component of the philosophy that has directed

development within the primary care field of family medicine. Recognition of this commonality leads to a commitment to do everything possible to "marry" these two areas of clinical practice—applied psychophysiology and primary care (Moss & Davies, 1999).

## PRIMARY CARE MEDICINE AND FAMILY MEDICINE

As discussed in the foreword to this volume, primary care as an academic discipline is a relatively recent phenomenon. Before the 1960s, physicians who chose general practice had no standardized pathway of graduate training. The most common process was to perform one year of rotating in-hospital internship following graduation from medical school and then either link up with one or more established general practitioners or go it alone and simply open up an office in the community. Subsequently, most GPs "learned on the job"—under ideal circumstances, as partners or apprentices to more experienced colleagues, but in most instances, as neophyte physician empiricists. Clearly, this training process led to wide variations in levels of knowledge and skill. The best practitioners became legends within the communities that benefited from their dedicated attention, and the worst achieved a notoriety within the medical profession as a whole that led to general practice being regarded as inferior. Consequently, when family medicine was created in 1968 as the 20th medical specialty, there was a deep commitment on the part of the physician founding fathers to demonstrate intellectual rigor, high clinical standards, and educational excellence. One illustration of this idealistic philosophy was the decision to require all board-certified family physicians to be recertified by examination every seven years—an unprecedented standard within the entire field of medicine (and one that is emulated even now by few other disciplines).

Family medicine also elected to rededicate itself to "the whole person" and specifically emphasized the need for behavioral medicine training and skills. One guideline of the American Academy of Family Practice (1995) stipulates the following:

> Knowledge and skills in this area should be acquired through a program in which behavioral science and psychiatry are integrated with all disciplines throughout the resident's total educational experience. Training should be accomplished primarily in an outpatient setting through a combination of longitudinal experiences and didactic sessions. Intensive short-term experiences in the facilities devoted to the care of chronically ill patients should be limited. Instruction must be provided by faculty who have the training and experience necessary to apply modern behavioral and psychiatric principles to the care of the undifferentiated patient. Family physicians, psychiatrists, and behavioral scientists should be involved in teaching this curricular component. (p. 1,599)

As a consequence, academic family medicine has had some three decades of experience in attempting to integrate behavioral medicine practice and teaching into its primary care outpatient clinical programs. To date, its success in this endeavor has been debatable, but its belief in and commitment to the goal of a truly holistic mind-body clinical practice remains unshakable. Perhaps it is not overly simplistic to characterize family medicine as a primary care discipline in search of a method that will enable it to be fully effective at the mind-body interface. The magnitude of the mental health problem in primary care practice would certainly justify such a prioritized goal.

## EXACTITUDE VERSUS AMBIGUITY IN PRIMARY CARE PRACTICE

Currently, evidence-based medicine and outcomes research have become lodestars for primary care practitioners and researchers. To a significant degree, this reflects the influence of managed care programs and health care administrative policies regarding cost-containment , but it also represents a continuation of the commitment made by family medicine to legitimize the intellectual integrity of primary care as a discipline. Major new publications, such as *Clinical Evidence*, sponsored by the United Health Foundation in Minnesota and published by the British Medical Journal Publishing Group, are promoting an international effort to disseminate the best available evidence for effective health care. This represents a quantum leap for the credibility of the primary care knowledge base, but it simultaneously ignores some of the compelling realities of primary care practice.

For example, some studies have shown that as much as 90 percent of the most common symptoms encountered in the primary care setting end up being unexplained in terms of a physical diagnosis. The list of such complaints includes chest and back pain, headache, dizziness, insomnia, abdominal pain, and sensory disturbances (Kroenke & Mangelsdorff, 1989). Many of these etiologically obscure presentations are examples of somatization, which has been described by Barsky and Borus (1995) as "the propensity to experience and report somatic symptoms that have no pathophysiological explanation, to misattribute them to disease, and to seek medical attention for them" (p. 1,931). The data relating to such somatizing patients are profoundly significant for primary care practitioners. Overall, they constitute between 25 percent and 75 percent of primary care patient visits and generate health care costs that are 14 times higher than those of other patients. Unless some kind of effective intervention strategy is implemented, 82 percent of these patients may stop working because of their perceived health problems (McCahill, 1995). There is evidence that specially designed behavioral modification programs such as the Personal Health Improvement Program developed by Harvard Pilgrim Health Care can have a high degree of success with patients who demonstrate chronic somatizing behavior (Johnson, Staubach, & Millar, 1997), but it takes a considerable degree of organization and interdisciplinary collaboration to implement such a program. It would certainly not be feasible for the majority of primary care practices to introduce such programs under the currently prevailing circumstances.

## PRIMARY CARE AND PSYCHIATRY

The psychiatrist George Engel introduced a new paradigm for medical practice in 1977 when he described the biopsychosocial model. This concept was eagerly embraced by family medicine but failed to make a significant impact on the field of psychiatry itself. Engel later commented that "as long as physicians are imbued with the reductionism and dualism of Western science, there is no way in which the conflict between psychiatry and the rest of medicine can be resolved" (Engel, 1979, p. 78). Ironically, it could be argued that in the intervening time, psychiatry, as a discipline, has become even more reductionistic in its orientation. The advent of sophisticated new diagnostic technology has been accompanied by major innovations in the area of psychopharmacy. Thus, psychiatry has moved increasingly into line with the majority of other fields of medicine, which is to say that it has become specialized to the point of assuming the character of a tertiary care discipline.

Partly as a consequence of what has been described, primary care physicians end up treating around 50 percent of the 13 most commonly defined mental disorders compared with 20 percent cared for by psychiatrists (Regier, Narrow, Rae, Manderscheidt, Locke, & Goodwin, 1993). As Mack Lipkin

(1999) pointed out, "primary care is the foundation of the mental health system in the United States, as it accounts for the most patients seen, drugs prescribed, hospital admissions, and cases of mental disorder treated" (p. 7). Lipkin went on to observe that tensions between primary care physicians and psychiatrists are real and often result in counterproductive consequences. Matters are not helped by the fact that "multiple data sets suggest that primary care physicians miss about 33 percent of cases of major depression, over half of substance abuse, and at first pass, 90 percent of panic disorder" (p. 10). This is not surprising in view of the wide variations in quality and quantity of mental health instruction provided to primary care physicians in training. Whereas family practice residency programs are expected to dedicate approximately 15 percent of the curriculum to mental health topics, the average internal medicine residency program devotes less than two hours per year to behavioral health training (Lipkin, 1996). In addition to the potential inadequacies in behavioral medicine educational background, primary care physicians have to cope with the stress of high-volume practices and 15-minute appointments, neither of which is conducive to the time and effort needed to explore the complexities that accompany a usually covert diagnosis of mental health dysfunction.

If the number of somatizing patients is combined with the number of patients who have definable mental maladies, it becomes clear that the primary care physician requires a high level of behavioral medicine knowledge and expertise to function effectively. The reason that Engel's biopsychosocial paradigm had such appeal to primary care family physicians is that it provided them with a contextual frame of reference that at least led to an understanding of the source of the patient's complaints. As Engel himself described the paradigm, "it provides a conceptual framework which enables the physician to act rationally in areas now excluded from a rational approach" (Engel, 1981, p. 121). Thus, family physicians were often able to make a behavioral diagnosis in definitive terms rather than via a process of exclusion. Unfortunately, having arrived at a diagnostic understanding, they still—most of the time—lacked effective management strategies, including ready access to and collaboration with a mental health professional. A survey conducted by the Center for Studying Health System Change and published in 1996 revealed that about 70 percent of primary care physicians report that they have difficulty finding high-quality inpatient and outpatient mental health services for their patients (*Primary Care Docs Report Poor Access,* 1997).

## PRIMARY CARE IN EVOLUTION

As previously discussed, primary care has finally achieved a hard-won level of academic respectability—and even grudging acceptance by the rest of the medical establishment. However, it may now be at a critical juncture in terms of its future role and identity. Its designation as the "gatekeeper" for managed care organizations, its current love affair with the evidence-based approach to clinical practice, and its failure to fully recognize and meet the challenge of behavioral medicine are all troublesome issues that have the potential to distort its original commitment to whole-person medical care. This is not to deny the ongoing need for rigor and scholarship in the further development of primary care disciplines; it is rather an expression of concern that the system-oriented openness and spirit of innovation that characterized the early years of family medicine (for example) may be in the process of being replaced by the more conventional values and mind-set of so-called mainstream medicine.

There are alternative directions to choose, and they do not need to be exclusionary of the best that is happening currently. A study published in the *Journal of the American Medical Association* revealed that the public made more visits to alternative medical practitioners and spent more money for that care than they did to allopathic primary care clinicians (Eisenberg et al., 1998). Subsequently, a great deal of attention and a significant level of federal funding has been directed at CAM. It happens that biofeedback (and by implication the related field of applied psychophysiology) is included in the listing of methodologies and practices designated as CAM. For the past decade, Eastern Virginia Medical School has been teaching and applying biofeedback to primary care problems. Its effectiveness in a variety of common conditions is clearly established, and its potential for benefit in primary care practice is enormous. The same may very well be true for acupuncture and other CAM modalities. I believe that it is incumbent on the field of primary care to explore the potential of such CAM approaches. More than that, the public's future acceptance and level of satisfaction with primary care health services may depend, significantly, on these efforts being fruitful.

These are not original ideas of course. Some visionary pioneers have been leading the way for some time. Larry Dossey is among the most notable. In his 1982 book *Space, Time and Medicine,* Dossey gave a grippingly imaginative (but scientifically referenced) account of a man who self-regulates the management of a heart attack. Primary care practitioners would perform a major public health and community service if they would lobby for physiological self-regulation techniques to begin to be introduced at a preschool level and then taught at increasing levels of sophistication throughout the educational continuum. This has the potential to become the most effective strategy for preventive public health ever introduced into society and might ultimately merit recognition on a level with vaccination against specific diseases. There are nascent programs of collaboration between primary care and mental health within school systems that could provide the birthing ground for this truly evolutionary concept (Kubiszyn, 1999).

Melvyn Werbach (1986) used the term *third line medicine* to refer to the integration of CAM practices with conventional primary care. Most recently, Victor Sierpina (2001) published a volume titled *Integrative Health Care* that has the same goal of elaborating on the practice of primary care medicine with alternative methods. All these and similar efforts are leading us toward the same desired goal—namely, to address the health care needs of all patients who seek our services with any and every diagnostic or therapeutic resource that can be shown to be effective. To achieve this ambition, we cannot be restrained by the biases of entrenched medical dogmas. On the other hand, we must rigorously guard against the inherent human tendency toward uncritical acceptance of miraculous benefit. The witch doctor and the priest are powerful figures within the history of our healing tradition, and we are foolish to believe that we have nothing to learn from their examples. We would be equally foolish to succumb to the superstition and lack of critical appraisal that tolerated their excesses and failures.

## VISIONS FOR THE
## FUTURE OF PRIMARY CARE

Frank deGruy (1997), a leading U.S. (and family practice) proponent for the incorporation of mental health care into the primary care setting, has argued that the primary care arena is well suited to the provision of most mental health services and that the structure and operation of primary care can be modified to augment the provision of these services. He described a variety of efforts currently under way in the United States to reform the health care system along these lines. At a global level, the World Health Organization has initiated a strategy to base mental health services in a number of different countries within the primary care health delivery structure (Goldberg, Mubbashar, & Mubbasher, 2000). The volume of literature describing this trend worldwide continues to grow at an exponential rate, and it is now more a question of when this will happen in any given country rather than whether or not it is the right strategic health care policy (virtually all authorities having answered that latter question in the affirmative). What remains to be clearly defined is how such a system should be constituted, which health care professionals should be incorporated, and what role mainstream psychiatry should play in the future functioning of this evolving scenario.

Family physicians have made it clear that they regard behavioral medicine as an integral and indissoluble aspect of their primary care clinical role. Psychiatrists have experimented with their involvement in primary care, mainly via the consultation-liaison model of interaction and influence, but for the most part without impressive benefit (Bower & Sibbald, 2000). We must hope that it is not too late for meaningful and constructive dialogue and collaboration to occur between the two medical fields (Schuyler & Davis, 1999). Unless this happens soon, the increasing collaboration between primary care physicians and other nonpsychiatric mental health clinicians can be expected to dominate further developments.

For family practice (and, one would hope, for the entire field of primary care practice), the challenge in developing holistic health care is greater than that encompassed by the prevailing parameters of conventional therapeutic practices (and even the currently recognized varieties of unconventional practices). The person-oriented gurus of our time, ranging from Andrew Weil (1995) to talk-show hostess Oprah Winfrey, have demonstrated by their popularity and success that people are searching for self-enhancing and self-efficacious ways to take better control of their lives and states of well-being. This represents a direction and an opportunity that primary care practitioners would be foolish to neglect. Many of our patients are seeking to be as self-efficacious in the care of their health and symptomatic disease conditions as they possibly can.

Perhaps what is needed first is a new and refined definition of the purpose of medical practice. Some years ago, Eric Cassell (1982) shocked the medical community by asserting in a *New England Journal of Medicine* article that the relief of suffering was no longer the primary goal of medicine. His argument was so well constructed and persuasive that he was able to expand it into a successful book (Cassell, 1991). His perspective was dramatic and confrontational because it reflected a refutation of one of the most respected ancient aphorisms of medicine's purpose, namely "to cure sometimes but to offer relief always."

For the past half-century, medicine has been obsessed with the concept of cure. It has pursued this goal with a compulsion that can only be compared to the style of the knights of the Holy Grail. Anything less than cure has been regarded either as failure or as something to be "passed over" with as little time and attention as possible being spent in the process. This is admittedly stating the matter in the most extreme terms, but it is a fair representation of reality. Perhaps with the advent of AIDS, and the re-recognition of the importance of supportive care for the massive volume of patients who clearly cannot be cured, things have begun to gradually change. The emerging field of geriatrics and the concept of functional improvement (rather than curative) goals for chronic illness have also had an influence on refining the drive of medicine to be totally successful in its therapeutic endeavors. But all this leads us to the ultimate and predominant priority—the opinion and behavior of the patient.

Kaplan (1990) presented an eloquent argument for regarding behavior as the central outcome in health care. He stated his case as follows: "There are only two health outcomes that are of importance. First, there is life expectancy. Second, there is the function or quality of life during the years that people are alive. Biological and physical events are mediators of these behavioral outcomes" (p. 1,218). He reminded us that W. T. Kelvin was the proponent of a mind-set that made measurement a prerequisite to science. But Feinstein (1967) challenged Kelvin's doctrine, referring to it as the "curse of Kelvin" and drawing attention to the fact that "because there is a measure for some variable does not always mean that the measure is useful" (p. 61). For example, a high erythrocyte sedimentation rate in a patient diagnosed with rheumatoid arthritis has little significance if the patient is pain free and fully functional. On the other hand, a sedimentation rate of zero is not unusual in patients suffering from the profoundly behaviorally affecting condition of chronic fatigue syndrome. But if, as Kaplan asserted, the only important indicators of health and wellness are behavioral, then we have to find methods to track and validate behavioral outcomes. This is one of the major challenges facing primary care medical practice in the future, and it is relevant to take note of the fact that the field of nursing has addressed this item as a research priority for at least the past two decades (thus, the lesson: explore the nursing research literature).

## THE SHAPE OF THINGS TO COME: FUNCTIONAL INTEGRATION OF PRIMARY CARE AND MIND-BODY MEDICINE

Universal health care coverage of some kind in the United States is almost a certainty in the not-too-distant future. Primary care will be central within any such scheme, and therefore, as has been described in this chapter, integrated mental health care will become a key necessity at the primary care level. In my experience, so-called carve-out models of managed mental health care are an abomination that should be terminated. Close to 50 percent of primary care physicians report an almost total lack of interdisciplinary communication within carve-out arrangements. Moreover, the quality of care is perceived to be lower than that provided by individually selected mental health providers (Yuen, Gerdes, & Waldforgel, 1999). The only financial model that makes sense in terms of incentivizing all clinicians involved in patient health care outcomes is the shared-risk model of capitation (Goldberg, 1999). For such a model to operate effectively and efficiently, behavioral medicine practitioners have to be incorporated within the primary care clinical setting, according to Pruitt, Klapow, Epping-Jordan, and Dresselhaus (1998), who described a detailed and progressive model of how to achieve such an arrangement. Referred to as Med-Plus (medicine plus behavior), the model explained a three-step process that places heavy emphasis on the continuing mental health education of primary care physicians, as well as a collaborative clinical approach to presenting patient problems. Palsson and Davies (1999) offered a broad review of the issues and potential solutions involved in arranging a working marriage between behavioral medicine and primary care practitioners.

In the meantime, a quiet process of experimentation and often covert cooperation between primary care and CAM practice has been progressing. Eastern Virginia Medical School, for example, has been promoting biofeedback and the principles of applied psychophysiology to students and patients for at least the past 15 years (Wickramasekera, 1988; see also Chapter 32). As a family physician, I was inspired and taught by the example of Ian Wickramasekera over a decade ago. Two years ago, we gently introduced the availability of an acupuncture clinical service, which has now outgrown its "Saturday morning only" origins (and which is requiring referral of part of the volume of patients to external practitioners). With the greatest care and respect for our more traditional medical colleagues and their standards, we intend to continue to explore the ultimate limits of holistic, primary care medical practice. In the final analysis, whatever provides relief and improved quality of life for our patients is worthy of our academic attention.

## REFERENCES

American Academy of Family Physicians (AAFP). (1995). American Academy of Family Physicians recommended core educational guidelines for family practice residents: Human behavior and mental health. *American Family Physician, 51,* 1599–1603.

Barsky, A., & Borus, J. F. (1995). Somatization and medicalization in the era of managed care. *Journal of the American Medical Association, 274*(24), 1931–1934.

Bower, P., & Sibbald, B. (2000). Do consultation-liaison services change the behavior of primary care providers? A review. *General Hospital Psychiatry, 22*(2), 84–96.

Cassell, E. J. (1982). The nature of suffering and the goals of medicine. *New England Journal of Medicine, 306,* 639–645.

Cassell, E. J. (1991). *The nature of suffering and the goals of medicine.* New York: Oxford University Press.

Damasio, A. R. (1994). *Descartes' error: Emotion, reason and the human brain.* New York: Avon.

deGruy, F. V., III. (1997). Mental healthcare in the primary care setting: A paradigm problem. *Families, Systems & Health, 15*(1), 3–26.

Dossey, L. (1982). *Space, time and medicine.* Boulder, CO: Shambhala.

Eisenberg, D. M., Davis, R. B., Ettner, S., Appel, S., Wilkey, S., Van Rompay, M., et al. (1998). Trends in alternative medicine use in the United States, 1990–1997: Results of a follow-up national survey. *Journal of the American Medical Association, 280,* 1569–1575.

Engel, G. L. (1977). The need for a new medical model: A challenge for biomedicine. *Science, 196,* 129–136.

Engel, G. L. (1979). Resolving the conflict between medicine and psychiatry. *Research Staff Physician, 26,* 73–79.

Engel, G. L. (1981). The clinical application of the biopsychosocial model. *The Journal of Medicine and Philosophy, 6,* 101–123.

Feinstein, A. R. (1967). *Clinical judgment.* Huntington, NY: Kreiger.

Goldberg, D., Mubbashar, M., & Mubbashar, S., (2000). Development in mental health services—A world view. *International Review of Psychiatry, 12*(3), 240–248.

Goldberg, R. J. (1999). Financial incentives influencing the integration of mental health care and primary care. *Psychiatric Services, 50*(8), 1071–1075.

Jaynes, J. (1976). *The origin of consciousness in the breakdown of the bicameral mind.* Boston: Houghton Mifflin.

Johnson, P. B., Staubach, L. B., & Millar, A. P. (1997). High utilizers of health services: The purchaser perspective and experience with the personal health improvement program (PHIP). In J. D. Haber & G. E. Mitchell (Eds.), *Primary care meets mental health: Tools for the 21st century* (pp. 99–113). Tiburon, CA: CentraLink Publications.

Kaplan, R. M. (1990). Behavior as the central outcome in health care. *American Psychologist, 45*(11), 1211–1220.

Kroenke, K., & Mangelsdorff, A. D. (1989). Common symptoms in ambulatory care: Incidence, evaluation, therapy and outcomes. *American Journal of Medicine, 86,* 262–265.

Kubiszyn, T. (1999). Integrating health and mental health services in schools: Psychologists collaborating with primary care providers. *Clinical Psychology Review, 19*(2), 179–198.

Lipkin, M. (1996). Can primary care physicians deliver quality mental healthcare? *Behavioral Healthcare Tomorrow, 5,* 48–53.

Lipkin, M. (1999). Psychiatry and primary care: Two cultures divided by a common cause. In R. R. Goetz, D. A. Pollack, & D. L. Cutler (Eds.), *Advancing mental health and primary care collaboration in the public sector* (pp. 7–15). San Francisco: Jossey-Bass.

McCahill, M. E. (1995). Somatoform and related disorders: Delivery of diagnosis as first step. *American Family Physician, 52*(1), 193–203.

Moss, D., & Davies, T. C. (1999). Special issue: A vision of partnership: The marriage of clinical psychophysiology and primary care. *Biofeedback, 27*(1), 2.

Palsson, O. S., & Davies, T. C. (1999). Behavioral health providers and primary care: Innovative models for intervention and service delivery. *Biofeedback, 27*(1), 14–20.

*Primary care docs report poor access to quality mental health care.* (1997). Retrieved March 28, 2002, fromhttp://www.psych.org/pnews/97-11-07/primary.html

Pruitt, S. D., Klapow, J. C., Epping-Jordan, J. E., & Dresselhaus, T. R. (1998). Moving behavioral medicine to the front line: A model for the integration of behavioral and medical sciences in primary care. *Professional Psychology: Research and Practice, 29*(3), 230–236.

Regier, D. A., Narrow, W. E., Rae, D. S., Manderscheidt, R. W., Locke, B. Z., & Goodwin, F. K. (1993). The de facto U.S. mental and addictive disorders service system. *Archives of General Psychiatry, 50,* 85–93.

Schuyler, D., & Davis, K. (1999). Primary care and psychiatry: Anticipating an interfaith marriage. *Academic Medicine, 74*(1), 27–32.

Sierpina, V. S. (2001). *Integrative health care: Complementary and alternative therapies for the whole person.* Philadelphia: F. A. Davies.

Weil, A. (1995). *Spontaneous healing: How to discover and enhance your body's natural ability to maintain and heal itself.* New York: Knopf.

Werbach, M. R. (1986). *Third line medicine: Modern treatment for persistent symptoms.* New York: Routledge & Kegan Paul.

Wickramasekera, I. (1988). *Clinical behavioral medicine: Some concepts and procedures.* New York: Plenum.

Yuen, E. J., Gerdes, J. L., & Waldforgel, S. (1999). Linkages between primary care physicians and mental health specialists. *Families, Systems & Health, 17*(3), 295–307.

# CHAPTER 7

# Professional Ethics and Practice Standards in Mind-Body Medicine

SEBASTIAN STRIEFEL

**Abstract:** This chapter presents a framework for ethical professional conduct and exemplary practice that provides the foundation for conventional ethical principles and practice standards. The chapter stresses the importance of the practitioner's personal involvement, biases, and values and introduces the concept of aspirational ethics. Nine universal ethical principles, which help clarify many problem situations in mind-body practice, are introduced. The chapter also reviews core values and virtues to guide the professional. Five case studies highlight problem situations in mind-body practice.

## INTRODUCTION

Ethical principles and practice standards alone are insufficient for resolving the many ethical situations encountered by mind-body medicine practitioners (Jordan & Meara, 1990). It is easy to try to resolve a situation without taking into account the human issues involved—that is, one's own emotional involvement, biases, and values, or the client's pain and affect (Jordan & Meara, 1990). For example, Kitchener (2000) reported that because of personal biases, practitioners who are homophobic are more likely to violate the confidentiality of a client who is homosexual and HIV positive than they are of a client who is heterosexual and engaged in the same dangerous practices.

Losing sight of the context of a problem situation is easy, especially if resolving the problem is reduced to an abstract cognitive process by simply applying ethical principles. Since the ethical principles applicable in specific situations are often in conflict, it takes *something more* to resolve the situation. That something more is the moral character of the practitioner involved. Morally, what kind of person is involved in making the necessary decisions?

Someone with good moral values is likely to make better moral decisions than is someone who does not have them (Kitchener, 2000). For example, the ethical principles for most health care professions make clear that sexual intimacies with clients are prohibited, even if the client attempts to initiate a sexual encounter. Those of sound moral character are unlikely to get sexually involved with a client, whereas those who put their own needs ahead of the welfare of the client are more likely to behave unethically by getting sexually involved. Sound ethical decisions involve achieving a balance between figuring out what one ought to do and being willing to do it. Deciding what one ought to do should be based on an interaction of existing legal mandates, the universal foundational ethical principles that form the basis for codes of ethics and standards of practice, the codes of ethics and standards of practice themselves, and the virtuous character and values of the professional making the decision.

## THE ROLE OF A CODE OF ETHICS AND PRACTICE STANDARDS

Knowing and adhering to the professional ethics and practice standards for one's profession and to existing laws are critical for "doing what is in the best interests of the client," for maintaining one's reputation, for promoting a positive image for one's profession, and for avoiding legal and ethical difficulties (Striefel, in press). Each mind-body medicine profession has its own unique code of ethics, and most, if not all, also have their own standards of practice. Codes of ethics and standards of practice are developed by professional organizations to guide their members in terms of expectations and acceptable practices. Expectations across professions vary somewhat based on the unique aspects of the profession and may change over time.

During the last 10 to 15 years, most professionals have had either a specialized ethics course geared to their profession as a part of their university training program or have attended an ethics workshop for continuing education. Many states are mandating continuing education in ethics as a requirement for renewing one's professional practice license. Yet the training received has often ignored the role of core ethical

principles, moral values, and personal character as factors influencing ethical practice behaviors.

Is it ever permissible to deceive a client for the client's own good? If so, when? Under what conditions, if any, is it permissible to violate client confidentiality? Is it ever permissible to harm or permit harm to a client to protect the welfare of someone else? Is it ever acceptable not to obtain informed consent before using a risky treatment? These and similar questions are encountered by professionals on a regular basis and require professionals to make difficult and complex decisions. Making such decisions requires more than just adherence to ethical principles and standards of practice, because the guidance provided by codes of ethics and standards of practice is general and may or may not apply to a specific situation encountered (Corey, Corey, & Callanan, 2000). What is needed is a lifelong commitment by each professional to aspire both to develop a virtuous character and to develop and adhere to the highest standards of ethical behavior. This means going beyond the code of ethics and standards of practice for one's profession. Becoming an ethical professional requires one to develop a systematic basis for resolving ethical dilemmas, one that is based on understanding and applying both *core ethical principles* and *virtue ethics*. Doing so also involves developing a sound moral character. This chapter provides a foundation for understanding the core ethical principles and values and how they influence ethical decision making and the content of codes of ethics and practice standards.

The moral, ethical, and practice issues that arise within the health care professions tend to be similar across professions (Callahan, 1988), so this chapter will be organized around issues that cut across all such professions.

## ASPIRATIONAL VERSUS MANDATORY ETHICAL FUNCTIONING

Everyone is likely to be involved with the health care system at one time or another and is thus likely to be affected by health care providers and how they practice (Callahan, 1988). Everyone has a set of moral beliefs about how professionals should behave. "*Morals* are what people believe about what is right and wrong or good and bad about character or conduct" (Kitchener, 2000, p. 2). *Ethics* is concerned with deciding what is right and wrong and with what one's obligation is, in both general and specific sets of circumstances. Because the public believes that professionals should do what is right, professionals should strive to develop a sound moral character and an excellent moral sense of what is right, and they should adhere to the highest standards of conduct. This requires every professional to do more than simply comply with a code of ethics.

Aspiring to this highest level of conduct is called engaging in an *aspirational level of ethical functioning* (Corey, Corey, & Callanan, 2000; Striefel, 1995, in press). *Mandatory ethics* refers to a level of functioning where one simply does what is required to be in compliance with a code of ethics, that is, adhering to the "musts" and "must nots" (Corey, Corey, & Callanan, 2000; Striefel, 1995, in press). Those functioning at an aspirational level strive to do what is in the best interests of their clients while simultaneously maximizing benefits and minimizing harm. Such professionals often engage in proactive behavior; that is, they think about how they will deal with situations that are likely to happen in their practice before those situations arise (e.g., a suicidal client, suspected child abuse, an infectious disease), and thus they are able to develop a plan for dealing with those

situations proactively rather than reactively. Continuing education beyond the minimum required to maintain one's license, periodic consultation and/or supervision, reflective thinking, and keeping up with factors that might impact one's practice and one's clients are all part of aspirational ethical functioning. In essence, professionals should strive to refine and enhance their "ordinary" moral sense of what is right.

---

*Do you aspire to the highest level of professional conduct?*

---

A person's ordinary moral sense is based on everything learned over his or her lifetime about being moral and doing what is right, his or her ability to reason, and his or her moral character (Kitchener, 2000). Thus developing one's own moral character, gaining the right kinds of knowledge and experience about what is right and wrong, and learning how to engage in sound ethical reasoning should ideally predispose a person to make the right ethical choices in most situations. Developing a good moral sense is influenced by appropriate consultation and/or supervision.

---

*Ordinary moral sense = Lifelong learning + Reasoning ability + Moral character*

---

## THE UNIVERSAL BASIS FOR ETHICAL BEHAVIOR

Nine universal ethical principles form the basis for the codes of ethics and standards of practice developed by professional associations (Koocher, 1999; Koocher & Keith-Spiegel,

1998). These nine principles are described in this section.

*Nonmaleficence* means striving through acts of commission and omission to do no harm. It requires careful attention to all factors in assessment and treatment to minimize or eliminate the potential for harm or injury. Generally, not harming others is a "stronger ethical obligation than benefiting them" (Kitchener, 2000, p. 22). As such, failing to maximize one's efforts to stop the physical or psychological pain and suffering of clients would be harming them and thus would be a violation of this core principle. Short-term harm or discomfort sometimes accompanies treatment that will eliminate or minimize more severe or long-term harm or discomfort. Such harm or discomfort would not be unethical if the client has given informed consent (Kitchener, 2000). Misdiagnosis, negligence (practicing below what is considered a reasonable standard of care or being careless), not terminating a treatment that is not working, or using treatments that cause more long-term harm than what was experienced by the client before treatment would all be considered violations of the principle of nonmaleficence. Informed consent provides a basis for a client to make reasonable choices and can help practitioners identify the level of risk or harm that a client is willing to experience in order to get better.

*Respecting autonomy* means respecting the right of clients to choose how to live their lives, as long as their behavior does not severely interfere with the rights or welfare of others (Koocher, 1999). Autonomy is a core goal in health care. One ideal goal of treatment in mind-body medicine is for a client to enhance or maintain his or her independence and self-reliance. As such, the principle of autonomy provides the basis for several client rights, including informed consent, privacy, and confidentiality.

*Beneficence* refers to service providers' ethical responsibility to make decisions that have the potential for having positive effects on those served. Contributing to the health and welfare of those served is at the core of why health care professions were developed, including those engaged in mind-body medicine (Kitchener, 2000). The codes of ethics for specific helping professions are based on the expectation that professionals will act in ways that will, in all probability, benefit those served. Thus professionals must balance the potential beneficial consequences of a specific action against the potential harmful ones, while simultaneously resolving potential conflicts with other ethical principles, such as autonomy (Kitchener, 2000). Deciding when and if it is acceptable to override a client's right to autonomy to achieve a beneficial treatment result can be difficult.

*Being just* means treating all clients fairly and equitably—that is, in the same way that an ethical professional would want to be treated under similar circumstances (Koocher, 1999). This principle applies to both the individual relationship that the mind-body practitioner has with a client and, more broadly, to how services are distributed in the community. What is fair and equitable to an individual client being treated and what is fair and equitable to other potential clients? For example, is it just to provide services only to those who have insurance or the ability to pay, or should everyone have access to treatment? Society and government entities generally struggle with this issue, but professional groups also struggle with and may even address the issue partially in their code of ethics. The American Psychological Association (1995) suggests that psychologists consider providing some services for no fee or for a reduced fee to help make services available to those who might otherwise not have access to needed services. The creation of a nationwide, federally subsidized system of mental health centers during the 1970s was based on the principle of justice, making services available to people who might not otherwise receive needed services—for example, those with chronic mental illnesses who cannot afford to pay because of the ongoing expense. Being just is the basis for not discriminating against any client because of gender, age, race, ethnicity, religion, national origin, sexual orientation, disability, or socioeconomic status (American Psychological Association, 1995).

*Fidelity* has two meanings in reference to mind-body medicine. It refers to the obligation of professionals first to be loyal and faithful to those served, and second to be honest and trustworthy (Kitchener, 2000). Both meanings reflect aspects of human trust and relate to the core fiduciary relationship that a professional has with those served (Kitchener, 2000). A meaningful relationship with a client is based on the client's belief that the professional will keep the promises that he or she makes (e.g., maintaining confidentiality) and that the professional will be truthful (e.g., informing the client of any significant risks). The professional must also be faithful and loyal to the relationship and to meeting the client's needs. If the professional violates these core components of the bond with his or her clients, trust and the relationship between the client and the professional may well be damaged beyond the point of being able to work together. In addition, when a client believes that he or she was injured because the professional was dishonest or did not keep his or her promises, the client is more likely to file a lawsuit or ethical complaint against the professional (Zuckerman, 1997). A professional who violates the principle of fidelity may also damage the reputation of that profession or even of other helping professions. Fidelity also serves as a basis for meaningful informed consent, confidentiality, truth in advertising, and avoidance of problematic conflicts of interest and multiple-role relationships, as expressed in professional codes of ethics.

*According dignity* refers to the professional obligation to view those served with respect and thus increases the likelihood that

the professional makes decisions that are ethical and in the client's best interests (Koocher, 1999). The personal values, history, and biases of professionals can interfere with according dignity equally to all persons who seek services. A professional should strive to become aware of his or her values and biases and how they might interfere with working with a specific group of clients. Once the professional is aware of factors that might potentially interfere with according a client dignity, he or she has the option of not accepting such clients for treatment, obtaining additional education and/or supervision, or obtaining personal treatment for overcoming such issues. For example, a professional who was severely abused as a child may have difficulty according dignity to clients with a history of abusing children. Thus the professional should consider referring such clients elsewhere and should consider obtaining personal treatment to overcome any unresolved issues. According dignity to a client also means accepting the client's right to hold values that are different from those of the professional or even values with which the professional does not agree (Corey, Corey, & Callanan, 2000).

*Treating others with care and compassion* means being kind and considerate to those being served within the boundaries of the profession (Koocher, 1999). Being kind and considerate directly affects the quality of the professional relationship developed with clients, thus professionals should attend to these variables. Being kind and considerate begins with the first client contact and includes, and goes beyond, normal courtesies, directions for getting to your office, where to park, and appointments scheduled at times convenient for the client.

*Pursuing excellence* refers to the obligation of a professional to maintain competence, do his or her best, and take pride in his or her work (Koocher, 1999). It means that a professional should be aware of his or her limits of competence and should, through continuing education, both maintain and expand his or her areas of competence to better meet the needs of those served. Pursuing excellence helps ensure high-quality services that are legal, professional, and ethical.

*Accepting accountability* means that a professional considers the potential consequences of both what he or she does or fails to do, accepts responsibility for both acts of commission and omission, and avoids trying to shift the blame or make excuses when things go wrong (Koocher, 1999). It includes sharing the responsibility for the actions or inactions of those one supervises. Being accountable directly affects one's integrity, self-respect, and reputation with others. It also means that the professional is serious in terms of learning his or her responsibilities, being competent, and attending to details. Acting responsibly is not something that can be totally imposed by an external authority. Rather, it is due to the development of an inner quality or value (Corey, Corey, & Callanan, 2000).

These nine core principles form the basis for professional codes of ethics, but unfortunately they have often been overlooked in courses on ethics. Reflecting on the impact these core ethical principles have on what one does or does not do, and why one does or does not do something, is important to enhancing one's skills for behaving ethically.

---

*Core ethical principles form the basis for developing codes of ethics.*

---

## VALUES

Moral values are beliefs and attitudes that provide direction in everyday living or in everyday professional activities (Corey, Corey, & Callanan, 2000). They comprise one's moral sense of what is right and are the things that one morally prizes, esteems, likes, or desires (Kitchener, 2000). There are some values that mind-body medicine practitioners should hold and some that they should not have because they are immoral. For example, it is desirable to believe that a client has the right to make choices that affect him or her, whereas it is not desirable to reveal confidential information about a client to those not involved in the client's treatment. One function of professional training is to implicitly or explicitly socialize trainees regarding acceptable values and to "weed out" those who do not have or do not develop the right moral values. After all, professionals have specific moral and ethical responsibilities that are often value driven (Kitchener, 2000). What one morally values tends to shape one's moral character, and professionals, by definition, hold themselves out to the public as having specialized knowledge and skills that exceed those of the general public (Striefel, 1995). Professionals are thus expected to behave ethically at a level that exceeds that of the general public.

What are the values that mind-body professionals should hold? Based on a national survey of members of various mental health disciplines, a set of commonly accepted values that are important for fostering client mental health and for guiding the actions of practitioners was identified (Jensen & Bergin, 1988). These values also seem very appropriate for those providing mind-body services and include the following (Corey, Corey, & Callanan, 2000; Jensen & Bergin, 1988):

- Pursuing self-determination
- Developing effective strategies for dealing with stress
- Developing the ability to give and receive affection
- Enhancing one's ability to be sensitive to the feelings of others
- Having a sense of purpose for living
- Developing the ability to practice self-control

- Being genuine, honest, and open
- Finding satisfaction in what one does for a living
- Developing a sense of identity and self-worth
- Becoming skilled at interpersonal relationships
- Enhancing one's self-awareness and motivation for personal growth
- Practicing good habits of physical and mental health

A code of ethics is a list of common values adopted by members of a professional association to help guide them in their practice activities. The values listed in a code of ethics are not optional but represent the core values of that profession (Kitchener, 2000). The values listed in codes of ethics across professions engaged in mind-body medicine have many similarities; for example, all support client confidentiality, respect for clients, and the importance of continuing education. They also have differences; for example, some do not explicitly prohibit sexual intimacies with clients. Professional codes of ethics do not list all the values that members of that profession should have and should promote. Training and supervision are part of the process used to help professionals acquire both the values listed in the codes of ethics and those not listed. What are your values and how do they affect clients? How do your values compare with those of other members of your profession? If you do not know your own values, it is important for you to find out what they are. This can be accomplished by taking a values clarification course or workshop, reading, engaging in discussions with members of your profession, and reflecting. Professionals must be aware of their own values to avoid unwittingly imposing their values on clients (Corey, Corey, & Callanan, 2000).

Professional standards of practice also include values and often provide much more direct guidance in terms of the "minimum standard of care" expected by members of a profession. The standards of care should also be known and adhered too. Every professional is encouraged to put together a three-ring binder in which to place useful documents that might be needed at a moment's notice. The binder should contain the code of ethics and practice standards for the professional's discipline and those of other groups to which she or he belongs; the laws governing professional activities such as licensing, child abuse and neglect, duty to warn and protect, involuntary commitment, insurance and billing, and records retention; and relevant Web sites (e.g., professional associations), e-mail addresses, and telephone numbers (Striefel, 1995). A library of relevant books on ethics, practice standards, laws, and so on can also be useful (Striefel, 1995).

A computerized Internet search can readily help find the Web site for one's profession, which usually includes a copy of the profession's code of ethics and standards of practice. The Web site for the Center for the Study of Ethics in Professions (http://www.iit.edu/departments/csep/PublicWWW/codes) includes copies of the codes of ethics for many associations, such as the American Chiropractic Association and the American Occupational Therapy Association.

## VIRTUES

Answering the question "What kind of person and professional do I want to be?" is essential if one aspires to the highest level of ethical functioning. The effort requires reflection, reading, discussion with colleagues, and continuing education, as well as a lifelong commitment to developing a virtuous moral character. Developing a virtuous character means learning about and adhering to *virtue ethics*, which focus on motivation, emotion, character, and ideals (Kitchener, 2000). The word *virtue* comes from the Greek concept of *arete*, which means excellence (Callahan,

1988). A virtue is a specific moral quality that is generally regarded as meritorious or good. May (1984) considers virtues to represent the ideal traits that professionals should acquire. These ideals are not optional; rather, it is imperative for professionals to strive to achieve these character ideals.

A virtue is a predisposition to do what is morally right (Kitchener, 2000). Having a virtuous character means that one is generally characterized as having specific moral qualities or virtues and behaving morally. Someone with an excellent moral character is more likely to understand the ethical principles and rules on which she or he bases her or his actions than is someone with a bad moral character (Kitchener, 2000). Professionals who have virtuous characters strive to achieve excellence in their ethical behavior, in their practice activities, and in their lives. Principle ethics focus on obligation, duty, and following the rules. Principle ethics focus on the question, "What should I do?" while virtue ethics focus on "What kind of person should I be?" or "How do I go about doing what is right?" (Kitchener, 2000). Principles provide guidance for resolving ethical dilemmas, and virtue ethics help provide the motivation to do what one knows is right. The two work hand-in-hand. Professionals who have virtuous characters have developed an attitude toward clients that motivates them to behave ethically. There are many virtues that can be useful in guiding ethical behavior. A few of them that mind-body practitioners should consider adopting and developing are discussed in the following sections.

## Prudence

A prudent professional has practical wisdom and is able to reason well about the moral and ethical issues that arise in daily practice and apply that reasoning to resolving those issues in a flexible manner (Kitchener, 2000). Prudence includes knowing when, if, and how to apply the ethical principles in specific circumstances. A prudent professional is capable of exercising sound judgment within the framework of being cautious and discrete and deliberately reflecting on what moral action to take, understanding the consequences of the choices made, and doing what is right. A prudent professional acts with care and wisdom and gives due consideration to the feelings and perceptions of others (Kitchener, 2000).

## Integrity

*Integrity* refers to having good core values; being honest, fair, and sincere; keeping promises; and being reliable in behaving ethically and morally. Professionals who have integrity can be counted on to adhere firmly to their ethical codes in their striving to do what is morally best (Kitchener, 2000). *Behaving with integrity* means upholding the code of ethics and standards of practice even when that is difficult to do or unpopular, such as reporting the unethical behavior of a friend or colleague. Does the sanctity of human life override an individual's right to have an abortion or to commit suicide? When does integrity become rigidity that prevents a professional from compromising when compromise is in fact the best solution to the situation? Integrity refers to one's commitment to moral values and adherence to those values. How does one behave with integrity when two moral principles are in conflict? Those who lack integrity cannot be counted on to do what is right and clients and colleagues often do not trust them.

## Respectfulness

Respectfulness is a willingness to consider the particular concerns of others, especially if one's actions will affect them (Kitchener, 2000). What does the client want to happen in this particular situation? How might I help the client get what he or she wants within acceptable ethical guidelines and law? Being respectful restricts the way a professional acts toward clients. It prohibits discrimination of any kind, including sexism or racism (Kitchener, 2000). *Respectfulness* means knowing about the culture of those served and providing services in a culturally sensitive and appropriate manner, such as understanding that eye contact is not an acceptable practice with some Native American tribes or that family is more important than the individual in some Asian cultures. Respectfulness is more than just tolerance of individual differences. It includes taking these individual differences into account in selecting assessment instruments and treatment approaches to ensure that they fit the value system and cultural needs of those served. Respectfulness includes protecting all the rights of a client—for example, the right to confidentiality, autonomy, and informed consent—and simultaneously recognizing that there are exceptions to each right—for example, times when confidentiality must be breached to preserve life and limb.

## Compassion and Caring

Compassion for others should be a component of the character of mind-body medicine practitioners. Clients expect health care practitioners to be caring, gentle, and concerned about their personal welfare (Drane, 1994). *Compassion* means showing empathy and concern for another's welfare and sympathy and concern for another's suffering or misfortune (Kitchener, 2000). It is an obligation to alleviate suffering and enhance the well-being of clients purely and simply because they are human. Humans have intrinsic value just because they are human.

Professionals are expected to be caring in their relationships with clients (Kitchener, 2000). Caring is at the core of helping others and means reflecting and acting in the best

interests of those served (Kitchener, 2000). It includes being tough enough to advocate on behalf of clients with managed care organizations that try to restrict or prevent clients from receiving needed services. In following the rules, professionals should not sacrifice the client for a principle (Kitchener, 2000). Caring and compassion remind professionals that they have a responsibility to protect the welfare of all clients, even the clients they do not like. For example, rather than abandoning a difficult client, a professional strives to find a way to work with the client in a productive manner or helps the client access appropriate services from another qualified professional. It is important not to take caring to an extreme—for example, violating a client's right to autonomy by becoming paternalistic out of concern for the client. A caring and compassionate professional seeks to answer, "How would I want to be cared for if I were in the client's situation?"

## Trustworthiness

Trust is essential for a mind-body practitioner to establish and maintain a good working relationship with clients. Clients must be able to trust that the practitioner will look out for their interests, will keep the promises made (e.g., to maintain confidentiality), will be truthful (e.g., during the informed-consent process), and will act within the accepted code of ethics and standards of practice. When a practitioner is trustworthy, clients are more willing to take the risks inherent in sharing intimate information. Without accurate and complete information from clients, practitioners may find it difficult to make the correct diagnosis or provide the appropriate treatment. Trustworthiness includes not being deceptive, not engaging in problematic dual relationships, not falsifying advertisements, not promising cures, and not accepting clients for treatment one cannot competently provide.

---

*What virtues are you developing as part of your character?*

---

Kitchener (2000) reported that every universal ethical principle has a corresponding character trait or virtue that helps predispose those who have it to act in accordance with the principle. Although the specific virtues related to practicing mind-body medicine have not yet been identified, they surely include those previously discussed here and others, including courage, perseverance, humility, benevolence, discretion, and hope. It is important to reflect on what kind of moral character you have now and what you would like to do to develop it further. Doing so is part of striving for the highest level of ethical functioning.

## ETHICAL DECISION-MAKING MODELS

Many different ethical decision-making models exist, such as those developed by Haas and Malouf (1989); Kentsmith, Salladay, and Miya (1986); Kitchener (2000); Schwartz and Striefel (1987); and Striefel (1999). They all have common characteristics and differences. Most importantly, an ethical decision-making model should be thought about, refined, and used over time to help one systematically consider a number of factors in making decisions that are in the best interests of the client and of other relevant stakeholders. Client outcomes often improve as practitioners learn from the process (Striefel, 1999).

## EXAMPLES OF PROBLEMATIC SITUATIONS

A few examples of potentially problematic situations and some of the issues raised by these situations follow.

### Case 1: Advanced Planning

A psychiatrist, Dr. Ben King, formed an alternative medicine clinic and invited Dr. Harry Johnson, a psychologist; Mary Fine, a physical therapist; Judy Smith, a chiropractor; and John Strain, a nutritionist, to join his group. Each person was to pay 50 percent of his or her collections for the cost for space, utilities, billing, secretarial services, computers, and other expenses. After six months, Harry realized that the number of referrals he was receiving from within the practice group was very small, and these referrals were not generating enough income to pay expenses and to make a living. He decided to move to a location nearby that was less expensive. After notifying Dr. King of his decision, Harry was informed that he could not take any current clients or files of his past clients with him. He filed a complaint with the appropriate ethics committee.

Dr. King's behavior is both unethical and in many states illegal (Koocher & Keith-Spiegel, 1998). Clients always maintain the right to choose whom to see or not to see for treatment (principle of autonomy). Dr. Johnson has an obligation to his clients based on the universal principles of fidelity, benificence, according dignity, treating others with caring and compassion, and accepting accountability. His clients should be given the option of continuing to receive services from him or receiving services from other appropriate providers, including Dr. King. Once a client has entered treatment with a particular professional, it can be disruptive and detrimental to have to start over with another professional. The principle of non-maleficence or do no harm is thus also relevant. In addition, if any client was in crisis, Dr. Johnson could be charged with abandonment, and if harm occurred to the client, Dr. Johnson and the group practice could be sued for negligence.

A fair, legal, and ethical option might be that Dr. Johnson would pay the group practice a reasonable number of dollars for each client that he took with him. This amount cannot include any costs for services not yet provided (i.e., future services) because that would be considered fee splitting, which is both unethical and illegal in many states. Nor can the cost be passed on to the client. The possibility of costs related to practitioners leaving the practice and taking clients with them should have been part of the original agreement.

Prior planning could have avoided problems by specifying how the practice group will deal with anyone who chooses to leave the practice (informed consent). In addition, there is the issue of fairness and justice for all concerned in regards to costs. A more equitable basis for paying for costs would be to determine what the actual cost of the space and services used by each member of the group is or will be and to charge accordingly. Another option would have been for Dr. King to hire everyone based on a fixed salary.

### Case 2: Boundary Issues

Betty Doital, a mind-body medicine practitioner whose primary specialty is psychotherapy, also offers nutritional services to her psychotherapy clients in her office. She is a licensed professional counselor (LPC) but is not licensed as a nutritionist (her state does not license nutritionists). Betty is contacted by the state LPC licensing board and informed that she is practicing beyond the scope of practice allowed by her license. The state in which she practices has a Licensing Practice Act that defines what is included in the practice of LPCs. The act does not include nutritional services. Betty is informed that she is to cease offering nutritional services in her LPC practice or her license will be rescinded. She is also informed that if

she wishes to offer nutritional services, it must be done in a different location. It is unclear if this means a different office in the same building or a different location altogether.

The universal ethical principle of pursuing excellence raises the expectation that practitioners will strive to do their best. This includes continuing education and knowing the limits of one's competence. Being competent includes being aware of relevant laws and abiding by them, and if appropriate striving to change laws with which one does not agree.

If a client comes to see Betty because of her LPC practice, he or she must be given appropriate referral options if nutritional services might also be helpful. This includes being given several options in terms of nutritionists who might provide the appropriate assessment and other nutritional services. The referral options can include Betty and at least two other nutritionists. When a client comes to a practitioner expecting to receive one kind of service (in this case, psychotherapy) and then is also given or offered another service (nutritional services) without being offered a choice, it raises the issue of conflict of interest and violates the client's right to autonomy. If a client is referred to Betty for nutritional services and it appears that psychotherapy might also be appropriate, the client must again be given choices. If a client chooses to go elsewhere for the additional services needed or chooses not to pursue those other services, there should be no recriminations for having made that choice.

### Case 3: Appropriate Supervision

Dr. Steve Huber has a reasonably successful medical practice. Many of his patients have problems that appear to be caused by excessive stress. After attending a presentation on the benefits of biofeedback, he decides to expand his practice to include biofeedback services. In his state, biofeed-back is restricted to those who are licensed in a health care discipline or who are supervised by someone so licensed. Because Dr. Huber has no training in biofeedback, he hires a BCIA-certified but unlicensed assistant, Mary Concerned, and then his office begins to offer biofeedback services. Mary soon finds that she is receiving referrals from Dr. Huber for clients needing services that go beyond her areas of competence. She makes several attempts to refer these clients for services elsewhere and is berated by Dr. Huber for doing so. She is also unsuccessful in her attempt to educate Dr. Huber about the legal and ethical issues involved, including not operating beyond one's limits of competence, potential harm to clients, and the possibility of litigation if harm occurs to a client.

Mary approaches other biofeedback practitioners in the community for guidance on how to proceed in the treatment of clients whose needs exceed her limits of competence. One of these practitioners files a complaint with the state medical licensing board. After considerable time and review of the situation, the licensing board informs Dr. Huber that he should either cease offering biofeedback services or hire a licensed practitioner competent in biofeedback to either supervise or provide the biofeedback services. He hires a licensed psychologist competent in biofeedback part-time to supervise Mary's activities.

It is important not to offer services, including supervision, that go beyond your areas of competence because harm could occur to clients (nonmaleficence), and there could be financial consequences if sued, ethical consequences if a complaint is filed, and damage to one's reputation if others learn about the situation.

When clients have needs that go beyond one's own areas of expertise, it is important to resolve the situation in a way that prevents harm to clients. This includes receiving supervision or consultation if that will be sufficient for providing services that at least meet the minimal standard of expected care, referring clients elsewhere, and becoming competent in those areas via continuing education and supervised practice.

It is also important to not accept or stay in a job that puts your clients at risk or where you are at risk because you are expected to serve clients whose needs go beyond your limits of competence without appropriate supervision and/or consultation being available. Check into the options available for making referrals and receiving supervision before you accept a position working for others, especially if they are not competent in the areas of service that you would be expected to provide.

Supervisors need to remember that they share legal and ethical responsibility for what those they supervise do or fail to do. This includes those that one should be supervising, even if one is not doing so. In this case, Mary could provide services only under the supervision of Dr. Huber. He is accountable for what she does or does not do. His risk is especially high if he fails to arrange for appropriate supervision and prevents Mary from making appropriate referrals to other practitioners.

### Case 4: Conflict of Interest

Robert Dollar is a wealthy man who has been diagnosed as having major depression and a substance abuse problem. He seeks treatment from Christine Double, a social worker. The treatment is very successful, and Robert suggests to Christine that he become her business partner. He will provide the business expertise and funds for purchasing some nice space in a medical complex and she will provide the treatment to clients. She agrees and they enter business together. Soon they are disagreeing about financial matters and frequently argue bitterly about the business. Robert again becomes depressed and, without realizing it, Christine brings up issues from his past treatment. This is a violation of his right to confidentiality.

Christine realizes that she is involved in a serious conflict-of-interest situation. With Robert's consent, she discusses the situation with another licensed social worker. She helps Robert to get treatment for his depression from another practitioner, and with his agreement they negotiate an end to their partnership.

Christine learned that dual relationships can be very problematic. She was lucky in that she was able to resolve the situation before a lawsuit or ethics complaint was filed against her. Being someone's business partner is always potentially problematic because of the financial concerns. These concerns are magnified if one partner also has intense personal information about the other partner because of the difference in perceived power. By entering into a business partnership with Robert, Christine removed Robert's option of receiving treatment from her again when he got depressed. This impacted his right to autonomy. Many courts have ruled that once a patient, always a patient.

Such conflict-of-interest situations often affect one's professional reputation with other professionals in the community, and they may well stop making referrals. Professionals often evaluate such situations as being examples of a professional exploiting a patient who is vulnerable and in need. Most often they are right.

## SUMMARY

All mind-body medicine practitioners should make a lifelong commitment to developing a virtuous character and to striving to develop and adhere to the highest level of ethical functioning. This can be accomplished through various forms of continuing education, reflection, and discussion with others. In addition, it is important to have available, understand, reflect on, and appropriately apply the universal ethical principles, appropriate virtues and values, all relevant laws, codes of ethics, and standards of practice.

## REFERENCES

American Psychological Association. (1995). *Ethical principles of psychologists and code of conduct.* Washington, DC: Author.

Callahan, J. C. (1988). *Ethical issues in professional life.* New York: Oxford University Press.

Corey, G., Corey, M. S., & Callanan, P. (2000). *Issues and ethics in the helping professions.* Pacific Grove, CA: Brooks/Cole.

Drane, J. F. (1994). Character and moral life: A virtue approach to biomedical ethics. In E. R. DuBose, R. P. Hamel, & L. J. O'Connell (Eds.), *A matter of principles? Ferment in U.S. bioethics* (pp. 284–300). Valley Forge, PA: Trinity Press International.

Haas, L. J., & Malouf, J. L. (1989). *Keeping up the good work: A professional's guide to mental health ethics.* Sarasota, FL: Professional Resource Exchange.

Jensen, J. P., & Bergin, A. E. (1988). Mental health values of professional therapists: A national interdisciplinary survey. *Professional Psychology: Research and Practice, 21*(2), 290–297.

Jordan, A. E., & Meara, N. M. (1990). Ethics and the professional practice of psychologists: The role of virtues and principles. *Professional Psychology: Research and Practice, 21,* 107–114.

Kentsmith, D. K., Salladay, S. A., & Miya, P. A. (Eds.). (1986). *Ethics in mental health practice*. Orlando, FL: Grune & Stratton.

Kitchener, K. S. (2000). *Foundations of ethical practice, research, and teaching in psychology*. Mahwah, NJ: Lawrence Erlbaum.

Koocher, G. P. (1999). *Ethical dilemmas and decisions in psychological practice*. Salt Lake City, UT: Utah Psychological Association.

Koocher, C. P., & Keith-Spiegel, P. (1998). *Ethics in psychology: Professional standards and cases*. New York: Oxford University Press.

May, W. F. (1984). The virtues in a professional setting. *Soundings, 67,* 245–266.

Schwartz, M. S., & Striefel, S. (1987, Fall). A pound of prevention is worth a ton of cure: Biofeedback ethics. *Biofeedback, 15*(3), 3–4.

Striefel, S. (1995). Professional ethical behavior for providers of biofeedback. In M. S. Schwartz (Ed.), *Biofeedback: A practitioner's guide* (2nd ed., pp. 685–705). New York: Guilford.

Striefel, S. (1999, Summer). Making the right choice is not always easy. *Biofeedback, 27*(2), 4–5.

Striefel, S. (in press). The application of ethics and law in daily practice. In M. S. Schwartz & F. Andrasik (Eds.), *Biofeedback: A practitioner's guide* (3rd ed.). New York: Guilford.

Zuckerman, E. L. (1997). *The paper office* (2nd ed.). New York: Guilford.

# Part II

# BASIC CLINICAL TOOLS

# CHAPTER 8

# Biofeedback and Biological Monitoring

## CHRISTOPHER GILBERT AND DONALD MOSS

**Abstract:** Biofeedback is a mind-body therapy using electronic instruments to help individuals gain awareness and control over physiological processes. The instruments used in biofeedback measure muscle activity, skin temperature, electrodermal activity, respiration, heart rate, blood pressure, brain electrical activity, and brain blood flow. Research shows that biofeedback is effective for treating a variety of medical and mental disorders. Used by physicians, nurses, psychologists, physical therapists, occupational therapists, and others, biofeedback therapies guide the individual to facilitate the learning of voluntary control over body and mind and to take a more active role in maintaining personal health.

## ORIGINS

Biofeedback uses electronic devices to measure and provide an individual with information about fluctuations in physiological processes. The goal is to extend conscious influence over normally automatic bodily functions. Biofeedback is a unitary mind-body therapeutic approach, emphasizing the following psychophysiological principle:

Every change in the physiological state is accompanied by an appropriate change in the mental emotional state, conscious or unconscious, and conversely, every change in the mental emotional state, conscious or unconscious, is accompanied by an appropriate change in the physiological state. (Green, Green, & Walters, 1970, p. 3)

The 1960s provided the technological, philosophical, and cultural context for the emergence of biofeedback. Biological monitoring was advanced at that time by miniaturization and portability. At the same time, interest in yoga and Eastern meditation proliferated. Three trends were present that, in retrospect, seemed to make biofeedback inevitable: (1) the challenge to Freudian psychoanalysis by behavior therapy based on theories of conditioning, (2) the application of cybernetic principles to biological systems, and (3) the humanistic and transpersonal psychology movements that urged individuals and society to reach higher levels of human potential.

Notable early contributions to the emerging field of biofeedback included the research of Neal Miller (1969) on conditioning visceral responses in laboratory animals, the work of Elmer Green (Green, Green, & Walters, 1970) on self-regulation and voluntary controls, and investigations of Charles Tart (1969) into altered states of consciousness. Yogis from India submitted to study by Western scientists and endured electrodes as they demonstrated their self-regulation skills. Elmer and Alyce Green's book *Beyond Biofeedback* (1977) depicts the early feeling of boundless potential, as does Barbara Brown's *New Mind, New Body* (1974).

Biofeedback was officially named in 1969 at a Santa Monica, California, conference marking the formation of the Biofeedback Research Society. The principle of voluntary controls, however, appeared sporadically in much earlier research and clinical work. In the 1920s and 1930s, Edmund Jacobson (1938) developed a device to detect muscle tension and a technique to reduce this tension; this was the beginning of progressive relaxation (McGuigan, 1984). Jacobson taught patients to enhance awareness of skeletal muscle tension by the methodical tensing and relaxing of various muscle groups. (This approach was successful with many physiological problems outside the voluntary muscle system.) Meanwhile, Johannes Schultz in Germany developed his autogenic training technique for promoting self-regulation of various body processes, though without biofeedback instruments (Schultz & Luthe, 1959).

Progressive relaxation and autogenic training, both Western-based therapies, provided systematic methods for learning to influence the autonomic nervous system, which was still considered "off limits" to the Western world (see Chapter 10). Yoga practitioners had already developed sophisticated voluntary control of blood flow, heart rate, skin circulation, and brain waves, all without the aid of instruments, so scientists were finally convinced it was possible. But the times were not ripe for Westerners *en masse*

to learn from yogis without translation into mechanistic, data-based Western terms. Thus Elmer Green titled his influential film about his trip to India to document yogis in action *Biofeedback—The Yoga of the West.*

A conceptual basis for the idea of biofeedback was provided by the field of cybernetics, originally developed by engineers for designing self-guiding missiles. Feeding information back to the guidance system creates a feedback loop, permitting ongoing, intelligent adjustment. This paradigm typifies organic motor control and is already programmed into our bodies. The possibility of using electronic instruments to create external feedback loops and to facilitate augmented physiological control caught the imaginations of theorists. These early pioneers declared biofeedback possible based on machine analogues of organic nervous systems (Mulholland, 1977).

Meanwhile, John Basmajian (1967, 1989) began to explore the limits of voluntary control over the skeletal muscles, using needle and surface electrodes with oscilloscope and audio feedback. He demonstrated that almost anyone could gain control of single motor units of a muscle within a brief time, given proper feedback for discrimination. His early work formed the basis for many applications of neuromuscular rehabilitation.

Joe Kamiya (1969) demonstrated that humans could learn to switch their alpha brain waves on and off at will. The key was accurate feedback of their current brain states. Sufficient information permitted discrimination, and discrimination permitted control. Since long-time meditators often had a higher proportion of alpha wave activity, biofeedback was touted as a "shortcut to enlightenment."

Thus by the early 1970s, the three major bodily systems had all been shown to be subject to voluntary control: the autonomic nervous system, the skeletal muscle system, and the central nervous system. These "conquests" were sufficient for practitioners, researchers, and the popular press to begin promising remarkable clinical applications "just around the corner." An enormous outpouring of clinical reports and research studies followed, applying biofeedback to disorders ranging from headache to blood pressure to anxiety.

## INSTRUMENTATION AND PROCEDURES

Current biofeedback instrumentation has advanced far beyond early prototypes, which sometimes consisted of simply turning around an existing physiological monitor or chart recorder so that the learner could see what the scientist usually sees. Instrumentation complexity does not necessarily speed or enhance the learning process, because the most essential ingredients are still within the learner's mind. Small thermometers costing less than a dollar, calibrated to the proper range, can provide enough information for subjects to learn self-regulation of peripheral temperature. Biofeedback instruments can reflect success but do not create success. The learning process depends on mental operations such as imagery, selective remembering, muscle relaxation, controlled breathing, repetition of words, or creation of a different state of consciousness.

Nevertheless, the biofeedback process has been aided by computer processing. Today, the electronic equivalent of an entire laboratory can be carried in a briefcase. Computer-interfaced biofeedback systems make possible instantaneous and sophisticated analysis of biological signals, so subjects can see computer displays of instantaneous spectral (frequency) analyses of their heart rhythms or brain waves.

The main biofeedback modalities are described briefly in the following sections.

## Electromyograph

The electromyograph (EMG) uses surface electrodes placed on the skin over any muscle of interest. The most common placements are forehead, neck, shoulder, arms, jaw, and back muscles. Surface electrodes detect fluctuating voltage through the skin and transduce the raw signals into a visual display on a meter, a moving LED bar, or a computer screen. Audio feedback is also provided. Using this continuous stream of information, in effect like a magnifying electronic mirror, an individual gains control of a muscle or muscle group—for instance, learning to relax the jaw muscle to counteract a destructive repetitive clenching. A handheld scanning device can be applied to various muscle sites to obtain immediate readouts of muscle tension. This can be either self-contained, with an indicator built in, or extended from a larger system for processing and display of the information. EMGs can be small, stand-alone, battery-powered instruments priced under $1,000 or part of a multimodal computer system priced between $3,000 and $10,000.

## Skin Temperature

In temperature biofeedback (TEMP), a thermistor taped to the skin detects temperature and a processor transforms it into a visual or audio signal (see Figure 8.1). The information is updated once every few seconds or faster, giving the learner clear information about local changes in blood flow with a precision of one-tenth of a degree or less, beyond conscious discrimination. The most common placement is on a finger or toe. Changes in blood flow are linked with emotional tension; cooler fingers usually indicate vasoconstriction, which correlates with anxiety, caution, or hypervigilance. Temperature devices are less expensive than other biofeedback devices, and a small alcohol thermometer taped to the finger will suffice as a home

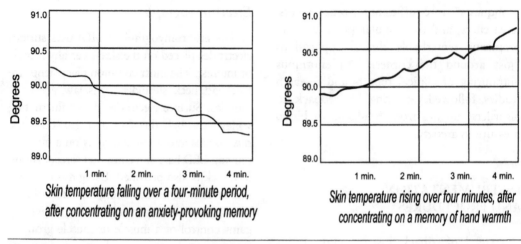

Skin temperature falling over a four-minute period, after concentrating on an anxiety-provoking memory

Skin temperature rising over four minutes, after concentrating on a memory of hand warmth

**Figure 8.1**    Temperature Biofeedback (TEMP)

trainer. Temperature-sensitive liquid crystal adhesive spots and rings are also available and can be worn for continuous monitoring.

### Skin Conductance

Skin conductance (SC) is also called electrodermal response (EDR), or galvanic skin response (GSR). Sensors are applied to the palm or fingers, and the fluctuating conductance is converted by a processor into a visual or audio signal. This biofeedback mode reflects changes in the electrical conductance of the skin on the palmar surface of the hand. Increases in conductance correlate with greater sweat gland activity, which is roughly correlated with changes in arousal and orientation related to transient mental events. Worry or anxiety quickly induces changes in skin electrical activity. These devices are not expensive and, like thermometers, are widely available. Their response to emotional change is faster by a few seconds than skin temperature.

### Electroencephalograph

As with other biofeedback modalities, systems for detecting and displaying electrical brain activity existed for decades before the idea caught on of displaying the output to the person being measured. Feeding back cortical activity establishes a loop of information, allowing the brain to witness its own operations from the outside. The necessary equipment is complex, expensive, and subject to many artifacts but offers a potential tool for self-regulation of the entire nervous system. A single channel of EEG information can be useful, but montages of 19 or more electrodes monitoring many sites and many frequencies simultaneously are sometimes used. Alpha-wave feedback began this biofeedback area, but many different frequencies are now routinely monitored and analyzed. Digital real-time processing allows analysis of complex aspects of the brain-wave signal using computers. A current synonym for *EEG biofeedback* is *neurofeedback* (see Chapter 9).

### Heart Rate and Blood Pressure Feedback

Compared with the EEG, acquiring and feeding back information about cardiovascular variables is simple. Heart rate can be obtained on a continuous basis, updated every few seconds, averaged to a beats-per-minute rate, and displayed on a screen or meter or transformed into sound or shifting colors. An electrocardiogram (EKG) detects the electrical activity of the heart and provides the most precise measurement of cardiac activity. Alternatively, a photoplethysmograph (PPG) detects the perfusion of blood optically with a sensor on the skin of the thumb. New software also makes possible a display of a spectral analysis of heart rate. The display shows dominant frequencies evident in the moment-to-moment variation of heart rate, making possible a new training modality called heart rate variability (HRV) biofeedback. Chapter 26 discusses the application of HRV biofeedback to the anxiety disorders. Blood pressure is more difficult to obtain continuously, but intermittent measurements from an autoinflating cuff can provide enough information to be useful for feedback.

## Respiration Feedback

In recent years, biofeedback practitioners have paid increasing attention to breath training for anxiety, asthma, and many other conditions. Respiration feedback (RESP) training uses a pneumograph with bands that measure the expansion and contraction across the chest or abdomen during breathing. The instrument displays a waveform depicting inhalation and exhalation, and a continuously updated estimate of breaths taken per minute. The heart rate and respiration signals are combined to produce respiratory sinus arrhythmia (RSA) biofeedback, which displays the relationship between heart rhythm and breathing. At a particular breathing rate (usually around six per minute), a synchrony is established between the cardiovascular and respiratory systems. This is called the resonant frequency and is related to regulation of the autonomic nervous system, promoting homeostasis by balancing the sympathetic and parasympathetic branches.

## ANATOMY AND PHYSIOLOGY

Identifying the relevant psychophysiological mechanisms involved in biofeedback learning is an ongoing challenge that drives research. Thoughts and emotions transduce into observable physiological changes and physical symptoms.[1] Biofeedback draws on this mind-body linkage; the individual learns a variety of strategies to produce positive physiological changes and a reduction in symptoms. Understanding this process is essential to the therapeutic power of biofeedback. This principle applies to the voluntary muscle system as well as to autonomic control. Each biofeedback modality monitors a specific system and offers a path for introducing conscious "steering" into the regulation of that system. Current instrumentation facilitates voluntary control over peripheral blood flow and blood pressure, sweat and gastrointestinal activity, heart rate, brain waves, muscular activity, respiration, and other physiological processes.

Early conceptualizations of biofeedback emphasized a global understanding of the stress response, including mass action by the autonomic system, through the hypothalamic-pituitary-adrenal (HPA) axis. The limbic system of the brain responds to threat and signals a fight-or-flight response to the HPA axis. This generalized emergency response sends a flood of neurohormones and neurochemicals into the bloodstream; increases blood flow to the skeletal muscles; increases blood pressure, heart rate, and respiration; and causes a variety of other changes that enable the body to face or flee danger (Benson, 1975; Selye, 1976). Biofeedback in turn enables the individual to cultivate a relaxation response, reversing each aspect of the stress response. Muscles relax; heart rate, blood pressure, and respiration decrease; and the individual experiences a quieting within the nervous system (Moss, 2001; Schwartz & Associates, 1995; Schwartz & Andrasik, in press).

This stress response model has been supplemented in recent years by the recognition that the human body can respond differentially to stress. Both physical symptoms and emotional disorders can reflect excessive sympathetic or parasympathetic dominance within the autonomic nervous system. Some individuals are musculoskeletal responders, others cardiovascular, respiratory, gastrointestinal, or cognitive responders.

In addition, there is a greater emphasis today on the effects of biofeedback on both central and peripheral mechanisms in the body. Early models of biofeedback intervention for headache and back pain, for example, emphasized the reduction of muscle tension and a concomitant reduction in pain: "Relax the muscle, hurt less." Now it is clear that the brain mediates a *hyperalgesia*—an extremely sensitive readiness to feel pain (Bendtsen & Ashina, 2000; Bernstein, 2000; Flor, Birbaumer, et al., 1993; Flor, Braun, Elbert, & Birbaumer, 1997). The slightest strain in or pressure on a muscle triggers pain. Recent research reports that patients with recurrent pain show modifications in the well-known *homunculus*—the representation of the body's outline in the sensorimotor cortex. Those parts of the body with pain are overrepresented in the sensorimotor cortex and quicker to signal pain (Flor, 2000). Successful biofeedback training probably affects central neurophysiological mechanisms and cognitive processes, as well as the tension levels in the specific muscle trained (Rokicki et al., 1997).

General relaxation is valuable to most people, but biofeedback can do more than assist relaxation. Biofeedback interventions can be used strategically if the physiological mechanisms active in a disorder are understood. Biofeedback can guide an individual to activate specific muscle groups, increase specific wave activity in an area of the brain, or alter circulation in hands and fingers. For example, Sterman (1986) reduced the occurrence of seizures by training patients with epilepsy to increase the production of a specific wave frequency (the sensorimotor rhythm, at 13 to 15 Hz) over the sensorimotor strip of the brain.

Research is clarifying the circuits that allow conscious control over the body. The brain contains numerous incoming and outgoing connections between the cerebral cortex, frontal lobes, and lower motor and sensory systems. Tracing signals from either direction to the edge of conscious awareness would be helpful, and brain-imaging techniques are a potential tool for this purpose. Complete reliance on such a mechanistic approach violates the holistic principle espoused by yogis, who have demonstrated their skills in bodily manipulation and generally explain their methods with reference to imagery plus erasing mind-body distinctions (Jonas, 1973). Similarly, today's research on the placebo response shows the powerful role of hope and expectation in healing (Ader & Cohen, 1993; Wickramasekera, 1999; see Chapter 5 of this text). Understanding the neurophysiology and neurochemistry of the imagination and of hope is an important research challenge for understanding biofeedback.

## LEARNING PRINCIPLES

The learning processes underlying biofeedback probably cannot be captured in a single description or conceptual model. In some cases, feedback provides an artificial information conduit, replacing destroyed afferent nerve pathways. This model applies to the recovery of motor function in a post-stroke flaccid muscle. In other cases, feedback provides information about internal processes that was never available. This model applies to biofeedback-induced reductions in blood pressure, because we have no direct sensory perception of blood pressure changes. The degree of preexisting control of the target system makes a difference: We can learn better control of a shoulder muscle, for instance, because the efferent pathways are already part of the voluntary motor system. But altering bowel activity or blood vessel diameter involves extending conscious control to an entirely new realm.

Providing a visual or auditory signal of ongoing physiological activity to the conscious mind seems to complete a loop that can be seen as cybernetic. Feedback is essential for self-control within a system, as in a thermostat within a building's heating system or in the biological thermoregulation of the body. When we apply this cybernetic model to human beings, however, greater emphasis needs to be placed on consciousness and volition.

The biofeedback procedure can also be described in operant conditioning terms: A desired change in the signal reinforces whatever is occurring. Reinforcement is operationally defined as anything that increases the occurrence of some event. The "reward value" of a line moving up on a screen or a sound getting dimmer may seem abstract, but a drive to excel or the anticipation of relief from symptoms can enable an individual to learn quickly.

Control of autonomic functions with the aid of biofeedback is imprecise and slow compared with voluntary muscle control, and the mechanism is less clear. Through association with a particular psychophysiological state, certain images and memories (seashore, lake, forest, etc.) may develop the power to evoke that state at will. Many autonomic functions respond naturally to conscious relaxation, so the appearance of "control" is frequently a simple consequence of the relaxation process.

In any case, the biofeedback learning process usually proceeds from difficult to easy, from a smaller effect to a larger one, from slower to faster, from more gross effects (in the case of voluntary muscles) to

more precise, and from fully conscious to more automatic. The behavioral principle of shaping guides much of biofeedback learning. Shaping duplicates the progression of an infant's gradually acquiring control over muscles. Because biofeedback is usually done with the help of an instructor rather than in isolation, interpersonal factors enter the learning process. The personality of the practitioner, including such traits as warmth, encouragement, patience, and sensitivity, has been found to influence speed of learning (Taub & School, 1978). These qualities influence the learning of anything in anyone at any age and suggest the essential role not only of consciousness but attitude and emotional state in the delicate process of learning bodily control.

## DOCUMENTED APPLICATIONS OF BIOFEEDBACK

This section summarizes applications of biofeedback to common disorders for which adequate outcome research is available. Comprehensive compilations of empirical support for biofeedback's efficacy can be found in Amar and Schneider (1995); Shellenberger, Amar, Schneider, and Turner (1994); and Schwartz and Associates (1995).[2]

### Global Effects of Biofeedback

It should be kept in mind that biofeedback often has an impact on the entire organism, with both central and peripheral effects, beyond the target symptom. Describing specific "applications" of biofeedback suggests that the target disorders are separate entities, but self-regulation (and dysregulation) also has general effects because of the interaction of various bodily systems and the consequences of homeostasis. For instance, relaxation of neck muscles to reduce tension headaches may also improve digestion, blood pressure, or anxiety, presumably because of a generalized relaxation component. Self-regulation using any mode of biofeedback easily crosses the borders among various physiological, cognitive, and affective systems, causing many positive "side effects" (Sovak, Kunzel, Sternbach, & Dalessio, 1981). Chapter 15 addresses the probable central mediation of biofeedback effects.

Nonspecific or placebo effects are also important in biofeedback. Many patients report symptomatic improvement that is not correlated with their mastery of physiological control. The experience of gaining "some" control over one's own body appears to generalize into a broader hopefulness about recovery and wellness. In an important early study, Holroyd et al. (1984) showed that reduction in headache pain during biofeedback treatment was more closely related to cognitive changes induced by feedback training than to measurable changes in muscle tension. Today's sophisticated biofeedback instrumentation with computer interfaces and colorful visual displays are in themselves a powerful placebo, eliciting patients' faith in the healing process. Research shows that hope and positive expectation have neurophysiological consequences, and these nonspecific effects should be regarded as a positive element within biofeedback treatment.

## Headaches

General medical guidelines for headache treatment often recommend biofeedback. Research support is strong for alleviation of tension-type headaches (presumed to involve chronic muscle tension in the head and neck, as well as the development of trigger points) as well as for migraines (Kroner-Herwig, Mohn, & Pothmann, 1998; Moss, Andrasik, McGrady, Perry, & Baskin, 2001). Current emphasis in headache research on the role of central (brain) processes driving headache suggests that biofeedback training may also

affect these central neural mechanisms. The evidence in many headache studies is often equally good for relaxation with or without biofeedback, suggesting that the active ingredient of change may not require actual monitoring. Treating pediatric headaches with biofeedback, using either temperature or EMG biofeedback, has also shown good success (Blanchard, Taylor, & Dentinger, 1992). Chapter 15 provides more specific information on biofeedback interventions for headache, training modalities, electrode placement, home practice, and the role of preexisting medical illness and psychopathology.

## Raynaud's Disease

While less common than headaches, Raynaud's disease has been well studied and found responsive to temperature biofeedback, especially with the use of a "cold stress challenge" (Freedman, 1987; Freedman, Ianni, & Wenig, 1983). The essence of Raynaud's disease is a hyperresponsivity of blood vessels in the hands and feet. The digits change colors, becoming dramatically white, red, or blue with changes in blood supply to tissue. The condition is painful, and in the extreme, the patient may suffer loss of a digit due to failed circulation. Learning to prevent, limit, or reverse vasospasms in response to cold stimuli is facilitated by temperature biofeedback.

## Essential Hypertension

Fluctuations in blood pressure are multidimensional in origin. Emotional stress contributes in many individuals to either momentary (phasic) or long-term (tonic) rises in systolic or diastolic pressure. Biofeedback is a reasonable complementary therapy, along with the usual lifestyle modifications such as weight, diet, and exercise. Medication regimens involve both negative side effects and expense. Reducing dependence on medication is possible for some,

---

**Box 8.1**    Documented Applications of Biofeedback to Common Disorders

| | |
|---|---|
| Anxiety disorders | Irritable bowel syndrome |
| Asthma | Motion sickness |
| Attention deficit disorder | Nocturnal enuresis (bed-wetting) |
| Bruxism | Phantom-limb pain |
| Chronic pain | Raynaud's disease |
| Epileptic seizures | Temporomandibular joint dysfunction |
| Functional nausea and vomiting | Tinnitus |
| Headache (migraine and tension) | Urinary and fecal incontinence |
| Essential hypertension | Various muscle and dermatological disorders |

---

given sufficient practice and discipline. GSR, EMG, and temperature biofeedback have all been found useful in helping to reduce blood pressure. Goebel, Viol, and Orebaugh (1993) compared various feedback conditions over several years in a group of hypertensives and showed consistent long-term decreases compared with a control group. McGrady and Higgins (1989) developed a profile of those individuals most likely to benefit from biofeedback for essential hypertension. Schwartz and Associates (1995, pp. 445–467) reviewed the area thoroughly.

## Methodological Problems in Outcome Research on Biofeedback

There are inherent methodological challenges to creating the double-blind situation that many regard as the epitome in efficacy research. Biofeedback is a procedure that rests its effectiveness on using feedback to increase the subject's awareness and control over his or her own body. How does one "blind" a subject or an experimenter to a procedure that rests on awareness? It is simple to blind participants as to who is getting a placebo and who is getting an antianxiety medication, but not so simple to disguise who receives biofeedback and who receives a pill or cognitive therapy.

La Vaque and Rossiter (2001a, 2001b) have identified ethical issues arising from the use of placebos when known treatments exist. Today, withholding treatment for experimental purposes is at least questionable given the World Medical Association's Declaration of Helsinki. La Vaque and Rossiter suggested that we need to examine alternative designs and statistical analyses that may be more appropriate to clinical psychophysiology as well as complementary and alternative medicine. Shellenberger and Green (1987) suggested that a mastery model was a more appropriate research model for biofeedback than the double-blind model.

Nevertheless, a large body of empirical studies has accumulated on the efficacy of biofeedback: many controlled studies without blinding, wait-list control studies, and ABA crossover-type studies, where a group serves as its own control. In an ABA crossover study, the subjects may be trained to modify a physiological parameter consecutively in opposite directions (e.g., Lubar & Shouse, 1976).

Disorders with adequate research support to justify the use of biofeedback are listed in Box 8.1. In addition, there are many specialized applications in neuromuscular rehabilitation, where biofeedback is used by physical therapists not for relaxation but for restoring function when either motor or sensory pathways have been damaged (see Basmajian, 1989). Finally, EEG neurofeedback and its applications are covered in Chapter 9 of this book.

## TREATMENT
## PROTOCOL FOR HEADACHE

The following is a brief description of the application of EMG biofeedback to muscle-tension headaches.

*1. Information Gathering.* An intake interview collects information about the details of the headaches: frequency, duration, intensity, location, headache triggers, remedies, current medications, and the results of recent medical evaluation. The interviewer also inquires about life history and explores psychological factors such as depression, life stress, suppressed anger, and negative thinking.

*2. Demonstration.* After giving the patient a brief explanation of biofeedback principles, EMG electrodes are applied over a muscle group. It is helpful to start with a neutral muscle, such as the forearm, to demonstrate how relaxation changes the screen or instrument display and the audio feedback. Attention is directed to how muscle sensations vary with measured tension level. The patient may also be asked to visualize stressful job or family situations she or he is experiencing or engage in worrisome or negative thinking and watch the impact on the biofeedback display. This procedure dramatically demonstrates the effect of mind on body.

*3. Static and Dynamic Muscle Scan.* The initial muscular assessment is ideally conducted with a combination of fixed bilateral electrode placements and a handheld scanning unit. A scanning module is a handheld

EMG, either self-contained or a cabled extension of the main instrument. The scanner enables the practitioner to acquire several quick readings of resting muscle tension in a number of locations. This can help pinpoint areas of chronic bracing, but recorded tension will not always correlate with pain reports. Detection of right-left asymmetries may correlate with pain patterns.

The patient is also instructed to engage in activities straining the muscles relevant to the current problem. An electrician with headache may be asked to reach overhead as though working on overhead wiring. The practitioner gains information on the magnitude of muscle tension during such motions and then observes the recovery process in each muscle group. Tension headache patients typically show upper torso and head musculature with high baseline muscle tension, asymmetric elevations of tension on the left or right side, slowness to recover after activity, and a co-contraction of adjacent muscle groups not functionally involved in a motion (Middaugh, 2000; Middaugh, Kee, Nicholson, & Allenback, 1995).

*4. First Biofeedback Session.* The practitioner applies electrodes to relevant muscles. For muscle tension headache, the most common electrode placements are some combination of forehead, neck, jaw, and shoulder muscles, with one or two areas used in training. The initial muscle scan guides the selection of specific training sites. The patient is guided through a deliberate tensing and relaxing of the muscle groups, to further orient him or her to the display screen and audio signals.

Many therapists initially emphasize general relaxation. Various suggestions can be offered to promote the general release of muscle tension. The feedback is tailored to the patient's preferences (soft audio feedback permits an eyes-closed condition). This stage involves helping the patient discover how to relax certain muscles, if not the entire body, and always has a psychological component. Images such as lying in the sun, floating in water, or lying in a bathtub can evoke relaxation. Some people prefer intermittent (occasional glance) access to the feedback information, and others like continuous awareness of the signal.

Once general muscle relaxation is achieved, the therapist sets goals that are more specific and guides the patient in a shaping procedure. Most equipment allows the therapist to set a threshold so the patient can hear an auditory tone or musical phrase whenever a muscle group is relaxed below the threshold. If there is clear muscle asymmetry, the patient may be encouraged to balance the tension levels in the two muscle groups. If there is co-contraction of left-sided shoulder musculature when the patient raises the right arm, a training goal may include keeping the left shoulder relaxed while lifting the right arm.

*5. Home Practice.* The therapist encourages regular practice between sessions to develop skill in relaxing, and to deemphasize dependence on the biofeedback instrument and the clinical setting. Regular practice of relaxation reinforces what is learned during clinic sessions and facilitates generalization of the relaxation response. An audiotape of muscle relaxation instructions can guide home practice.

*6. Record Keeping.* The therapist offers the patient forms for recording headache occurrence and intensity and the headache context or triggers. Most therapists also provide a form for the patient to record relaxation practice times and results.

*7. Subsequent Sessions.* In uncomplicated cases, several office sessions may be enough

to develop good relaxation skills, defined as reaching and holding a criterion microvolt level. Various types of feedback display can be offered for their information and novelty value. Weekly progress in muscle relaxation ability is examined along with any improvement in headache.

Over time, the therapist introduces additional goals, such as decreasing reliance on the biofeedback instrument, improving ability to sense muscle tension internally, maintaining relaxation while carrying out simple tasks (perhaps during a sample stressor such as mental calculation), and generalizing relaxation outside the office. By this time, something is usually known about the context in which the headaches occur, and the therapeutic focus can turn to coping with stressors using an array of cognitive-behavioral therapy techniques. The patient is also encouraged to sharpen her or his awareness of headache warning signs, whether they are sensations, particular feelings, or something in the environment.

## CONCLUSION

Biofeedback is normally the centerpiece of a larger mind-body intervention plan that includes several techniques aimed at pain or anxiety control, emotional self-regulation, and mastery of relaxation.[3] The patient may be challenged to make simultaneous behavioral and lifestyle changes, to journal emotions, and to modify diet and exercise. The treatment normally requires two to four months of weekly sessions along with home practice. The instrumentation is a prominent part of the procedure, but the heart of the patient's progress is the development of greater self-regulation skills. Self-mastery is not automatic but requires active engagement by the patient and skillful communication and finesse on the part of the therapist.

## NOTES

    1. The high risk model of threat perception identifies a number of factors influencing which individuals transduce thoughts and feelings into symptoms. Chapter 2 introduced this model.

    2. An updated edition of Schwartz and Associates (1995) is under way.

    3. Emotional self-regulation includes increasing awareness and identification of emotions and moods and improving personal control over emotions and moods.

## REFERENCES

Ader, R., & Cohen, N. (1993). Psychoneuroimmunology: Conditioning and stress. *Annual Review of Psychology, 44,* 53–85.

Amar, P. B., & Schneider, C. (Eds.). (1995). *Clinical applications of biofeedback and applied psychophysiology.* Wheat Ridge, CO: Association for Applied Psychophysiology and Biofeedback.

Basmajian, J. V. (1967). *Muscles alive: Their functions revealed by electromyography.* Baltimore: Williams and Wilkins.

Basmajian, J. V. (Ed.). (1989). *Biofeedback: Principles and practice for clinicians* (3rd ed.). Baltimore: Williams & Wilkins.

Bendtsen, L., & Ashina, M. (2000). Sensitization of myofacial pain pathways in tension-type headache. In J. Olesen, P. Tfelt-Hansen, & K. M. A. Welch (Eds.), *The headaches* (2nd ed., pp. 573–577). Philadelphia: Lippincott Williams & Wilkins.

Benson, H. (1975). *The relaxation response.* New York: Morrow.

Bernstein, R. (2000). Central sensitization and headache. In J. Olesen, P. Tfelt-Hansen, & K. M. A. Welch (Eds.), *The headaches* (2nd ed., pp. 125–136). Philadelphia: Lippincott Williams & Wilkins.

Blanchard, E. B., Taylor, A. E., & Dentinger, M. P. (1992). Preliminary results from the self-regulatory treatment of high-medication-consumption headache. *Biofeedback & Self-Regulation, 17*(3), 179–202.

Brown, B. (1974). *New mind, new body.* New York: Harper & Row.

Flor, H. (2000). The functional organization of the brain in chronic pain. *Progress in Brain Research, 129,* 313–322.

Flor, H., Birbaumer, N., Furst, M., Lutzenberger, W., Elbert, T., & Braun, C. (1993). Evidence of enhanced peripheral and central responses to painful stimulation in chronic pain. *Psychophysiology, 30,* 9.

Flor, H., Braun, C., Elbert, T., & Birbaumer, N. (1997). Extensive reorganization of primary somatosensory cortex in chronic pain patients. *Neuroscience Letters, 224,* 5–8.

Freedman, R. R. (1987). Long-term effectiveness of behavioral treatment for Raynaud's disease. *Behavior Therapy, 18,* 337–399.

Freedman, R., Ianni, P., & Wenig, P. (1983). Behavioral treatment of Raynaud's disease. *Journal of Consulting and Clinical Psychology, 51,* 539–549.

Goebel, M., Viol, G. W., & Orebaugh, C. (1993). An incremental model to isolate specific effects of behavioral treatments in essential hypertension. *Biofeedback & Self-Regulation, 18*(4), 255–280.

Green, E., & Green, A. (1977). *Beyond biofeedback.* San Francisco: Delacorte Press.

Green, E., Green, A. M., & Walters, E. D. (1970). Voluntary control of internal states: Psychological and physiological. *Journal of Transpersonal Psychology, 2,* 1–26.

Holroyd, K. A., Penzien, D. B., Hursey, K. G., Tobin, D. L., Rogers, L., Holm, J. E., et al. (1984). Change mechanisms in EMG biofeedback training: Cognitive changes underlying improvements in tension headache. *Journal of Clinical and Consulting Psychology, 512*(6), 1039–1053.

Jacobson, E. (1938). *Progressive relaxation.* Chicago: University of Chicago Press.

Jonas, G. (1973). *Visceral learning: Toward a science of self-control.* New York: Viking.

Kamiya, J. (1969). Operant control of the EEG alpha rhythm and some of its reported effects on consciousness. In C. Tart (Ed.), *Altered states of consciousness* (pp. 489–501). New York: Wiley.

Kroner-Herwig, B., Mohn, U., & Pothmann, R. (1998). Comparison of biofeedback and relaxation in the treatment of pediatric headache and the influence of parent involvement on outcome. *Applied Psychophysiology and Biofeedback, 23*(3), 143–157.

La Vaque, T. J., & Rossiter, T. (2001a). The ethical use of placebo controls in clinical research: The Declaration of Helsinki. *Applied Psychophysiology and Biofeedback, 26*(1), 25–38.

La Vaque, T. J., & Rossiter, T. (2001b). Response to Striefel and Glaros. *Applied Psychophysiology and Biofeedback, 26*(1), 69–73.

Lubar, J. F., & Shouse, M. N. (1976). EEG and behavioral changes in a hyperkinetic child concurrent with training of the sensorimotor rhythm (SMR): A preliminary report. *Biofeedback & Self-Regulation, 3,* 293-306.

McGrady, A., & Higgins, J. T., Jr. (1989). Prediction of response to biofeedback assisted relaxation in hypertensives: Development of a hypertensive predictor profile (HYPP). *Psychosomatic Medicine, 51,* 277–284.

McGuigan, F. J. (1984). Progressive relaxation: Origins, principles, and clinical applications. In R. L. Woolfolk & P. M. Lehrer (Eds.), *Principles and practice of stress management* (pp. 12–42). New York: Guilford.

Middaugh, S. (2000). Combining EMG feedback with physical therapy for treatment of headache. *Biofeedback Newsmagazine, 28*(1), 16-20.

Middaugh, S. J., Kee, W. G., Nicholson, J. A., & Allenback, G. (1995). Upper trapezius overuse in chronic headache and correction with EMG biofeedback training. *Proceedings of the Association for Applied Psychophysiology and Biofeedback, 1995,* 89–92. Abstract, *Biofeedback & Self-Regulation, 20,* 303.

Miller, N. E. (1969). Learning of visceral and glandular responses. *Science, 163,* 434–445.

Moss, D. (2001). Biofeedback. In S. Shannon (Ed.), *Handbook of complementary and alternative therapies in mental health.* San Diego, CA: Academic Press.

Moss, D., Andrasik, F., McGrady, A., Perry, J. D., & Baskin, S. M. (2001). Biofeedback can help headache sufferers. *Biofeedback, 29*(4), 11–13.

Mulholland, T. (1977). Biofeedback as scientific method. In G. E. Schwartz & J. Beatty (Eds.), *Biofeedback: Theory and research* (pp. 9–28). New York: Academic Press.

Rokicki, L. A., Holroyd, K. A., France, C. R., Lipchik, G. L., France, J. L., & Kvaal, S. A. (1997). Change mechanisms associated with combined relaxation/ EMG biofeedback training for chronic tension headache. *Applied Psychophysiology and Biofeedback, 22,* 21–41.

Schultz, J., & Luthe, W. (1959). *Autogenic therapy.* New York: Grune & Stratton.

Schwartz, M., & Andrasik, F. (in press). *Biofeedback: A practitioner's guide* (3rd ed.). New York: Guilford.

Schwartz, M., & Associates. (1995). *Biofeedback: A practitioner's guide* (2nd ed.). New York: Guilford.

Selye, H. (1976). *The stress of life* (rev. ed.). New York: McGraw-Hill.

Shellenberger, R., Amar, P., Schneider, P., & Turner, J. (1994). *Clinical efficacy and cost effectiveness of biofeedback therapy. Guidelines for third party reimbursement.* Wheat Ridge, CO: Association for Applied Psychophysiology and Biofeedback.

Shellenberger, R., & Green, J. (1987). Specific effects of biofeedback versus biofeedback-assisted relaxation training. *Biofeedback & Self-Regulation, 12*(3), 185–209.

Sovak, M., Kunzel, M., Sternbach, R. A., & Dalessio, D. J. (1981). Mechanism of the biofeedback therapy of migraine: Volitional manipulation of the psychophysiological background. *Headache, 21,* 89–92.

Sterman, M. B. (1986). Epilepsy and its treatment with EEG feedback therapy. *Annals of Behavioral Medicine, 8,* 21–25.

Tart, C. (1969). *Altered states of consciousness.* New York: Wiley.

Taub, E., & School, P. J. (1978). Some methodological considerations in thermal biofeedback training. *Behavior Research Methods and Instrumentation, 10,* 617–622.

Wickramasekera, I. (1999). The faith factor, the placebo, and AAPB. *Biofeedback, 27*(1), 1A–3A.

# CHAPTER 9

# Neurofeedback, Neurotherapy, and Quantitative EEG

## Theodore J. La Vaque

**Abstract:** Neurofeedback is the use of electroencephalograph (EEG) biofeedback to modify cortical (brain) activity, alter states of consciousness, and affect cortically mediated physical and psychological functioning. Neurotherapy is the clinical application of neurofeedback to modify cortical functioning in clinically beneficial ways. Neurotherapy can include the use of audiovisual stimulation as well as operant feedback procedures. Research provides at least moderate support for applying neurotherapy to a variety of disorders, including seizures, attention deficit hyperactivity disorder, depression, anxiety disorders, addictive disorders, and closed head injuries. Quantitative EEG (QEEG) involves the diagnostic use of multisite digital EEG to sample cortical electrical activity recorded at 19 to 128 different electrode sites. In cases where adequate normative databases are available, the QEEG data can be subjected to statistical analysis for comparison to age-specific population norms. QEEG results can improve the effectiveness of neurotherapy by identifying areas of abnormal cortical function, which can become the focus for intervention.

## ORIGINS

The emergence of operant or instrumental conditioning procedures using brain-wave technology (electroencephalography, or EEG) for research and clinical applications has been made possible largely by advances in computer technology.[1] Technical fundamentals such as quantitative electroencephalography (QEEG), brain mapping, and normative databases have existed conceptually and factually for many years (Berger, 1932; Gibbs & Knott, 1949; John, Karmel, et al., 1977; John & Prichep, 1993; Matousek & Petersen, 1973; Walter, 1943, 1954). Certainly, the operant conditioning principles used to acquire control of physiological states (biofeedback) are well understood. The computational power of the personal computer has permitted the practical integration of EEG technology with operant conditioning procedures to develop EEG biofeedback, now often referred to as neurofeedback.

Neurotherapy is a clinical intervention based on neurofeedback that uses the technical principles of operant conditioning to facilitate specific corrective changes in the brain state assumed to underlie particular clinical disorders. We implicitly assume that neurotherapy ameliorates the symptoms by "normalizing" the underlying dysfunctional brain state, but that critical assumption has not been well tested (La Vaque, 1999). In the case of attention deficit hyperactivity disorder (ADD/HD), for instance, the goal of neurotherapy is to "change cortical functioning" by "establishing a 'cortical template' that responds, in terms of its EEG signatures, similarly to that of non-ADD/HD individuals in those circumstances and situations that cause problems for the ADD/HD child, adolescent, or adult" (Lubar, 1995). In other words, the ADD/HD subject is trained to produce cortical activity more similar to that of a normal, more attentive individual, in any given situation.

Thus, neurofeedback is a particular application of an operant conditioning paradigm in which selected features of brain activity are recorded, amplified, and displayed back to the subject in visual and/or auditory form at a speed very close to "real time." Successful changes in those EEG features are rewarded and reinforced to facilitate acquisition of voluntary control over the brain activity that generates those signals. The electrophysiological signals may be components of the QEEG (e.g., frequency, coherence, etc.) or evoked potentials.

A variant of the typical EEG biofeedback procedure is audiovisual stimulation (AVS), which "drives" the desired EEG frequency using photic stimulation (Frederick, Lubar, Rasey, Brim, & Blackburn, 1999; Kumano et al., 1996). In AVS, the subject is exposed to strobing light and sound at preselected frequencies, and this exposure entrains the brain to emulate, in its dominant frequency, the frequency of the light and sound.

## INSTRUMENTATION AND PROCEDURES

To understand neurotherapy, it is necessary to acquire an appreciation of the sometimes arcane world and vocabulary of EEG and QEEG. QEEG analyses are used to assist in differential diagnosis and to guide the individual neurotherapy protocol. QEEG refers to the mathematical and statistical analysis of the complex waveform of the standard, or analog, EEG, which is recorded as the changes in electrical potential created by electrochemical events of the brain (cortex) and measured from the human scalp (Fisch, 1991; Speckman & Elger, 1993). The complex waveform is analyzed using a mathematical Fourier analysis or fast Fourier transform (FFT) to reveal the component frequencies resulting in the QEEG. Then neurofeedback training parameters are based on features derived from the QEEG analysis.

## TERMINOLOGY

*Spectral Analysis.* The spectral analysis of EEG signals is accomplished in the frequency domain (with frequency on the X axis, amplitude on the Y axis), as opposed to the more familiar time domain ("strip chart" recording, with time on the X axis and amplitude on the Y axis).

*Compressed Spectral Analysis.* Multiple frequency domain graphs present? as a three-dimensional figure, with time on the Z axis (see Figure 9.1). A single active electrode permits only an analysis of frequency (cycles per second, or Hz) and magnitude as microvolts ($\mu V$) or power ($\mu V^2$). Multiple electrode recording (such as the 19-channel International 10-20 System configuration (see Figure 9.2) allows further analysis of additional between-channel features of the EEG, defined by the following terms:

*Phase.* The degree of waveform offset between channels that indicates *transmission time* between cortical areas in milliseconds.

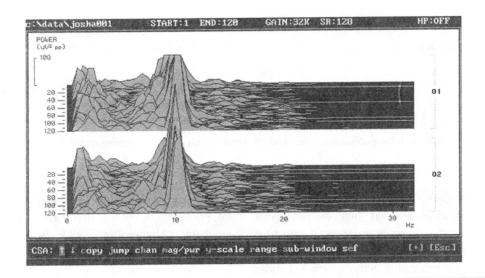

**Figure 9.1    Compressed Spectral Analysis (CSA)**

Notes: Frequency (Hz) is represented on the horizontal (X) axis, power ($\mu V^2$) on the vertical (Y) axis, and time by epoch number on the Z axis. Electrode location is identified on the right ($O_1$ and $O_2$). This CSA, from an eyes-closed EEG, shows a specific dominant frequency at about 10 Hz (alpha) at locations $O_1$ and $O_2$. The EEG was monitored with a Lexicor Neurosearch 24, using Lexicor version 151 software to process the signal.

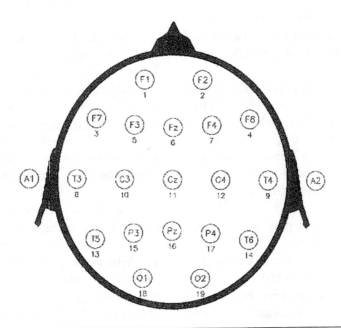

**Figure 9.2    Locations and Labels for the International 10-20 System**

SOURCE: Hudspeth (1998). Used with permission from Grey Matters, Inc.

Notes: C = central, P = parietal, T = temporal, O = occipital, F = frontal. All midline sites are designated with z (e.g., Cz). Sites to the left of midline are odd numbered (e.g., C3), and sites to the right of midline are even numbered (e.g., C4).

**Table 9.1**    Classic Designations of Cortical Frequency Bands

| Frequency Bands (Hz) | Label | Subjective State (Cycles/Second) |
|---|---|---|
| 0–4 | Delta (δ) | Sleep states |
| 4–8 | Theta (θ) | Daydreaming, imagery, working memory |
| 8–12 | Alpha (α) | Awake, receptive, meditative |
| 12–20 | Beta (β) | Activated, focused |

Note: The exact numerical specification of the frequency bands varies considerably among specialists.

*Coherence.* A cross-correlation function between channels that suggests *functional connectivity* among brain areas. If two sites are highly coherent with a minimal phase delay, the processing activity between those sites is highly synchronized (Nunez et al., 1997; Thatcher, Krause, & Hrybyk, 1986).

*Amplitude Asymmetry.* Magnitude differences between channels.

*Brain Map.* A graphical display, usually in color, showing the topographic distribution of particular EEG features across the head.

*Frequency Band.* A particular frequency range. The classic bands are delta (δ, 0 to 4 Hz); theta (θ, 4 to 8 Hz); alpha (α, 8 to 12 Hz); and beta (β, 12 to 20 Hz). Each of these classic frequency bands is associated with a typical state of alertness, vigilance, consciousness, or cognitive activity (see Table 9.1).

EEG waveforms can now easily be analyzed down to single hertz "bins," or even fractions of a hertz, and might be designated as $\delta_1$ (0 to 2 Hz), $\delta_2$ (2 to 4 Hz), and so forth. Other frequency bands have been recognized, such as the sensorimotor rhythm (SMR) recorded from the sensory motor strip of the cortex (11 to 15 Hz); the Mu rhythm, also recorded from the sensory motor cortex, and consisting of an arch-shaped wave (7 to 11 Hz); and gamma (γ), a designation typically reserved for very high frequencies of 40 Hz and above. Slow cortical potentials (SCPs) below 1 Hz are also used in neurofeedback (Altenmüller, 1993; Birbaumer, 1997; Birbaumer & Flor, 1999).

*Ratios.* Standardized values in QEEG are often expressed as magnitude or power ratios between bands. For example, the *theta/beta ratio* shows the ratio between the magnitude or power of theta activity and the magnitude or power of beta activity.

*Epoch.* An EEG sample size is specified as a time range, as in a 1-second epoch, a 2-second epoch, and so forth. The epoch is also used to identify a particular point in the record, as in epochs 27 and 256. The most common epoch length used for quantitative analysis is 1 second, and a minimum of about 60 seconds of artifact-free EEG (60 epochs) should be available for analysis.

*Montage.* The particular combination of electrodes used to define a channel. The most frequent montage used in neurofeedback is the referential montage, using the earlobes as the electrical reference sites. One considerable advantage of the computer-acquired EEG is that the EEG can be "remontaged" within the computer to examine the EEG in a variety of different ways (Goldensohn, Legatte, Koszer, & Wolf, 1999).

Once the vocabulary and associated concepts are understood, a (theoretical) neurofeedback protocol might be described as "increasing theta$_2$ coherence between C3 and C4 using a linked ear reference" or "decreasing F1–F2 delta amplitude asymmetry." (The labels C3, C4, F1, and F2 refer to locations on the scalp designated in the International 10-20 System, as shown in Figure 9.2.)

## NORMATIVE DATABASES

Once it became practical to digitize and mathematically analyze the EEG, the way was opened for the development of normative databases. Since the EEG features change dramatically with maturation, the EEG of a child must be interpreted differently from that of an adolescent, and the adolescent EEG is not the same as that of the adult (Epstein, 1980; Gasser, Jennen-Steinmetz, Sroka, Verleger, & Mochs, 1988; Gasser, Verleger, Bocher, & Sroka, 1988; Hudspeth, 1985; Hudspeth & Pribram, 1992; Knott & Gibbs, 1939). Reliable diagnostic conclusions about the QEEG of a child at various ages are only possible when an age-specific normative database is available. As a very general description, maturation in the EEG is reflected as a gradual decrease in slow wave (theta and delta bands) dominance, increased presence of faster activity (alpha and beta), and increased cortical differentiation. Developmental equations allow the QEEG to be interpreted according to age-specific norms (John, Ahn, et al., 1980; Matousek & Petersen, 1973). The equations have been shown to be stable across cultures (Alvarez, Valdez, & Pasquale, 1987; Matsuura et al., 1993).

Further, the technology of neurometric analysis developed by John and colleagues (John, Ahn, et al., 1980) uses mathematically derived *discriminant functions* to assist in differential diagnosis of certain psychiatric disorders and postconcussion syndrome (John, 1989; John, Karmel, et al., 1977;

John, Prichep, et al., 1994; Thatcher, Walker, Gerson, & Geisler, 1989), and of developmental disorders such as ADD/HD (Chabot, Merkin, Wood, Davenport, & Serfontein, 1996; Chabot, Orgill, Crawford, Harris, & Serfontein, 1999; Chabot & Serfontein, 1996; Monastra et al., 1999; Suffin & Emory, 1995). The development of generally accepted discriminant functions as "laboratory tests" for such disorders is an important aid in differential diagnosis.

## LEARNING PRINCIPLES

Research demonstrates that neurofeedback methods follow the known characteristics of operant conditioning, and, using these principles, voluntary control of brain-wave activity can be acquired in both animals and humans. Operant conditioning of the auditory-evoked potential has also been demonstrated in humans. In one of the earliest such experiments, the subjects were given a monetary reward for increasing a segment of the evoked potential (a negative-going peak at 200 msec.) by one standard deviation above baseline (Rosenfeld, Rudell, & Fox, 1969). Although the percentage of responses was modest (30 percent of the responses reached the criterion as a function of the operant procedure), the principle was clearly demonstrated.

The early research that ultimately led to EEG operant procedures for seizure disorder and attention disorders began with animal studies examining the toxic effects of hydrazine compounds used as rocket fuel. There was a serendipitous observation that cats operantly trained to produce sensorimotor rhythm (in a previous sleep study) were unaccountably resistant to chemically induced seizures at doses that produced a 100 percent seizure rate in "SMR-naïve" cats. This research led to human trials of SMR training for seizure control with remarkable results (Sterman, 2000). Other studies have demonstrated equally successful operant control of the slow cortical potentials (SCP) for seizure control (Kotchoubey, Strehl, et al., 1999). Later studies using SMR neurofeedback for control of hyperactivity in children ultimately led to studies of theta-suppression neurofeedback for the treatment of ADD/HD (Lubar, 1991; Lubar & Shouse, 1976). Lubar and his colleagues, examining the ability to decrease theta, demonstrated that there are "good learners" and "poor learners" in neurofeedback settings. Of 17 children entered into a theta-suppression/beta-enhancement study using a bipolar midline montage, 11 demonstrated the ability to alter the theta/beta ratio, while 6 did not (Lubar, Swartwood, Swartwood, & Timmermann, 1995).

Recent research in brain-computer interface (BCI) technology has been directed to operant conditioning of the Mu rhythm and SCP as a voluntary, controlled-signal source that would allow people with severe motor diseases to control a neuroprosthesis or communication device that would help "unlock" them from their disorder (Birbaumer, Kubler, et al., 2000; McFarland, McCane, David, & Wolpaw, 1997; McFarland, McCane, & Wolpaw, 1998; Vaughan, Miner, McFarland, & Wolpaw, 1998; Wolpaw, Birbaumer, et al., 2000). Subjects operantly trained to control the Mu rhythm repeatedly demonstrate the ability to control the direction of movement of a cursor on a computer screen with a high degree of accuracy (Wolpaw, Flotzinger, Pfurtscheller, & McFarland, 1997). An EEG-driven spelling device for completely paralyzed patients is under development (Birbaumer, Ghanayim, et al., 1999).

The demonstration of learned, voluntary EEG control is compelling. However, the necessary relationship between specific neurotherapy interventions and symptom relief has not been demonstrated as clearly in other applications, as some critics have pointed out (Birbaumer & Flor, 1999; Duffy, 2000; La Vaque, 1999). Clinical studies rarely report pre- or posttreatment QEEG changes related to the treatment protocol. A clear exception is the research on seizure control. A further step in this direction was recently accomplished in a limited study of neurotherapy for brain trauma; this study showed a direct relationship among the specific training parameters of the neurotherapy protocol, changes in the brain-wave features in the predetermined direction and the degree of improvement in the brain trauma symptoms (Thornton, 2000).

## DOCUMENTED APPLICATIONS

The case for neurotherapy efficacy has been made for several disorders. The definition of *efficacy* can be difficult, and the criteria should be as explicit as possible. The Association for Applied Psychophysiology and Biofeedback (AAPB) and Division 12 of the American Psychological Association (APA) adopted similar criteria for the definition of *validated treatments*. The Society of Clinical Psychology (APA Division 12) Task Force on Promotion and Dissemination of Psychological Procedures published "Criteria for Empirically Validated Treatments" (Chambless, 1995; Chambless & Hollon, 1998), which the AAPB Board adopted *in toto* in 1997 (Striefel, 1998). The criterion for well-established treatments is at least one of the following:

• A minimum of two good group design studies, conducted by different investigators, that demonstrate efficacy by *superiority* of the investigative treatment (neurotherapy, in this instance) to pill, placebo, or other treatment, or *equivalence* to an established treatment in studies with adequate statistical power.

• A large series of single case design studies that demonstrate efficacy, have good experimental designs, and compare the intervention to another treatment.

Both criteria require that the characteristics of the client samples be clearly specified and that the studies be carried out with treatment manuals. Conclusions based on less rigorous standards, such as waiting-list controls, evidence by same investigator, group studies flawed by heterogeneity of the patient samples, or a small series of single case studies that meet the criteria for well-established treatments, would be considered as preliminary evidence or, at best, probably efficacious. Neurotherapy studies seem to rely on historical controls rather than group designs incorporating internal research controls such as sham feedback or active (other treatment) controls. A direct comparison to drug treatment or to other accepted therapies constitutes a treatment equivalence or noninferiority design. Historical controls are generally regarded as suspect unless the course of the disorder is very well established. The issue of placebo controls versus active controls is rife with statistical and ethical controversy (Glaros, 2001; La Vaque & Rossiter, 2001a, 2001b; Striefel, 2001; Temple & Ellenberg, 2000). Most published reports in neurofeedback come from clinical studies in which large samples and standard control designs are not feasible. The conditions under which clinical psychophysiological studies can or should follow the same experimental design requirements established for pharmacological and/or biomedical studies to establish treatment efficacy are currently unclear (La Vaque, 2001; La Vaque & Rossiter, 2001a).

## Seizure Disorder

Evidence for the efficacy of operant EEG procedures for the control of intractable epilepsy is strong. In a review of the relevant research, Sterman (2000) examined the neurophysiological substrates of SMR operant procedures as they relate to seizure control and reviewed much of the extensive literature that supports this intervention. In a meta-analysis of the literature, Sterman identified 19 peer-reviewed articles from 1972 to 1996 covering 174 subjects treated using the SMR paradigm. A total of 142 (82 percent) of the patients demonstrated clinical improvement and, where measured, 66 percent of the cases exhibited EEG improvement according to pre- and posttreatment EEG measures.

SCP biofeedback has also been remarkably successful for improved control of drug-resistant, intractable epilepsy. The literature is too expansive for this chapter, hence a brief discussion will have to suffice. Kotchoubey, Busch, Strehl, and Birbaumer (1999) noted that both SMR and SCP feedback studies report similar success rates, with improvement observed in about two-thirds of the patients. They examined changes in EEG power spectra as a function of SCP biofeedback in 34 patients in an attempt to determine whether the two approaches affect different cortical mechanisms or whether both approaches actually produce the same cortical response. The patients were trained to produce either SCP positivity or negativity in response to discriminative stimuli (the letter *A* or *B* presented on the screen) during feedback trials, and they were required to perform the discrimination task in the absence of feedback later during transfer trials. EEG was simultaneously recorded at Cz (the vertex or cortical center in the International 10-20 System). The main consistent finding was increased power of $theta_2$ (6.0 to 7.9 Hz) activity and decreased power in all other bands only during transfer trials. They hypothesized that the increased $theta_2$ power may reflect either the high degree of internal awareness (autocentric attention) required in the absence of external feedback when patients concentrated on their internal state or the cortical inhibitory processes associated with slow positive shifts. The relationship between SCP and SMR thus remains unclear. However, the improved control over even "intractable" seizures is so compelling that "to continue to single out EEG operant conditioning as 'experimental' seems neither rational, objective, or in the best interest of these patients" (Sterman, 2000, p. 53).

## Attention Deficit Hyperactivity Disorder

Perhaps the most recognized clinical application of neurotherapy is the treatment of ADD/HD. The increasing popularity of the treatment has been paralleled by increasing controversy about its efficacy. See Chapter 25 for a detailed discussion of neurotherapy and ADD/HD.

In one of the larger studies, 98 children and 13 adults attended forty 50-minute sessions using the Lubar protocol of theta suppression combined with metacognitive strategies aimed toward improving academic skills (Thompson & Thompson, 1998). The number of children taking Ritalin declined from 30 percent at the beginning of treatment to 6 percent after treatment. Objective pre- and posttreatment measures demonstrated significantly increased ($p<.001$) intelligence scores, with increases averaging 12 points (attributed to improved attention to the test tasks), normalized scores on the computerized continuous performance task (Test of Variable Attention, or TOVA), and improved academic performance based on the Wide Range Achievement Test (WRAT 3). The adult theta/beta microvolt ratios declined from 2.6 to 1.8 ($p<.08$), and the child ratios declined from 3.3 to 2.3 ($p<.0001$).

A large medical-center study carried out from May 1994 through March 1997 examined QEEG differences between 209 normal and 165 ADHD children (Camp, 1999). As part of that study, 48 children also participated in a study comparing EEG biofeedback (theta suppression) to cognitive-behavioral therapies. Pre- and posttherapy change scores were measured using the TOVA, teacher and parent behavior rating scales (ACTeRS), and ADD/HD scales taken from the *DSM-IV* (SNAP-IV). Camp concluded that "behavioral improvement following biofeedback training is comparable to the best and somewhat better than the best efforts achieved with the cognitive behavior modification program" (p. 71). Camp further noted that EEG biofeedback led to greater cognitive performance and "parent enthusiasm" than did cognitive behavior modification.

Similar results are demonstrated in an active control (treatment equivalence) study directly comparing the benefits of psychostimulant medication (MEDS group, $N = 23$) to EEG biofeedback for theta suppression (EEG group, $N = 23$) (Rossiter & La Vaque, 1995). The purpose of the study was to determine whether it was possible to identify treatment response at approximately the halfway point of therapy. The groups were closely matched for age, intelligence level, gender, diagnosis, and pre- and post-TOVA. Repeated TOVA measures were obtained from both groups halfway into EEG therapy (session 20). Both the EEG (19 of 23) and MEDS (20 of 23) groups showed significant improvement in measures of attention, impulsivity, processing speed, and response variability; there were no significant differences between groups in the change scores.

## OTHER APPLICATIONS

Other clinical applications for neurofeedback have exciting potential but have not yet developed to the point of demonstrated efficacy. Frontal alpha asymmetry feedback for affective disorders (Rosenfeld, 2000; Rosenfeld, Cha, Blair, & Gotlib, 1995) is an application with exciting prospects. The theoretical underpinnings derived from the affective sequelae of frontal lobe stroke and electrophysiological studies of depression point the way. Chapter 27 discusses the asymmetry training protocol for depression in more detail.

Several additional applications are under investigation, including neurotherapy for clinical disorders such as schizophrenia using SCP (Gruzalier, 2000); alpha enhancement or reduction for anxiety disorders (Moore, 2000; Rice, Blanchard, & Purcell, 1993); and alpha enhancement, alpha-theta feedback, or SMR-beta neurofeedback for addictive disorders (Trudeau, 2000; Trudeau, Thuras, & Stockley, 1999). More research needs to be done to satisfactorily demonstrate clinical efficacy for these applications.

## CONCLUSION

The full potential of neurofeedback and neurotherapy remains to be seen. Modern neuroscience is uncovering the extraordinary plasticity of the brain—its ability to change function and microstructure in some fundamental ways based on experience. Neurofeedback offers us a vision of human beings modifying brain function to exert at least some control over a host of brain-mediated medical and emotional disorders. Neurofeedback is already a useful clinical tool and offers a brighter future.

## NOTE

1. In this case, *operant conditioning* means a learning process that proceeds by positive reinforcement for desired behaviors and no reinforcement (no reward) for undesired behaviors. The individual receives positive reinforcement (reward) in the form of visual feedback and auditory tones whenever his or her brain waves move closer to the criterion brain pattern. The individual receives no reward when certain other undesired physiological states occur, such as an increase in muscle tension or an increase in a brain-wave frequency incompatible with the criterion pattern.

## REFERENCES

Altenmüller, E. O. (1993). Psychophysiology and EEG. In E. Niedermeyer & F. Lopes Da Silva (Eds.), *Electroencephalography: Basic principles, clinical applications, and related fields* (3rd ed., pp. 597–614). Baltimore: Williams & Wilkins.

Alvarez, A., Valdez, P., & Pasquale, R. (1987). EEG developmental equations confirmed for Cuban schoolchildren. *Electroencephalography and Clinical Neurophysiology, 67*, 330–332.

Berger, H. (1932). Über das Elektrenkephalogramm des Menschen [Concerning the electroencephalogram of the human being]. Vierte Mitteilung. *Archiv für Psychiatrie und Nervenkrankheiten, 97*, 6–26.

Birbaumer, N. (1997). Multiple functional effects of biofeedback with slow cortical potentials. *Biofeedback, 25*(1), 12–13, 22.

Birbaumer, N., & Flor, H. (1999). Applied psychophysiology and learned physiological regulation. *Applied Psychophysiology and Biofeedback, 24*(1), 35–37; discussion, 43–54.

Birbaumer, N., Ghanayim, N., Hinterberger, T., Iversen, I., Kotchoubey, B., Kubler, A., et al. (1999). A spelling device for the paralysed. *Nature, 398 (6725),* 297–298.

Birbaumer, N., Kubler, A., Ghanayim, N., Hinterberger, T., Perelmouter, J., Kaiser, J., et al. (2000). The thought translation device (TTD) for completely paralyzed patients. *IEEE Transactions in Rehabilitation Engineering, 8*(2), 190–193.

Camp, B. W. (1999). *Attention deficit hyperactivity disorders: Studies of EEG patterns and biofeedback training* (Final Report, Grant No. H113G40130). Washington, DC: U.S. Office of Education.

Chabot, R. J., Merkin, M., Wood, L. M., Davenport, T. L., & Serfontein, G. (1996). Sensitivity and specificity of QEEG in children with attention deficit or specific developmental learning disorders. *Clinical Electroencephalography, 27,* 26–34.

Chabot, R. J., Orgill, A. A., Crawford, G., Harris, M. J., & Serfontein, G. (1999). Behavioral and electrophysiologic predictors of treatment response to stimulants in children with attention disorders. *Journal of Child Neurology, 14*(6), 343–351.

Chabot, R. J., & Serfontein, G. (1996). Quantitative electroencephalographic profiles of children with attention deficit disorder. *Biological Psychiatry, 40*(10), 951–963.

Chambless, D. L. (1995). Task force on promotion and dissemination of psychological procedures. *Clinical Psychologist, 48*(1).

Chambless, D. L., & Hollon, S. D. (1998). Defining empirically supported therapies. *Journal of Consulting and Clinical Psychology, 66*(1), 7–18.

Duffy, F. H. (2000). The state of EEG biofeedback therapy (EEG operant conditioning) in 2000: An editor's opinion. *Clinical Electroencephalography, 31*(1), v–viii.

Epstein, H. (1980). EEG developmental stages. *Developmental Psychobiology, 13,* 629–631.

Fisch, B. J. (1991). *Spehlman's EEG primer* (2nd ed.). New York: Elsevier.

Frederick, J., Lubar, J., Rasey, H., Brim, S., & Blackburn, J. (1999). Effects of 18.5 Hz auditory and visual stimulation on EEG amplitude at the vertex. *Journal of Neurotherapy, 3,* 23–28.

Gasser, T., Jennen-Steinmetz, C., Sroka, L., Verleger, R., & Mochs, J. (1988). Development of the EEG of school-age children and adolescents. II. Topography. *Electroencephalography and Clinical Neurophysiology, 69,* 100–109.

Gasser, T., Verleger, R., Bocher, P., & Sroka, L. (1988). Development of the EEG of school-age children and adolescents. I. Analysis of band power. *Electroencephalography and Clinical Neurophysiology, 69,* 91–99.

Gibbs, F. A., & Knott, J. R. (1949). Growth of the electrical activity of the cortex. *Electroencephalography and Clinical Neurophysiology, 1,* 223–229.

Glaros, A. G. (2001). A comment on La Vaque and Rossiter. *Applied Psychophysiology and Biofeedback, 26*(1), 61–65.

Goldensohn, E. S., Legatte, A. D., Koszer, S., & Wolf, S. M. (1999). *Goldensohn's EEG Interpretation: Problems of overreading and underrreading* (2nd ed.). Armonk, NY: Futura.

Gruzalier, J. (2000). Self-regulation of electrocortical activity in schizophrenia and schizotypy: A review. *Clinical Electroencephalography, 31*(1), 23–29.

Hudspeth, W. (1985). Developmental neuropsychology: Functional implications of quantitative EEG maturation [Abstract]. *Journal of Clinical and Experimental Neuropsychology, 7,* 606.

Hudspeth, W. (1998). *Neurorep: QEEG analysis and report system.* Reno, NV: Grey Matters.

Hudspeth, W., & Pribram, K. (1992). Psychophysiological indices of cerebral maturation. *International Journal of Psychophysiology, 12,* 19–29.

Jasper, H. H. (1958). The ten-twenty electrode system of the International Federation. *Electrophysiology and Clinical Neurology, 10,* 371–375.

John, E. R. (1989). The role of quantitative EEG topographic mapping or "neurometrics" in the diagnosis of psychiatric and neurological disorders: The pros. *Electroencephalography and Clinical Neurophysiology, 73,* 2–4.

John, E. R., Ahn, H., Prichep, L. S., Trepetin, M., Brown, D., & Kaye, H. (1980). Developmental equations for the electroencephalogram. *Science, 210,* 1255–1258.

John, E. R., Karmel, B. Z., Corning, W. C., Easton, P., Brown, D., Ahn, H., et al. (1977). Neurometrics: Numerical taxonomy identifies different profiles of brain functions within groups of behaviorally similar people. *Science, 196,* 1393–1410.

John, E. R., & Prichep, L. S. (1993). Principles of neurometric analysis of EEG and evoked potentials. In E. Niedermeyer & F. Lopes Da Silva (Eds.), *Electroencephalography: Basic principles, clinical applications, and related fields* (3rd ed., pp. 989–1003). Baltimore: Williams & Wilkins.

John, E. R., Prichep, L. S., Alper, K. R., Mas, F. G., Cancro, R., Easton, P., et al. (1994). Quantitative electrophysiological characteristics and subtyping of schizophrenia. *Biological Psychiatry, 36*(12), 801–826.

Knott, J. R., & Gibbs, F. A. (1939). A Fourier analysis of the electroencephalogram from one to eighteen years. *Psychological Bulletin, 36,* 512–513.

Kotchoubey, B., Busch, S., Strehl, U., & Birbaumer, N. (1999). Changes in EEG power spectra during biofeedback of slow cortical potentials in epilepsy. *Applied Psychophysiology and Biofeedback, 24*(4), 213–233.

Kotchoubey, B., Strehl, U., Holzapfel, S., Schneider, D., Blankenhorn, V., & Birbaumer, N. (1999). Control of cortical excitability in epilepsy. *Advances in Neurology, 81,* 281–290.

Kumano, H., Horie, H., Shidara, T., Kuboki, T., Suematsu, H., & Yasushi, M. (1996). Treatment of a depressive disorder patient with EEG-driven photic stimulation. *Biofeedback & Self-Regulation, 21*(4), 323–334.

La Vaque, T. J. (1999). Neurotherapy and clinical science. *Journal of Neurotherapy, 3*(3&4), 29–31.

La Vaque, T. J. (2001). Pills, politics, and placebos. *Journal of Neurotherapy, 5*(1), 73–86.

La Vaque, T. J., & Rossiter, T. R. (2001a). The ethical use of placebo controls in clinical research: The Declaration of Helsinki. *Applied Psychophysiology and Biofeedback, 26*(1), 23–37.

La Vaque, T. J., & Rossiter, T. R. (2001b). Response to Striefel and Glaros. *Applied Psychophysiology and Biofeedback, 26*(1), 67–71.

Lubar, J. F. (1991). Discourse on the development of EEG diagnostics and biofeedback for attention deficit/hyperactivity disorders. *Biofeedback & Self-Regulation, 16,* 202–225.

Lubar, J. F. (1995). Neurofeedback for the management of attention-deficit/hyperactivity disorder. In M. S. Schwartz & Associates (Eds.), *Biofeedback: A practitioners guide* (2nd ed., pp. 493–522). New York: Guilford.

Lubar, J. F., & Shouse, M. N. (1976). EEG and behavioral changes in a hyperkinetic child concurrent with training of the sensorimotor rhythm (SMR): A preliminary report. *Biofeedback & Self-Regulation, 3,* 293–306.

Lubar, J. F., Swartwood, M. O., Swartwood, D. I., & Timmermann, D. L. (1995). Quantitative EEG and auditory event-related potentials in the evaluation of attention-deficit/hyperactivity disorder: Effects of methylphenidate and implications for neurofeedback training. *Journal of Psychoeducational Assessment* [ADHD Special], 143–160.

Matousek, M., & Petersen, I. (1973). Automatic evaluation of EEG background activity by means of age-dependent EEG quotients. *Electroencephalography and Clinical Neurophysiology, 35*, 603–612.

Matsuura, M., Okubo, Y., Toro, M., Kojima, T., He, Y., Hou, Y., Shen, Y., & Lee, C. K. (1993). A cross-national EEG study of children with emotional and behavioral problems: A WHO collaborative study in the western Pacific region. *Biological Psychiatry, 34*, 59–65.

McFarland, D. J., McCane, L. M., David, S. V., & Wolpaw, J. R. (1997). Spatial filter selection for EEG-based communication. *Electroencephalography and Clinical Neurophysiology, 103*, 386–394.

McFarland, D. J., McCane, L. M., & Wolpaw, J. R. (1998). EEG-based communication and control: Short-term role of feedback. *IEEE Transactions in Rehabilitation Engineering, 6*(1), 7–11.

Monastra, V. J., Lubar, J. F., Linden, M., Van Deusen, P., Green, G., Wing, W., et al. (1999). Assessing attention deficit hyperactivity disorder via quantitative electroencephalography: An initial validation study. *Neuropsychology, 13*(3), 424–433.

Moore, N. C. (2000). A review of EEG biofeedback treatment of anxiety disorders. *Clinical Electroencephalography, 31*(1), 1–6.

Nunez, P. L., Srinivasan, R., Westdorp, A. F., Tucker, D. M., Silberstein, R. B., & Cadusch, P. J. (1997). EEG coherency. I: Statistics, reference electrode, volume conduction, Laplacians, cortical imaging, and interpretation at multiple scales. *Electroencephalography and Clinical Neurophysiology, 103*(5), 499–515.

Rice, K. M., Blanchard, E. B., & Purcell, M. (1993). Biofeedback treatments of generalized anxiety disorder: Preliminary results. *Biofeedback & Self-Regulation, 18*(2), 93–105.

Rosenfeld, J. P. (2000). An EEG biofeedback protocol for affective disorders. *Clinical Electroencephalography, 31*(1), 7–12.

Rosenfeld, J. P., Cha, G., Blair, T., & Gotlib, I. H. (1995). Operant (biofeedback) control of left-right frontal alpha power differences: Potential neurotherapy for affective disorders. *Biofeedback & Self-Regulation, 20*(3), 241–258.

Rosenfeld, J. P., Rudell, A., & Fox, S. (1969). Operant control of neural events in humans. *Science, 165*, 821–823.

Rossiter, T. R., & La Vaque, T. J. (1995). A comparison of EEG biofeedback and psychostimulants in treating attention deficit hyperactivity disorders. *Journal of Neurotherapy, 1*, 48–59.

Speckman, E.-F., & Elger, C. E. (1993). Introduction to the neurophysiological basis of the EEG and DC potentials. In E. Niedermeyer & F. Lopes Da Silva (Eds.), *Electroencephalography: Basic principles, clinical applications, and related fields* (3rd ed., pp. 15–26). Baltimore: Williams & Wilkins.

Sterman, M. B. (2000). Basic concepts and clinical findings in the treatment of seizure disorders with EEG operant conditioning. *Clinical Electroencephalography, 31*(1), 45–55.

Striefel, S. (1998). Is EEG biofeedback *per se* experimental? *Biofeedback, 26*(4), 4–6, 12.

Striefel, S. (2001). Ethical research issues: Going beyond the Declaration of Helsinki. *Applied Psychophysiology and Biofeedback, 26*(1), 39–59.

Suffin, S. C., & Emory, W. H. (1995). Neurometric subgroups in attentional and affective disorders and their association with pharmacotherapeutic outcome. *Clinical Electroencephalography, 26*, 76–83.

Temple, R., & Ellenberg, S. S. (2000). Placebo-controlled trials and active-control trials in the evaluation of new treatments. Part 1: Ethical and scientific issues. *Annals of Internal Medicine, 133*(6), 455–463.

Thatcher, R. W., Krause, P. J., & Hrybyk, M. (1986). Cortico-cortical associations and EEG coherence: A two-compartment model. *Electroencephalography and Clinical Neurophysiology, 64,* 123–143.

Thatcher, R. W., Walker, R. A., Gerson, I., & Geisler, F. H. (1989). EEG discriminant analysis of mild head trauma. *Electroencephalography and Clinical Neurophysiology, 73,* 94–106.

Thompson, L., & Thompson, M. (1998). Neurofeedback combined with training in metacognitive strategies: Effectiveness in students with ADD. *Applied Psychophysiology and Biofeedback, 23*(4), 243–263.

Thornton, K. (2000). Improvement/rehabilitation of memory functioning with neurotherapy/QEEG biofeedback. *Journal of Head Trauma Rehabilitation, 15*(6), 1285–1296.

Trudeau, D. L. (2000). The treatment of addictive disorders by brain wave biofeedback: A review and suggestions for future research. *Clinical Electroencephalography, 31*(1), 13–22.

Trudeau, D. L., Thuras, P., & Stockley, H. (1999). Quantitative EEG findings associated with chronic stimulant and cannabis abuse and ADHD in an adult male substance use disorder population. *Clinical Electroencephalography, 30*(4), 165–174.

Vaughan, T. M., Miner, L. A., McFarland, D. J., & Wolpaw, J. R. (1998). EEG-based communication: Analysis of concurrent EMG activity. *Electroencephalography and Clinical Neurophysiology, 107*(6), 428–433.

Walter, W. G. (1943, June). An automatic low frequency analyzer. *Electronic Engineering,* 9–13.

Walter, W. G. (1954, June). The electrical activity of the brain. *Scientific American,* 54–63.

Wolpaw, J. R., Birbaumer, N., Heetderks, W. J., McFarland, D. J., Peckham, P. H., Schalk, G., et al. (2000). Brain-computer interface technology: A review of the first international meeting. *IEEE Transaction in Rehabilitation Engineering, 8*(2), 164–173.

Wolpaw, J. R., Flotzinger, D., Pfurtscheller, G., & McFarland, D. J. (1997). Timing of EEG-based cursor control. *Journal of Clinical Neurophysiology, 14*(6), 529–538.

# CHAPTER 10

# Progressive Relaxation, Autogenic Training, and Meditation

PAUL LEHRER AND PATRICIA CARRINGTON

**Abstract:** Most widely used relaxation methods produce both a generalized relaxation response and specific effects related to particular characteristics of the method. This chapter reviews the effects of three of the most widely used relaxation techniques: progressive muscle relaxation, autogenic training, and clinically standardized meditation. Progressive relaxation most directly affects muscular systems; autogenic training produces the greatest autonomic effects; and mantra meditation methods have the most cognitive effects. The chapter outlines the pathways by which each method addresses muscular, autonomic, and cognitive manifestations of stress.

## ORIGINS

It has long been known that rest and relaxation are beneficial for promoting peace of mind and health and for treating various diseases, particularly those specifically identified as caused or exacerbated by stress. Stress appears to play a role in more than 70 percent of all outpatient physician visits in the United States as well as in many debilitating and life-threatening illnesses, from hypertension and heart disease to cancer. It is thus clearly a widespread problem of major proportions. Just as many factors can contribute to stress, many approaches are available to treat it. Differentiable behavioral, cognitive, and psychophysiological dimensions of stress have previously been identified (Lehrer & Woolfolk, 1993), each of which may have

independent causes and may be specifically targeted by particular treatments. For example, poor coping skills (e.g., job skills, social skills, assertiveness skills, etc.) can produce stress, so development of these skills can play an important role in inoculating people against its ill effects. The psychophysiological effects of stress are most directly targeted by various relaxation techniques. A number of such techniques have been used. Medical applications for relaxation were developed by Edmund Jacobson (1938) in the United States in the 1920s and 1930s and by Johannes Schultz in Germany in the 1930s (Schultz & Luthe, 1969). In the 1970s, Herbert Benson (1975) in the United States established the medical benefits of meditation methods. The relaxation techniques with the greatest empirical validation include progressive relaxation, biofeedback, autogenic training, various meditation methods, and several cognitive interventions. Considerably less empirical data are available to evaluate the relative effectiveness of other commonly used procedures, such as listening to relaxing music or doing aerobic exercises, controlled breathing, or postural relaxation methods (such as those described by F. M. Alexander, 1974, and Moshe Feldenkrais, 1977).

## DOCUMENTED APPLICATIONS: SPECIFIC EFFECTS

For almost three decades, an unresolved question for stress management practitioners has been whether these techniques all elicit a single "relaxation response," as proposed by Benson (1975). An alternative hypothesis is that they have specific effects, as proposed by Davidson and Schwartz (1976): specific cognitive effects for cognitively oriented methods, autonomic effects for autonomically oriented methods, and muscular effects for musculoskeletal-oriented methods. Davidson and Schwartz hypothesize that progressive relaxation therapy has predominantly somatic effects because it emphasizes development of a muscular skill. Autogenic training, on the other hand, generates both cognitive and somatic effects (Linden, 1993). It emphasizes achieving body homeostasis through self-suggestion and involves repeating an internal verbal formula (a cognitive process) that has a specific somatic focus— for example, "My arms are warm," and "My forehead is cool."

Assessing the specific cognitive effects of various stress management techniques requires definition of the term *cognitive*. Used broadly, the term denotes either (1) the act of thinking about something or (2) the content of a thought—for example, that an event is stressful. The specific-effects theory would predict greater effects for cognitively focused treatments on both types of cognitive activity. Meditation methods target the first of these activities (Carrington, 1993). They can also affect the latter by providing an alternative activity through which the practitioner can block generic "worry" activity that could reinforce a negative or catastrophic interpretation of events. Mental focus on a verbal mantra, according to this hypothesis, inhibits any other type of verbal activity, including worry. Therefore, mantra meditation's greatest and most direct effect is a reduction in verbal thought. Cognitive therapy (Beck, 1993) is more specifically focused on modifying the *content* of cognitions. It therefore has greater effect on this aspect of cognition than does meditation therapy.

The research literature has revealed considerable evidence for specific effects, although these sometimes are superimposed on a more generalized relaxation response (Lehrer & Woolfolk, 1993). Progressive relaxation tends to have the greatest muscular effects (e.g., for treating tension headaches, muscular spasms, etc.), autogenic training the greatest autonomic effects (for treating migraine headaches, hypertension, etc.), and mantra meditation the greatest cognitive effects (for treating anxiety conditions, etc.).

## ANATOMY, PHYSIOLOGY, AND PSYCHOPHYSIOLOGY

The overlap among these relaxation methods is most striking when people have become expert at them. Thus Jacobson (1938) reports cases of patients given extensive training only in muscle relaxation who concomitantly produce significant decreases in blood pressure, improvement in various gastrointestinal problems, and decreased anxiety levels. At extraordinarily low levels of muscle tension throughout the body, people appear not even to be able to think. The research of

Jacobson and McGuigan (Lusebrink & McGuigan, 1989) found that visual imaging inevitably involves tension in the muscles of the eyes, while verbal thoughts involve sub-vocalization and tension in the mouth and throat. Kinesthetic thoughts involve muscle tension throughout the body, particularly including the eyes and the area of the body targeted by thoughts. Therefore, like mantra meditation, blocking muscle tension in the facial muscles may have the direct effect of blocking cognitive activity. In addition, because of a direct connection between the reticular arousal system and muscle efferents (Gellhorn, 1958), a dramatic decrease in muscle activity throughout the body can produce a major decrease in sympathetic arousal and, presumably, vice versa. More recently, it has also been determined that skeletal muscle activity is closely related to sympathetic activation (Passatore, Deriu, Grassi, & Roatta, 1996; Potts, Hand, Li, & Mitchell, 1998), so more direct pathways may exist between muscle relaxation and decreased sympathetic arousal. Jacobson instructed patients that anxiety was inevitably accompanied by muscle tension and that elimination of muscle tension directly reduced anxiety. Jacobson claimed that even low levels of muscle tone can be eliminated by learning the most subtle level of muscle control.

Similarly, autonomic changes mediated by autogenic training may produce muscular and cognitive relaxation. In each autonomic exercise, the individual mentally repeats a specific verbal formula. This activity may thus block cognitive activity by a pathway similar to that of mantra meditation. Also, changes in cognitive activity produce related changes in physiological functioning. Worry, preparation for activity, hopelessness, and the assessment of danger all produce physiological changes. Any method that effectively blocks maladaptive mental activity should also produce correlated psychophysiological effects.

Novices at any of these methods might be expected to experience less *generalized* effects, and it is presumably among these people that the specific effects of various methods are evident most clearly. Deeper levels of relaxation usually are not achieved until the individual has become relatively expert at a method. The literature on these various approaches to relaxation must be interpreted with this consideration in mind, because almost all relaxation studies have involved only relatively brief exposure to a procedure compared with the many months (or even years) of training undertaken by serious meditators and by serious students of Jacobson's progressive relaxation (1938) and disciples of Schultz's autogenic training (Schultz & Luthe, 1969).

Other factors besides strength of effect may also be important in deciding the type of intervention to use in any particular case. Whether a person *likes* practicing a particular method may be critically important. A technique that is taught but not practiced has no therapeutic effect.

In addition, Smith (1999) hypothesized that these relaxation methods are best taught in a specific order, beginning with the most physical (progressive relaxation), gradually progressing toward more mental and abstract (autogenic training), and finally to the most abstract (meditation). In support of this recommendation, he notes that Eastern meditative disciplines begin training with physical exercises and then progress gradually to methods that are more specifically directed toward experiencing mental states (sense of "oneness," enlightenment, etc.).

Also worth noting is the fact that all relaxation techniques involve multiple response components. Meditation methods are the most complex. Stemming from Eastern religious traditions, they all involve physical as well as mental foci, although the major "goal" is usually more of a subjective state. In addition to achieving a sense of immediacy, mental clarity, and sometimes bliss, these methods are often accompanied by a world-view, lifestyle, and system of values that also would promote such a mental (and through it, physiological) effect. Hence some of these methods may train people in self-manage-ment through many converging pathways simultaneously. Even the methods focused more narrowly on physical effects have some mental effects, as mentioned earlier.

## TREATMENT PROTOCOLS

Stress management and relaxation methods have been incorporated in the treatment of most diseases and disorders involving auto-nomic, emotional, and immune system dysfunction because of the well-known relationship between stress and vulnerability to these disorders (Critelli & Ee, 1996).

### Progressive Relaxation

Progressive relaxation has been applied within several quite different muscle relax-ation methods. This chapter emphasizes the work of Edmund Jacobson (1938) because it provides the most intensive physiological training. Specific contrasts between Jacobson's method and other progressive relaxation methods have been described elsewhere (Lehrer and Woolfolk, 1993).

#### General Protocol and Procedural Points

Wasting energy in muscle tension and ner-vous habits can cause fatigue. By learning to switch off when tense, the trainee not only feels more relaxed but also saves energy that can be used more efficiently for other things. Jacobson (1938) uses the term *switching off* as analogous to running a machine: When the power switch is off, the machine is com-pletely inactive. This is the goal of muscle relaxation. To switch off is to remain completely relaxed, without doing *anything*.

The treatment protocol for progressive relaxation is as follows:

1. Ask the trainee to tense each muscle just enough to feel the "control sensations" (i.e., the sensations accompanying muscle tension) and to distinguish these from other sensations that also might accompany a par-ticular muscular maneuver (e.g., straining a joint or passive stretching of a muscle).

2. Use the *method of diminishing ten-sions*, whereby the individual detects tension at progressively lower levels of contraction, until the individual is just imagining the contraction.

3. Instruct the trainee to switch off to achieve zero tension in each muscle, as mea-sured either subjectively or by surface elec-tromyography (SEMG).

4. Ask the trainee if any residual tension is felt in the muscle. This is the sensation that the trainee should try to detect in the body at other times when tension may be a problem.

5. Explain that the relaxation, *not the tensing*, is the most important activity of the session. Help the trainee understand the need to achieve a state of complete passivity, because *doing* anything inevitably involves muscle tension.

By individually tensing and relaxing vari-ous muscles throughout the body, the trainee will learn to notice and control tension. Tensing muscles does not automatically *pro-duce* relaxation. It just teaches the trainee to recognize and control feelings of muscle ten-sion. The trainee must develop control over the muscles to make voluntary relaxation possible.

The therapist should use the following procedural principles throughout training:

- Train awareness of muscle tension in spe-cific muscles, and simultaneous training in control of this tension.

- Avoid external methods for "producing" relaxation (such as use of suggestion, "relaxing" environments, etc.).
- Train muscles or muscle groups one at a time, until the trainee learns awareness and control of each muscle individually.
- By tensing and relaxing muscles throughout the body, the trainee learns to notice and control tension.
- Relaxing is the opposite of *doing*. *Trying* too hard will *prevent* relaxation.
- Learning relaxation is a gradual process. It may take several days or several weeks before the trainee notices any benefits.
- Relaxation is called switching off or "going negative" to indicate that no effort is required to relax. An effort to relax is a failure to relax.

## Troubleshooting Problem Muscles

At any point during training, a trainee may experience difficulty in recognizing tension, may find it difficult to discriminate tension from other interoceptive stimuli (such as the stretching of counterposing muscles), or may just not "get it." Here are five strategies to assist the trainee in recognizing and acquiring control of muscle tension:

1. The therapist instructs the trainee to carry out a specific movement, and uses his or her own hands to offer resistance to the movement. This increases muscle sensations and makes them easier to perceive.

2. The trainee touches the place where she or he should be feeling a control signal, and the therapist then has the trainee make the movement, asking if any sensation of tension can be felt there.

3. The therapist can lightly touch the spot where the trainee should be feeling a control signal and then have the trainee make the movement, asking if any sensation of tension can be felt there.

4. The therapist can tell the trainee that this area may be an individual trouble spot, and if so, with practice, the perception of

sensations from it should become easier. The more generally relaxed the trainee is, the easier it will be to feel the tension.

5. EMG biofeedback can be used on occasion to verify whether the trainee's perceptions of tension are in fact valid.

### Home Practice

The trainee should practice the technique for one hour every day to learn how to detect and control tension and to add each muscle group to those learned in previous sessions. Minimum muscle tension should be used, just enough to allow the trainee to recognize the sensations of tension. In addition, the trainee should apply relaxation skills 24 hours a day, checking her or his muscles several times during the day and releasing tension, particularly when experiencing emotional or physical tension. This continuous method is called *differential relaxation*. The therapist can teach the trainee how to perform differential relaxation by practicing relaxing while doing everyday activities in the office, such as reading and conversing. The goal is to notice muscle tension automatically throughout the day and to be able to relax at will during daily activities. Feelings of anxiety are related to muscle tension. Nervousness, tension, or even thinking about an anxious situation inevitably produces muscle tension. The goal of training is to recognize tension and to relax it away voluntarily.

### Specific Protocol

*Session 1: Progressive Relaxation of the Arms.* For each step of the following instructions, the trainee should start with the dominant arm and then repeat for the other arm after several minutes of relaxation. Try not to tell the trainee where the sensations of tension should be felt, unless the trainee appears to become frustrated. Let the trainee discover this through repeated tensing. If the trainee cannot perceive the sensations after several attempts and some counterforce, move to another muscle group. Eventually, however, the therapist may point out the correct spot.

1. Keeping the arm relaxed on the arm of a chair, bend the hand back at the wrist at a 45-degree angle. Observe tension in the back of the upper part of the forearm.

After the trainee carries out step 1, the instructor should point out the differing sensations of tension in this muscle (the forearm extensor muscle, on the back of the forearm approximately two thirds of the distance to the elbow). Have the trainee contrast this sensation with the more easily perceived sensation of strain in the wrist joint and the passive stretching of the opposing muscle (on the underside of the arm). Actual muscle tension is usually perceived as a slight squeezing sensation, whereas joint strain may actually be painful, and passive sensations may appear as qualitatively different stretching sensations.

2. Switch off, relaxing for several minutes, after each step involving tensing.

3. Repeat step 1 with the other arm, and then again switch off.

4. Bend the hand forward from the wrist. Observe tension in the inside (ventral) surface of the forearm (the flexor). Sensations of stretching may occur in the extensor, as may strain in the wrist.

5. Keeping the forearm relaxed, bend the arm back at the elbow to about 45 degrees, as if moving to touch the shoulder with the back of the hand. Observe tension in the biceps. Turn the palm up for stronger sensations.

6. Press the hand and forearm down on the surface of the armrest or couch (use a book under the wrist if the tension is difficult to feel and more bending is needed). Observe tension in the back of the upper arm (triceps).

*Session 2: Progressive Relaxation of the Legs.* Relaxation of the leg muscles is best done with the trainee in a reclining position on a bed, couch, or reclining chair. The trainee should perform each step with one leg and then repeat for the other leg.

1. Bend the foot at the ankle, pointing the toes toward the head. Observe tension along the front of the lower leg (leg extensor), and stretching sensations in the flexor.

2. Bend the foot down at the ankle, pointing the toe away from the body. Observe tension in the calf (flexor).

3. Extend the lower leg, straightening the knee. Observe tension on the top of the lap.

4. Press the heel down, bending at the knee, as if trying to kick the buttocks. Observe tension along the back of the thigh.

5. Lying supine with one leg dangling off the side of the couch (bed, chair), raise the knee of the dangling leg. Observe tension in muscles deep in the abdomen, toward the back and near the hip.

6. Place a pillow under the back of the knee. Press the back of the knee and upper leg down onto the pillow. Observe tension in the buttock.

*Session 3: Progressive Relaxation of the Trunk*

1. Squeeze the abdomen in. Observe tension all over the abdomen.

2. Arch the back. Observe tension on both sides of the lower spine.

3. Bend the shoulders back. Observe tension in the back between the shoulder blades.

4. Bring the left arm over and across the chest, pointing to the opposite wall. Let the arm just fall over the chest and relax when a tension signal is noticed. Observe tension in the front of the chest, near the left arm (pectoral muscles).

5. Raise the shoulders as if in a shrug. Observe the tension along the top of the shoulders and in the back of the neck.

6. Concentrate on breathing. Feel the sensation of tension in the chest when inhaling. When exhaling, switch off. If the tension is not noticeable, take a slightly deeper breath. Observe a vague tenseness all over the chest and/or abdomen while inhaling.

*Session 4: Progressive Relation of the Neck.* This training is sometimes combined with the training in session 3.

1. Bend the head back so that the chin points to the ceiling. Observe the tension in the back of the neck.

2. Raising the head slightly, bend the chin down to the chest. Observe the tension in the sides of the neck towards the front.

3. Facing forward, bend the head to the left as if trying to touch the left ear to the shoulder. Observe the tension on the left side of the neck and the stretching on the right.

*Session 5: Progressive Relaxation of the Eye Muscles*

1. Wrinkle the forehead by raising the eyebrows. Feel the tension diffusely over the entire forehead.

2. Frown or bring the eyebrows together. Observe tension in the forehead, above the nose.

3. Close the eyes tightly. Observe tension all over and around the eyelids.

4. With eyelids closed, look up and notice tension toward the top of the eyeball. Look down and notice tension toward the bottom of the eyeball. Look to the right and notice tension on the right of the eyeball, and stretching to the left. Then repeat this looking to the left, and feel the tension on the opposite side.

5. With the eyes closed and without deliberately moving the eyeballs, imagine being at a tennis game, sitting at the net. Visualize the ball as it goes from side to side. Observe the tension inside the eyeballs from side to side. Thereafter, notice tension in the eyeball whenever a visual thought occurs.

*Session 6: Progressive Relaxation of the Speech Region*

1. Clench the teeth. Observe the tension in the jaw and temples.

2. Open the mouth and jaws. Observe the tension under the chin and stretching in the jaw.

3. As if smiling, show the teeth. Observe tension in the cheeks.

4. Push the tongue against the front teeth. Observe tension in the tongue.

5. Press the tip of the tongue down to the bottom of the mouth and pull it backward toward the throat. Observe tension in the tongue and in the floor of the mouth.

6. Purse the lips. Observe tension in and around the lips

7. Count out loud from 1 to 10, observing tension in the area of the vocal cords as well as in the tongue, lips, chest, and so on. Muscle tension should be differentiated from the vibrations of the cords. Then say the alphabet. Begin in a normal speaking voice, and gradually speak more softly, reaching a whisper by the letter *E,* and only *thinking* the alphabet by the time you reach the letter *L.* It is helpful for the therapist to speak along with the trainee at first. Tension also may be observed in the cheeks, lips, tongue, jaw muscles, throat, chest, and perhaps abdomen. If perceiving this tension is difficult, count and speak in a high-pitched voice to increase the tension.

*Session 7: Differential Relaxation and Using Progressive Relaxation in Daily Life.* Give the trainee a book to read, with instructions to continue relaxing even while reading. Give feedback, instructions, and encouragement. Talk with the trainee about situations or circumstances that may arouse some feelings of stress or emotion. Note generalized tension, particularly in the arms, legs, and facial muscles, and remind the trainee to try to keep relaxed while talking. Give feedback immediately on noticing tension. Speak with the trainee about applications of differential relaxation in daily life and the use of scheduled relaxation periods during times of stress.

### Autogenic Training

Autogenic training was developed by the German physician Johannes Schultz, who lived and worked contemporaneously with Edmund Jacobson, in the first part of the 20th century. In developing this technique, he was heavily influenced by European applications of hypnosis and hypnotic phenomena and by Japanese methods of Zen meditation. Elements of both are combined in the technique. More complete descriptions of the method and its effects are available elsewhere (Schultz & Luthe, 1969).

Although autogenic training is essentially a self-hypnotic technique, there is some debate among practitioners whether it should be considered a type of hypnosis, primarily because formal hypnotic induction does not take place and because no hypnotist is involved.

The autogenic method is taught while the trainee sits or lies in the autogenic position— that is, supine with arms at the sides and legs uncrossed—or sits on a chair, with the head's center of gravity balanced on the neck so the head does not tilt, with the arms on the lap and the muscles relatively relaxed. As in progressive relaxation, the trainee learns a

skill during the practice and training sessions that he or she can apply at any time, even while doing other activities.

Some practitioners (Norris & Fahrion, 1993) use biofeedback methods, particularly hand warming, along with autogenic training. However, Freedman (1991) found that the effects of brief exposure to autogenic training tend to differ somewhat from the effects of hand-warming biofeedback. The latter method tends to produce warmer hands, while autogenic training produces a deeper sense of relaxation. Freedman pointed out that the physiological mechanism for hand warming is rather complex, involving both a decrease in alpha and an increase in beta sympathetic activation. Relaxation, which tends to reduce sympathetic arousal, may have mixed effects on hand temperature.

Indeed, Schultz did not classify autogenic training as a relaxation technique (Schultz & Luthe, 1969). He argued that improved self-regulation, not deep relaxation, is the goal of autogenic training. He conceptualized the method as freeing the body from inappropriate blocks in psychophysiological energy, enabling the body to regulate itself more effectively.

The method begins with the six standard exercises, during which the trainee performs mental repetitions of autogenic formulas involving specific body sensations. As in progressive relaxation, the trainee is advised not to try to achieve a particular sensation but to engage only in "passive concentration" on it—that is, to *imagine* what the sensation might be like but not to try to achieve it. Schultz pointed out that the act of doing the autogenic exercise produces beneficial effects, whether the specific sensations are experienced or not, and that, indeed, about half of trainees do not experience the suggested sensations during the early stages of treatment.

The exercises are usually given one at a time at approximately equal intervals. The trainee is instructed to practice them initially for very brief periods (30 seconds to 1 minute) several times each day and to increase the practice time gradually.

The six standard exercises are as follows:

1. Heaviness in the limbs.
   My right arm is heavy.
   My left arm is heavy.
   My right leg is heavy.
   My left leg is heavy.

2. Warmth in the limbs.
   My right leg is warm.
   My left leg is warm.
   My right leg is warm.
   My left leg is warm.

3. My heartbeat is calm and regular.

4. It breathes me (automatic breathing). Although this phrase sounds awkward in English, it conveys the meaning of a passivity regarding breathing. The trainee is instructed to allow breathing to occur automatically, without any voluntary effort.

5. My solar plexus is warm (warmth in the area slightly in front of the spine, below the sternum).

6. My forehead is cool.

These formulas are often interspersed with the formula, "My mind is at peace."

Each exercise is followed by a specific termination instruction: Squeeze the fists two times, take a slow deep breath, slowly let it out, and then open the eyes.

Practicing autogenic exercises can be accompanied by unanticipated and often unpleasant side effects. Although all methods of relaxation training can produce relaxation-induced anxiety on occasion, autogenic training tends to produce these sensations more frequently than progressive relaxation (Heide & Borkovec, 1983), for reasons that are unknown. Although this experience occurs even to the most experienced autogenic training practitioners, it is most common among novices to the method. Schultz described these events as "autogenic discharges," caused by a sudden discharge of pent-up nervous energy (Schultz & Luthe, 1969). This hydraulic model of emotional regulation is not accepted in modern psychology. Alternatively, the phenomenon could be ascribed to disinhibition and consequent lapses in self-regulation. Other forms of disinhibition frequently occur during autogenic training, including a dream-like uncritical stream of consciousness, similar to that described in psychoanalytic terminology as "primary process thinking." Physical sensations are common experiences, particularly pain or discomfort related to previous illnesses, injuries, or surgeries. Intense emotion, fear, and/or tearfulness are not uncommon. Perhaps these sensations are normally inhibited by higher neural circuitry that is temporarily disabled during autogenic exercises.

Although autogenic discharges can sometimes cause sufficient discomfort to necessitate termination of training, they also can have beneficial effects. Schultz argued that release of pent-up energy allows the body to regain its equilibrium. Alternatively, the beneficial effects could be interpreted as similar to those commonly prescribed by behavior therapists for treating panic disorder and other conditions involving fear and avoidance of particular sensations. Exposure and response prevention (deliberate experience of the unpleasant sensations or stimuli and blocking of the usual methods of avoiding them) are considered critical components in treating a variety of psychological ailments (Lang, Craske, & Bjork, 1999). Autogenic discharges may produce just such an effect. Through autogenic discharges, the trainee reexperiences unpleasant sensations, sometimes repeatedly. Either through extinction of a classically conditioned emotional response or by cognitive restructuring in response to deliberate thought about them, the sensations no longer produce as great an emotional response.

Considering the specific hypnotic aspects of autogenic training can be helpful to the clinician. In inducing a hypnotic trance, the hypnotist commonly instructs the subject only to experience what the subject is, in fact, experiencing anyway. This is a well-known method for overcoming resistance to hypnotic suggestion. In autogenic training, this is done by avoiding any instructions to experience anything that will not, in fact, occur. The standardized nature of the autogenic training situation allows the experienced practitioner to predict the full variety of responses to the autogenic situation and provide appropriate instructions. Thus in passive concentration instructions, the vast majority of trainees can easily *imagine* specific body sensations, although actually experiencing them may be more difficult. Hence the trainee is specifically instructed *not* to try to experience them; and even the unpleasant side effects of autogenic training are reinterpreted as a beneficial part of the therapeutic process. Also, thinking about a particular sensation can, at times, bring the sensation about. Often a trainee may feel frightened about various physical sensations, including those associated with relaxation, and may avoid thinking about them. Autogenic training raises awareness of these sensations and allows the trainee to habituate to them. Because fear of one's body can contribute to anxiety, habituation to physical sensations can increase the sense of well-being. This further reinforces the hypnotic power of the autogenic instructions.

After learning the standard exercises, trainees often use autogenic methods to induce physiological changes in specific areas using "organ-specific formulas" and to produce self-hypnotically induced behavioral changes.

## Clinically Standardized Meditation

Among the clinically oriented meditation techniques, clinically standardized meditation, or CSM (Carrington, 1999); the respiratory one method, or ROM (Benson, 1975); and mindfulness meditation (Kabat-Zinn, 1982) have been the most widely used to date. These techniques were devised with clinical objectives in mind.

Optimal use of meditation in a clinical setting depends on teaching the trainee to manage the technique successfully—a consideration that can easily be overlooked. Unless routine problems arising during the practice of meditation are handled correctly, the likelihood of obtaining satisfactory compliance is poor. If the technique is adjusted to meet the needs of the particular trainee, however, compliance is often excellent (Carrington et al., 1980).

It is doubtful that meditation can ever be taught effectively through written instructions, because correct learning of the technique relies on the communication of the "meditative mood"—a subtle atmosphere of tranquility best transferred through nuances of voice and tonal quality (Carrington, 1998). Meditation can be taught successfully by means of tape recordings, providing they effectively convey this elusive meditative mood (Carrington et al., 1980). In addition, the recorded teaching system should be thorough so the trainee learns to handle any minor problems that may arise on the way to mastery of the technique.

The CSM method (which incorporates ROM as an alternative form of meditation) is a total training program in meditation that can be learned either through cassette tapes and a programmed instruction text or in person with trained instructors. Because of these advantages, the following discussion on meditation method is confined to CSM.

Whatever the method of instruction (recorded or in person), close clinical supervision of the meditation practice is strongly recommended. Clinicians are in a strategic position to introduce the idea of learning CSM to patients with previously identified difficulties or symptoms. Given the absence of any validated predictive measures (Carrington et al., 1980), a clinician attempting to assess the suitability of meditation for a particular trainee must seek to determine whether this patient shows one or more meditation-responsive symptoms or difficulties, such as anxiety or physical discomfort.

Training should occur in a quiet, uncluttered room where the trainee can be alone. This room should contain two comfortable straight-backed chairs and a visually pleasant object such as a plant or vase on which the trainee can gaze when entering and exiting meditation. While these arrangements seem simple, they should be carefully followed for maximum effect.

A trainee receiving personal instruction first selects a soothing sound, or mantra, from the 16 listed in the CSM workbook or may make up a mantra according to simple instructions. The mantras used in CSM are resonant sounds (often ending in the nasal consonants *m* or *n*) that have no meaning in the English language but that, in pretesting, have been shown to have a calming effect on many people—for example, "Ah-nam," "Shi-rim," and "Ra-mah." After the trainee has selected a mantra, training is conducted in a peaceful setting removed from any disturbances that may detract from the meditative mood. The instructor walks quietly, speaks in low tones, and typically conveys by his or her behavior a respect for the occasion of learning meditation.

When teaching meditation, the instructor first repeats the trainee's mantra out loud in a rhythmical manner to demonstrate how this is done. The trainee then repeats the mantra out loud in unison with the instructor, and finally alone. Next the instructor asks the trainee to whisper it and then simply to think it silently, with eyes closed. Instructor and trainee then meditate together for 10 minutes, after which the trainee remains seated for a minute or two with eyes closed, allowing the

mind to return to everyday thoughts. The trainee is then asked to open his or her eyes very slowly. At this point, the instructor answers any questions the trainee may have about the technique and corrects any misconceptions. Then the instructor leaves the room so that the trainee can meditate alone for a stated period of time (10 to 20 minutes). The experience of meditating on one's own is included to "wean" the trainee as soon as possible from dependency on the instructor's presence when meditating and allow for generalization of the experience to the trainee's life outside the instructor's office.

Immediately following the instruction session, the trainee completes a postinstruction questionnaire and reviews his or her responses with the instructor. In a postinstruction interview, the instructor clarifies procedures for home meditation practice and teaches the trainee the meditation program for the next week. The trainee is then told about possible side effects of meditation (Carrington, 1999) and is taught how to handle these should they occur. The trainee is usually instructed to practice meditating for approximately 20 minutes, twice daily, although shorter periods are prescribed when the trainee experiences transitory unpleasant effects.

Individual follow-up interviews are held at intervals. Alternatively, group meetings are scheduled where new meditators can gather to share experiences, meditate in a group, or pick up new ideas on handling any problems that may have arisen in their practice. Trainees then learn to adjust their techniques to suit their own individual needs and lifestyles. A careful follow-up program leads to much more satisfactory compliance with a continued program of meditation.

## CONCLUSION

Relaxation methods play a large role in treating the stress-related components of disease, emotional discomfort, and disability. They primarily target the psychophysiological component of the stress response, although some components may also influence behavioral and cognitive effects of stress. In this chapter, we have reviewed the three relaxation methods with the greatest empirical validation. Each has specific effects, although it also may produce more generalized relaxation. All involve subtle training in the body's ability to manage the effects of stress. Jacobson's (1938) progressive relaxation method involves learning to recognize and control very subtle levels of muscle tension that are always activated in the stress response. Schultz's method of autogenic training tends to focus initially on autonomic effects of stress (Schultz & Luthe,

1969). Suggestion and hypnosis are seen very differently in the two methods. Although Jacobson's method rejects suggestion and hypnosis as producing ephemeral results (sometimes defined as not measurable in the musculoskeletal system), Schultz's method is based on them. These differences may account for some of the initial differences in therapeutic effects. Mantra meditation, on the other hand, uses concentration on a particular word with minimal prior meaning to the individual. Its initial specific effects on blocking anxiety and worry may derive from mental focus on the mantra, which could preclude thinking about various stress-related concerns and worries. More serious longer-term practice of these methods may produce more generalized effects.

## REFERENCES

Alexander, F. M. (1974). *The resurrection of the body.* New York: Delta.

Beck, A. T. (1993). Cognitive approaches to stress. In P. M. Lehrer and R. L. Woolfolk (Eds.), *Principles and practice of stress management* (2nd ed., pp. 333–372). New York: Guilford.

Benson, H. (1975). *The relaxation response.* New York: William Morrow.

Carrington, P. (1993). The clinical use of meditation. In P. M. Lehrer and R. L. Woolfolk (Eds.), *Principles and practice of stress management* (2nd ed., pp. 139–168). New York: Guilford.

Carrington, P. (1998). *The book of meditation.* London: Element Books.

Carrington, P. (1999). *Clinically standardized meditation (CSM) instructor's kit.* Kendall Park, NJ: Pace Educational Systems.

Carrington, P., Collings, G. H., Benson, H., Robinson, H., Wood, L. W., Lehrer, P. M., et al. (1980). The use of meditation-relaxation techniques for the management of stress in a working population. *Journal of Occupational Medicine, 22*, 221–231.

Critelli, J. W., & Ee, J. S. (1996). Stress and physical illness: Development of an integrative model. In T. W. Miller (Ed.), *Theory and assessment of stressful life events* (pp. 139–159). Madison, CT: International Universities Press.

Davidson, R. J., & Schwartz, G. E. (1976). The psychobiology of relaxation and related states: A multiprocess theory. In D. I. Mostofsky (Ed.), *Behavior control and modification of physiological activity* (pp. 399–442). Englewood Cliffs, NJ: Prentice Hall.

Feldenkrais, M. (1977). *Awareness through movement: Health exercises for personal growth.* New York: Harper & Row.

Freedman, R. R. (1991). Physiological mechanisms of temperature biofeedback. *Biofeedback and Self-Regulation, 16*, 95–116.

Gellhorn, E. (1958). The physiological basis of neuromuscular relaxation. *Archives of Internal Medicine, 102,* 392–399.

Heide, F., & Borkovec, T. D. (1983). Relaxation-induced anxiety: Paradoxical anxiety enhancement due to relaxation training. *Journal of Consulting and Clinical Psychology, 51,* 171–182.

Jacobson, E. (1938). *Progressive relaxation.* Chicago: University of Chicago Press.

Kabat-Zinn, J. (1982). An outpatient program in behavioral medicine for chronic pain patients based on the practice of mindfulness meditation: Theoretical considerations and preliminary results. *General Hospital Psychiatry, 4,* 936–943.

Lang, A. J., Craske, M. G., & Bjork, R. A. (1999). Implications of a new theory of disuse for the treatment of emotional disorders. *Clinical Psychology—Science and Practice, 6,* 80–94.

Lehrer, P. M., & Woolfolk, R. L. (Eds.). (1993). *Principles and practice of stress management* (2nd ed.). New York: Guilford.

Linden, W. (1993). The autogenic training method of J. H. Schultz. In P. M. Lehrer & R. L. Woolfolk (Eds.), *Principles and practice of stress management* (2nd ed., pp. 205–230). New York: Guilford.

Lusebrink, V. B., & McGuigan, F. J. (1989). Psychophysiological components of imagery. *Pavlovian Journal of Biological Science, 24,* 58–62.

Norris, P. A., & Fahrion, S. (1993). Autogenic biofeedback in psychophysiological therapy and stress management. In P. M. Lehrer & R. L. Woolfolk (Eds.), *Principles and practice of stress management* (2nd ed., pp. 231–262). New York: Guilford.

Passatore, M., Deriu, F., Grassi, C., & Roatta, S. (1996). A comparative study of changes operated by sympathetic nervous system activation on spindle afferent discharge and on tonic vibration reflex in rabbit jaw muscles. *Journal of the Autonomic Nervous System, 57,* 163–177.

Potts, J. T., Hand, G. A., Li, J., & Mitchell, J. H. (1998). Central interaction between carotid baroreceptors and skeletal muscle receptors inhibits sympathoexcitation. *Journal of Applied Physiology, 84,* 1158–1165.

Schultz, J. H., & Luthe, W. (1969). *Autogenic therapy: Vol. 1. Autogenic methods.* New York: Grune & Stratton.

Smith, J. C. (1999). *ABC relaxation theory: An evidence-based approach.* New York: Springer.

# CHAPTER 11

# Hypnotherapy

IAN WICKRAMASEKERA

**Abstract:** Hypnotherapy combines hypnotic techniques with standard medical, psychological, and dental treatments. Empirical research shows a high efficacy for hypnotherapy with many conditions commonly found in primary care. The chapter presents an integrative, psychophysiological model for understanding the effects of hypnosis and hypnotherapy and reviews the empirical research showing positive outcomes with hypnosis for a number of medical and psychological conditions. The author emphasizes the measurable personality factor of hypnotizability and its role in shaping the individual patient's response to hypnotherapies in a specific sense. Hypnosis also has a nonspecific, or placebo, effect that can amplify clinical response in any hypnotic treatment.

## INTRODUCTION

Hypnotherapy can be defined as the addition of a major or minor component of hypnosis to a standard psychological, medical, or dental treatment. The addition of a hypnotic induction can be a powerful catalyst of any standard psychological or medical (drug, surgical, etc.) therapy (Bennett, 1986; "Integration of Behavioral and Relaxation Approaches," 1996; Kirsch, Montgomery, & Sapirstein, 1995; Lang, Benotsch, et al., 2000; Lang, Joyce, Spiegel, Hamilton, & Lee, 1996; Smith, Glass, & Miller, 1980; Spiegel, 1991). It is puzzling, but at least for some chronic conditions, efficacy appears to increase with time (see Figure 11.1). Accessing the hypnotic mode of information processing can speed up many types of emotional and physical healing (Ewer & Stewart, 1986; Harvey, Hinton, & Gunary, 1989; Patterson, Goldberg, & Ehde, 1996; Whorwell, 1989; Whorwell, Prior, & Colgan, 1987; Whorwell, Prior, & Faragher, 1984; Zachariae, 2001; Zachariae, Bjerring, & Arendt-Nielsen, 1989). Hypnosis can also speed up negative mind-body effects (Wickramasekera, 1979, 1988, 1998). People who are high on trait hypnotic ability appear to have a hypersensitivity to mind-body effects (Barber 1984; Szechtman, Woody, Bowers, & Nahmias, 1998; Wickramasekera, 1979, 1988, 1998; Woody & Szechtman, 2000), and people who are low on trait hypnotic ability have a hyposensitivity to mind-body effects (Barber, 1984; Wickramasekera, 1979, 1988, 1998). Hence, the measurement of baseline hypnotic ability is crucial to all mind-body therapies. As the scientific specification of the neuroendocrine and immune links between mind and body proceeds

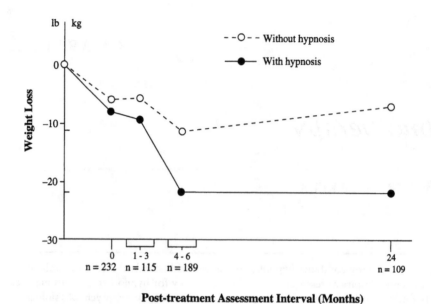

**Figure 11.1**    Weight Loss as a Function of Assessment Interval and Inclusion of Hypnosis in Treatment

SOURCE: Adapted with permission from Kirsch, Montgomery, and Sapirstein (1995).

(Damasio, 1999; Institute of Medicine, 1989; Rose & Sternberg, 2001), the recognition grows that the majority of diseases are psychophysiological in nature.

The last 75 years of experimental research have clearly established that the bulk of hypnotic phenomena reside in the hypnotized persons' natural hypnotic ability, and not in any projection from the hypnotist (Hilgard, 1965). In 1979, I proposed a new model of *mind-body incongruence* to account for psychophysiological disease. The central component of the model is hypnotic ability interacting with negative affect (Watson & Tellegen, 1985). Also critical is the hypothesis that beliefs have biological consequences (Wickramasekera, 1979, 1986, 1988, 1993, 1995, 2000), based on the accumulating neuroscience evidence that negative emotions, beliefs, and hypnosis have biological consequences through neuroendocrine and immune mechanisms (Wickramasekera, 1979, 1988, 1993, 1995; Zachariae, 2001).

Many physicians and psychologists are unaware of the fact that the teaching of hypnosis in medical schools and its use in clinical practice was recommended in 1955 by the British Medical Association and in 1960 by the American Medical Association. In 1960, the American Psychological Association officially recognized the American Board of Psychological Hypnosis and its authority to examine and certify diplomates with advanced competence in either experimental or clinical hypnosis. There are similar national boards identifying advanced competence in medical and dental hypnosis (Hilgard, 1965).

## HYPNOSIS AND THE HIGH RISK MODEL OF THREAT PERCEPTION

Hypnosis is a form of information processing in which peripheral awareness and critical analytic cognition are suspended, readily leading to apparently involuntary changes in perception, memory, and mood that have profound behavioral and biological consequences (Wickramasekera, 1988, 1993, 1995, 1998). There appears to be a correlation between a patient's measured hypnotic ability and the clinical efficacy of hypnotherapy for several somatic and psychological symptoms (Brown, 1992; Levitt, 1993; Wadden & Anderton, 1982; Zachariae, 2001). There is evidence from the high risk model of threat perception (HRMTP) that high and also low hypnotic ability in interaction with conscious or *unconscious* negative affect may be risk factors for several psychophysiological disorders and some psychological disorders (Wickramasekera, 1979, 1986, 1988, 1993, 1995, 1998; Wickramasekera, Pope, & Kolm, 1996; see Chapter 2 of this text for an introduction to the HRMTP). High measured baseline hypnotic ability has been related to migraine pain intensity (Andreychuk & Skriver, 1975), experimental pain intensity (DeBenedittis, Paneral, & Villamirqa, 1989), facial pain intensity (Stam, McGrath, Brooke, & Cosire, 1986), intensity of chronic urticaria (Shertzer & Lookingbill, 1987; Zachariae, 2001), atopic eczema (H'ajek, Jakoubek, & Radil, 1990; Zachariae, 2001), severity of clinical and dental phobias (John, Hollander, & Perry, 1983; Kelly, 1984), negative moods (Crowson, Conroy, & Chester, 1991; Velten, 1968) major depression (Pettinati, Kogan, et al., 1990), posttraumatic stress disorder (Spiegel, Hunt, & Dondershine, 1988; Stutman & Bliss, 1985), dissociative disorders (Braun & Sachs, 1985; Putnam, 1989), predisposition to nightmares (Belicki & Belicki, 1986), EEG-defined insomnia (Perlstrom & Wickramasekera, 1998; Wickramasekera, Ware, & Saxon, 1992), musical performance anxiety (Zinn, McCain, & Zinn, 2000), substance abuse and bulimia (Perlstrom & Wickramasekera, 1998; Pettinati, Horne, & Staats, 1985), moderate obesity (Wickramasekera & Atkinson, 1992),

nausea and vomiting during pregnancy (Apfel, Kelly & Frankel, 1986), and chronic somatic symptoms (Gick, McLeod, & Hulihan, 1997; McGrady, Lynch, Nagel, & Zsembik, 1999). High hypnotizability also appears related to alterations in immune function (Ruzyla-Smith, Barabasz, Barabasz, & Warner, 1995; Zachariae, 2001), and there is evidence that low hypnotic ability may be a risk factor for somatic symptoms associated with pathophysiology, including chronic pain, morbid obesity, cardiac disease, response to cardiac surgery, chest pain, and chronic insomnia (Greenleaf, Fisher, Miaskowski, & DuHamel, 1992; Kermit, Devine, & Tatman, 2000; Saxon & Wickramasekera, 1994; Wickramasekera, 1995, 1998; Wickramasekera & Price, 1997). In summary, a subset of patients presenting chronic somatic complaints unresponsive to standard medical or surgical therapy are high or low on hypnotic ability (Wickramasekera, 1995, 1998).

## HYPNOTIZABILITY, PHYSIOLOGY, AND PSYCHOLOGY

The degree of an individual's hypnotic ability has electrophysiological correlates. Hypnotic ability varies directly with EEG alpha at baseline and there are systematic EEG theta differences between carefully selected high and low hypnotizables (Graffin, Ray, & Lundy, 1995; Paskewitz, 1977). It is worth noting that these electrophysiological features exist in the frontal and temporal cortex, and they distinguish between high and low hypnotizable subjects at baseline *before hypnotic induction*. High hypnotic responsivity may also be related to 40-Hz EEG activity that is task related (DePascalis, 1999). Klein and Spiegel (1989) and Whorwell, Houghton, Taylor, and Maxton (1992) showed that hypnotizability or hypnosis could stimulate and inhibit gastric acid secretion and affect a colonic motility index. In a controlled study, Ruzyla-Smith et al. (1995) showed that hypnotizability was related to alterations in B cells and helper T cells of the immune system. Black (1963) and Zachariae et al. (1989) showed that high hypnotic ability was related to the inhibition of the Mantoux reaction to tuberculin and that the Mantoux reaction could be selectively increased in one arm and reduced in the other. For high hypnotizables, it has been shown that hypnotic analgesia is as effective as morphine and more effective than acupuncture (Knox, Gekoski, Shum, & McLaughlin, 1981; Stern, Brown, Ulett, & Sletten, 1977). It has also been shown that naloxone does not block the mechanism of hypnotic analgesia (Barber & Mayer, 1977; Goldstein & Hilgard, 1975). Several physiological research studies have shown that hypnotically suggested visual hallucinations alter cortical EEG-event-related potentials and not simply the subjects' verbal reports (Blum & Nash, 1981; Spiegel & Barabasz, 1988; Spiegel, Cutcomb, Ren, & Pribram, 1985). High hypnotic ability can increase the rate of acquisition of learning in both operant conditioning (King & McDonald, 1976; Webb, 1962; Weiss, Ullman, & Krasner, 1960; Wickramasekera, 1970b, 1976) and Pavlovian conditioning (Wickramasekera, 1988) situations. Hence, it is not surprising to find that superior hypnotic subjects respond more rapidly to various types of short-term psychotherapy and credible instructions (Larsen, 1966; Nace, Warwick, Kelley, & Evans, 1982; Wickramasekera, 1971b) and appear to learn both *adaptive* and *maladaptive* responses rapidly and unconsciously (Wickramasekera, 1979, 1986, 1988, 1993, 1994).

### Tests of Hypnotizability

There is general agreement that the gold standard in the measurement of hypnotic ability is the Stanford Hypnotic Susceptibility Scale Form C (Kurtz & Strube, 1996). But its use in a clinical practice requires a skilled clinician, and use of the Stanford scale can generate a high rate of negative side effects (29 percent to 31 percent), even with normal college students (Crawford, Hilgard, & Macdonald, 1982; Hilgard, 1974).

For clinical research, there are several reasons to use the Harvard Group Scale of Hypnotic Susceptibility Form A (Shor & Orne, 1962) with congruent subjective validation (Kirsch, Council, & Wickless, 1990). The Harvard scale was found to correlate 0.68 ($p<.0001$) with the gold standard in a recent study (Kurtz & Strube, 1996), and other studies have found correlations as high as 0.84 (Green, Lynn, & Carlson, 1992). The Harvard scale has norms on large cross-cultural normal samples (Perry, Nadon, & Button, 1992) and patient samples (Jupp, Collins, & McCabe, 1985; Pettinati, Horne, & Staats, 1985; Pettinati, Kogan, et al., 1990; Wickramasekera, 1995). With subjective scoring, the Harvard scale has many merits as a first test of hypnotizability. The score indicates the patient's risk for certain disorders and the mean rate of therapeutic response to learning-based treatments. The Hypnotic Induction Profile (Spiegel & Spiegel, 1978) has many merits, including its brevity (10 minutes), but its limited acceptance by the research community is a constraint on its use in clinical research.

### The Absorption Test

The absorption test does not involve a hypnotic induction or an actual behavioral measure of response to standardized suggestions. It is a short (10-minute) paper-and-pencil test that correlates moderately ($r = .2$ to $.4$) with the Harvard and Stanford tests (Nadon, Hoyt, Register, & Kihlstrom, 1991; Roche & McConkey, 1990; Tellegen & Atkinson, 1974; Woody, Bowers, &

Oakman, 1992). Absorption is a personality trait that is normally distributed, stable (30-day retest, $r = .91$) and appears to be partly genetically based, as shown in studies of monozygotic twins reared apart (Tellegen et al., 1988). Like hypnotic ability, absorption has also been shown to be a risk factor for several stress-related disorders (Wickramasekera, 1988, 1995, 2000), such as nonorganic chest pain (Saxon & Wickramasekera, 1994), somatic complaints in family medicine patients (Lynch, McGrady, Scherger, & Nagel, 1996), morbid obesity (Wickramasekera & Price, 1997), nightmares (Belicki & Belicki, 1986), and anticipatory nausea and vomiting secondary to chemotherapy (Challis & Stam, 1992).

In summary, hypnotic ability and absorption are influenced by genetic predisposition and serve as important indicators of risk. Absorption appears to provide a nonintrusive measure of hypnotic ability, particularly at the high (above 75 percent) and low (below 25 percent) ends of the scale. It can be given to a patient before a clinical session to obtain a primitive estimate of the patient's hypnotic ability.

## THERAPY AND OUTCOMES: CLINICAL EFFICACY AND HYPNOTIZABILITY

Hypnotherapy is the addition of hypnosis to some established form of psychosocial therapy (Wickramasekera, 1988, 1993), such as psychodynamic psychotherapy (Smith et al., 1980), behavior therapy (Bolocofsky, Spinter, & Coulthard-Morris, 1985; Wickramasekera, 1976), or biofeedback therapy (Wickramasekera, 1976, 1988). After a hypnotic induction, a variety of psychological techniques—for example, age regression (psychodynamic therapy), guided imagery, systematic desensitization (behavior therapy), or the feedback of biological information (biofeedback) may

reduce specific clinical symptoms. The clinical efficacy of blocking or recovering memories or altering pain perception is related to hypnotic ability (Hilgard, 1977; Hilgard & Hilgard, 1975). Hypnotic ability appears to be a normally distributed stable trait (Hilgard, 1965; Piccione, Hilgard, & Zimbardo, 1989) with a 0.71 test-retest correlation after 25 years. It also appears to be partly genetically based (Morgan, 1973; Morgan, Hilgard, & Davert, 1970). Hypnotizability is not compliance, conformity, gullibility, or social desirability (Hilgard, 1965; Wickramasekera, 1995), and it is *not* correlated significantly with known personality factors, except for absorption.

### Hypnotizability and the Empirical Efficacy of Specific Hypnotherapy

The use of hypnosis with people who have high measured hypnotizability can be called *specific hypnotherapy*. Several empirical studies have shown a correlation between measured hypnotizability and the clinical efficacy of hypnosis for asthma, acute and chronic pain, nausea and vomiting of pregnancy, obesity, and warts (Apfel et al., 1986; Barabasz & Barabasz, 1989; Barabasz & Spiegel, 1989; Collison, 1975; Ewer & Stewart, 1986; Hilgard & Hilgard, 1975; Levitt, 1993; Murphy et al., 1989; Stam et al., 1986; Wadden & Anderton, 1982). Hypnotizability has also been found to be related to the clinical efficacy of hypnotherapy for severe itching with chronic urticaria (Shertzer & Lookingbill, 1987), the pain of atopic eczema (H'ajek et al., 1990), obesity (Andersen, 1985), smoking cessation (Barabasz, Baer, Sheehan, & Barabasz, 1986), allergic skin reactions (Black, 1963), and migraine headaches (Cedercreutz, 1978).

### Empirical Efficacy of Nonspecific Hypnotherapy

It is likely that the label "hypnosis" and the relaxation and sensory restriction components of the hypnotic induction ritual can elicit a temporary increase in state hypnotic ability in some people of low or moderate trait hypnotic ability (Wickramasekera, 1970a, 1970c, 1970d, 1971a, 1971b, 1977b). It has been found that in some people, the label "hypnosis," operating as a placebo, can activate cognitive motivations, positive attitudes, and expectancies independent of baseline trait hypnotic ability (Kirsch, 1990). Lang, Benotsch, et al. (2000) reported that patients receiving hypnosis experienced reduced pain, anxiety, drug use, and time in surgery more than did patients in a standard medical control group. Kirsch, Montgomery, and Sapirstein (1995) conducted a meta-analysis of eight studies (see Figure 11.1) and found that hypnosis can *double* the efficacy of cognitive behavior therapy for obesity and that efficacy *increases* during a two-year follow up. A well-known earlier meta-analysis by Smith et al. (1980) found that the addition of hypnosis to psychodynamic psychotherapy significantly increased its efficacy above all other types of nonhypnotic therapies. A hypnotic induction has been shown to potentiate the effects of psychodynamic psychotherapy and cognitive behavior therapy for pain, insomnia, and hypertension, and most notably and surprisingly for obesity (Kirsch, 1996; Kirsch, Montgomery, & Sapirstein, 1995; Smith et al., 1980). Long-term weight loss is rare except with surgery (Brownell & Rodin, 1994). The Kirsch (1996) and Levitt (1993) studies challenged a previous literature review (Wadden & Anderton, 1982), which concluded that the efficacy of hypnosis would be limited to involuntary or autonomically mediated symptoms (e.g., pain, asthma, warts). In controlled studies, a hypnotic induction and therapy effectively reduced the aversiveness of medical procedures (Lang, Benotsch, et al., 2000; Wall & Womack, 1989). The same combination reduced insomnia (Stanton, 1989), severe nausea and vomiting secondary to chemotherapy (Walker, Dawson, Pollet,

Ratcliffe, & Hamilton, 1988), refractory irritable bowel syndrome (Harvey et al., 1989; Whorwell, Prior, & Colgan, 1987; Whorwell, Prior, & Faragher, 1984), fibromyalgia (Haanen et al., 1991), allergy relief (Madrid, Rostel, Pennington, & Murphy, 1995), and severe burn pain (Patterson et al., 1996). But the most important finding was from a randomized prospective study of breast cancer patients (Spiegel, Bloom, Kraemer, & Gottehil, 1989). Half of the women received self-hypnosis training for pain control added to standard medical management, and half received standard medical management alone. A 10-year follow-up showed that adjunctive hypnotherapy and group therapy for pain reduction was associated with a survival time of 36.6 months for the hypnotherapy group compared with 18.9 months for the standard medical management group (see Figure 11.2).

Hypnosis may be effective in uncovering unconscious threatening perceptions and memories that drive somatization and autonomic nervous system dysregulation (Wickramasekera, 1988, 1993, 1994; Wickramasekera & Wickramasekera, 1997). Although simply putting out symptomatic "fires" without finding the "matches" (the underlying causes) may be ineffective therapy (Wickramasekera, 1988, 1993), reducing symptoms makes the patient more comfortable and improves communication with the patient. Generally, the response of acute clinical symptoms (acute pain, anxiety) to hypnosis has a rapid onset (within a few minutes). But more recent randomized controlled prospective studies of adjunctive hypnotherapy suggested that for chronic diseases like metastatic breast cancer (Spiegel, Bloom, et al., 1989) and obesity (Kirsch, Montgomery, & Sapirstein, 1995; Levitt, 1993), positive effects from hypnotherapy could be delayed for several weeks or months.

In summary, measured hypnotic ability contributes in a *specific* way to the clinical

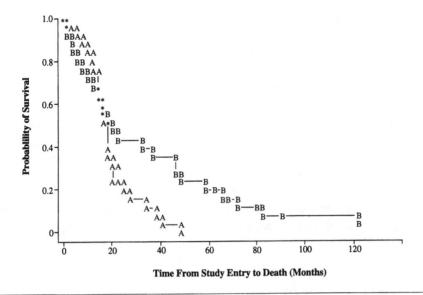

**Figure 11.2**   Kaplan-Meier Survival Plot of Metastatic Breast Cancer Patients in Psychosocial Treatment Study

SOURCE: Adapted with permission from Spiegel, Bloom, et al., 1989.

efficacy of hypnosis, and hypnotic induction alone functions in a *nonspecific* way as a placebo, serving as the basis for the clinical efficacy of hypnotherapy in individuals of low or moderate hypnotic ability.

## INDICATIONS AND CONTRAINDICATIONS FOR THE ADDITION OF HYPNOSIS TO A STANDARD FORM OF PSYCHOTHERAPY

Hypnosis is particularly indicated if the patient has high hypnotic ability and a positive attitude toward hypnosis. For example, a chronic pain patient with high hypnotic ability and a positive attitude toward hypnosis will profit from suggestions that alter present or future pain perception, blur the memory of past pain, and provide ego-strengthening suggestions to elevate mood and increase patient self-efficacy perception. Hypnosis appears to be particularly effective for involuntary or autonomically mediated symptoms

like acute pain, asthma, warts, and irritable bowel syndrome. Hypnosis may be effective for patients with moderate or even low hypnotic ability on a nonspecific (placebo) basis if they have very positive but realistic attitudes toward hypnosis. Subjects with moderate and low trait hypnotic ability are more likely to profit from hypnosis if adjunctive methods are used to temporarily increase "state" hypnotic responsivity. Adjunctive methods include theta and alpha EEG biofeedback, heart rate variability biofeedback (HRV), frontal EMG biofeedback, or sensory restriction (Barabasz & Barabasz, 1989; Engstrom, London & Hart, 1970; Wickramasekera, 1970a, 1971a, 1976, 1977a, 1977b, 1988). If there is a need to increase rapport and intensify positive transference reactions, hypnosis may be indicated (Fromm & Nash, 1992; Wickramasekera, 1970a, 1970c, 1970d).

The major contraindications for hypnosis are poor diagnostic and psychotherapeutic skills in the therapist, and particularly, countertransference problems. In people with high hypnotic responsivity, hypnosis can mask organic disease (e.g., the pain of a brain tumor) and objective psychopathology (*DSM-IV*). Everything that occurs in psychotherapy occurs with more rapid onset in hypnotherapy (Wickramasekera, 1988). Is the patient's ego stable and integrated enough to do abreactive, regressive, or uncovering psychodynamic work? Patients with borderline personality disorder, major dissociative disorders, and paranoid reactions need to be approached with caution even by highly trained and experienced hypnotherapists.

## CLINICAL APPLICATIONS OF HYPNOTIZABILITY MEASURES

A patient who has high hypnotic ability but is technologically and quantitatively minded and skeptical of hypnosis should get "delayed biofeedback" (Wickramasekera, 1988, 1993). Delayed biofeedback involves verbally instructing the patient to relax with eyes closed and withholding immediate biological feedback (e.g., EMG). The feedback can be provided after 4 or 5 minutes of passive relaxation to confirm the objective changes in physiology. This objectively builds the high hypnotizable patients' faith in their ability to alter their physiology. It is a replicated finding that immediate auditory EMG feedback initially interferes with relaxation learning of high hypnotic subjects (Qualls & Sheehan, 1981). Labeling the procedure "delayed biofeedback" rather than "hypnosis" enables the skilled therapist to still access instructionally the patient's hypnotic ability, but to bypass the patient's skepticism. People with low hypnotic ability learn to decrease the frontal EMG signal (relaxation) most rapidly with immediate EMG biofeedback (Qualls & Sheehan, 1981). If a patient with low hypnotic ability has a

strongly positive attitude toward hypnosis, hypnotic suggestions can be given along with the immediate biofeedback training procedure, thus capitalizing on the separate placebo or nonspecific components of both biofeedback and hypnosis (Wickramasekera, 1976, 1977a, 1977b, 1988). Hence, there are good clinical and scientific reasons (matching cognitive styles to therapy procedures) to unobtrusively measure every patient's hypnotic ability in routine clinical practice, especially with chronic stress-related disease (Wickramasekera, 1988, 1993, 1998).

If a patient is found to have low hypnotic ability but has a positive attitude toward hypnosis, certain biofeedback procedures may temporarily increase "state" hypnotic responsivity. In fact, pretreatment procedures such as sensory restriction, HRV, EMG, and EEG alpha-theta biofeedback training (Wickramasekera, 1976, 1977a, 1977b, 1988, 1993) are required for 90 percent of patients to respond to hypnosis, because only 10 percent of the population have high hypnotic ability. These pretreatments can temporarily disable security operations perhaps encoded in muscular bracing and vascular constriction (Wickramasekera, 1976, 1977b, 1988).

## PROFESSIONAL ORGANIZATION

Candidates to be trained for clinical hypnotic training must be licensed professionals in psychology, medicine, or other state-licensed health professions. The Society for Clinical and Experimental Hypnosis and the International Society of Hypnosis have established codes of ethics that define and limit the persons who can be taught hypnosis. The American Boards of Hypnosis identify clinicians with advanced competence in psychological (ABPH), medical (ABMH), and dental (ABDH) hypnosis.

## CONCLUSION

Hypnosis and hypnotherapy are powerful interventions with many applications in primary care medicine and dentistry. Hypnotherapy can be combined with many medical, psychological, and dental treatments. Measuring the hypnotic ability of patients is important in selecting those individuals who will benefit best from hypnotic interventions, as well as in customizing a hypnotherapy protocol for a specific patient. Positive patient attitudes toward hypnosis increase the efficacy of hypnotherapy, even in individuals of lower hypnotic ability. Adjunctive interventions such as biofeedback and neurofeedback can be useful in initially increasing hypnotic responsiveness and can be used in tandem with hypnotherapy for many patients throughout treatment. The absorption test is a paper-and-pencil test that can serve as a time-efficient identification of good candidates for hypnotherapy. The availability of well-trained hypnotherapists who are also skilled in psychotherapy is critical in delivering effective hypnotic interventions in any clinical setting. Severely unstable patients, with diagnoses such as borderline personality and dissociative disorders, should undergo hypnotherapy only with great caution. Several professional organizations provide ethical guidelines and certification programs for professionals using hypnosis and hypnotherapy.

## REFERENCES

Andersen, M. S. (1985). Hypnotizability as a factor in the hypnotic treatment of obesity. *International Journal of Clinical and Experimental Hypnosis, 33,* 150–159.

Andreychuk, T., & Skriver, C. (1975). Hypnosis and biofeedback in the treatment of migraine headaches. *International Journal of Clinical and Experimental Hypnosis, 13*(3), 172–183.

Apfel, R. J., Kelley, S. F., & Frankel, F. H. (1986). The role of hypnotizability in the pathogenesis and treatment of nausea and vomiting of pregnancy. *Journal of Psychosomatic Obstetrics and Gynecology, 5,* 179–186.

Barabasz, A. F., Baer, L., Sheehan, D. V., & Barabasz, M. (1986). A three year clinical follow-up of hypnosis and restricted environmental stimulation therapy for smoking. *International Journal of Clinical and Experimental Hypnosis, 34,* 169–181.

Barabasz, A. F., & Barabasz, M. (1989). Effects of restricted environmental stimulation: Enhancement of hypnotizability for experimental and chronic pain control. *International Journal of Clinical and Experimental Hypnosis, 37,* 217–231.

Barabasz, M., & Spiegel, D. (1989). Hypnotizability and weight loss in obese subjects. *International Journal of Eating Disorders, 8,* 335–341.

Barber, J., & Mayer, D. J. (1977). Evaluation of the efficacy and neural mechanism of a hypnotic analgesia procedure in experimental and clinical dental pain. *Pain, 4,* 41–48.

Barber, T. X. (1984). Changing "unchangeable" bodily processes by (hypnotic) suggestion: A new look at hypnosis, cognitions, imagining, and the mind-body problem. *Advances, 1*(2), 6–40.

Belicki, K., & Belicki, D. (1986). Predisposition for nightmares: A study of hypnotic ability, vividness of imagery, and absorption. *Journal of Clinical Psychology, 42,* 714–718.

Bennett, H. L. (1986). Preoperative instruction for decreased bleeding during spine surgery. *Anesthesiology, 65,* A245.

Black, S. (1963). Inhibition of immediate-type hypersensitivity response by direct suggestion under hypnosis. *British Medical Journal, vi,* 925–929.

Blum, G. S., & Nash, J. (1981). Posthypnotic attenuation of a visual illusion as reflected in perceptual reports and cortical event-related potentials. *Academic Psychology Bulletin, 3,* 251–271.

Bolocofsky, D. N., Spinter, D., & Coulthard-Morris, L. (1985). Effectiveness of hypnosis as an adjunct to behavioral weight management. *Journal of Clinical Psychology, 41,* 35–41.

Braun, G. G., & Sachs, R. G. (1985). The development of multiple personality disorder: Predisposing, precipitating, and perpetuating factors. In R. P. Kluft (Ed.), *Childhood antecedents of multiple personality* (pp. 37–64). Washington, DC: American Psychiatric Press.

Brown, D. P. (1992). Clinical hypnosis research since 1986. In E. Fromm & M. R. Nash (Eds.), *Contemporary hypnosis research* (pp. 427–458). New York: Guilford.

Brownell, K. D., & Rodin, J. (1994). The dieting maelstrom: Is it possible and advisable to lose weight? *American Psychologist, 49(9),* 781–791.

Cedercreutz, C. (1978). Hypnotic treatment of 100 cases of migraines. In F. H. Frankel & H. S. Zamansky (Eds.), *Hypnosis at its bicentennial* (pp. 122–133). New York: Plenum.

Challis, G. B., & Stam, H. J. (1992). A longitudinal study of the development of anticipatory nausea and vomiting in cancer chemotherapy patients: The role of absorption and autonomic perception. *Health Psychology, 11(3),* 181–189.

Collison, D. A. (1975). Which asthmatic patients should be treated by hypnotherapy? *Medical Journal of Australia, 1,* 776–781.

Crawford, H. J., Hilgard, J. R., & Macdonald, H. (1982). Transient experiences following hypnotic testing and special termination procedures. *International Journal of Clinical and Experimental Hypnosis, 30,* 117–126.

Crowson, J. J., Conroy, A. M., & Chester, T. D. (1991). Hypnotizability as related to visually induced affective reactivity. *International Journal of Clinical and Experimental Hypnosis, 39(3),* 140–144.

Damasio, A. R. (1999). *The feeling of what happens: Body and emotion in the making of consciousness.* New York: Harcourt Brace Jovanovich.

DeBenedittis, G., Paneral, A. A., & Villamirqa, M. A. (1989). Effects of hypnotic analgesia and hypnotizability on experimental ischemic pain. *International Journal of Clinical and Experimental Hypnosis, 37(1),* 55–69.

DePascalis, V. (1999). Psychophysiological correlates of hypnosis and hypnotic susceptibility. *International Journal of Clinical and Experimental Hypnosis, 47(2),* 117–143.

Engstrom, D. R., London, P., & Hart, J. T. (1970). Hypnotic susceptibility increased by EEG alpha training. *Nature, 227,* 1261–1262.

Ewer, T. C., & Stewart, D. E. (1986). Improvement in bronchial hyperresponsiveness in patients with moderate asthma after treatment with a hypnotic technique. *British Medical Journal, i,* 1129–1132.

Fromm, E., & Nash, M. R. (Eds.). (1992). *Contemporary hypnosis research.* New York: Guilford.

Gick, M., McLeod, C., & Hulihan, D. (1997). Absorption, social desirability, and symptoms in a behavioral medicine population. *Journal of Nervous and Mental Disease, 815(7),* 454–458.

Goldstein, A., & Hilgard, E. R. (1975). Lack of influence of the morphine antagonist naloxone on hypnotic analgesia. *Proceedings of the National Academy of Sciences USA, 72,* 2041–2043.

Graffin, N. F., Ray, W. J., & Lundy, R. (1995). EEG concomitants of hypnosis and hypnotic susceptibility. *Journal of Abnormal Psychology, 104(1),* 123–131.

Green, J., Lynn, S., & Carlson, B. (1992). Finding the hypnotic virtuoso—Another look. *International Journal of Clinical and Experimental Hypnosis, 50,* 68–73.

Greenleaf, M., Fisher, S., Miaskowski, C., & DuHamel, K. (1992). Hypnotizability and recovery from cardiac surgery. *American Journal of Clinical Hypnosis, 35*(2), 119–128.

Haanen, H. C. M., Hoenderdos, T. W., Romunde, L. K. J., Hop, W. C. J., Mallee, C., Terwiel, J. P., & Hekster, G. B. (1991). Controlled trial of hypnotherapy in the treatment of refractory fibromyalgia. *Journal of Rheumatology, 18*(1), 72–75.

H'ajek, P., Jakoubek, B., & Radil, T. (1990). Gradual increase in cutaneous threshold induced by repeated hypnosis of healthy individuals and patients with atopic eczema. *Perceptual and Motor Skills, 70,* 549–550.

Harvey, R. F., Hinton, R. A., & Gunary, R. M. (1989). Individual and group hypnotherapy in treatment of refractory irritable bowel syndrome. *Lancet, 1,* 424–425.

Hilgard, E. R. (1965). *Hypnotic susceptibility.* New York: Harcourt, Brace & World.

Hilgard, E. R. (1974). Sequelae to hypnosis. *International Journal of Clinical and Experimental Hypnosis, 22,* 281–298.

Hilgard, E. R. (1977). *Divided consciousness: Multiple controls in human thought and action.* New York: Wiley.

Hilgard, E. R., & Hilgard, J. R. (1975). *Hypnosis in the relief of pain.* Los Altos, CA: William Kaufmann.

Institute of Medicine. (1989). Behavioral influences on the endocrine and immune systems. Research briefing from the Division of Health Sciences Policy and the Division of Mental Health and Biobehavioral Medicine. Washington, DC: Author.

Integration of behavioral and relaxation approaches into the treatment of chronic pain and insomnia. NIH technology assessment panel on integration of behavioral and relaxation approaches in the treatment of chronic pain and insomnia. (1996). *Journal of the American Medical Association, 276*(4), 313–318.

John, R., Hollander, B., & Perry, C. (1983). Hypnotizability and phobic behavior: Further supporting data. *Journal of Abnormal Psychology, 92*(3), 390–392.

Jupp, J. J., Collins, J. K., & McCabe, M. P. (1985). Estimates of hypnotizability: Standard group scale versus subjective impression in clinical populations. *International Journal of Clinical and Experimental Hypnosis, 33*(2), 140–149.

Kelly, S. F. (1984). Measured hypnotic response and phobic behavior. A brief communication. *International Journal of Clinical and Experimental Hypnosis, 32*(1), 1–5.

Kermit, K., Devine, D. A., & Tatman, S. M. (2000). HRMTP in chronic pain patients: Implications for primary care and chronic pain programs. *The Journal of Nervous and Mental Disease, 188*(9), 577–582.

King, D. R., & McDonald, R. D. (1976). Hypnotic susceptibility and verbal conditioning. *International Journal of Clinical and Experimental Hypnosis, 24,* 29–37.

Kirsch, I. (1990). *Changing expectations: A key to effective psychotherapy.* Pacific Grove, CA: Brooks/Cole.

Kirsch, I. (1996). Hypnotic enhancement of cognitive-behavioral weight loss treatments—Another meta-reanalysis. *Journal of Consulting and Clinical Psychology, 64*(3), 517–519.

Kirsch, I., Council, J. R., & Wickless, C. (1990). Subjective scoring for the Harvard Group Scale of Hypnotic Susceptibility, Form A. *International Journal of Clinical and Experimental Hypnosis, 38,* 112–124.

Kirsch, I., Montgomery, G., & Sapirstein, G. (1995). Hypnosis as an adjunct to cognitive-behavioral psychotherapy: A meta-analysis. *Journal of Consulting and Clinical Psychology, 63*(2), 214–220.

Klein, K. B., & Spiegel, D. (1989). Modulation of gastric acid secretion by hypnosis. *Gastroenterology, 96,* 1383–1387.

Knox, V. J., Gekoski, W. L., Shum, K., & McLaughlin, D. M. (1981). Analgesia for experimentally induced pain: Multiple sessions of acupuncture compared to hypnosis in high- and low-susceptible subjects. *Journal of Abnormal Psychology, 90,* 28–34.

Kurtz, R. M., & Strube, M. J. (1996). Multiple susceptibility testing: Is it helpful? *American Journal of Clinical Hypnosis, 38*(3), 172–184.

Lang, E. V., Benotsch, E. G., Fick, L. J., Lutgendorf, S., Berbaum, M. L., Berbaum, K. S., et al. (2000). Adjunctive non-pharmacological analgesia for invasive medical procedures: A randomized trial. *Lancet, 355,* 1486–1490.

Lang, E. V., Joyce, J., Spiegel, D., Hamilton, D., & Lee, K. K. (1996). Self-hypnotic relaxation during interventional radiological procedures: Effects on pain perception and intravenous drug use. *International Journal of Clinical and Experimental Hypnosis, 44*(2), 106–119.

Larsen, S. (1966). Strategies for reducing phobic behavior. *Dissertation Abstracts International, 26,* 6850.

Levitt, E. E. (1993). Hypnosis in the treatment of obesity. In J. W. Rhue, S. J. Lynn, & I. Kirsch (Eds.), *Handbook of clinical hypnosis* (pp. 511–532). Washington, DC: American Psychological Association.

Lynch, D. J., McGrady, A., Scherger, C., & Nagel, R. (1996). Somatization in family practice. Paper presented at the annual meeting of the American Psychological Association, Toronto, Ontario.

Madrid, A., Rostel, G., Pennington, D., & Murphy, D. (1995). Subjective assessment of allergy relief following group hypnosis and self-hypnosis: A preliminary study. *American Journal of Clinical Hypnosis, 38*(2), 80–86.

McGrady, A., Lynch, D., Nagel, R., & Zsembik, C. (1999). Application of the high risk model of threat perception to a primary care patient population. *The Journal of Nervous and Mental Disease, 187,* 369–375.

Morgan, A. H. (1973). The heritability of hypnotic susceptibility in twins. *Journal of Abnormal Psychology, 82,* 55–61.

Morgan, A. H., Hilgard, E. R., & Davert, E. C. (1970). The heritability of hypnotic susceptibility in twins: A preliminary report. *Behavior Genetics, 1,* 213–224.

Murphy, A. I., Lehrer, P. M., Karlin, R., Swartzman, L., Hochron, S., & McCann, G. (1989). Hypnotic susceptibility and its relationship to outcome in the behavioral treatment of asthma: Some preliminary data. *Psychological Reports, 65*(2), 691–698.

Nace, E. P., Warwick, A. M., Kelley, R. L., & Evans, F. J. (1982). Hypnotizability and outcome in brief psychotherapy. *Journal of Clinical Psychiatry, 43,* 129–133.

Nadon, R., Hoyt, I. P., Register, P. A., & Kihlstrom, J. F. (1991). Absorption and hypnotizability: Context effects reexamined. *Journal of Personality and Social Psychology, 60,* 144–153.

Paskewitz, D. A. (1977). EEG alpha activity and its relationship to altered states of consciousness. Conceptual and investigative approaches to hypnosis and hypnotic phenomena. *Annals of the New York Academy of Sciences, 296,* 154–161.

Patterson, D. R., Goldberg, M. L., & Ehde, D. M. (1996). Hypnosis in the treatment of patients with severe burns. *American Journal of Clinical Hypnosis, 38*(3), 200–212.

Perlstrom, J. R., & Wickramasekera, I. E. (1998). Insomnia, hypnotic ability, negative affectivity, and the high risk model of threat perception. *Journal of Nervous and Mental Disease, 186,* 437–440.

Perry, C., Nadon, R., & Button, J. (1992). The measurement of hypnotic ability. In E. Fromm & M. R. Nash (Eds.), *Contemporary hypnosis research* (pp. 459–490). New York: Guilford.

Pettinati, H. M., Horne, R. L., & Staats, J. M. (1985). Hypnotizability in patients with anorexia nervosa and bulimia. *Archives of General Psychiatry, 42,* 1014–1016.

Pettinati, H. M., Kogan, L. G., Evans, F. J., Wade, J. H., Horne, L., & Staats, J. M. (1990). Hypnotizability of psychiatric inpatients according to two different scales. *American Journal of Psychiatry, 147*(1), 69–75.

Piccione, C., Hilgard, E. R., & Zimbardo, P. G. (1989). On the degree of stability of measured hypnotizability over a 25-year period. *Journal of Personality and Social Psychology, 56*(2), 289–295.

Putnam, F. W. (1989). *Diagnosis and treatment of multiple personality disorder.* New York: Guilford.

Qualls, P. J., & Sheehan, P. W. (1981). Electromyograph biofeedback as a relaxation technique. A critical appraisal and reassessment. *Psychological Bulletin, 90*(1), 21–42.

Roche, S. M., & McConkey, M. (1990). Absorption: Nature, assessment, and correlates. *Journal of Personality and Social Psychology, 59*(1), 91–101.

Rose, R., & Sternberg, E. (2001, March). *Vital connections: Science of mind-body interactions: A report on the interdisciplinary conference.* Conference held at the National Institutes of Health, Bethesda, MD.

Ruzyla-Smith, P., Barabasz, A., Barabasz, M., & Warner, D. (1995). Effects of hypnosis on the immune response: B-cells, T-cells, helper and suppressor cells. *American Journal of Clinical Hypnosis, 38*(2), 71–79.

Saxon, J., & Wickramasekera, I. (1994, October). Discriminating patients with organic disease from somatizers among patients with chest pain using factors from the high risk model of threat perception. Presentation to the Society for Experimental and Clinical Hypnosis, San Francisco, CA.

Shertzer, C. I, & Lookingbill, D. P. (1987). Effects of relaxation therapy and hypnotizability in chronic urticaria. *Archives of Dermatology, 123,* 913–916.

Shor, R. E., & Orne, E. C. (1962). *Harvard group scale of hypnotic susceptibility, form A.* Palo Alto, CA: Consulting Psychologists Press.

Smith, M. L., Glass, G. V., & Miller, T. I. (1980). *The benefits of psychotherapy.* Baltimore: Johns Hopkins University Press.

Spiegel, D. (1991). Uses of hypnosis in managing medical symptoms. *Psychiatric Medicine, 6*(3), 521–533.

Spiegel, D., & Barabasz, A. F. (1988). Effects of hypnotic instructions on P300 event-related-potential amplitudes: Research and clinical applications. *American Journal of Clinical Hypnosis, 31,* 11–17.

Spiegel, D., Bloom, J. R., Kraemer, H. C., & Gottehil, E. (1989). Effect of psychosocial treatment on survival of patients with metastatic breast cancer. *Lancet, 2,* 888–891.

Spiegel, D., Cutcomb, S., Ren, C., & Pribram, K. (1985). Hypnotic hallucination alters evoked potentials. *Journal of Abnormal Psychology, 94,* 249–255.

Spiegel, D., Hunt, T., & Dondershine, H. (1988). Dissociation and hypnotizability in post-traumatic stress disorder, *American Journal of Psychiatry, 145,* 301–305.

Spiegel, H., & Spiegel, D. (1978). *Trance and treatment: Clinical uses of hypnosis.* New York: Basic Books.

Stam, H., McGrath, P., Brooke, R., & Cosire, F. (1986). Hypnotizability and the treatment of chronic facial pain. *International Journal of Clinical and Experimental Hypnosis, 34,* 182–191.

Stanton, H. E. (1989). Hypnotic relaxation and the reduction of sleep onset insomnia. *International Journal of Psychosomatics, 35*(1–4), 64–68.

Stern, J. A., Brown, M., Ulett, A., & Sletten, I. (1977). A comparison of hypnosis, acupuncture, morphine, Valium, aspirin, and placebo in the management of experimentally induced pain. *Annals of the New York Academy of Sciences, 296,* 175–193.

Stutman, R. K., & Bliss, E. L. (1985). Post-traumatic stress disorder, hypnotizability, and imagery. *American Journal of Psychiatry, 142*(6), 741–743.

Szechtman, H., Woody, E., Bowers, K. S., & Nahmias, C. (1998). Where the imaginal appears real: A positron emission tomography study of auditory hallucinations. *Proceedings of the National Academy of Sciences, 95,* 1956–1960.

Tellegen, A., & Atkinson, G. (1974). Openness to absorbing and self-altering experiences ("absorption"), a trait related to hypnotic susceptibility. *Journal of Abnormal Psychology, 83,* 268–277.

Tellegen, A., Lykken, D. T., Bouchard, T. J., Jr., Wilcox, K. J., Segal, N. L., & Rich, S. (1988). Personality similarity in twins reared apart and together. *Journal of Personality and Social Psychology, 54*(6), 1031–1039.

Velten, E. (1968). A laboratory task for induction of mood states. *Behavior Research and Therapy, 18,* 79–86.

Wadden, T. A., & Anderton, C. H. (1982). The clinical use of hypnosis. *Psychological Bulletin, 91,* 215–243.

Walker, L. G., Dawson, A. A., Pollet, S. M., Ratcliffe, M. A., & Hamilton, L. (1988). Hypnotherapy for chemotherapy side effects. *British Journal of Experimental and Clinical Hypnosis, 5*(2), 79–82.

Wall, V. J., & Womack, W. (1989). Hypnotic versus active cognitive strategies for alleviation of procedural distress in pediatric oncology patients. *American Journal of Clinical Hypnosis, 31*(3), 181–189.

Watson, D. & Tellegen, A. (1985). Toward a consensual structure of mood. *Psychological Bulletin, 98*(2), 219–235.

Webb, R. A. (1962). Suggestibility and verbal conditioning. *International Journal of Clinical and Experimental Hypnosis, 10,* 275–279.

Weiss, R. L., Ullman, L. P., & Krasner, L. (1960). On the relationship between hypnotizability and response to verbal operant conditioning. *Psychological Reports, 6,* 59–60.

Whorwell, P.J. (1989). Hypnotherapy in irritable bowel syndrome. *Lancet, 1*(8638), 622.

Whorwell, P. J., Houghton, L. A., Taylor, E. E., & Maxton, D. G. (1992). Physiological effects of emotion: Assessment via hypnosis. *Lancet, 340*(8811), 69–72.

Whorwell, P. J., Prior, A., & Colgan, S. M. (1987). Hypnotherapy in severe irritable bowel syndrome: Further experience. *Gut, 28,* 423–425.

Whorwell, P. J., Prior, A., & Faragher, E. B. (1984). Controlled trial of hypnotherapy in the treatment of severe refractory irritable bowel syndrome. *Lancet, 2*(8414), 1232–1234.

Wickramasekera, I. (1970a). Effects of sensory restriction on susceptibility to hypnosis. *Journal of Abnormal Psychology, 76,* 69–75.

Wickramasekera, I. (1970b). The effects of hypnosis and a control procedure on verbal conditioning. Paper presented at the annual meeting of the American Psychological Association, Miami, FL.

Wickramasekera, I. (1970c, October). Goals and some methods in psychotherapy: Hypnosis and isolation. *The American Journal of Clinical Hypnosis, 13(2),* 95–100.

Wickramasekera, I. (1970d). Reinforcement and/or transference in hypnosis and psychotherapy: A hypothesis. *The American Journal of Clinical Hypnosis, 12(3),* 137–140.

Wickramasekera, I. (1971a). Effects of EMG feedback training on susceptibility to hypnosis: Preliminary observations (summary). *Proceedings, 79th Annual Convention of the American Psychological Association, 6,* 783–784.

Wickramasekera, I. (1971b). Effects of "hypnosis" and task motivational instructions in attempting to influence the "voluntary" self-deprivation of money. *Journal of Personality and Social Psychology, 19(3),* 311–314.

Wickramasekera, I. (1976). *Biofeedback, behavior therapy and hypnosis.* Chicago: Nelson Hall.

Wickramasekera, I. (1977a). The placebo effect and medical instruments in biofeedback. *Journal of Clinical Engineering, 2(3),* 227–230.

Wickramasekera, I. (1977b). On attempts to modify hypnotic susceptibility: Some psychophysiological procedures and promising directions. *Annals of the New York Academy of Sciences, 296,* 143–153.

Wickramasekera, I. (1979). A model of the patient at high risk for chronic stress related disorders: Do beliefs have biological consequences? Paper presented at the annual convention of the Biofeedback Society of America, San Diego, CA.

Wickramasekera, I. (1986). A model of people at high risk to develop chronic stress related somatic symptoms: Some predictions. *Professional Psychology: Research and Practice, 17(5),* 437–447.

Wickramasekera, I. (1988). *Clinical behavioral medicine: Some concepts and procedures.* New York: Plenum.

Wickramasekera, I. (1993). Assessment and treatment of somatization disorders: The high risk model of threat perception. In J. W. Rhue, S. J. Lynn, & I. Kirsch (Eds.), *Handbook of clinical hypnosis* (pp. 587–621). Washington, DC: American Psychological Association.

Wickramasekera, I. (1994). Somatic to psychological symptoms and information transfer from implicit to explicit memory: A controlled case study with predictions from the high risk model of threat perception. *Dissociation, 7(3),* 153–166.

Wickramasekera, I. (1995). Somatization: Concepts, data and predictions from the high risk model of threat perception. *Journal of Nervous and Mental Disease, 183(1),* 15–23.

Wickramasekera, I. (1998). Secrets kept from the mind but not the body or behavior: The unsolved problems of identifying and treating somatization and psychophysiological disease. *Advances: The Journal of Mind-Body Medicine, 14,* 81–132.

Wickramasekera, I. (2000). On the interaction of two orthogonal risk factors, (1) hypnotic ability and (2) negative affect (threat perception) for psychophysiological dysregulation (sympathetic and parasympathetic) in somatization disorders. In V. DePascalis, V. A. Gheorghiu, P. W. Sheehan, & I. Kirsch (Eds.), *Suggestion and suggestibility—Theory and research* (pp. 245–252). Munich, Germany: Hypnosis International Monograph.

Wickramasekera, I., & Atkinson, R. (1992, August). Obesity, hypnotic ability and the psychophysiology of cognitive threat. In I. Wickramasekera (Chair, with H. Spiegel & A. Tellegen), *Hypnotic ability as a risk factor for psychopathology and pathophysiology.* Symposium conducted at the annual meeting of the American Psychological Association, Washington, DC.

Wickramasekera, I., Pope, A. T., & Kolm, P. (1996). On the interaction of hypnotizability and negative affect in chronic pain: Implications for the somatization of trauma. *Journal of Nervous and Mental Disease, 184,* 628–635.

Wickramasekera, I., & Price, D. (1997). Morbid obesity, absorption, neuroticism and the high risk model of threat perception. *American Journal of Clinical Hypnosis, 34*(4), 291–302.

Wickramasekera, I., Ware, C., & Saxon, J. (1992, August). EEG defined insomnia and hypnotic ability with pathophysiology excluded. In I. Wickramasekera (Chair, with H. Spiegel & A. Tellegen), *Hypnotic ability as a risk factor for psychopathology and pathophysiology.* Symposium conducted at the annual meeting of the American Psychological Association, Washington, DC.

Wickramasekera, I., & Wickramasekera, I., II. (1997). EMG correlates in hypnosis: Recall of a repressed memory: A case report. *Dissociation, 10*(1), 11–20.

Woody, E. Z., Bowers, K. S., & Oakman, J. M. (1992). A conceptual analysis of hypnotic responsiveness: Experience, individual differences, and context. In E. Fromm, & M. Nash (Eds.), *Contemporary hypnosis research* (pp. 3–33). New York: Guilford.

Woody, E., & Szechtman, H. (2000). Hypnotic hallucinations: Towards a biology of epistemology. *Contemporary Hypnosis, 17*(1), 4–14.

Zachariae, R. (2001). Hypnosis and immunity. In R. Ader, D. L. Felton, & N. Cohen (Ed.), *Psychoneuroimmunology* (3rd ed., vol. 2, pp. 133–160). San Diego: Academic Press.

Zachariae, R., Bjerring, P., & Arendt-Nielsen, L. (1989). Modulation of type I immediate and type IV delayed immunoreactivity using direct suggestion and guided imagery during hypnosis. *Allergy, 44*(8), 537–542.

Zinn, M., McCain, C., & Zinn, M. (2000). Musical performance anxiety and the high-risk model of threat perception. *Medical Problems of Performing Artists, 15*(2), 65–71.

# CHAPTER 12

# Cognitive-Behavioral Therapies for the Medical Clinic

MARK A. LAU, ZINDEL V. SEGAL, AND ARI E. ZARETSKY

---

**Abstract:** Many common medical conditions—for example, chronic pain, chronic fatigue, atypical chest pain, and irritable bowel syndrome—and many medical conditions with unknown etiology have very strong psychological underpinnings. Regardless of the specific disease entity, cognitive factors play an important role in determining how people cope with illness. Cognitive-behavioral therapy (CBT) was originally developed to treat depression and anxiety. Over the last two decades, empirical research has shown that CBT can be successfully applied to treat an array of different medical conditions, and several standard CBT protocols now exist. This chapter describes the basic principles of CBT and illustrates specific cognitive and behavioral strategies for medical disorders. Further, the chapter emphasizes customizing CBT techniques to the individual patient and structuring treatment based on a comprehensive cognitive formulation.

---

## ORIGINS OF COGNITIVE-BEHAVIOR THERAPY FOR MEDICAL DISORDERS

The huge variation in the subjective effects of medical conditions of equal objective severity is now well accepted. People display marked differences in how much they complain about physical symptoms, how they respond to treatment, and how they cope with medical conditions. One explanation for this variation emphasizes the *illness representation* held by the patient—that is, the patient's cognitive (mental) schema or paradigm of the illness (Weinman, Petrie, Moss-Morris, & Horne, 1996). There is evidence that these representations are disease-specific in nature and

that they can explain differences in self-care behaviors (Petrie, Weinman, Sharpe, & Buckley, 1996) and in emotional reactions to symptoms (Prohaska, Keller, Leventhal, & Leventhal, 1987). Moreover, understanding the types of meanings patients ascribe to their illnesses may depend in large part on the cognitive representations they hold (Buick, 1997). These representations may influence patients' emotional reactions (e.g., depression, anxiety) to their symptoms, patients' adaptation to the limits imposed by their illnesses, and/or patients' compliance with treatment regimens for their disorders.

Cognitive-behavioral interventions, which focus on identifying and modifying cognitive representations, are therefore well suited to the treatment of medical problems. Many approaches can be classified as cognitive-behavioral in nature, including cognitive therapy (DeRubeis, Tang, & Beck, 2001), rational emotive behavior therapy (Dryden & Ellis, 2001), self-management therapy (Rokke & Rehm, 2001), and problem-solving therapy (D'Zurilla & Nezu, 2001).

All these cognitive-behavioral interventions share three fundamental assumptions: (1) Cognition mediates an individual's response to the environment; (2) change can be effected through an exploration and alteration of idiosyncratic, dysfunctional ways of thinking; and (3) cognitive-behavioral therapies draw on a combination of cognitive and behavioral principles and techniques to effect change (Dobson & Dozois, 2001).

Of several cognitive-behavioral interventions, the approach advocated by Aaron T. Beck has received the greatest amount of empirical validation and acceptance (A. T. Beck, 1967; J. S. Beck, 1995; Clark & Beck, 1999). A. T. Beck developed cognitive therapy in the early 1960s as a structured, short-term, symptom-focused treatment for depression. Although he initially adopted a traditional psychoanalytic perspective on the repetitive, negative, and self-defeating nature of depressed patients' thinking styles, Beck found little support for the view that these thoughts reflected important symbolic processes related to introjected anger. He began to work more directly with the overt thoughts that patients were reporting and focused less on interpreting patients' thoughts and behavior in terms of their deeper symbolic meanings. With time, Beck described the content and processes of cognition, which seemed unique to depression, and developed several clinical interventions that improved patients' moods by directly addressing their ways of thinking.

Since that time, numerous outcome studies have established cognitive-behavioral therapy as an empirically validated therapy for a wide range of psychological disorders, including depression and the anxiety disorders (DeRubeis & Crits-Christoph, 1998). The applications of CBT have also been expanded to include it as a sole or adjunctive treatment for a variety of medical disorders. As early as the 1970s, CBT was modified to specifically address medical problems such as chronic pain (Holzman, Turk, & Kerns, 1986). Subsequent research has established CBT as an effective treatment for the management of chronic pain (Morley, Eccleston, & Williams, 1999) as well as for other health-related conditions, including chronic fatigue syndrome (Price & Couper, 2000) and irritable bowel syndrome (Payne & Blanchard, 1995). In addition, CBT has been established as an empirically validated treatment for the management of the psychological effects of cancer and for smoking cessation (Compas, Haaga, Keefe, Leitenber, & Williams, 1998). Research exploring a potential role for CBT in the treatment of other medical disorders is ongoing. There is good reason to believe that CBT can be successfully adapted to a wide range of medical difficulties, including diabetes and cardiac problems (White, 2001).

## PRINCIPLES OF COGNITIVE-BEHAVIORAL THERAPY

Cognitive-behavioral therapy is an intensive, short-term psychotherapy that focuses on how patients make use of the available information to arrive at the meanings they assign to particular events and how these interpretations affect patients' emotions and behaviors. Cognitive-behavioral therapists ask patients to assess and evaluate their thoughts, attitudes, and beliefs, especially those accessed in the midst of problematic situations. Patients with chronic low-back pain, for example, might be asked to monitor what they say to themselves when experiencing

---

**Box 12.1**    Principles of Cognitive Behavioral Therapy

CBT is based on an ever evolving formulation of the patient's problems in cognitive terms.

CBT requires a sound therapeutic alliance and emphasizes a collaborative relationship.

CBT is goal oriented and problem focused.

CBT initially emphasizes a here-and-now focus.

CBT is educational.

CBT is structured and aims to be time limited.

CBT teaches patients to identify, evaluate, and respond to their problematic automatic thoughts.

CBT uses a range of behavioral and cognitive techniques to change thinking, mood, and behavior.

---

SOURCE: Adapted from J. S. Beck (1995).

---

painful sensations. Therapists encourage patients to treat these beliefs as hypotheses and to devise strategies for subjecting these views to empirical testing. In doing so, patients may come to recognize the powerful, but often selective, ways in which they choose to interpret these painful sensations. Bringing unrecognized biases to light enhances the possibility of addressing habitual patterns of thinking through explicit cognitive and behavioral interventions.

Although CBT must be customized to the individual patient, there are fundamental principles that underlie the application of CBT for all patients. These principles are listed in the accompanying Box 12.1 and briefly described in the following paragraphs.

*CBT is based on an ever evolving formulation of the patient's problems in cognitive terms.* A CBT formulation is based on the cognitive model, which holds that cognitions mediate an individual's emotional, physiological, and behavioral responses to their environment. Furthermore, there is good support for the notion that there are three levels of cognition—automatic thoughts,

underlying assumptions, and core beliefs (Hollon & Kriss, 1984; Segal, 1988)—and that there is some specificity to the processes affected by different treatments (DeRubeis, Evans, et al. 1990; Imber et al., 1990).

Automatic thoughts are cognitions or visual images that occur in a seemingly involuntary fashion as part of an individual's ongoing stream of consciousness. They exist at the most manifest, symptomatic level of thinking and are characterized by (1) their instantaneous appearance in response to a stimulus; (2) their unquestioned plausibility; and (3) the fact that, though not always in the patient's focal awareness, they can be detected by shifting attention to how the patient is interpreting a given situation. For example, a therapist might ask a patient who experiences anxiety associated with painful sensations to recall what he or she was thinking at the moment the anxious feelings began. The patient might report the automatic thought, "I will never get better."

The content of automatic thoughts is hypothesized to arise from intermediate beliefs or assumptions. These beliefs typically reflect a person's "rules of living." Although typically not spontaneously or explicitly expressed in therapy, these beliefs can be elicited from the patient. Examples of intermediate beliefs include "There is nothing I can do to help with the pain" or "I don't need to worry about diabetes" (White, 2001).

At the third and final level of abstraction, underlying assumptions are thought to arise from the core beliefs or *schemas,* which are enduring structural components of the information processing system. A person's core beliefs reflect experientially derived abstractions about that individual's view of her- or himself, the future, or the world. Individuals can possess a number of different core beliefs, which remain latent until activated by thematically related events. For example, suppose in many different situations, a patient presents with the automatic thought "I must succeed . . . I must be perfect." On a deeper level, it may become apparent that the patient is operating from the following conditional assumptions: "If I succeed or am perfect, I'm not worthless or inadequate. However, if I am not perfect or don't totally succeed, then I am worthless." The conditional assumptions that become "personal rules for living" can be understood as essentially ways to compensate for deeper negative core beliefs, such as "I am worthless" or "I am inadequate." The deeper core beliefs remain latent but still lead to harsh self-evaluations regarding performance and a tendency to dismiss any achievements as being minor or marginal.

Because core beliefs guide the processing of incoming data and facilitate the retrieval of information congruent with the core beliefs, the danger is that a vicious cycle is established whereby patients, guided by their core beliefs, behave in ways that influence their perceptions, thereby confirming their initial views. From a clinical vantage point, core beliefs are important because they are largely unspoken, abstract regulators of behavior; are often inferred from a set of automatic thoughts; and may be maladaptive by disrupting more adaptive responses in patients' repertoires (Shaw & Segal, 1988).

*CBT requires a sound therapeutic alliance and emphasizes a collaborative relationship.* As in other psychotherapies, cognitive therapists need to establish sound therapeutic alliances by demonstrating warmth, empathy, caring, genuine regard and competence. Studies evaluating the importance of empathy in CBT have confirmed that patients' perceptions of therapist empathy are related to symptomatic improvement (Persons & Burns, 1985), independent of compliance with technical CBT interventions (Burns & Nolen-Hoeksema, 1992).

CBT is distinguished from many other psychotherapeutic approaches, however, in its insistence on collaborative empiricism and the patient's active participation. Therapists and patients work together to identify and track target problems, generate and execute strategies for change, and evaluate the strategies. For example, therapists encourage patients to treat their beliefs as hypotheses and to use their behaviors to test the accuracy of those beliefs. As such, cognitive change requires patients, in collaboration with their therapists, to compare and contrast their thoughts (expectations, assumptions, beliefs, etc.) with actual behavioral outcomes. This evidence-gathering approach contrasts with other cognitively oriented therapies, notably rational emotive behavior therapy (Ellis, 1989), which emphasizes the role of logical disputation and persuasion in promoting cognitive change.

*CBT is goal oriented and problem focused.* In CBT, patients are encouraged to specify their problems and establish specific goals. For example, a patient who would like to cope better with a chronic pain problem is encouraged to state a goal in behavioral terms, such as engaging in a recreational activity three times a week. Therapy involves helping the patient to evaluate and respond to the thoughts that interfere with this goal, such as, "Being active will make my pain worse." Thus, the therapist pays attention to the obstacles that prevent the patient from solving problems and reaching goals. While patients who functioned well before the onset of their difficulties may not need direct training in problem solving, other patients may need specific instruction to learn these strategies.

*CBT initially emphasizes a here-and-now focus.* Cognitive therapy focuses predominantly on the here and now. This stance does not imply a view of historical material as irrelevant or unimportant. Indeed, there is convergent evidence that dysfunctional attitudes and beliefs may arise from negative early experiences (Herman, 1992; Kovacs & Beck, 1978). Nevertheless, the emphasis in short-term cognitive therapy is on identifying and addressing the thoughts and beliefs related to the problems that brought the patient to treatment.

*CBT is educational.* CBT emphasizes educating patients early in therapy about the nature, course, and management of their disorders as well as about the process of cognitive therapy. In many cases, patients' maladaptive responses to their medical disorders or their poor adherence with treatment regimes are a direct result of inaccurate facts and erroneous beliefs about their disorders.

*CBT is structured and aims to be time limited.* Irrespective of the problem being addressed, the therapist tends to follow a defined session structure. This includes working with the patient to set an agenda for the session, checking on the patient's progress with respect to the presenting problem, eliciting feedback on the previous session, reviewing homework, working on the

agenda items, deciding on new homework, and eliciting feedback at the end of the session. In addition, cognitive-behavioral treatment protocols for several medical disorders provide across-session structure. Adhering to a structured treatment helps the patient and therapist maintain a problem-centered focus and has been shown to positively influence outcome (Shaw et al. 1999). In addition, structure helps limit the number of treatment sessions; many CBT protocols are shorter than 20 weeks long, with some as short as six to eight sessions.

*CBT teaches patients to identify, evaluate, and respond to their problematic automatic thoughts.* One of the primary methods for challenging automatic thoughts is the use of Socratic questioning. A question-asking orientation facilitates the process of translating patients' personal axioms into tentative hypotheses, thereby setting the stage for considering self-generated alternatives and subsequent experimentation. In addition, questioning (rather than indoctrination or aggressive disputation) can promote collaborative, respectful therapeutic alliances in which therapists help patients focus their concerns, explore the evidence for their beliefs, identify the criteria for their evaluations, and examine the consequences of their actions.

*CBT uses a range of behavioral and cognitive techniques to change thinking, mood, and behavior.* Each of these techniques has been shown to be effective (e.g., Jacobson et al., 1996; Zang & DeRubeis, 1999). A few representative techniques are described in the next section. Regardless of the technique, once the therapist has demonstrated the effectiveness of a particular modality in session, the patient is encouraged to carry out and practice the technique as homework between sessions. In early sessions, homework may involve the maintenance of daily records of mood, behavior, and dysfunctional

Box 12.2    Behavioral Interventions

Activity scheduling
Graded task assignment
Reinforcement
Role play
Social skills training
Distraction
Relaxation (controlled breathing, progressive muscle relaxation)
Exposure
Exercise

thoughts. Homework assignments may later take the form of behavioral experiments, designed to test the validity of the patient's thoughts, beliefs, or assumptions. When the patient is developing a new behavioral skill (e.g., assertiveness), homework may involve the strategic real-life application of these skills (Swallow & Segal, 1995). Whatever their form, homework assignments constitute an integral component of CBT. Indeed, patient adherence to homework assignments has been linked to superior therapeutic response (DeRubeis & Feeley, 1990; Neimeyer & Feixas, 1990). Further, therapists who regularly review homework assignments with patients obtain better clinical outcomes than those who fail to do so (Burns & Nolen-Hoeksema, 1991; Williams, 1992).

## DOCUMENTED APPLICATIONS

CBT uses a wide range of behavioral and cognitive intervention strategies. This section describes some of the most frequently used strategies as they might apply to medical disorders. Readers interested in learning more about these and other interventions should consult J. S. Beck (1995) and White (2001).

### Behavioral Intervention Strategies

Behavioral interventions are particularly helpful in addressing difficulties with initiating or maintaining goal-directed behaviors; for example, changing activity levels or increasing compliance with medication or treatment regimens. In general, behavioral interventions in CBT are implemented to attain the larger goal of cognitive change. For example, the immobilization typical of a chronic-pain patient may be related to negative expectancies about the consequences of exercise: "If I do something when I am in pain, I may cause harm to myself." Behavioral activation can provide evidence that the patient can marshal against self-defeating thoughts: "I can't do anything." Similarly, when a patient maintains inactivity by avoidant patterns (e.g., social withdrawal), behavioral interventions (e.g., exposure tasks) serve to provide evidence against catastrophic expectations (e.g., "Others will reject me because they see me as a burden"). Box 12.2 lists several common behavioral interventions. The following sections discuss four of these techniques in some detail: activity scheduling, graded task assignment, reinforcement, and exposure.

## Activity Scheduling

Activity scheduling is helpful for individuals who experience significant disruptions in their activity level, daily routine, and/or ability to experience pleasure or a sense of achievement in their activities. This strategy is particularly helpful for patients who suffer from reduced functioning (e.g., chronic fatigue syndrome), must incorporate new treatment regimens into their daily routine (e.g., to comply with antiretroviral therapy), or suffer from depression.

The first step in activity scheduling involves obtaining baseline measures of patients' activities, moods, and/or physical symptoms. This helps patients recognize the association between activity levels and symptoms. Some patients learn that inactivity intensifies their symptoms, and others learn that a sudden increase in their activity levels when they begin to feel good actually increases their symptoms (e.g., chronic fatigue syndrome). In the next phase, patients enumerate the activities they want to add to or delete from their schedule. Following this, a daily schedule can be worked out in which patients designate specific time slots for engaging in selected activities. Both pleasure- and mastery-related events should be included in the schedule. Mastery-related events are those that provide a sense of accomplishment when completed. At this point, it can be helpful to have patients actually predict the amount of pleasure and/or mastery they expect to derive from each scheduled activity. In addition, obstacles to the successful completion of these activities should be anticipated and addressed and contingency plans made when possible. Finally, patients should be instructed to monitor their behavior, noting the actual degree of pleasure and/or mastery they derived from the scheduled activities. These actual pleasure and mastery ratings can be compared to patients' earlier ratings to obtain an index of the accuracy of their predictions (Lewinsohn, Muñoz, Youngren, & Zeiss, 1978).

## Graded Task Assignment

In selecting and scheduling pleasant events and mastery tasks, therapists attempt to maximize patients' chances of success. This intervention strategy is particularly helpful for those who are depressed, are overwhelmed, or have diminished functional abilities. In many cases, patients set unrealistic expectations for their performance. Graded task assignment involves breaking a task down into smaller units so a patient can start with the easiest and move on to greater challenges (Williams, 1992). For example, whereas housecleaning may represent an overwhelming prospect for a severely depressed patient, smaller components of the task, like making the bed, may be more manageable. After the patient has made the bed successfully, she or he can try doing other components of the larger task.

## Reinforcement

The principles of operant conditioning hold that the frequency of a given behavior can be modified by the consequences that follow. A positive consequence or removal of an aversive consequence leads to an increase in the frequency of behavior. Thus, rewarding oneself for successfully accomplishing certain goals can be an effective means of increasing levels of behavioral activation and of maintaining these gains. In addition, for individuals who view themselves as unworthy, self-reinforcement represents counterattitudinal behavior and as such promotes change at the cognitive level. Therapists can encourage self-reinforcement by (1) providing a compelling rationale; (2) encouraging patients to establish specific, attainable goals with clearly defined performance criteria; (3) identifying activities that patients construe as reinforcing; (4) instructing patients to engage in reinforcing activities immediately after

---

**Box 12.3**     Cognitive Strategies

Thought records
"Pie" technique
Identifying cognitive distortions
Behavioral experiments
Cognitive continuum to modify beliefs
Rational-emotional role play
Cost-benefit analysis of beliefs
Downward arrow technique
Core belief log
Historical test of core belief

---

meeting their goals; and (5) monitoring patients' progress (Lewinsohn et al., 1978; Rehm, Kaslow, & Rabin, 1987).

### Exposure

Anxiety and avoidance experienced by patients with medical disorders can interfere with treatment compliance, prevent adaptation to illness, and increase sensitivity to medical symptoms. Whatever the source of the anxiety, exposure-based strategies are effective in reducing anxiety and related avoidances that are cognitive (e.g., thinking about the illness and the need to take medication) and behavioral (e.g., seeking medical treatment). The goal of exposure therapy is to reduce or eliminate the patient's anxiety response when exposed to the anxiety-provoking stimulus. The anxiety-provoking stimulus can be *in vivo,* imaginal (that is, the patient is exposed to the anxiety-provoking stimulus through imagery or his or her imagination), or interoceptive (the patient is exposed through internal sensations). All these exposure strategies involve having the patient face the feared stimuli in a structured way to disconfirm her or his catastrophic predictions. For example, a patient with non-cardiac chest pain may fear that an increase in heart rate signals an imminent heart

attack. Having the patient experience increased heart rate in a controlled setting can serve to disconfirm this belief.

### Cognitive Strategies

Cognitive intervention strategies exist that specifically target the three different levels of cognition: automatic thoughts, underlying assumptions, and core beliefs. These strategies are listed in Box 12.3 and described in the following sections.

#### Targeting Automatic Thoughts

One of the most commonly used techniques for targeting automatic thoughts is a thought record that helps organize the monitoring, evaluation, and modification of automatic thoughts. Two of the most popular versions of thought records are the Automatic Thought Record (Greenberger & Padesky, 1995) and the Dysfunctional Thought Record (J. S. Beck, 1995). However, therapists often modify thought records to meet the specific needs of the patient population in their practice. For example, when working with a physically ill patient, an extra column could be added to record physical symptoms.

Self-monitoring is fundamental to many cognitive interventions. Patients are encouraged to write down their thoughts, images, and feelings in problematic situations. Thought records are preferable to retrospective accounts of events because they are a more direct data source and less subject to mood-related biases in recall. In addition, the act of monitoring their thinking may help patients to begin the critical task of "stepping back" or "distancing themselves" from negative thought streams (Teasdale, Segal, & Williams, 1995).

Therapists encourage patients to regard their automatic thoughts as scientific hypotheses that they can subject to empirical examination. Using Socratic questioning and guided discovery, therapists help patients evaluate their automatic thoughts. This process may help patients consider self-generated alternative interpretations of their problematic situations and encourage subsequent experimentation. Alternatively, the process may validate patients' interpretation of their situations and generate new solutions to their problems. If patients find this evaluation process helpful, therapists then teach them how to complete thought records, which help patients organize the evaluation process on their own. For example, the Automatic Thought Record (Greenberger & Padesky, 1995) includes prompts or questions to guide patients through a systematic process of collecting evidence that supports and does not support automatic thoughts.

### Targeting Intermediate Beliefs

Intermediate beliefs or conditional assumptions are more difficult to modify than automatic thoughts. These beliefs can be identified by looking for recurring themes in patients' thought records or repetitious patterns in their behaviors. Patients may have beliefs about their symptoms, their disorders, the effectiveness of their treatments, and even their doctors. The basic form of a conditional assumption is an if-then statement; therefore,

one way to elicit these assumptions is to present the patient with an if-then clause to complete. For example, a patient may complete the following clause: "If I do something when I am in pain, then . . ." with the phrase "I may cause harm to myself."

The next step is to help the patient identify the benefits and costs of holding the belief in question. It is important to keep in mind that patients' rules often represent a way to protect themselves from negative consequences. However, further questioning often reveals that adhering to particular beliefs over the long term yields the same negative consequences patients were trying to avoid in the first place. Quite often, recognition of the costs of maintaining particular beliefs motivates patients to work on changing their beliefs. Once patients have identified new assumptions or rules that will better serve them in attaining their goals, patients can begin conducting behavioral experiments to learn more about the usefulness of the alternative approaches.

Designing effective experiments can require a good deal of creativity and ingenuity on the part of both therapist and patient. One means of generating ideas for experiments involves operationalizing, a priori, the kind of evidence that could either support or refute the hypothesis in question. For example, to test the assumption "If I do something when I am in pain, then I may cause harm to myself," therapist and patient might first consider specific measures that might be harmful. Next, an experiment could be designed in which the patient would gradually increase her or his activity level and take note of the health impacts. A series of such experiments could help weaken the subjective plausibility of the patient's old assumption and may strengthen her or his belief in the alternative assumption of "If I do something when I am in pain, then I sometimes feel better."

### Targeting Core Beliefs

The patient does not typically spontaneously articulate core beliefs. Core beliefs can be identified, however, using the downward arrow technique. This strategy involves asking questions like, "What does this situation mean about me/other people/the world and how it operates?" or "If this were true, what would be so bad about . . . ?" Negative core beliefs about the self can be broadly classified as either helpless (e.g., "I am powerless" or "I am vulnerable") or unlovable (e.g., "I am uncared for" or "I am unworthy"; J. S. Beck, 1995).

One method of targeting core beliefs is to begin by recording evidence that the core belief is not 100 percent true under all circumstances. This process may involve examining the historical underpinnings of the core belief and considering the possibility that although the core belief may have been somewhat valid in a previous context, it may no longer be applicable in many current situations. As evidence accumulates that is inconsistent with the core belief, the patient might consider an alternative belief that is less absolute and negative. The patient can then maintain a log of evidence that supports the new belief. It is important to recognize, however, that changing core beliefs can often take many months.

## STRUCTURING TREATMENT

The goal of CBT is to teach patients new strategies or techniques so they can better deal with their medical disorders and essentially become their own therapists. In general, adhering to a structured format facilitates this objective. Specific treatment protocols have been created for a number of psychological disorders, including depression (Beck, Rush, Shaw, & Emery, 1979) and panic disorder (e.g., Barlow & Craske, 2000). In addition, CBT protocols exist for

the management of a growing number of medical disorders. More recent texts include treatment protocols for irritable bowel syndrome (Toner, Segal, Emmott, & Myran, 2000), psychosomatic illness (Warwick & Salkovskis, 2001), and chronic medical disorders (White, 2001).

Whether there is a preexisting CBT protocol for a patient's presenting problem or not, CBT unfolds in a relatively standard and systematic manner. In the early phase of therapy, the therapist needs to accomplish a number of tasks (J. S. Beck, 1995). First, the therapist conducts a diagnostic interview and assesses the patient's presenting problems, current functioning, symptoms, and history to begin formulating the case from a cognitive perspective. This early formulation is essential for generating a treatment plan that is specific to the patient's problems. In addition, the therapist must establish trust and rapport with the patient; orient the patient to the cognitive model; educate the patient about his or her disorder, the cognitive model, and the process of cognitive therapy; and construct a list of concrete therapeutic goals.

The treatment plan is implemented in the middle phase of therapy. During this phase, the patient learns the specific behavioral and/or cognitive strategies described in the treatment plan. For example, if cognitive strategies are necessary, the patient might begin by learning to identify and monitor automatic thoughts. The patient would then learn to evaluate these thoughts using an Automatic Thought Record (Greenberger & Padesky, 1995). The patient might follow this work by testing self-generated alternative responses using behavioral experiments.

The final phase of therapy is geared toward relapse prevention. In this phase, the therapist reviews therapy and addresses termination. Special emphasis is placed on helping the patient identify potential future triggers of his or her disorder, the warning signs that indicate a relapse is beginning, and the strategies the patient found most helpful in therapy as aids for dealing with future problems. During the relapse-prevention phase, the frequency of therapy sessions is often tapered to help the patient apply CBT coping skills independently. The patient may also be encouraged to formally set aside time to do "self-therapy sessions" (J. S. Beck, 1995) during the weeks between sessions with the therapist. The goal is to experientially reinforce that the patient can now become his or her own therapist and has the skills to cope independently. After completing an acute phase of CBT, many patients continue to have booster sessions (at frequencies ranging from every month to every three months) to strongly reinforce the application of CBT coping skills and to further prevent relapse.

## CONCLUSION

Cognitive-behavioral therapy initially proved to be an effective intervention in the management of anxiety and depressive disorders. Applied to medical illnesses, this treatment paradigm can improve patients' emotional response to illness, assist patients to adapt to their illness and limitations, and increase their compliance with treatment regimens. The cognitive approach has shown efficacy in treating such diverse medical conditions as chronic pain, chronic fatigue syndrome, and irritable bowel disorder, as well as in conducting such health promoting interventions as smoking cessation.

The cognitive-behavioral approach focuses on patients' cognitive schema of their illnesses, and seeks to modify patients' beliefs at several levels. A wide range of specific techniques and strategies have emerged, many with strong empirical support, including behavioral intervention strategies, cognitive techniques, and protocols structuring treatment. This research-based approach offers promise for applications throughout the field of mind-body medicine, alone and in combination with both traditional medical approaches and other mind-body approaches.

## REFERENCES

Barlow, D. H., & Craske, M. G. (2000). *Mastery of your anxiety and panic, III.* Albany, NY: Graywind.

Beck, A. T. (1967). *Depression: Causes and treatment.* Philadelphia: University of Pennsylvania Press.

Beck, A. T., Rush, A. J., Shaw, B. F., & Emery, G. (1979). *Cognitive therapy of depression.* New York: Guilford.

Beck, J. S. (1995). *Cognitive therapy: Basics and beyond.* New York: Guilford.

Buick, D. L. (1997). Illness representations and breast cancer: Coping with radiation and chemotherapy. In K. J. Petrie & J. A. Weinman (Eds.), *Perceptions of health and illness* (pp. 379–409). Singapore: Harwood Academic Publishers.

Burns, D. D., & Nolen-Hoeksema, S. (1991). Coping styles, homework assignments and the effectiveness of cognitive behavioral therapy. *Journal of Consulting and Clinical Psychology, 59,* 564–578.

Burns, D. D., & Nolen-Hoeksema, S. (1992). Therapeutic empathy and recovery from depression in cognitive-behavioral therapy: A structured equation model. *Journal of Consulting and Clinical Psychology, 59,* 305–311.

Clark, D. A., & Beck, A. T. (1999). *Scientific foundations of cognitive theory and therapy of depression.* New York: Wiley.

Compas, B. E., Haaga, D. A. F., Keefe, F. J., Leitenber, H., & Williams, D. A. (1998). Sampling of empirically supported psychological treatments from health psychology: Smoking, chronic pain, cancer, and bulimia nervosa. *Journal of Clinical and Consulting Psychology, 66,* 89–112.

DeRubeis, R. J., & Crits-Christoph, P. (1998). Empirically supported individual and group psychological treatments for adult mental disorders. *Journal of Clinical and Consulting Psychology, 66,* 37–52.

DeRubeis, R. J., Evans, M. D., Hollon, S. D., Garvey, M. J., Grove, W. M., Tuason, V. B. (1990). How does cognitive therapy work? Cognitive change and symptom changes in cognitive therapy and pharmacotherapy for depression. *Journal of Consulting and Clinical Psychology, 58,* 862–869.

DeRubeis, R. J., & Feeley, M. (1990). Determinants of change in cognitive therapy for depression. *Cognitive Therapy and Research, 14,* 469–482.

DeRubeis, R. J., Tang, T. Z., & Beck, A. T. (2001). Cognitive therapy. In K. S. Dobson (Ed.), *Handbook of cognitive-behavioral therapies* (2nd ed., pp. 349–392). New York: Guilford.

Dobson, K. S., & Dozois, D. J. A. (2001). Historical and philosophical bases of the cognitive-behavioral therapies. In K. S. Dobson (Ed.), *Handbook of cognitive-behavioral therapies* (2nd ed., pp. 3–39). New York: Guilford.

Dryden, W., & Ellis, A. (2001). Rational emotive behavior therapy. In K. S. Dobson (Ed.), *Handbook of cognitive-behavioral therapies* (2nd ed., pp. 295–348). New York: Guilford.

D'Zurilla, T. J., & Nezu, A. M. (2001). Problem-solving therapies. In K. S. Dobson (Ed.), *Handbook of cognitive-behavioral therapies* (2nd ed., pp. 211–245). New York: Guilford.

Ellis, A. (1989). The history of cognition in psychotherapy. In A. Freeman, K. Simon, L. Beutler, & H. Arkowicz. (Eds.), *Comprehensive handbook of cognitive therapy* (pp. 5–20). New York: Plenum.

Greenberger, D., & Padesky, C. A. (1995). *Mind over mood: A cognitive therapy treatment manual for clients.* New York: Guilford.

Herman, J. (1992). *Trauma and recovery.* New York: Basic Books.

Hollon, S. D., & Kriss, M. R. (1984). Cognitive factors in clinical research and practice. *Clinical Psychology Review, 4,* 38–78.

Holzman, A. D., Turk, D. C., & Kerns, R. D. (1986). The cognitive-behavioral approach to the management of chronic pain. In A. D. Holzman & D. C. Turk (Eds.), *Pain management: A handbook of psychological treatment approaches* (pp. 31–50). Elmsford, NY: Pergamon Press.

Imber, S. D., Pilkonis, P. A., Sotsky, S. M., Elkin, I., Watkins, J. T., Collins, J. F., et al. (1990). Mode-specific effects among three treatments for depression. *Journal of Consulting and Clinical Psychology, 58,* 352–359.

Jacobson, N. S., Dobson, K. S., Truax, P. A., Addis, M. E., Koerner, K., Gollan, J. K., Gortner, E., & Prince, S. E. (1996). A component analysis of cognitive-behavioral treatment for depression. *Journal of Consulting and Clinical Psychology, 64,* 295–304.

Kovacs, M., & Beck, A. T. (1978). Maladaptive cognitive structures in depression. *American Journal of Psychiatry, 135,* 525–533.

Lewinsohn, P. M., Muñoz, R. F., Youngren, M. A., & Zeiss, A. M. (1978). *Control your depression.* Englewood Cliffs, NJ: Prentice Hall.

Morley, S., Eccleston, C., & Williams, A. (1999). Systematic review and meta-analysis of randomized controlled trials of cognitive behavior therapy and behavior therapy for chronic pain in adults, excluding headache. *Pain, 80,* 1–13.

Neimeyer, R., & Feixas, G. (1990). The role of homework and skill acquisition in the outcome of group cognitive therapy for depression. *Behavior Therapy, 21,* 281–292.

Payne, A., & Blanchard, E. B. (1995). A controlled comparison of cognitive therapy and self-help support groups in the treatment of irritable bowel syndrome. *Journal of Consulting and Clinical Psychology, 63,* 779–786.

Persons, J. B., & Burns, D. D. (1985). Mechanism of action of cognitive therapy: Relative contribution of technical and interpersonal intervention. *Cognitive Therapy and Research, 12,* 557–575.

Petrie, K. J., Weinman, J., Sharpe, N., & Buckley, J. (1996). Roles of patients' view of their illness in predicting return to work and functioning after myocardial infarction: Longitudinal study. *British Medical Journal, 312,* 1191–1194.

Price, J. R., & Couper, J. (2000). Cognitive behavior therapy for adults with chronic fatigue syndrome. *Cochrane Database of Systematic Reviews,* CD001027.

Prohaska, T. R., Keller, M. L., Leventhal, E. A., & Leventhal, H. (1987). Impact of symptoms and aging attribution on emotions and coping. *Health Psychology, 6,* 495–514.

Rehm, L. P., Kaslow, N. J., & Rabin, A. S. (1987). Cognitive and behavioral targets in a self-control therapy program for depression. *Journal of Consulting and Clinical Psychology, 55,* 60–67.

Rokke, P. D., & Rehm, L. P. (2001). Self-management therapies. In K. S. Dobson (Ed.), *Handbook of cognitive-behavioral therapies* (2nd ed., pp. 173–210). New York: Guilford.

Segal, Z. V. (1988). Appraisal of the self-schema construct in cognitive models of depression. *Psychological Bulletin, 103,* 147–162.

Shaw, B. F., Elkin, I., Yamaguchi, J., Olmsted, M., Vallis, M., Dobson, K. S., et al. (1999). Therapist competence ratings in relation to clinical outcome in cognitive therapy of depression. *Journal of Consulting and Clinical Psychology, 67,* 837–846.

Shaw, B. F., & Segal, Z. V. (1988). Introduction to cognitive theory and therapy. In A. J. Frances & R. E. Hales (Eds.), *American Psychiatric Press review of psychiatry: Vol. 7* (pp. 538–553). Washington, DC: American Psychiatric Press.

Swallow, S. R., & Segal, Z. V. (1995). Cognitive therapy for unipolar depression. In K. D. Craig & K. S. Dobson (Eds.), *Anxiety and depression in adults and children* (pp. 209–229). Thousand Oaks, CA: Sage.

Teasdale, J. D., Segal, Z. V., & Williams, J. M. G. (1995). How does cognitive therapy prevent relapse and why should attentional control (mindfulness) training help? *Behavior Research and Therapy, 33,* 25–39.

Toner, B. B., Segal, Z. V., Emmott, S. D., & Myran, D. (2000). *Cognitive-behavioral treatment of irritable bowel syndrome: The brain-gut connection.* New York: Guilford.

Warwick, H. M. C., & Salkovskis, P. M. (2001). Cognitive-behavioral treatment of hypochondriasis. In V. Starcevic & D. R. Lipsitt (Eds.), *Hypochondriasis: Modern perspectives on an ancient malady* (pp. 314–328). New York: Oxford University Press.

Weinman, J., Petrie, K. J., Moss-Morris, R., & Horne, R. (1996). The illness perception questionnaire: A new method for assessing the cognitive representation of illness. *Psychology and Health, 11,* 431–455.

White, C. A. (2001). *Cognitive behavior therapy for chronic medical problems: A guide to assessment and treatment in practice.* New York: Wiley.

Williams, J. M. G. (1992). *The psychological treatment of depression.* New York: Routledge.

Zang, T. Z., & DeRubeis, R. J. (1999). Sudden gains and critical sessions in cognitive-behavioral therapy for depression. *Journal of Consulting and Clinical Psychology, 67,* 894–904.

# CHAPTER 13

# Acupuncture

## EMANUEL STEIN

**Abstract:** Acupuncture evolved within millennia-old Traditional Chinese Medicine and is now slowly being integrated into Western medicine for a variety of medical conditions ranging from pain to allergies to cardiovascular conditions. The chapter reviews the origins of acupuncture, its conceptual model, and current applications in acupuncture practice. The author, a cardiologist and licensed acupuncturist in the state of Virginia, presents two case studies illustrating positive outcomes with medical patients and closes with a perspective on Western acupuncture practice.

## ORIGINS

"Acupuncture has been used by millions of American patients and performed by thousands of physicians, dentists, acupuncturists and other practitioners for relief or prevention of pain and for a variety of health conditions" (National Institutes of Health, 1997, p. 3). Acceptance of acupuncture therapy as part of mainstream Western medicine has been developing in stages.

In stage 1, acupuncture was clearly outside the boundaries of Western medicine. The U.S. Food and Drug Administration categorized acupuncture needles as "experimental medical devices" (National Institutes of Health, 1997, p. 3). Now in stage 2, acupuncture is moving into the mainstream of primary care. Educational opportunities for the physician and nonphysician acupuncturist are expanding rapidly, some associated with universities. No longer are acupuncture needles "experimental medical devices." The Food and Drug Administration now regulates them just as it does other devices, such as surgical scalpels and hypodermic syringes, under good manufacturing practices and single-use standards of sterility (National Institutes of Health, 1997, pp. 3–4). Stage 3, visible on the horizon, will witness the full integration of acupuncture into primary care practice. The typical medical practice will consist of a physician using acupuncture directly or in close association with a well-trained acupuncturist.

This chapter is divided into three main parts. The first part reviews the history of acupuncture in America since the 1970s. The second part is an overview of some of the

AUTHOR'S NOTE: The author acknowledges the assistance of his associates: James Fletcher, medical student, Eastern Virginia Medical School; Allison Lynn, physician's assistant student, EVMS; and Viki Lorraine, assistant professor, Family and Community Medicine, EVMS.

details of acupuncture treatment, including definitions of *Qi* and the meridians and a list of conditions responding to acupuncture. Space limitations do not permit discussion of the development of acupuncture beyond the traditional model. The third part describes the acupuncture treatments given to two patients diagnosed with Bell's palsy.

## EMERGENCE OF ACUPUNCTURE IN THE UNITED STATES

Acupuncture came to the attention of Americans with the experience of James Reston (1971), a journalist who underwent emergency surgery while in China. Reston described his experience as follows:

> I was in considerable discomfort, if not pain, during the second night after the operation. . . . [The] doctor . . . inserted three long thin needles into the outer part of my right elbow and below my knees and manipulated them in order to stimulate the intestine and relieve the pressure and distention of the stomach. . . . Meanwhile . . . [the doctor] lit two pieces of an herb which looked like burning stumps of a broken cheap cigar and held them close to my abdomen while occasionally twirling the needles into action. . . . Although this took about twenty minutes . . . there was a noticeable relaxation of the pressure and distention within an hour and no recurrence of the problem thereafter. (pp. 1, 6)

Concerned about disbelief among his readers, he stated further,

> It has been suggested that maybe the whole accidental experience of mine, or at least the acupuncture part of it, was a journalistic trick to learn about needle anesthesia. This is not only untrue but greatly exaggerates my gifts of imagination, courage and self-sacrifice. There are many things I will do for a good story, but getting slit open in the night or offering myself as an experimental porcupine is not among them. (pp. 1, 6)

A group of distinguished American physicians then visited China to become familiar with acupuncture anesthesia (Dimond, 1971). Further interest in acupuncture continued following the visit to China by President Richard Nixon in 1972. The president's personal physician, Walter R. Tkach (1972), who accompanied the president, was invited to witness the use of acupuncture during several surgeries. He used the word *astonished* to describe his reaction when he saw that the patients were ambulatory immediately after surgery. One hour later they were drinking tea and answering questions.

## CONCEPTUAL MODEL AND TECHNOLOGY OF TRADITIONAL CHINESE MEDICINE

### *Qi, the Life Energy*

Acupuncture was viewed by the Chinese as part of a complete system of medical care for the mind and body influencing the psychological, emotional, and physiological functions. In Traditional Chinese Medicine, Qi (pronounced "chee"), the life energy, is vital for good health. Helms (1995) defines *Qi* as "the basic constituent of the body that represents the finest material aspect of the nourishment obtained from eating, drinking and breathing; the vivifying force circulating through the acupuncture channels to protect, nourish and animate living beings. In contemporary texts, *Qi* is commonly translated as energy or energetic influences" (p. 694).

### *The Meridians*

Qi circulates throughout the body in channels called meridians. These channels may be envisioned as a railroad system or a system of rivers traversing the body, providing a route for Qi, the life energy, to nourish the tissues along the way. Freely flowing Qi is essential for good health, while blockage of Qi leads to illness and pain. The appropriate

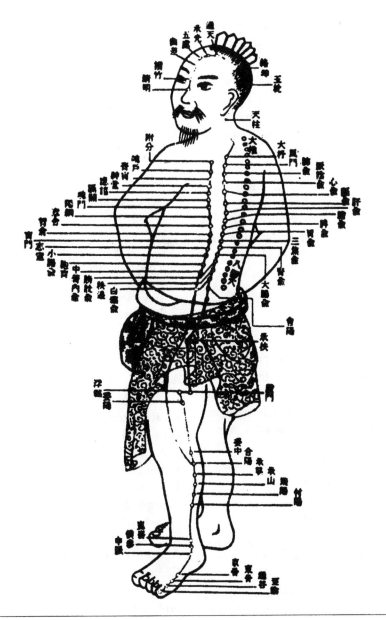

**Figure 13.1**    Ancient Chart Illustrating Points on the Bladder Meridian

placement of needles may relieve the blockage, restore the flow, and correct imbalances in Qi. The needles may be placed in the neutral position or manipulated for tonification or sedation.

The meridian system comprises 14 meridians. Twelve are bilateral and are associated with organs or tissues: the small intestine, bladder (see Figure 13.1), kidney, heart, triple heater, gallbladder, liver, master of the heart (pericardium), large intestine, stomach, spleen, and lung. The remaining 2 meridians, the conception vessel and the governor vessel, are unilateral and follow the midline over the front and back of the body, respectively.

To clarify, a meridian named for an organ may not appear to pass through that organ. For example, the small intestine meridian is on the upper part of the body. Nevertheless, a needle in an acupuncture point along the small intestine meridian will influence the energy of the small intestine. Needles in other meridians may also influence the small intestine. In summary, both Qi and the meridians introduce novel paradigms of energy and pathways into Western science.

With the insertion of very fine needles into the skin at precise points, acupuncture encourages natural healing and improved function. Manipulation of the needles, heat, and electricity may be added. Acupuncture needles are solid, thin, and made of stainless steel. Disposable needles are available to minimize infection.

Aldous Huxley noted that "the notion that a needle which is introduced into the foot can somehow improve liver function sounds absurd in the light of commonly accepted physiological theories. . . . Anomalous phenomena, like Chinese acupuncture, have often been ignored precisely by those whose duty it is to study them" (Pomeranz, 1997).

### Applications of Acupuncture

Acupuncture is often viewed solely in the context of pain management. The scope is actually much broader, encompassing promotion of health and prevention of disease. Both the National Institutes of Health (1994) and the World Health Organization (1990) encouraged the clinical evaluation of acupuncture. The World Health Organization report names several body systems, conditions, and medical specialty areas for which acupuncture can be applied:

#### Body Parts and Systems

Cardiac and cardiovascular
Dental
Ear, nose, and throat
Musculoskeletal
Respiratory
Sexual
Skin

#### Disorders

Allergies
Infectious diseases
Pain
Substance abuse

#### Medical Specialty Areas

Endocrinology and immunology
Gastroenterology
Neurology
Psychology
Obstetrics and gynecology
Ophthalmology
Urology

Research reports documenting the effects of acupuncture for these physiological systems and conditions are accumulating, including studies in the following areas: alcohol, smoking, and cocaine (Bullock, Culliton, & Olander, 1989; Clavel-Chapelon, Paoletti, & Banhamou, 1997; He, Berg, & Hostmark, 1997; Konefal, Duncan, & Clemence, 1995; Margolin, Avants, Chang, & Kosten, 1993); gastroenterology (Dundee, Chestnut, Ghaly, & Lynas, 1986; He et al., 1997; Li, Tougas, Chiverton, & Hunt, 1992); neurology (Naeser, 1996); and pain (Ter Riet, Kleijnen, & Knipschild, 1990).

### Issues Regarding Acupuncture Practice

Questions frequently asked by patients about acupuncture include the following:

1. Does acupuncture work?

2. How many treatments will I need?

3. Will it hurt?

4. What are the side effects?

5. What are the possible complications?

6. Do I have to believe that it works?

Each of these concerns will be addressed in the following discussion.

1. Acupuncture has been used for thousands of years in China and more recently in Europe and North America, both as the sole treatment and in conjunction with conventional Western medicine.

2. The number of treatments varies with the chronicity and complexity of the illness and the patient's response. Serious chronic conditions require more treatments.

3. Although reported levels of pain vary from patient to patient, most patients feel minimal or no pain with acupuncture treatment. The pain is usually associated with the insertion of the disposable needles and quickly abates.

4. Side effects following acupuncture treatments are usually minimal. Deep relaxation commonly occurs following the early treatments. However, a rebound phenomenon may occur for several days, with the original symptoms worsening. Following treatment, the original symptoms either get better or get worse. If there is no change, treatment should be reassessed.

5. Because needles enter the body, lists of possible complications have been published. As noted by Helms (1995, pp. 294–296), because the body is pierced with needles, three main complications can occur: piercing a large vessel, puncturing an organ, and infection. A well-trained acupuncturist can minimize these uncommon complications and is prepared to treat vasovagal reflex, which may occur, usually in the first few acupuncture treatments.

6. Acupuncture has also been used increasingly by veterinary physicians. When a limping horse, which has no set opinion about acupuncture, gallops away following treatment, success is evident.

## CASE STUDIES

Two cases, both involving Bell's palsy, illustrate effective acupuncture treatment. Bell's palsy cases were chosen because outcomes can be shown pictorially.

### Case One: C. B.

C. B., a 47-year-old man, presented with classic Bell's palsy. Flaccid paralysis of his right facial muscles was apparent involving the distribution of the facial nerve. His skin was smooth, with a widened palpebral fissure and depressed angle of the mouth. On expiration, his cheek was noted to balloon. The upper lid remained open and the lower lid was everted, with tears running down his face. In trying to close the lids, both eyes rolled upward, with the right eye remaining open. The facial muscles were paralyzed to both voluntary and involuntary movements with loss of facial reflexes. He complained of numbness, tingling, heaviness, and aching on the right side of his face (see Figure 13.2). He described the symptoms of hyperacusis, which involves the nerve to the stapedius muscle. Any loud sound elicited sharp pain in his right ear; this symptom was especially disturbing as he was the father of two children, the younger an infant.

The onset of symptoms was first noted four months earlier. Medical therapy was started early in the course of the illness with systemic as well as local medication. The symptoms, however, continued to progress. He was told that not much more could be done for him.

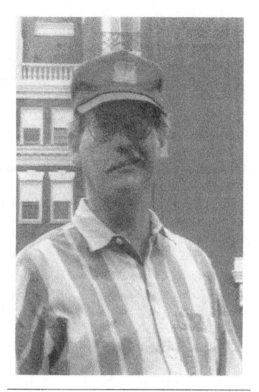

**Figure 13.2** C. B. 10 Days Before Start of Acupuncture Treatment for Bell's Palsy

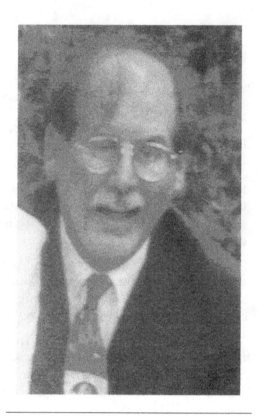

**Figure 13.3** C. B. After Series of Acupuncture Treatments

Acupuncture treatment was started immediately and included meridian treatment with electricity and local treatment. Symptoms started to abate immediately, with virtually complete recovery within several weeks (see Figure 13.3).

### Case Two: J. W.

A more acute case of Bell's palsy is illustrated in Figures 13.4 and 13.5. J. W., a 41-year-old man, was treated early in the course of his illness. The results of the treatment were similar to those of C. B., with fewer treatments.

Because many patients with Bell's palsy recover spontaneously, especially in the acute state, the case of a chronic patient (C. B.),

whose recovery did not appear likely, was elaborated. The experiences of C. B. and J. W. were similar to those of other patients treated in our acupuncture clinic. Although many cases of Bell's palsy are labeled idiopathic, a viral basis is becoming accepted. Specific causes include herpes zoster, sarcoid, and Lyme disease.

### TRAINING RESOURCES AND CERTIFICATION OF ACUPUNCTURE PRACTITIONERS

The regulation of the practice of acupuncture differs from state to state. For information on training, certification, and licensing contact

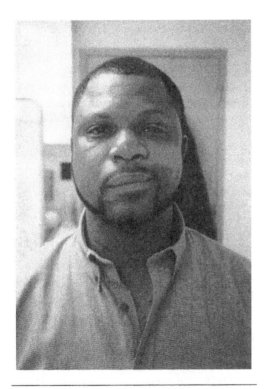

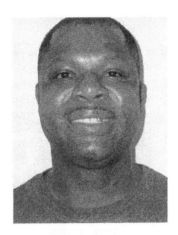

**Figure 13.5** J. W. After Series of Acupuncture Treatments

**Figure 13.4** J. W. on Day One of Acupuncture Treatments for Bell's Palsy

Duke, Kaplan, Coulter, Olik, and Hurwitz (1997); Hoizey and Hoizey (1988); Kaptchuk (1983); Lao (1996); Liao, Lee, and Ng (1994); Lu and Needham (1980); Stux and Pomeranz (1995); and Vincent and Richardson (1986).

The National Certification Commission for Acupuncture and Oriental Medicine
11 Canal Center Plaza, Suite 300
Alexandria, VA 22314
Telephone: 703-548-9004

Physicians can also contact

The American Academy of Medical Acupuncture
4929 Wilshire Blvd., Suite 428
Los Angeles, CA 90010
Telephone: 323-937-5514

Additional source materials on acupuncture and its clinical applications include

## CONCLUSION

Many patients request acupuncture as a last resort, after having been told that medicine can do nothing more. As acupuncture comes into the mainstream of medicine, patients will seek acupuncture earlier, and physicians will refer patients earlier in the disease process. It is fitting to conclude with the final comment of the National Institutes of Health Consensus Statement on Acupuncture (1997): "There is sufficient evidence of acupuncture's value to expand its use into conventional medicine and to encourage further studies of its physiology and clinical value" (p. 19).

## REFERENCES

Bullock, M. L., Culliton, P. D., & Olander, R. T. (1989). Controlled trial of acupuncture for severe recidivist alcoholism. *Lancet, 1,* 1435–1439.

Clavel-Chapelon, F., Paoletti, C., & Banhamou, S. (1997). Smoking cessation rates four years after treatment by nicotine gum and acupuncture. *Preventive Medicine, 26*(1), 25–28.

Dimond, E. G. (1971). Acupuncture anesthesia: Western medicine and Chinese traditional medicine. *Journal of the American Medical Association, 218,* 1558–1563.

Duke, D. L., Kaplan, G., Coulter, I., Olik, D., & Hurwitz, E. L. (1997). Use of acupuncture by American physicians. *Journal of Alternative and Complementary Medicine, 3*(2), 119–126.

Dundee, J. W., Chestnut, W. N., Ghaly, R. G., & Lynas, A. G. (1986). Traditional Chinese acupuncture: A potentially useful antiemetic? *British Medical Journal (Clinical Research), 293*(6547), 583–584.

He, D., Berg, J. E., & Hostmark, A. T. (1997). Effects of acupuncture on smoking cessation or reduction for motivated smokers. *Preventive Medicine, 26*(2), 208–214.

Helms, J. M. (1995). *Acupuncture energetics: A clinical approach for physicians.* Berkeley, CA: Medical Acupuncture Publishers.

Hoizey, D., & Hoizey, M. J. (1988). *A history of Chinese medicine.* Edinburgh, Scotland: Edinburgh University Press.

Kaptchuk, T. J. (1983). *The web that has no weaver: Understanding Chinese medicine.* New York: Congdon & Weed.

Konefal, J., Duncan, R., & Clemence, C. (1995). Comparison of three levels of auricular acupuncture in an outpatient substance abuse program. *Alternative Medicine Journal, 2*(5), 8–9.

Lao, L. (1996). Acupuncture techniques and devices. *Journal of Alternative and Complementary Medicine, 2*(1), 23–25.

Li, Y., Tougas, G., Chiverton, S. G., & Hunt, R. H. (1992). The effects of acupuncture on gastrointestinal function and disorders. *American Journal of Gastroenterology, 87*(10), 1372–1381.

Liao, S. J., Lee, M. H. M., & Ng, N. K. Y. (1994). *Principles and practice of contemporary acupuncture.* New York: Marcel Dekker.

Lu, G. D., & Needham, J. (1980). *Celestial lancets. A history and rationale of acupuncture and moxa.* New York: Cambridge University Press.

Margolin, A., Avants, S. K., Chang, P., & Kosten, T. R. (1993). Acupuncture for the treatment of cocaine dependence in methadone-maintained patients. *American Journal of Addictions, 2,* 194–201.

Naeser, M. A. (1996). Acupuncture in the treatment of paralysis due to central nervous system damage. *Journal of Alternative and Complementary Medicine, 2*(1), 211–248.

National Institutes of Health. (1994). *Alternative Medicine, Newsletter of the Office of Alternative Medicine, 2*(2).

National Institutes of Health. (1997, November). Acupuncture. *NIH Consensus Statement, 15*(5), 1–34.

Pomeranz, B. (1997). Audiocassette recording of lecture by Aldous Huxley. Toronto, Ontario: University of Toronto.

Reston, J. (1971, July 26). Now about my operation in Peking. *New York Times,* pp. 1, 6.

Stux, G., & Pomeranz, B. (1995). *Basics of acupuncture.* Berlin: Springer Verlag.

Ter Riet, G., Kleijnen, J., & Knipschild, P. (1990). Acupuncture and chronic pain: A criteria-based meta-analysis. *Journal of Clinical Epidemiology, 43,* 1191–1199.

Tkach, W. (1972). I have seen acupuncture work. *Today's Health, 50,* 50–56.

Vincent, C. A., & Richardson, P. H. (1986). The evaluation of therapeutic acupuncture: Concepts and methods. *Pain, 24,* 1–13.

World Health Organization. (1990, October). *Traditional medicine and modern health care.* Executive board 87th session, Geneva, Switzerland, WHO EB87/11, 5–6.

# CHAPTER 14

# Spirituality and Healing

STANLEY KRIPPNER

**Abstract:** Modern Western biomedicine, nursing, social work, counseling, and psychological therapy address people's physical, mental, emotional, and social problems but rarely their spiritual concerns. Spirituality is, however, an integral part of the healing models of indigenous healers, who respond to the health care needs of some 70 percent of the current world population. The chapter provides examples of the role of spirituality in non-Western practices. It concludes that allopathic practitioners need to integrate a concern for the spiritual aspects of life into their practice and collaborate with indigenous healers in areas of the world where Western practitioners are virtually absent or are regarded with suspicion.[1]

## SPIRITUALITY, TRANSCENDENT EXPERIENCES, AND HEALING

The word *spiritual* can be used to describe the aspects of human behavior and experience that reflect an alleged transcendent intelligence or process that inspires devotion and directs behavior. The spiritual dimension of human life is evident to any person who becomes aware of a life meaning that extends beyond the immediacy of everyday expediency and concerns (Krippner & Welch, 1992). Elkins (1998) views spirituality as "indefinable" but approaches it from multiple angles—for example, as a hunger for psychological health (and for imagination, passion, and depth); as a search for the sacred; and as the yearning of one's soul for "the more." In the Western world, biomedicine, nursing, social work, counseling, and psychological therapy focus on physical, mental, emotional, and/or social problems but rarely address spiritual concerns.

When 1,400 California clinical psychologists were asked by mail whether or not they felt that spirituality was relevant in their personal lives and their clinical work, only 406 responded. Although the majority answered positively, fewer affirmed the personal relevance of spirituality than did the population in general. Behavioral psychologists were the least likely to affirm the relevance of spirituality in psychological therapy, and Jungian analysts were the most likely. The therapists who felt that spirituality was relevant to their personal lives were the most likely to use it in their clinical practice (Shafranske, 1984).

The difference between religion and spirituality has been described as a distinction between adherence to the beliefs and practices of an organized religious institution and a person's relationship to a purported transcendent reality without regard to religion or creed (Lukoff, Lu, & Turner, 1996, p. 234). From this distinction, it follows that many people are spiritual without being religious, in the sense of participating in organized religion. Likewise, it follows that many people are religious without being spiritual; that is, they perform the rituals and accept the creeds of religious institutions (at least superficially), but their ethics, morals, and opportunities for daily practice of their religion do not match their professed beliefs (Krippner & Welch, 1992).

A significant number of patients, when asked how they cope with life stressors and health problems (both physical and psychological), mention spiritual and religious attitudes, beliefs, and practices. In some parts of the United States, the proportion reaches between 33 percent and 50 percent, according to some surveys, especially among African Americans, women, and the elderly. Furthermore, a surprisingly large number of patients would like their physicians to address religious or spiritual issues in the context of medical visits (Koenig, McCullough, & Larson, 2001, p. 94).

In his survey of 47 societies, Winkelman (1992) studied the records of "religious and magical practitioners" who claimed to have access to spiritual entities (e.g., deities, ghosts, spirits). These practitioners alleged that they used special powers (e.g., casting spells, bestowing blessings, exorcising demons) to influence the course of human affairs or natural phenomena in ways not possible by other members of their social group. Underlying the procedures of each practitioner was an explicit or implicit model of healing that arranged, structured, and systematized the practitioner's beliefs and assumptions. Many of these models resembled that proposed by Seaward (2000), who proposed that stress is a disruption in "coherence between the layers

of consciousness in the human energy field" and that stress management procedures need to address the union of "mind, body, and spirit" (p. 241).

## INSTRUMENTATION AND PROCEDURES OF INDIGENOUS HEALERS

Indigenous healers, native healers, traditional healers, and similar practitioners manage the health care needs of roughly 70 percent of the world's population (Mahler, 1977). These practitioners often use signs (concrete representations of something else) and symbols (images that represent something more complex) in their work. Numbers, letters, and directional marks are signs; mandalas, totem poles, and abstract stone formations are symbols. An understanding of a culture's spiritual signs and symbols is essential to mental health practitioners who intend to relieve distress and facilitate recovery in settings different from their own.

For example, in the healing ceremonies of the Navajo and other tribes in the American Southwest, the central element is the sand painting, a symbolic design created in the soil by the tribal shamans. The painting represents the spiritual and physical landscape in which the client and her or his sickness exist, as well as the cause of the problem and the meaning of the procedure chosen by the practitioner for its cure. The practitioner often places stones, plants, and sacred objects inside the painting, with colored sand images symbolizing the relationships among the various elements. The sand figures may be clouds, snakes, or whatever is needed to portray the path of the sickness as it proceeds through time and space. Chanting and community vigils are typical procedures that bring the elements of a sand painting together. The indisposed person then becomes aware of the relationship between the sickness and the rest of his or her life. Usually, friends, neighbors, and relatives surround the client, singing and praying for a recovery (Sandner, 1979).

Levi-Strauss (1955) proposed that the kind of logic developed by tribal people is as rigorous and complete as that of modern individuals. Both use signs and symbols in highly sophisticated ways, but their modes of expression and application differ. For example, the cultural myths of pre-Columbian Mexican and Central American societies were not only comprehensive guides to daily conduct but also explanations for the mysteries of the universe. Mythic symbols were manipulated with such economy that each served a wide range of philosophical and religious ideas. Quetzalcoatl was the "feathered serpent" (who symbolized the transformation of matter into spirit), as well as the god of the winds, the lord of the dawn, the spirit of the sacred ocelot (a fierce jungle cat), the last king of the Toltecs, and (following the Spanish conquest) Jesus Christ.

The Christian cross, often used in healing ceremonies, is a symbol of Christ's crucifixion. In Buddhism, a white elephant often symbolizes the Buddha. The six-pointed Star of David is the symbol of Judaism. The swastika was a sacred symbol in Hinduism, in the Eastern Orthodox Church, and among the Maya in Central America and the Navajos of the American Southwest, long before its use by the Nazis in the 20th century.

For several decades, social and behavioral scientists have been collecting data that reflect the wide variety of healing systems. Sicknesses and injuries are universal experiences, but each society implicitly or explicitly classifies them according to cause and cure. These explanations include the spiritual dimension if the social context is supportive. For example, Mexican American *curanderos* and *curanderas* often attribute an illness to an agent whose existence must be taken on faith because it cannot be detected with medical instruments (Trotter & Chavira, 1981). The *mal ojo,* or "evil eye," has no place in allopathic biomedicine, but *curanderismo* practitioners claim it is caused by a person staring intently at someone else, usually with envy or desire. Treatment may include forming three crosses on the victim's body with an egg while the practitioner recites the Apostle's Creed.

An Apache disease, *nitsch,* purportedly results from the neglect of entities in nature. If an Apache does not properly salute an owl, he or she may suffer from heart palpitations, anxiety, sweating, and shaking. Apache shamans use spiritual prayers and songs to treat this illness that, it is believed, can lead to suicide if not carefully managed.

Frank and Frank (1991) conjectured that the first healing model was built around the belief that the etiology of illness was either supernatural (e.g., possession by a malevolent spirit) or magical (e.g., the result of a sorcerer's curse). Treatment consisted of appropriate rituals that supposedly undid or neutralized the cause. The rituals typically required the active participation of not only the sufferer but also family and community members. Both allopathic and indigenous models of healing are inclusive, yet each presents its adherents with a very different worldview. The native models are spiritual because they demonstrate an awareness of a broader life meaning that transcends the immediacy of everyday physical expediency, as well as an "otherworldly" transcendent reality that interfaces with ordinary reality.

The influence of indigenous healers can be seen in the practices of the Spiritual Emergence Network (Grof & Grof, 1990). The network consists of practitioners who claim expertise in working with such phenomena as purported spirit communication ("channeling," "visitations," etc.), unusual mental imagery (visions, voices, etc.), shifts in body sensations (out-of-body experiences, stigmata, etc.), dramatic religious experiences (encounters with Jesus Christ, the Buddha, etc.), and mystical experiences ("dissolving" into the cosmos or into "ineffable love"). The network's purpose is to offer a process that enables persons undergoing spiritual transformation to find the support and guidance they need to work through and then integrate their experiences.

Spiritual crises were conceptualized quite differently in the past, especially by Western religious and psychiatric institutions. The Roman Catholic Church's manual on exorcism lists many spiritual crises as symptoms of possession by satanic forces; for example, "the facility of divulging future and hidden events" is considered potentially "demonic" (Karpel, 1975). More recently, such claims have been labeled "magical thinking" or are considered symptoms of emotional disturbance by many conventional psychiatrists (American Psychiatric Association, 1980). Neither of these stances recognizes the potential for growth inherent in a spiritual crisis.

Those who would like to inform counselors and psychological therapists that unusual experiences are not necessarily pathological might consult a book published by the American Psychological Association titled *Varieties of Anomalous Experience* (Cardeña, Lynn, & Krippner, 2000), which draws attention to a number of meaningful human experiences too long neglected, ignored, or even derided. This resource does not debate the veridicality or "reality" of anomalous experiences, focusing instead on the nature of the descriptive reports and how these accounts can inform psychological therapists, counselors, psychiatrists, and related professionals who want to be informed about the full range of the human condition.

The contributors to this book, however, agree with David Lukoff (1985) that "differentiating psychotic from spiritual experience is not easy" (p. 155). The task requires familiarity with psychopathological perspectives as well as the religious, cultural, and ethnic background of the client. To facilitate the process of psychological therapy in his practice, Lukoff used creative writing and painting. In working with a client (diagnosed as suffering from manic psychosis) who claimed that he had been abducted by "space aliens," Lukoff (1988) tried to understand the client's underlying personal mythology and its accompanying metaphors. Eventually, the client was able to understand his mythic framework as well, communicating it in art and writing that was of such a high quality that it was displayed and published. Although the client continued to insist that he actually had been abducted, he dropped his preoccupation with the incident and was able to get on with his life.

Psychological therapists and counselors, when faced with a spiritual crisis, have several critical decisions to make. They need to determine whether the experience has psychotic components. They must decide whether the crisis is basically an *emergency* that has little growth potential, a spiritual *emergence* in which the client could gain something of value if the crisis is handled well, or an *emergency* that can lead to spiritual *emergence*. A recurring issue is whether the reported experience (e.g., abduction by "aliens," possession by a "demonic entity," or recollection of a "past life" episode) is a metaphor for an internal process, a trauma that has been forgotten, or an account that should be taken literally.

The American Psychological Association has also published two books on spirituality in psychological therapy. In *Integrating Spirituality into Treatment* (Miller, 1999), the authors assert that spirituality is of integral importance to psychology and offers practitioners practical ways of incorporating spiritual issues into therapy. Among the topics addressed are prayer, meditation, forgiveness, hope, serenity, 12-step programs, and diversity issues. Richards and Bergin (1997), in *A Spiritual Strategy for Counseling and Psychotherapy*, argue that when diagnosing and assessing a client, practitioners need to routinely assess the client's religious and spiritual status to obtain a richer and more accurate diagnostic picture. The authors insist that spirituality is susceptible to scientific investigation and offer a series of case studies that illustrate their point of view.

A related book, *Faith and Health: Psychological Perspectives* (Plante & Sherman, 2001) provides additional resources for practitioners who are considering applying spiritual perspectives in their work. However, the issue of adequate training must not be neglected as therapists and counselors jump on the spirituality bandwagon (Simmons, 2001). For example, Karasu (1999), in his call for a "spiritual psychotherapy," carefully described the therapeutic relationship and how it differs from religious counseling (p. 158).

An individual allopathic practitioner might work spiritual aspects into his or her worldview and medical practice, but this effort is not intrinsic to the Western biomedical model as it is widely taught and promulgated. Spirituality, however, is part and parcel of Apache shamanism and *curanderismo*, models of healing that would change radically if they were to lose their spiritual components.

These issues are important because they allow the differentiation between *disease* and *illness*. Several writers have conceptualized *disease* as a bodily dysfunction resulting from infections, inadequate diet, or poor sanitation. *Illness* is a broader term incorporating social constructs that imply dysfunctional behaviors, mood disorders, or inappropriate thoughts and feelings. These behaviors, moods, thoughts, and feelings can accompany diseases (as well as injuries), but are not the focus of treatment (e.g., Stoudemire, 1998, pp. 70–71).

## DOCUMENTED APPLICATIONS OF SPIRITUAL HEALING

More than 100 studies focusing on "spiritual wellness" rather than "illness" appear in the literature (Koenig et al., 2001, pp. 214–219). Westgate (1996), in summarizing some of the literature, identified four dimensions:

1. Meaning and purpose in life.
2. Intrinsic values.
3. Transcendent beliefs and experiences.
4. Community relationships.

In 16 empirical studies reviewed by Westgate, nine yielded statistically significant results demonstrating lower levels of depression in individuals who manifested one or more of the four dimensions. Of special interest was the fourth dimension; Westgate noted that "the spiritually well person also lives in the community—praying, chanting, worshiping, or meditating with others. This community not only provides a sense of shared values and identity but also offers mutual support and an avenue for community outreach" (p. 33). In commenting on young members of African American churches in the United States, Howd (1999) observed, "There's something about a faith community that seems to make a difference in their lives, and that seems to be the church" (p. 18). Given the high rate of hypertension among African Americans (40 percent in some studies), there has been increasing interest in the effectiveness of churches as blood pressure control centers and social support systems (Koenig et al., 2001, p. 262).

Indeed, there is some evidence that, in general, individuals with internalized spiritual and religious values score higher on measures of mental health than those who do not consider themselves religious, those who only give lip service to religious values, or those whose religious commitment takes the form of adherence to fanatical cults or uncompromising belief systems (Wulff, 1991, pp. 504–505, 635). A great deal of this value appears to emanate from the social support and community activities generated by fellow believers and participants.

After reviewing the research literature, Koenig (1999) concluded that the thoughts and actions of religious orientation seem to enhance health. Individuals who attend religious services at least once a week live longer than those who go less often, even after such factors as alcohol consumption and social support are accounted for. As they grow older, people who worship weekly are more likely to live on their own and be free of disabilities. High blood pressure and heart attacks are less common and hospitalizations less frequent and shorter among religiously oriented people.

The data on heart disease and hypertension are especially provocative. The interplay of biological and psychological factors in the development of chronic heart disease has long been suspected, but only recently has scientific evidence supported these speculations. A growing number of research studies has provided compelling evidence of a strong link between psychosocial factors such as stress, personality, and lifestyle and the development of heart disease (Bishop, 1994, p. 355). Treatment procedures including a spiritual component have been especially provocative. The best known of these regimens, designed by Ornish (1991), combines stress reduction procedures, moderate aerobic exercise, and a modified diet. Several controlled studies have demonstrated the program's effectiveness in improving coronary function. Cardiovascular disease (including chronic heart disease, hypertension, peripheral vascular disease, and stroke) accounts for about one million deaths in the United States alone, nearly double the number caused by cancer. The existing data support a hypothetical link between spirituality

and heart disease, both in terms of preventive variables and in treatment procedures (Koenig et al., 2001, p. 249). Nonlocal healing procedures involve people who send positive thoughts or prayers to patients at a distance; the results of this controversial treatment are mixed but are worth exploring if the procedures are not seen as substitutes for more established treatments (Koenig et al., 2001, pp. 248–249; Krippner & Achterberg, 2000).

These data refute scoffers (e.g., Ellis & Yeager, 1989) who claim that religious beliefs, spiritual practices, and transcendent experiences endanger one's mental health. Barron (1963) pointed out that religion, at its best, "is not a dogma, not a set of forever-prescribed particularities, not static abstraction at all, but a formative process with faith as its foundation and vision as its goal—faith in the intelligibility and order of the universe, leading through necessary difficulties of interpretation and changing meanings to moments of spiritual integration which are themselves transient" (p. 169). Nevertheless, the living situations of some groups studied prevent them from engaging in such lifestyle behaviors as smoking, alcohol consumption, and psychosocial stress, making it difficult to draw conclusions regarding causation. Finally, some religiously oriented people feel "abandoned" by God when they become sick. Sloan, Bagiella, and Powell (1999) conclude that it is premature to promote faith and religion as adjunctive medical treatments.

These considerations point out the necessity to consider the relationship between spiritual attitudes, religious involvement, and immune function (the mobilization of immunoglobins in a living system). The emerging field of psychoneuroimmunology explores the relationship between psychological and physiological factors in the onset of sickness. Pert and her associates (Pert, Ruff, Weber, & Herkenham, 1985) have identified the receptor sites for neuropeptides, hypothesizing that they serve as "messengers" or bridges that link emotions and attitudes with bodily processes. Preliminary studies have observed an association between improved immune functioning and spiritual experiences, with specific applications to breast cancer and AIDS patients. Future research is needed to identify the components of the immune system most directly influenced by spiritual activity (Koenig et al., 2001, p. 290). For example, a prospective, randomized study of 86 women with breast cancer indicated that patients who received group therapy with an emphasis on social support survived about twice as long as those who were not in therapy groups (Spiegel, Bloom, Kraemer, & Gottheil, 1989).

## CLASSIFICATION AND DIAGNOSTIC ISSUES

Such variables as age, gender, education, ethnicity, and socioeconomic status have not been given adequate consideration in most of the studies that have been conducted. The ways in which spirituality manifests itself differs from culture to culture. At its best, spiritual experience can be an impetus for growth, development, and the expression of an individual's or a group's full capacity for love and service. In one survey, those who reported having had deep "mystical" experiences scored higher than any other group on a standard test of psychological well-being (Greeley, 1975). At its worst, however, spiritual experience can lead to rigid, self-righteous attitudes and the persecution of those whose beliefs and behaviors deviate from a particular dogma or creed. The doctrines of some Western and non-Western religious groups oppose allopathic biomedical care; in several documented cases, patients, including children, have died because of this harsh dictum (Asser & Swan, 1998).

The fourth edition of the *Diagnostic and Statistical Manual of Mental Disorders* (*DSM-IV*; American Psychiatric Association, 1994) has attempted to enhance its universal validity not only with a brief mention of "dissociative trance disorder" but with a supplemental category of "religious or spiritual problem" and a glossary of "culture-bound syndromes." Lewis-Fernandez and Kleinman (1995) admitted that this aspect of *DSM-IV* is the "main clinical development in current cultural psychiatry in North America" (p. 437), even though they judged the overall attempt to have been less than successful (p. 439).

Why did Lewis-Fernandez and Kleinman judge the *DSM-IV* so harshly? They pointed out many cross-cultural limitations in *DSM-IV*. For example, Hopi Indians identify five distinct indigenous categories related to "depression," only one of which shares significant parameters with the depressive disorders defined in *DSM-IV*. Such disorders as those involving eating behavior and sexual behavior "show such pervasive Western cultural determinants that they cannot, as presently formulated, be compared across different cultures" (p. 437). Along with anorexia nervosa and chronic fatigue syndrome, they considered dissociative identity disorder to be a Western "culture-bound disorder." Many mental health practitioners prefer to use the *International Statistical Classification of Diseases and Related Health Problems* (e.g., Garcia, 1990), which includes a category for trance and possession disorders they feel to be more culture sensitive.

From an anthropological perspective, the differences among what Bourguignon (1973) called trance, possession, and possession trance depend on several variables. These include consideration of what is deemed appropriate in a particular setting, the relationships between the people involved, the nature and status of the person having the experience, the human interactions occurring at the time of the manifestation, and the possible factors that provoked the condition.

However, *DSM-IV* categories rarely are contextual. For example, in 1996, I learned of a 70-year-old Native American woman who had been diagnosed as schizophrenic because she had answered affirmatively when a psychiatrist asked if she "heard voices." The psychiatrist had not asked whether her behavior was a result of her Native American culture, which includes listening to the earth's messages for signs sent by a higher power. The misdiagnosis kept this woman in the hospital until her inner voices told her what measures to take to obtain a release (Breasure, 1996).

In parts of the American Southwest, Navajo practitioners are allowed to enter hospitals to work with Native American patients, where they frequently rely on the use of herbs and healing chants. In the early 1970s, several Papago Indians were recruited and trained as mental health workers by the University of Arizona department of psychology in Tucson (Torrey, 1986, pp. 177–178). In 1969, a grant from the National Institutes of Mental Health was awarded to finance the training of Navajo shamans in Rough Rock, Arizona. The training program taught apprentice medicine men and women the intricate Navajo healing ceremonies and techniques, thus preserving and propagating these procedures for the well-being of the Navajo people (Topper, 1987). The Navajo ceremonies are based on the worldview that personality is a totality, a part of a family, and inseparable from the tribe. Navajo medicine is dedicated to restoring not only the health and harmony of the individual but also family ecology and any aspects of the tribe that have become disharmonious with nature.

Voss (1999) took a critical look at social work literature that views Native Americans as a "problem group" and fails to recognize the contributions that tribal, shamanic-based traditions can make in shaping social work theory, practice, and policy. Using the Lakota Sioux as an example, Voss pointed out the centrality of tribalism, which emphasizes the importance of kinship bonds and the interconnectedness of all life, as well as the spiritual role of shamans in fostering individual and community health. Voss argued that these two paths can restore *wicozani* (i.e., health) and enhance *wo'wa'bleza* (i.e., understanding) among peoples. The Lakota sense of self is permeable and can cross boundaries to include the natural world and other people; detached, autonomous individuals without these connections are viewed as flawed and misguided.

Traditional Lakota Sioux philosophy sees abuse, rejection, and neglect as affecting the child's *nagi* (i.e., soul), often causing it to detach from the body, resulting in "soul loss." A shaman must find the child's *nagi* and bring it back. Other shamanic procedures (e.g., sweat lodges, vision quests) purportedly lead to empowerment, regeneration, synergy, and inner healing. Voss provided examples of social services and treatment centers for alcoholism that have incorporated Native American practitioners and perspectives with beneficial results, concluding that social work could benefit from the shamanic insight that all beings, human as well as nonhuman, deserve respect.

Nonetheless, the services of traditional healers have not always been welcomed. Denny Thong (1993) is an Indonesian psychiatrist who organized the Bangli Mental Hospital, the first psychiatric facility on the island of Bali. One of his innovations was the introduction of a "family ward" where patients could request that a family member live with them, cook for them, and take an active role in their treatment. If the family requested it, shamans and other native healers were permitted to examine and treat the patient. Despite the success of this program in reducing the time a patient spent at the hospital, the opposition was persistent and intense. Thong was accused of dabbling in "superstition" and the "occult," and was transferred to another hospital in 1987.

## CONCLUSION

An investigation of various healing models strongly suggests that it would be foolish to abandon what is of value in allopathic bio-medicine and Western-oriented counseling and therapy. There is abundant evidence that these procedures can be practical and power-ful, especially as carried out by competent, caring practitioners. However, allopathic practitioners and conventional therapists need to integrate a concern for the spiritual aspects of life into their practice, and collaborate with indigenous healers in those areas of the world where Western practitioners are virtually absent or are regarded with suspicion.

Given that this territory is largely uncharted, what position should psychologi-cal therapists and counselors take in regard to spiritual issues with their clients? Mental health practitioners need to discern their posi-tions and communicate them to clients when the therapeutic situation requires it. Practi-tioners need to collaborate with clients in con-sidering spiritual issues and help them realize the likely consequences of their actions. The expertise of the therapist needs to shape the course of therapy, and this includes helping clients formulate a set of values, morals, and ethics that will guide them through life. Such critical life issues as abortion, birth control, sexual practices, competitive business activi-ties, and participation in military service are some in which therapists and clients might disagree, or which might cause the therapist to bring in a member of the clergy or a spiritual advisor as a co-counselor. The client's growth toward autonomy and maturity must be the therapeutic goal, not the conversion of the client to the therapist's religious orientation or lack of it.

Vaughan (1991) described the perils of spiritual addiction, spiritual ambition, and the "denial of the shadow" that sometimes characterize individuals subsumed with reli-giosity. Predominantly African American churches, representing some 20 million mem-bers, exemplify a more holistic approach; most congregations are active in providing community services ranging from child care to substance abuse prevention (Howd, 1999).

Spirituality implies an awareness of broader life meanings that transcend the immediacy of everyday life. If allopathic bio-medicine, nursing, social work, counseling, and psychological therapy could participate in this awareness, health care would more closely reflect the wholeness and integrity of individuals as well as interactions with their families and societies.

In Tantric Buddhism, truth is said to find its most practical expression in terms of heal-ing. As Western practitioners explore the com-plexities of the therapeutic process, they may also discover that its structure can accommo-date the spiritual dimension. Indeed, that dimension may well lead to the unfolding of awe and the flowering of wonder that will enhance the scope of contemporary medicine, nursing, social work, psychological therapy, and counseling, revitalizing their quest.

## NOTE

1. *Allopathic medicine* is a term used to describe most mainstream Western medicine, which treats diseases largely with agents producing effects quite differ-ent from the disease they treat. In contrast, homeopathic physicians rely on agents that mimic the effects of the disease they are treating.

## REFERENCES

American Psychiatric Association. (1980). *Diagnostic and statistical manual of mental disorders* (3rd ed., *DSM-III*). Washington, DC: Author.

American Psychiatric Association. (1994). *Diagnostic and statistical manual of mental disorders* (4th ed., *DSM-IV*). Washington, DC: Author.

Asser, S. M., & Swan, R. (1998). Child fatalities from religion-motivated medical neglect. *Pediatrics, 101,* 625–629.

Barron, F. X. (1963). *Creativity and psychological health: Origins of personal vitality and creative freedom.* Princeton, NJ: Van Nostrand.

Bishop, G. D. (1994). *Health psychology: Integrating mind and body.* Boston: Allyn & Bacon.

Bourguignon, E. (1973). *Religion, altered states of consciousness, and social change.* Columbus: Ohio State University Press.

Breasure, J. (1996, March). The mind, body and soul connection. *Counseling Today,* p. 5.

Cardeña, E., Lynn, S. J., & Krippner, S. (Eds.). (2000). *Varieties of anomalous experience: Examining the scientific evidence.* Washington, DC: American Psychological Association.

Elkins, D. N. (1998). *Beyond religion: A personal program for building a spiritual life outside the walls of traditional religion.* Wheaton, IL: Quest Books.

Ellis, A., & Yeager, R. J. (1989). *Why some therapies don't work—The dangers of transpersonal psychology.* Buffalo, NY: Prometheus Books.

Frank, J. D., & Frank. J. B. (1991). *Persuasion and healing* (3rd ed.). Baltimore: Johns Hopkins University Press.

Garcia, F. O. (1990). The concept of dissociation and conversion in the new edition of the International Classification of Disease (ICD-10). *Dissociation, 3,* 204–208.

Greeley, A. M. (1975). *The sociology of the paranormal: A reconnaissance.* Beverly Hills, CA: Sage.

Grof, C., & Grof, S. (1990). *The stormy search for the self.* Los Angeles: J.P. Tarcher.

Howd, A. (1999, October 18). The black church in the inner city. *Insight,* pp. 18–19, 39.

Karasu, T. B. (1999). Spiritual psychotherapy. *American Journal of Psychotherapy, 53,* 143–161.

Karpel, C. (1975). *The rite of exorcism.* New York: Berkley.

Koenig, H. G. (1999). *The healing power of faith: Science explores medicine's last great frontier.* New York: Simon & Schuster.

Koenig, H. G., McCullough, M. E., & Larson, D. B. (2001). *Handbook of religion and health.* New York: Oxford University Press.

Krippner, S., & Achterberg, J. (2000). Anomalous healing experiences. In E. Cardeña, S. J. Lynn, & S. Krippner (Eds.), *Varieties of anomalous experience: Examining the scientific evidence* (pp. 353–396). Washington, DC: American Psychological Association.

Krippner, S., & Welch, P. (1992). *Spiritual dimensions of healing: From native shamanism to contemporary health care.* New York: Irvington.

Levi-Strauss, C. (1955). The structural study of myth. *Journal of American Folklore, 78,* 428–444.

Lewis-Fernandez, R., & Kleinman, A. (1995). Cultural psychiatry: Theoretical, clinical, and research issues. *Cultural Psychiatry, 18,* 433–448.

Lukoff, D. (1985). Diagnosis of mystical experiences with psychotic features. *Journal of Transpersonal Psychology, 17,* 155–181.

Lukoff, D. (1988). Transpersonal perspectives on manic psychosis, creative, visionary, and mystical states. *Journal of Transpersonal Psychology, 20,* 111–139.

Lukoff, D., Lu, F., & Turner, R. (1996). A transpersonal clinical approach to religious and spiritual problems. In B. W. Scotton, A. B. Chinen, & J. R. Battista (Eds.), *Textbook of transpersonal psychiatry and psychology* (pp. 231–249). New York: Basic Books.

Mahler, H. (1977, November). The staff of Aesculapius. *World Health*, p. 3.

Miller, W. R. (Ed.). (1999). *Integrating spirituality into treatment: Resources for practitioners*. Washington, DC: American Psychological Association.

Ornish, D. (1991). *Dr. Dean Ornish's program for reversing heart disease: The only program scientifically proven to reverse heart disease without drugs or surgery*. New York: Ballantine Books.

Pert, C., Ruff, M., Weber, R., & Herkenham, M. (1985). Neuropeptides and their receptors: A psychosomatic network. *Journal of Immunology, 135*, 820–826.

Plante, T. G., & Sherman, A. C. (2001). *Faith and health: Psychological perspectives*. New York: Guilford.

Richards, P. S., & Bergin, A. E. (1997). *A spiritual strategy for counseling and psychotherapy*. Washington, DC: American Psychological Association.

Sandner, D. (1979). *Navajo symbols of healing*. New York: Harcourt, Brace, Jovanovich.

Seaward, B. L. (2000). Stress and human spirituality 2000: At the crossroads of physics and metaphysics. *Applied Psychophysiology and Biofeedback, 25*, 241–246.

Shafranske, E. P. (1984). Factors associated with the perception of spirituality in psychotherapy. *Journal of Transpersonal Psychology, 16*, 231–241.

Simmons, J. (2001, August). Facing Jewish issues. *Counseling Today*, pp. 14–15.

Sloan, R. P., Bagiella, E., & Powell, B. T. (1999, Feb. 20). Religion, spirituality, and medicine. *The Lancet*, pp. 664–667.

Spiegel, D., Bloom, J. R., Kraemer, H. C., & Gottheil, E. (1989, October 14). Effect of psychosocial treatment on survival of patients with metastatic breast cancer. *The Lancet*, pp. 888–890.

Stoudemire, A. (1998). *Human behavior: An introduction for medical students*. Philadelphia: Lippincott-Raven.

Thong, D. (with Carpenter, B., & Krippner, S). (1993). *A psychiatrist in paradise: Treating mental illness in Bali*. Bangkok, Thailand: White Lotus Press.

Topper, M. D. (1987). The traditional Navajo medicine man: Therapist, counselor, and community leader. *Journal of Psychoanalytic Anthropology, 10*, 217–249.

Torrey, E. F. (1986). *Witchdoctors and psychiatrists*. New York: Harper & Row.

Trotter, R. T., III, & Chavira, J. A. (1981). *Curanderismo: Mexican-American folk healing*. Athens: University of Georgia Press.

Vaughan, F. (1991). Spiritual issues in psychotherapy. *Journal of Transpersonal Psychology, 23*, 105–119.

Voss, R. W. (1999). Tribal and shamanic social work practice: A Lakota perspective. *Social Work, 44*, 228–241.

Westgate, C. E. (1996). Spiritual wellness and depression. *Journal of Counseling and Development, 75*, 26–35.

Winkelman, M. J. (1992). *Shamans, priests and witches: A cross-cultural study of magico-religious practitioners*. Tempe: University of Arizona.

Wulff, D. N. (1991). *Psychology of religion: Classic and contemporary views*. New York: Wiley.

# Part III

# APPLICATIONS
# TO COMMON DISORDERS

# CHAPTER 15

# The Biobehavioral Treatment of Headache

## STEVEN M. BASKIN AND RANDALL E. WEEKS

**Abstract:** Primary headache disorders are highly prevalent and significantly affect both individual sufferers and society. The most common disorders are migraine and tension-type headache in their various forms. Migraine is typically an episodic disorder often associated with disability, a pulsating quality, nausea and/or vomiting, and sensitivity to sensory stimuli. Tension-type headache is less intense and is not accompanied by throbbing or significant associated symptoms. Chronic daily headache is a clinical entity most often transforming from migraine and often associated with medication overuse. These disorders have significant psychiatric comorbidity, and some patients exhibit poor adherence to medication regimens. A behavioral headache interview and a headache diary are essential for informed diagnosis and treatment. A model of coping skills therapy, derived from empirically tested behavioral headache therapies, addresses and treats different dimensions of these disorders.

## PROFILE OF HEADACHE DISORDERS

The International Headache Society (IHS) describes two broad types of headache disorders: primary and secondary headache disorders (Headache Classification Committee, 1988). Secondary headache disorders result from underlying conditions such as a brain tumor or sinus disease. Primary headache disorders have no diagnosable underlying medical conditions that explain the headache pain and associated symptoms. The two most common primary headache disorders are migraine and tension-type headache. They exist in a variety of forms and are highly prevalent in the population. They are

associated with direct and indirect costs that have profound individual and societal effects (Castillo, Munoz, Guitera, & Pascual, 1999; Holroyd, Stensland, et al., 2000; Pryse-Phillips et al., 1992; Schwartz, Stewart, Simon, & Lipton, 1998; Stewart, 1993; Stewart, Lipton, Celentano, & Reed, 1992; Strang & Osterhaus, 1993).

Migraine is typically an intermittent headache of considerable severity, lasting from hours to days and causing at least some disability. In 60 percent to 70 percent of cases, it presents unilaterally, although many patients report bilateral pain. It is often reported as a throbbing, pulsating pain, usually located frontotemporally, retroorbitally, or generalized throughout the

---

**Box 15.1**    Diagnostic Criteria for Migraine with Aura

1. At least two attacks fulfilling criteria 2.
2. Headache has at least three of the following characteristics:
   a. One or more fully reversible aura symptoms indicating focal cerebral cortical and/or brain stem dysfunction.
   b. At least one aura symptom develops gradually over more than 4 minutes, or two or more symptoms occur in succession.
   c. No aura symptom lasts more than 60 minutes. If more than one aura symptom is present, accepted duration is proportionally increased.
   d. Headache follows aura with a free interval of less than 60 minutes. (It may also begin before or simultaneously with the aura.)
      In addition, organic disorder is ruled out by the initial evaluation or by imaging studies. If disease is present, migraine with aura attacks should not occur for the first time in close temporal relation to the disorder.

---

SOURCE: Adapted from Headache Classification Committee (1988).

---

cranium. Most individuals present with associated gastrointestinal symptoms, most notably nausea, and many also report sensitivity to light and/or sound. In migraine with aura, neurological symptoms, usually visual, occur before or at the same time as the headache. The aura typically lasts 20 to 30 minutes, develops gradually, and is completely reversible. The visual phenomena are typically scintillating scotoma or shimmering zig-zag lines around a growing black spot in the visual field. Some less common auras include neurological events such as aphasia, ataxia, paresthesias, or even hemiparesis resembling stroke symptoms. The headache that follows the aura is typically less severe than in migraine without aura. Migraine with aura occurs in approximately 10 percent to 15 percent of patients with migraine. (Diagnostic criteria for migraine with and without aura are shown in Boxes 15.1 and 15.2, respectively.). Many migraine sufferers have a prodrome (warning signal) phase, different from an aura, which typically consists of vague manifestations of a migraine that may precede the attack by hours to several

days. The usual prodromal symptoms include changes in energy level, irritability, mood changes, food cravings, repetitive yawning, heightened sensory perception, and fluid retention. Prodromal manifestations are most likely a result of excitation or inhibition of the cerebral neurons. Migraine begins with a neurological disturbance and evolves gradually into severe pain (Baskin, 1993; Silberstein, Lipton, & Dalessio, 2001).

Historically, migraine was called a vascular headache, reflecting the widespread belief that the pain was caused by vasodilatation of the extracranial arteries (Tunis & Wolff, 1953). Much research over the last 20 years has shown that migraine is generated from a hyperexcitable brain (Goadsby, 2001; Welch, D'Andrea, Tepley, Barkley, & Ramadan, 1990). This brain hyperexcitability leads to inappropriate firing of neurons in the brain stem and cortex, which activates the trigeminovascular system. This system is the important pathway of migraine pain and involves the trigeminal nerve and its relationship with the arteries in the meninges. There is hypothesized to be a central migraine

Box 15.2 Diagnostic Criteria for Migraine Without Aura

1. At least five attacks fulfilling criteria 2 through 4.
2. Headache lasting 4 to 72 hours (untreated or unsuccessfully treated).
3. Headache has at least two of the following characteristics:
   a. Unilateral location.
   b. Pulsating quality.
   c. Moderate or severe intensity (inhibits or prohibits daily activities).
   d. Aggravation by walking stairs or similar routine physical activity.
4. During headache, at least one of the following occurs:
   a. Nausea and/or vomiting.
   b. Photophobia and phonophobia.

In addition, organic disorder is ruled out by the initial evaluation or by imaging studies. If disease is present, the migraine attacks do not occur for the first time in close temporal relation to the disorder.

SOURCE: Adapted from Headache Classification Committee (1988).

generator around the dorsal raphe (serotonergic region), which then initiates trigeminal firing (Weiler et al., 1995). Activation of this system leads to vasodilatation in the arteries around the meninges and neurogenic inflammation where pain-producing peptides such as calcitonin gene-related peptide (CGRP) and substance P are released from the ends of the trigeminal nerve. Afferent pain pathways would then carry information back into the brain stem, to the trigeminal nucleus caudalis, thalamus, and cortex, where the pain signals are then processed. Hence, migraine is a brain disorder with neurovascular symptom expression.

The pathophysiology of episodic and chronic tension-type headache is not well understood. Historically, it was believed that abnormal and sustained contraction of pericranial muscles was the primary cause of pain (Ad Hoc Committee on Classification of Headache, 1962). However, a clear relationship between pericranial muscle activity and tension-type headache has not emerged (Hatch et al., 1992; Jensen & Rasmussen, 1996; Lipchik et al., 1996; Olesen & Jensen,

1991; Pikoff, 1984; Schoenen, Gerard, DePasqua, & Sainard-Gainko, 1991). More recently, the role of abnormalities to the central antinociceptive system have been hypothesized (Neufeld, Holroyd, & Lipchik, 2000). The International Headache Society in 1988 designed a diagnostic system that was operational and descriptive without etiologic considerations (Headache Classification Committee, 1988). The diagnostic criteria for episodic and chronic tension-type headache are shown in Boxes 15.3 and 15.4, respectively. The term *chronic daily headache* refers to a pattern of headache activity and is not an official IHS diagnostic category. Many headache specialists use the term and view chronic daily headache as a widespread clinical problem. Researchers have viewed chronic tension-type headache as one aspect of chronic daily headache. Most cases of chronic daily headache evolve from previous migraine, with a slow escalation of headache activity ending with daily or near daily head pain that resembles chronic tension-type headache. This is termed *chronic migraine* or *transformational*

---

**Box 15.3**      Diagnostic Criteria for Episodic Tension-Type Headache

1. Number of days with headache is less than 180 per year (15 per month).
2. At least 10 previous headache episodes fulfilling criteria 3 through 5.
3. Headache lasting from 30 minutes to 7 days.
4. At least two of the following pain characteristics.
    a. Pressing/tightening (nonpulsating) quality.
    b. Mild or moderate intensity (may inhibit but does not prohibit activities).
    c. Bilateral location.
    d. No aggravation by walking stairs or similar routine physical activity.
5. Both of the following:
    a. No nausea or vomiting (anorexia may occur).
    b. Photophobia and phonophobia are absent, or one but not the other is present.

In addition, organic disorder is ruled out by the initial evaluation or by imaging studies. If disease is present, the headaches should not have started in close temporal relationship to the disorder.

SOURCE: Adapted from Headache Classification Committee (1988).

---

**Box 15.4**      Diagnostic Criteria for Chronic Tension-Type Headache

1. Average frequency of headaches fulfilling criteria 2 and 3 exceeds 15 days per month (180 days per year) for 6 months.
2. At least two of the following characteristics:
    a. Pressing/tightening quality.
    b. Mild or moderate severity (may inhibit but does not prohibit activities).
    c. Bilateral location.
    d. No aggravation by walking stairs or similar routine physical activity.
3. Both of the following:
    a. No vomiting.
    b. No more than one of the following: nausea, photophobia, or phonophobia.

SOURCE: Adapted from Headache Classification Committee (1988).

---

*migraine.* Transformation often develops from overuse of immediate-relief medications, although transformation may occur without "rebound" phenomena (Mathew, 1994, 1997). Chronic migraine has been associated with lower response to treatment (Barton & Blanchard, 2001; Blanchard, Appelbaum, Radnitz, Jaccard, & Dentinger, 1989; Holroyd, 2001). Chronic daily headache may also begin abruptly without a process of evolution and is then called new daily persistent headache (Vanast, 1986). New diagnostic criteria for chronic daily headache have been proposed (Silberstein & Lipton, 2001; Silberstein, Lipton, & Sliwinski, 1996).

## A BIOBEHAVIORAL APPROACH

Biobehavioral considerations in the management of headache have become more broad based to more fully examine issues related to diagnosis, pathophysiology, and treatment. Comprehensive interdisciplinary treatment programs have emerged to address the diverse factors affecting the clinical picture of headache. This section reviews an integrated approach from a self-regulation and coping skills perspective. The biobehavioral model targets different problematic dimensions (physiological, emotional, behavioral, and cognitive) to better control chronic head pain.

The integrated biobehavioral approach has emerged from psychobiological models of headache (Bakal, 1982). It is based on the concept that psychobiological processes are interactive, with biology affecting behavior and environmental influences and learning modifying biology. Psychobiological models suggest that conditions controlling chronic headache are multidimensional and involve cognitive, emotional, and behavioral factors as well as biological processes. Psychobiological models suggest that as a headache disorder becomes more severe and chronic, complex processes, some involving faulty learning and behavior, serve to maintain the disorder. These models suggest that the neurobiological mechanisms underlying the disorder may change with chronicity (Lipchik et al., 1996). Many patients exhibit difficulty coping (both biologically and psychologically) with episodic headache, either migraine or tension type. This may be one reason that migraine, in some patients, gradually transforms to chronic daily headache. Behavioral and psychological events become important maintenance factors as headache frequency increases.

The first phase of biobehavioral treatment includes a thorough assessment with multiple types of data collection. During the second phase, intervention, the patient is encouraged to become an active participant in treatment and learns coping skills targeting different dimensions of the headache problem. Patient education is a strong component of the program.

### Assessment

#### Clinical Interview

The first phase of the behavioral assessment is an in-depth clinical interview (Baskin, 1993). A key aspect of the interview is education, because many patients have misconceptions about head pain. Even patients who are medically referred for biobehavioral treatment have fears of brain pathology or that a referral for behavioral intervention suggests a psychogenic etiology. During the initial phase of the interview, the clinician must abandon an "organic versus psychogenic" distinction and begin educating the patient to understand that psychological and behavioral factors influence head pain. Patients may distort their histories in relation to their own naïve conceptualizations of headache and may omit or distort certain key points. Often patients have consulted with many other professionals as well as family members and friends. Some are taking many medications, either self-prescribed or prescribed by physicians, that have paradoxical effects on their headache frequency and response to treatment. Often, these patients report "daily" migraine headaches that transform from intermittent to daily pain via rebound mechanisms secondary to overuse of analgesics, opioids, ergotamines, triptans, and/or caffeine (Diener & Wilkinson, 1988; Mathew, 1990; Saper, 1987). In tertiary care headache clinics in the United States, nearly 80 percent of chronic daily headache patients present with analgesic overuse (Rapoport, 1988; Solomon, Lipton, & Newman, 1992). Triptans are presently the treatment of choice to terminate acute migraine attacks. They activate

---

**Box 15.5**    Headache History

1. Grade the headache by its intensity
   Incapacitating          Moderate to severe       Dull         No headache
2. Note the characteristics of pain for each intensity headache
   Frequency                                Prodrome/aura
   Location/laterality                      Associated symptoms
   Character of pain                        Behavior during attack
   Medication use and relief                Time of onset/duration/pain patterns

---

5-HT 1B/1D receptors and have been reported to induce rebound headache when used more than three days per week (Gaist, Hallas, Sindrup, & Gram, 1996; Gobel, Stolze, Heinze, & Dworschak, 1996; Katsarava, Limmroth, Fritsche, & Diener, 1999; Suchowersky, 1993).

Assessing whether the patient is suffering from more than one type of headache is another critical element of this stage of treatment. Commonly, a patient refers to "my headache," without adequately differentiating two different headache types, and has had episodic migraine attacks over the years that increase in frequency and become complicated by daily constant headaches between migraine attacks. This type of patient often uses analgesics chronically and excessively, claiming, "If I don't take my pain pills, all my headaches will be incapacitating." Overuse of immediate-relief medications may be both a response to and a cause of chronic headache. During the interview, it is helpful to grade the headache by its intensity and disability using a four-point intensity scale, and the characteristics of pain and associated symptoms for each headache type should be recorded (see Box 15.5). The following questions also help differentiate headache types: What is the frequency of headache that is incapacitating? How often do you have a

headache that is moderate to severe in intensity? How often do you have a dull headache? How often are you completely clear-headed? Any prodromal symptoms (even if vague) should be noted because close observation of migraine prodromes can improve outcome.

It is important to establish the age and circumstances of onset for each headache type (e.g., menarche, physical/psychological trauma, stressors, etc.). Some patients recognize environmental factors that trigger migraine attacks, some report increased headache in association with biological rhythm changes, such as changes in sleep patterns or time zones, and some note dietary triggers. Psychological events may play a role in headache onset and maintenance. Careful questioning about recent life changes and quality-of-life issues may explain an increase in headache frequency. Major negative life events in the year before headaches began have been modestly related to both the onset and maintenance of frequent headache (DeBenedittis & Lorenzetti, 1992a; DeBenedittis, Lorenzetti, & Pieri, 1990). Diary studies have shown significant correlations between daily stress levels and attacks of migraine (Chabriat, Danchot, Michel, Joire, & Henry, 1999; Holm, Lokken, & Myers, 1997). Stress may also exacerbate chronic daily headache (DeBenedittis & Lorenzetti, 1992b; Holroyd, Stensland, et al., 2000; Spierings, Schroevers, Honkoop, & Sorbi, 1998). Levels of daily minor stress are associated with migraine (DeBenedittis & Lorenzetti, 1992a, 1992b). Many patients do not have the problem-solving and coping skills necessary to manage stress or recurrent headache. The patient should be carefully questioned about family and marital relationships, vocational history, social/environmental stressors, and recent life changes. It is helpful to gather information on activity level, coping skills, disability issues, and perceptions about headache.

The clinician should evaluate pain behaviors, including operant and classical conditioning factors. In operant conditioning, pain behavior is affected by its consequences. It is important to observe reinforcement contingencies (secondary gain) and avoidance behaviors that occur secondary to pain. The reinforcing consequences of certain medications should be noted. In classical conditioning, biological reactions are conditioned to stimuli that are associated with pain. Thus some headache sufferers develop fear reactions as conditioned responses to the occurrence of intermittent, unpredictable, severe pain such as migraine. They become almost phobic to headache and preemptively take medication to avoid the pain, a powerful conditioning process.

Taking an in-depth habit history, assessing alcohol, nicotine, and "recreational" drug use is another important part of the clinical interview. Some patients believe that because caffeine is contained in many abortive headache preparations, it has an antiheadache effect if taken as a prophylactic. On the contrary, however, high daily caffeine consumption may increase the frequency of headache because of caffeine withdrawal effects and headache rebound

mechanisms. A family history regarding psychiatric illness, alcohol/drug abuse, as well as headache should be obtained. The clinician must thoroughly but subtly evaluate the symptoms of major depression as well as those of anxiety disorders. Numerous epidemiological and clinical research studies have confirmed elevated risk of anxiety and mood disorders in migraine as well as chronic daily headache (Breslau, Davis, Schultz, & Peterson, 1994; Merikangas & Angst, 1993; Merikangas & Stevens, 1997; Silberstein, Lipton, & Breslau, 1995). In one study, 90 percent of the chronic daily headache patients studied had at least one comorbid psychiatric disorder (Verri et al., 1998). The risk for depressive disorder is bidirectional, with migraine increasing the risk for the first onset of major depression and major depression increasing the risk for the initial onset of migraine (Breslau et al., 1994). The presence of comorbid psychiatric illness often contributes to treatment refractoriness (Guidetti, Galli, Fabrizi, Napoli, & Bruno, 1998). Treatment often becomes even more complicated by the presence of an Axis II personality disorder. Therefore, the clinician should determine the patient's psychological background and psychiatric history.

Behavioral assessment also includes evaluating the patient's adherence to medication treatment and determining if he or she overuses immediate-relief agents. Paradoxically, these agents may maintain headache and interfere with prophylactic pharmacological and behavioral therapies (Blanchard, Taylor, & Dentinger, 1992; Kudrow, 1982). Studies have shown that more than 50 percent of headache patients fail to properly comply with drug treatment regimens (Packard & O'Connell, 1986). Reasons for not adhering include lack of insight, financial issues, poor instructions by the physician, inappropriate expectations, strong belief systems ("I don't need medicine"), helplessness and pessimism, and anger at health care providers. It is important to note that complex therapy regimens require changes in behavior. Problems also exist when evaluating psychological/biofeedback interventions. It is essential to inquire about the specifics of past therapy and determine whether or not the patient learned and regularly practiced the skills.

### Psychophysiological Evaluation

There is inconsistency and controversy in the literature concerning psychophysiological assessment of headache (Flor & Turk, 1989; Schoenen et al., 1991). During the psychophysiological evaluation, biofeedback equipment helps identify certain physiological and sensorimotor targets for intervention. A physiological stress profile assesses generalized arousal (some combination of electrodermal response, heart rate, and respiratory dynamics), skeletal muscle responses (frontotemporal, masseter, trapezius), and smooth muscle/vascular responses (temporal pulse amplitude, finger temperature). Evaluating a variety of conditions, including baseline, mental and physical stressors, recovery, and relaxation, provides a clinical measure of autonomic reactivity (Flor & Turk, 1989). This measure is helpful in designing treatment for psychophysiological stress-related aspects of the patient's head pain. Sometimes surface electromyography is used to assess the tension levels of the pericranial muscles in two positions, sitting and standing (Cram, 1990; Schoenen et al., 1991). Muscles typically evaluated include frontalis, temporalis, masseter, sternomastoid, cervical paraspinals, upper trapezius, and T1 paraspinals. These are compared with normative data. With this type of assessment, the clinician may notice "guarding" responses that are secondary to chronic headache as well as primary muscle

contraction in some patients. Some patients show diffuse hyperactivity of numerous muscles of the head and neck. The most reliable finding in tension-type headache sufferers is tenderness of the pericranial muscles (with or without EMG elevations) during palpation, which escalates with increasing frequency and severity of pain (Hatch et al., 1992; Jensen, 1999; Jensen & Rasmussen, 1996; Lipchik et al., 1996; Neufeld et al., 2000; Olesen & Jensen, 1991; Pikoff, 1984; Schoenen et al., 1991). The significance of these responses is unknown. Nevertheless, these findings are often useful in guiding a biofeedback-based relaxation program.

### Treatment

Intervention proceeds from the detailed initial assessment and is an amalgam of empirically validated psychophysiological and cognitive stress management therapies (McGrady et al., 1999). Psychological and pharmacological interventions are often combined in a comprehensive multifaceted biobehavioral program (see Box 15.6). A major component of this type of intervention is teaching the patient coping skills designed to alleviate both a sensory component and a reactive component within the total pain experience. The sensory component involves the perception of physical sensations, including pain, which can be altered through relaxation therapies and biofeedback. The reactive component consists of thoughts and feelings that accompany headache and may lower pain threshold, lead to problematic behaviors, heighten levels of sympathetic arousal, and possibly increase neuronal hyperexcitability. The patient may display a decreased sense of mastery and control (helplessness). Cognitive-behavioral interventions help modify the reactive component by emphasizing skills that increase the patients ability to cope and reduce headache-related

---

**Box 15.6    Biobehavioral Program**

- Time limited and goal oriented
- Components:
  - Education
  - Cognitive strategies to enhance coping
  - Relaxation and biofeedback to foster self-regulation
- Patient requirements:
  - Active participation and personal responsibility
  - Self-monitoring with headache diary
  - Dietary and behavior changes
  - Maximum adherence to drug regimens

---

distress. The program requires a series of sessions, typically between 6 and 15, depending on clinical considerations.

More than 100 empirical studies have examined the efficacy of biobehavioral therapies in headache. The American Academy of Neurology–U.S. Consortium recently published evidence-based guidelines for migraine headache treatment and concluded that relaxation training, thermal biofeedback combined with relaxation training, EMG biofeedback, and cognitive-behavioral therapy yielded a consistent pattern of findings and were recommended as treatment options for migraine (Silberstein, 2000). Meta-analytic reviews of migraine treatment have shown an approximate 50 percent improvement rate for behavioral treatment, which is almost identical to propranolol, a common preventative medication (Holroyd & Penzien, 1990). Another recent meta-analysis showed that EMG biofeedback, relaxation therapy, and cognitive-behavioral therapy were moderately effective (40 percent to 50 percent reduction in headache activity) in the management of tension-type headache, relative to wait-list controls (McCrory, Penzien, & Rains, 1996).

## Education

Patients benefit from a detailed education program that emphasizes that headache is determined by a complex group of factors. Explanations of the pathophysiology of headache improve patient understanding of the rationale for pharmacological and non-pharmacological treatment. Discussions may include biological predispositions; hormonal factors; diet; the human stress response; biological rhythm factors; and relevant cognitive, emotional, and behavioral issues.

After learning how to monitor frequency, intensity, duration, and disability issues related to headache, the patient keeps a headache diary and brings it to each session. The diary is a record of the type and amount of medication taken as well as relief factors, menstrual days, and environmental triggers. These calendars generate important data, increase accuracy, save time, and are easy and efficient to use given a simple format (Rapoport & Sheftell, 1996).

## Skills Acquisition

The factors that act as headache triggers vary from person to person. Among the many triggers are changes in sleep rhythm, diet, fasting and skipping meals, acute and chronic stress, overexertion, hormonal changes, weather changes, and sensory stimuli.

Patients are encouraged to empirically validate dietary factors as possible headache triggers. They learn about foods that have

---

**Box 15.7     Foods That Trigger Headache**

Begin with a total elimination of the following for one month. If you observe a decrease in frequency or severity of headache, slowly reintroduce foods one at a time and observe the result.

- Chocolate
- Canned figs
- Nuts
- Peanut butter
- Onions
- Pizza
- Sour cream
- Yogurt
- Herring
- Chicken livers
- Avocado
- Nutrasweet, Aspartame
- Ripened cheeses (e.g., Cheddar, Gruyere, Brie, Camembert)
  - Cheeses that are permissible: American, cottage, cream, and Velveeta
- Vinegar
  - White vinegar is permissible
- Anything that is fermented, pickled, or marinated
- Hot fresh breads, raised coffee cakes, and doughnuts (due to activated yeast)
- Pods of broad beans (lima, navy, and pea pods)
- Monosodium glutamate (MSG)
  - Any foods containing large amounts of MSG (e.g., Chinese food)
- Citrus fruits (e.g., no more than one orange per day)
- Bananas (no more than half a banana per day)
- Pork (limit intake)
- Tea, coffee, cola beverages (limit intake)
- Fermented sausage (e.g., bologna, salami, pepperoni, summer sausage, hot dogs)
- Alcoholic beverages (most frequently cited food triggers for migraine)

---

been most often reported as headache and migraine triggers (see Box 15.7). To monitor their diets, including caffeine and alcohol use, patients are taught to use their diaries and to discuss necessary changes in diet as needed. Much has been written about dietary factors in relation to migraine (Cornwell & Clarke, 1991; Hanington, 1980; Hasselmark, Malmgren, & Hannerz, 1987; Medina & Diamond, 1978; Radnitz, 1990; Radnitz & Blanchard, 1991; Salfield et al., 1987; Selzer,

1982; Zeigler & Stewart, 1977). However, these studies indicate that dietary modification might be of *some* benefit for *some* patients, and few research protocols are well designed; therefore, it appears that widespread efficacy has not been established.

Patients are taught some general "hints" to help with headache control, such as maintaining consistent biological rhythms. They are encouraged to keep to normal sleep/wake patterns, even on weekends;

**Table 15.1**    Pain Tolerance and Perception

| *Patients With High Pain Tolerance* | *Patients With Low Pain Tolerance* |
| --- | --- |
| Perceive pain as a controllable challenge. | Perceive pain as an ordeal with much helplessness and "catastrophizing." |
| Are task-specific, breaking down responses to manageable target behaviors. | Are fatalistic. |
| Exhibit action-oriented self-talk ("I have a plan of action") and set realistic goals. | Have negative outlook about themselves and their ability to deal with pain. Self-talk often mentions "suffering" or "hope" but lacks action orientation. |

avoid oversleeping; and maintain consistency in bedtime and time of awakening. Patients are also advised to eat nutritious meals at regular intervals.

Patients also learn behavioral strategies to help with headache control and begin setting behavioral goals such as improving time management, increasing aerobic exercise, and participating in more pleasurable activities. Patients who exhibit aspects of the Type A behavior pattern are taught how to better evaluate threat so they can avoid automatic physiological mobilization.

Clinicians teach patients ways to self-manage medication. Brief educational interventions increase adherence to abortive drug regimens (Holroyd, Cordingley, et al., 1989; Holroyd, Holm, et al., 1988). This is especially important in patients with chronic daily headache who also experience intermittent migraine attacks. Patients are taught to identify migraine onset accurately by self-monitoring interoceptive cues, to keep medication readily available, and to follow instructions regarding usage and repeated administration. Specific limits are set to prevent rebound from overuse of medications. Patients are also taught strategies for managing side effects for both preventative and abortive medications.

Patients learn to focus interventions on two related components of the total pain experience: sensory and reactive. The sensory component consists of the precursors and the sensation of pain. In this component, the patient learns to control physiological responses such as pericranial muscle contraction and finger temperature. The reactive component is cognitive and emotional and alerts the patient to thoughts and feelings that may generate a stress response and precede or accompany headache attacks. Strategies that treat the reactive component of the "pain experience" enhance pain tolerance and alter pain perception (see Table 15.1).

Initial treatment sessions are directed toward the sensory component, using relaxation training and biofeedback to teach physiological self-regulation. Relaxation therapies comprise several procedures that target the entire body, enabling patients to achieve an overall relaxed state. Biofeedback, on the other hand, targets specific physical responses believed to contribute to increased headache susceptibility. Instrumentation "feeds back" immediate objective information about biological processes that are normally beyond patients' awareness and control. The feedback may be visual or auditory. Patients learn to bring biologic processes under voluntary control and thereby lower arousal (Schwartz, 1995). Through training, the processes are "shaped" in a more adaptive direction (i.e., muscle tension decreased in pericranial muscles and finger temperature increased). The biofeedback program is a step-by-step approach that builds patients' skills over a

---

**Box 15.8**  Biofeedback Program

Step 1.  Clinical interview and assessment
- Patient begins headache diary

Step 2.  Teach body awareness of tension and overarousal
- Introduce diaphragmatic breathing
- Make progressive relaxation tape while EMG is monitored

Step 3.  Use EMG biofeedback to discriminate between relaxed and tense muscles

Step 4.  Introduce passive relaxation using imagery and breathing as relaxation cues

Step 5.  Continue EMG training until patient can reliably decrease muscle tension by approximately 50 percent
- Emphasize scalp, facial, neck, and shoulder relaxation

Step 6.  For migraine sufferers, use passive relaxation and autogenic training with thermal biofeedback
- Goal is to increase finger temperature to 95 °F, or 1 °F per minute

Step 7.  Conduct frequent short generalization exercises
- Identify prodromal signs and use techniques early

---

series of sessions (see Box 15.8). Patients must master each skill before moving on to the next and should be encouraged to use audiocassettes for home practice.

Electromyographic (EMG) feedback is most commonly used for tension-type headache. The clinician places sensors on the patient's forehead and at the back of the neck or shoulders, and the patient learns how to achieve a low arousal state via relaxation training and decreased muscle contraction. For migraine, the most common biofeedback technique combines EMG biofeedback and thermal biofeedback, or finger temperature training. With thermal biofeedback, the clinician attaches a superficial thermistor to the patient's index finger. Skin temperature is largely determined by the volume of blood flow to an area; blood flow and skin temperature usually change together. Training the patient in a low-arousal relaxation response to decrease muscle tension and increase finger temperature may relax a hyperexcitable central nervous system, decrease sympathetic outflow, and help "retrain" the autonomic nervous system.

Patients are encouraged to practice relaxation on a daily basis. By taking "mini" relaxation breaks throughout the day, patients learn to heighten body awareness and reduce physiologic arousal leading to more automatic relaxation (Andrasik, 1990).

The second part of the program focuses on the reactive component of the pain experience and consists of cognitive-behavior stress management therapy. Patients learn to identify and modify distress-related thoughts and maladaptive styles of thinking that can contribute to headache susceptibility (see Box 15.9). This type of therapy emphasizes the role of thoughts, perceptions, belief systems, self-evaluations and appraisals that influence emotional states, physiology, and behavior. Techniques are aimed at providing patients with a set of problem-solving and coping skills they can use in a wide range of situations that trigger and maintain headache. Distress-related thoughts and negative

---

**Box 15.9    Goals of Cognitive-Behavior Therapy**

- Foster an internal locus of control and modify distress-related thoughts
- Rehearse adaptive cognitive and behavioral responses to the development of a migraine
- Accurately interpret body signals
- Develop action plans
- Reduce anxiety and depression
- Recognize triggers

---

self-talk ("Why me? I can't believe I'm getting another migraine. It's no use") mediate poor outcome via a variety of mechanisms, including depressed mood, increased anxiety level, decreased pain threshold, poor treatment compliance, and overuse of pain medications.

Many patients magnify the negative aspects of their situations, becoming fatalistic and appearing helpless. They often have low tolerance for pain and, believing they are unable to control their pain, look to an external locus of control and a "magic pill." To develop alternative cognitive responses to the experience of recurrent severe pain, these patients are taught self-statements and to consider headaches as manageable components of a problem that can be solved rather than as "these awful headaches." Patients rehearse adaptive cognitive and behavioral responses to the development of a migraine and develop task-relevant management skills to reduce the anxiety that often magnifies symptoms.

Self-statements help patients (1) prepare for an attack, (2) manage initial symptoms, (3) handle critical moments, and (4) act during the post-headache phase (Bakal, 1982). Patients become keen observers, prepared to cope adaptively yet not hypervigilant to pain sensations. Many headache patients exhibit irrational ideation about the possibility of a migraine attack; they underestimate their coping skills. As a result of conditioned fear, some patients with frequent headache misinterpret bodily sensations and "catastrophize." In treating these anxiety-related features, it is critical to help patients accurately interpret perceived danger signals and react with rational self-statements. Patients are taught to use the following internal dialogue:

What is my plan?  Pause, don't panic. What does the situation require? What strategies can I use? I will follow my plan, one step at a time, without creating a catastrophe. I can handle the attack, use many strategies, and take appropriate medicines at the appropriate amount and time. I can use my relaxation skills, focus on what the situation requires and keep things under control. Remember, I have many strategies to use if I stay focused without worrying. I did well, used my skills, interpreted the situation accurately and only had a small amount of "down time." I am getting better at managing these migraines.

These cognitive coping strategies foster adherence to drug regimens, reduce headache-related distress, and result in better management of acute migraine attacks and exacerbations of pain in the chronic daily headache sufferer.

Some patients require cognitive therapy for depression. This is especially true for chronic daily headache patients who often exhibit affective distress (Holroyd, Malinoski,

Davis, & Lipchik, 1999). Cognitive therapy involves modifying a patient's automatic internal dialogue that predisposes the patient to helplessness, self-blame, and expectations of losing control of future events. This psychotherapeutic approach is time limited, is effective, and integrates well with pharmacological therapies for depression (Beck, 1976). Cognitive therapies are often useful in treating comorbid panic disorder and generalized anxiety disorder. In these cases, cognitive treatment focuses on correcting misappraisals of bodily sensations as dangerous. Targets of treatment intervention also include excessive, uncontrollable worry with accompanying persistent overarousal (Barlow, 2000).

## CONCLUSION

Effective biobehavioral treatment for headache begins with a thorough headache interview and use of a headache diary as a tool for self-monitoring. This approach emphasizes educating patients about headache mechanisms and providing skills and knowledge to enable patients to take an active role in managing their headache disorder. Behavioral strategies include lifestyle and nutritional changes, medication self-management, relaxation skills, biofeedback training, and cognitive therapy. Treatment also must address the depression and anxiety that frequently accompany headache.

Effective headache therapies help patients incorporate a variety of problem-solving skills, encouraging personal responsibility and collaboration with the health care professional. They expand the scope of treatment to include emotional, cognitive, behavioral, and self-regulation factors that have a bearing on outcome. The treatment should enable the headache patient to cope more effectively with headache pain and issues that trigger and maintain the headache problem.

## REFERENCES

Ad Hoc Committee on Classification of Headache. (1962). Classification of headache. *Journal of the American Medical Association, 179,* 717–718.

Andrasik, F. (1990). Psychological and behavioral aspects of chronic headache. In N. T. Mathew (Ed.), *Neurologic clinics: Advances in headache* (pp. 961–976). Philadelphia: W. B. Saunders.

Bakal, D. A. (1982). The psychobiology of chronic headache. New York: Springer.

Barlow, D. H. (2000). *Anxiety and its disorders: The nature and treatment of anxiety and panic.* New York: Guilford.

Barton, K. A., & Blanchard, E. B. (2001). The failure of intensive self-regulatory treatment with chronic daily headache: A prospective study. *Applied Psychophysiology and Biofeedback, 26*(4), 311–318.

Baskin, S. (1993). The headache history. In A. M. Rapoport & F. D. Sheftell (Eds.), *Headache: A clinicians guide to diagnosis, pathophysiology and treatment strategies* (pp. 25–33). Costa Mesa, CA: PMA.

Beck, A. T. (1976). *Cognitive therapy and the emotional disorders.* New York: International Universities Press.

Blanchard, E. B., Appelbaum, K. A., Radnitz, C. L., Jaccard, J., & Dentinger, M. P. (1989). The refractory headache patient: I. Chronic, daily, high intensity headache. *Behavior Research and Therapy, 27,* 403–410.

Blanchard, E. B., Taylor, A., & Dentinger, M. (1992). Preliminary results from the self-regulatory treatment of high-medication-consumption headache. *Biofeedback & Self-Regulation, 17,* 179–202.

Breslau, N., Davis, G. C., Schultz, L. R., & Peterson, Z. L. (1994). Migraine and major depression: A longitudinal study. *Headache, 34,* 387–393.

Castillo, J., Munoz, P., Guitera, V., & Pascual, J. (1999). Epidemiology of chronic daily headache in the general population. *Headache, 39,* 190–196.

Chabriat, H., Danchot, J., Michel, P., Joire, J., & Henry, P. (1999). Precipitating factors of headache: A prospective survey in migraineurs and nonmigraineurs. *Headache, 39*(5), 335–338.

Cornwell, N., & Clarke, L. (1991). Dietary modification in patients with migraine and tension-type headache [Abstract]. *Cephalalgia, 11*(Suppl. 2), 143–144.

Cram, J. R. (1990). EMG muscle scanning and diagnostic manual for surface recordings. In J. R. Cram (Ed.), *Clinical EMG for surface recordings* (Vol. 2, pp. 1–141). Seattle. WA: Clinical Resources.

DeBenedittis, G., & Lorenzetti, A. (1992a). The role of stressful life events in the persistence of primary headache: Major events vs. daily hassles. *Pain, 51,* 35–42.

DeBenedittis, G., & Lorenzetti, A. (1992b). Minor stressful life events (daily hassles) in chronic primary headache: Relationship with MMPI personality patterns. *Headache, 32,* 330–334.

DeBenedittis, G., Lorenzetti, A., & Pieri, A. (1990). The role of stressful life events in the onset of chronic primary headache. *Pain, 40,* 65–76.

Diener, H. C., & Wilkinson, M. (1988). *Drug-induced headache.* Berlin: Springer-Verlag.

Flor, H., & Turk, D. C. (1989). Psychophysiology of chronic pain: Do chronic pain patients exhibit symptom-specific psychophysiological responses? *Psychological Bulletin, 105,* 215–259.

Gaist, D., Hallas, J., Sindrup, S., & Gram, L. (1996). Is overuse of sumatriptan a problem? A population-based study. *European Journal of Clinical Pharmacology, 50,* 161–165.

Goadsby, P. J. (2001). The pathophysiology of headache. In S. D. Silberstein, R. B. Lipton, & D. J. Dalessio (Eds.), *Wolff's headache and other head pain* (pp. 57–72). New York: Oxford University Press.

Gobel, H., Stolze, H., Heinze, A., & Dworschak, M. (1996). Easy therapeutical management of sumatriptan-induced daily headache. *Neurology, 47,* 297–298.

Guidetti, V., Galli, F., Fabrizi, P., Napoli, L., & Bruno, O. (1998). Headache and psychiatric comorbidity: Clinical aspects and outcome in an 8-year follow-up study. *Cephalalgia, 18,* 455–462.

Hanington, E. (1980). Diet and migraine. *Journal of Human Nutrition, 34,* 175–180.

Hasselmark, L., Malmgren, R., & Hannerz, J. (1987). Effect of a carbohydrate-rich diet, low in protein-tryptophan, in classic and common migraine. *Cephalalgia, 7,* 87–92.

Hatch, J. P., Moore, P. J., Cyr-Provost, M., Boutros, N. N., Seleshi, E., & Borcherding, S. (1992). The use of electromyography and muscle palpation in the diagnosis of tension-type headache with and without pericranial muscle involvement. *Pain, 149,* 175–178.

Headache Classification Committee of the International Headache Society. (1988). Classification and diagnostic criteria for headache disorders, cranial neuralgia and facial pain. *Cephalalgia, 8*(Suppl. 7), 1–96.

Holm, J. E., Lokken, C., & Myers, T. C. (1997). Migraine and stress: A daily examination of temporal relationships in women migraineurs. *Headache, 37,* 553–558.

Holroyd, K. A. (2001). Learning from our treatment failures. *Applied Psychophysiology and Biofeedback, 26,* 319–323.

Holroyd, K. A., Cordingley, G. F., Pingel, J. D., Jerome, A., Theofanous, A. G., Jackson, D., et al. (1989). Enhancing the effectiveness of abortive therapy: A controlled evaluation of self-management training. *Headache, 29,* 148–153.

Holroyd, K. A., Holm, J. E., Hursey, K. G., Penzien, D. B., Cordingley, G. E., & Theofanous, A. G. (1988). Recurrent vascular headache: Home-based behavioral treatment vs. abortive pharmacological treatment. *Journal of Consulting and Clinical Psychology, 56,* 218–223.

Holroyd, K. A., Malinoski, P., Davis, M. K., & Lipchik, G. L. (1999). The three dimensions of headache impact: Pain, disability, and affective distress. *Pain, 83,* 571–578.

Holroyd, K. A., & Penzien, D. B. (1990). Pharmacological versus non-pharmacological prophylaxis of recurrent migraine headache: A meta-analytic review of clinical trials. *Pain, 42,* 1–13.

Holroyd, K. A., Stensland, M., Lipchik, G., Hill, K., O'Donnell, F., & Cordingley, G. (2000). Psychosocial correlates and impact of chronic tension-type headaches. *Headache, 40,* 3–16.

Jensen, R. (1999). Pathophysiological mechanisms of tension-type headache: A review of epidemiological and experimental studies. *Cephalalgia, 19,* 602–621.

Jensen, R., & Rasmussen, B. K. (1996). Muscular disorders in tension-type headache. *Cephalalgia, 16,* 97–103.

Katsarava, Z., Limmroth, V., Fritsche, G., & Diener, H. C. (1999). Drug-induced headache following the use of zolmitriptan or naratriptan. *Cephalalgia, 19,* 414.

Kudrow, L. (1982). Paradoxical effects of chronic analgesic use. *Advances in Neurology, 33,* 335–341.

Lipchik, G. L., Holroyd, K. A., France, C. R., Kvaal, S. A., Segal, D., Cordingley, G. E., et al. (1996). Central and peripheral mechanisms in chronic tension-type headache. *Pain, 64,* 467–475.

Mathew, N. T. (1990). Drug induced headache. *Neurologic Clinics, 8,* 903–912.

Mathew, N. T. (1994). Migraine transformation and chronic daily headache. In R. K. Cady & A. W. Fox (Eds.), *Treating the headache patient* (pp. 75–100). New York: Marcel Dekker.

Mathew, N. T. (1997). Transformed migraine, analgesic rebound, and other chronic daily headaches. In N. T. Mathew (Ed.), *Neurologic clinics: Advances in headache* (pp. 167–186). Philadelphia: W. B. Saunders.

McCrory, D. C., Penzien, D. B., & Rains, J. C. (1996). Efficacy of behavioral treatments for migraine and tension-type headache: Meta-analysis of controlled trials [Abstract]. *Headache, 36,* 272.

McGrady, A., Andrasik, F., Davies, T., Striefel, S., Wickramasekera, I., Baskin, S., et al. (1999). Psychophysiologic therapy for chronic headache in primary care. *Primary Care Companion Journal of Clinical Psychiatry, 1,* 96–102.

Medina, J. L., & Diamond, S. (1978). The role of diet in migraine. *Headache, 18,* 31–34.

Merikangas, K. R., & Angst, J. (1993). Headache syndromes and psychiatric disorders: Associations and familial transmission. *Journal of Psychiatric Research, 27,* 197–210.

Merikangas, K. R., & Stevens, D. E. (1997). Comorbidity of migraine and psychiatric disorders. In N. T. Mathew (Ed.), *Neurologic clinics: Advances in headache* (pp. 115–124). Philadelphia: W. B. Saunders.

Neufeld, J. D., Holroyd, K. A., & Lipchik, G. L. (2000). Dynamic assessment of abnormalities in central pain transmission and modulation in tension-type headache sufferers. *Headache, 40,* 142–151.

Olesen, J., & Jensen, R. (1991). Getting away from simple muscle contraction as a mechanism of tension-type headache. *Pain, 46,* 123–124.

Packard, R. C., & O'Connell, P. (1986). Medication compliance among headache patients. *Headache, 26,* 416–419.

Pikoff, H. (1984). Is the muscular model of headache still viable? A review of conflicting data. *Headache, 24,* 186–198.

Pryse-Phillips, W., Findlay, H., Tugwell, P., Edmeads, J., Murray, T. J., & Nelson, R. F. (1992). A Canadian population survey on the clinical, epidemiologic, and societal impact of migraine and tension-type headache. *Canadian Journal of Neurological Science, 19,* 333–339.

Radnitz, C. L. (1990). Food triggered migraine: A critical review. *Annals of Behavioral Medicine, 12,* 51–65.

Radnitz, C. L., & Blanchard, E. B. (1991). Assessment and treatment of dietary factors in refractory vascular headache. *Headache Quarterly, 3,* 214–220.

Rapoport, A. M. (1988). Analgesic rebound headache. *Headache, 28,* 662–665.

Rapoport, A. M., & Sheftell, F. D. (1996). *Headache disorders: A management guide for practitioners.* Philadelphia: W. B. Saunders.

Salfield, S. A., Wardley, B. L., Houlsby, W. T., Turner, S. L., Spalton, A. P., Beckles-Wilson, N. R., et al. (1987). Controlled study of exclusion of dietary vasoactive amines in migraine. *Archives of Disease in Childhood, 62,* 458–460.

Saper, J. R. (1987). Ergotamine dependency: A review. *Headache, 27,* 435–438.

Schoenen, J., Gerard, P., DePasqua, V., & Sainard-Gainko, J. (1991). Multiple clinical and paraclinical analyses of chronic tension-type headache associated or unassociated with disorder of pericranial muscles. *Cephalalgia, 11,* 135–139.

Schwartz, B. S., Stewart, W. F., Simon, D., & Lipton, R. B. (1998). Epidemiology of tension-type headache. *Journal of the American Medical Association, 279,* 381–383.

Schwartz, M. (1995). Headache: Selected issues in evaluation and treatment, Part A: Evaluation, and Part B: Treatment. In M. Schwartz and Associates (Eds.), *Biofeedback: A practitioner's guide* (2nd ed., pp. 313–410). New York: Guilford.

Selzer, S. (1982). Foods, and food and drug combinations, responsible for head and neck pain. *Cephalalgia, 2,* 111–124.

Silberstein, S. D. (2000). Practice parameter: Evidence-based guidelines for migraine headache (an evidence-based review): Report of the quality standards subcommittee of the American Academy of Neurology. *Neurology, 55,* 754–762.

Silberstein, S. D., & Lipton, R. B. (2001). Chronic daily headache, including transformed migraine, chronic tension-type headache, and medication overuse. In S. D. Silberstein, R. B. Lipton, & D. J. Dalessio (Eds.), *Wolff's headache and other head pain* (pp. 247–282). New York: Oxford University Press.

Silberstein, S. D., Lipton, R. B., & Breslau, N. (1995). Migraine: Association with personality characteristics and psychopathology. *Cephalalgia, 15,* 337–369.

Silberstein, S. D., Lipton, R. B., & Dalessio, D. J. (2001). Overview, diagnosis and classification of headache. In S. D. Silberstein, R. B. Lipton, & D. J. Dalessio (Eds.), *Wolff's headache and other head pain* (pp. 6–26). New York: Oxford University Press.

Silberstein, S. D., Lipton, R. B., & Sliwinski, M. (1996). Classification of daily and near-daily headaches: Field trial of revised IHS criteria. *Neurology, 47,* 871–875.

Solomon, S., Lipton, R. B., & Newman, L. C. (1992). Clinical features of chronic daily headache. *Headache, 32,* 325–329.

Spierings, E. L., Schroevers, M., Honkoop, P., & Sorbi, M. (1998). Presentation of chronic daily headache: A clinical study. *Headache, 38,* 191–196.

Stewart, W. F. (1993). Migraine in the United States: A review of epidemiology and health care use. *Neurology, 43*(Suppl. 2), 211–221.

Stewart, W. F., Lipton, R. B., Celentano, D. D., & Reed, M. L. (1992). Prevalence of migraine headache in the United States: Relation to age, income, race and other sociodemographic factors. *Journal of the American Medical Association, 267*, 64–69.

Strang, P. E., & Osterhaus, J. T. (1993). Impact of migraine in the United States: Data from the National Health Interview Survey. *Headache, 33*, 29–35.

Suchowersky, O. (1993). Rebound headaches due to sumatriptan. *Neurology, 43* (Suppl. 2).

Tunis, M. M., & Wolff, H. G. (1953). Studies on headache: Long term observation of the reactivity of the cranial arteries in subjects with vascular headache of the migraine type. *Archives of Neurology and Psychiatry, 70*, 551–557.

Vanast, W. J. (1986). New daily persistent headache: Definition of a benign syndrome. *Headache, 26*, 317.

Verri, A. P., Proietti Cecchini, A., Galli, C., Granella, F., Sandrini, G., & Nappi, G. (1998). Psychiatric comorbidity in chronic daily headache. *Cephalalgia, 18*(Suppl. 21), 45–49.

Weiler, C., May, A., Limmroth, V., Juptner, M., Kaube, H., Schayck, R. V., et al. (1995). Brain stem activation in spontaneous human migraine attacks. *Nature Medicine, 1*, 658–660.

Welch, K. M. A., D'Andrea, G., Tepley, N., Barkley, G., & Ramadan, N. M. (1990). The concept of migraine as a state of central neuronal hyperexcitability. *Neurologic Clinics, 8*, 817–828.

Zeigler, D. K., & Stewart, R. (1977). Failure of tyramine to induce migraine. *Neurology, 7*, 25–27.

# CHAPTER 16

# Temporomandibular Disorders and Facial Pain

## Alan G. Glaros and Leonard Lausten

**Abstract:** Temporomandibular disorders affect the muscles of mastication and the osseous and soft tissues of the temporomandibular joint. Anatomical, psychological, behavioral, neuromuscular, and social factors can influence the initiation and progression of these disorders. Temporomandibular disorders can produce changes in emotional and behavioral functioning as well as activities of daily living. Thorough assessment of these disorders therefore requires physical, psychosocial, and behavioral components. Behavioral and psychosocial interventions appear to have positive and lasting effects on the pain associated with temporomandibular disorders.[1]

## INTRODUCTION

The term *temporomandibular disorders (TMDs)* represents a heterogeneous group of maladies affecting the muscles of mastication as well as the osseous and soft tissues of the temporomandibular joint (TMJ). Clinical signs and symptoms of this group of disorders most frequently include pain in and around the TMJ and associated muscles, joint sounds on movement of the jaw, and restrictions of jaw movement (most typically, limited opening or deviations in the jaw's opening or closing path). Researchers who investigate TMD publish primarily in the dental and psychological literatures, with additional work appearing in the neurosciences. It is not the intent of this chapter to present a comprehensive review of the literature. Instead, our goal is to provide sufficient information so that a primary care provider can posses a fundamental understanding of the complexity of the disorder, appreciate the overlap between TMD and other medical conditions, and offer appropriate treatment options to patients who present with TMD.

## MEDICAL PROFILE

The temporomandibular joint consists of the mandibular condyle, the articular fossa, an articular disc composed of fibrous connective tissue, synovial fluids, membranes, and ligaments that connect the joint to masticatory muscles (see Figure 16.1). Collectively these components are often called the articular capsule.

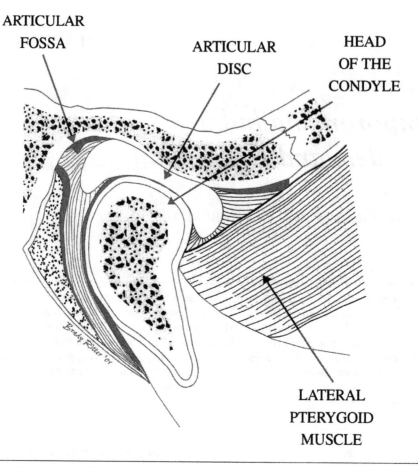

**Figure 16.1**    Temporomandibular Joint and Associated Structures

Opening and closing functions of the joint involve a complicated two-stage movement. In the initial phase of opening, the joint functions as a ball and socket in which the condyle rotates within the articular fossa. During this phase of movement, the articular disc remains positioned between the condyle and the articular fossa of the temporal bone. As opening proceeds, the condyle translates, or moves, anteriorly down the osseous articular eminence, with the articular disc positioned between the condyle and the eminence. The disc appears to act as a cushion between the condyle and the articular surfaces of the temporal bone. The result is a smooth, pain-free transition between the initial and secondary phases of mandibular opening.

Many conditions can affect the functioning of the joint. The disc can be displaced by damage to or stretching of the ligaments and membranes that support it. Temporary displacement of the disc during function, or disc displacement with reduction, can cause popping or clicking noises. In many instances, the patients recognize these noises. In other cases, joint auscultation is necessary to identify them. In less frequent circumstances, the displaced disc can limit mandibular movement due to its entrapment in the capsular space. This condition, termed disc displacement without reduction with limited opening according to the *Research Diagnostic Criteria (RDC)* for temporomandibular disorders (Dworkin & LeResche, 1992), is not associated with clicking or popping noises.

Degenerative changes can result in eroded or flattened condylar heads. Bony spurs may appear on the articular surfaces of either the condyle or the articular fossa. The disc itself can function abnormally due to tears or perforations in the disc itself or due to internal calcifications or deposits within the disc. According to the *RDC* (Dworkin & LeResche, 1992), clear evidence of degenerative changes can result in a diagnosis of either arthritis or arthrosis, depending on whether pain is present or not.

Most patients who present to tertiary care clinics for assessment and management of TMD complain of masticatory muscle pain that may be accompanied by joint soreness or tenderness (Fricton & Schiffman, 1995). Masticatory muscle pain may also be accompanied by difficulty in opening the mouth wide. Unlike disc displacement without reduction, with limited opening (which also involves difficulty opening wide caused by entrapment of the articular disc), patients limit mouth opening to avoid increased muscle pain. Patients who report pain on palpation in three or more of 20 muscle or tendon sites (i.e., 10 sites palpated bilaterally) receive a diagnosis of myofascial pain (with or without limited opening). Patients who also report joint pain on palpation but have no sign of degenerative change in the joint receive a diagnosis of arthralgia (Dworkin & LeResche, 1992).

While 65 percent of the general population exhibits one or more clinical signs of TMD (Rugh & Solberg, 1985), only 5 percent to 10 percent of the population seeks or needs treatment (Carlsson & LeResche, 1995). Because TMD is a heterogeneous group of disorders, the etiologies of the disorders also appear to be multifactorial. Anatomical, psychological, behavioral, neuromuscular, and social factors may all influence the initiation and progression of TMD. Because these factors may interact with one another, a biopsychosocial approach to TMD may be a most appropriate form of assessment and management (Greene & Laskin, 2000). In this approach to the management of illness, the clinician integrates biological, social, behavioral, and psychological findings in the development of a management strategy most suited to the patient.

Epidemiological studies of TMD show significant gender and age effects. Women are at least three times more likely (and more commonly, eight or more times as likely) to seek treatment for TMD than are men (Glaros, Glass, & Williams, 1998; Rieder, Martinoff, & Wilcox, 1983). Population studies, however, suggest that the ratio of women to men with symptoms of TMD may be 1:1 or 2:1 (Duckro, Tait, Margolis, & Deshields, 1990). Joint and muscle pain, limitations in opening the mouth, joint noise, and deviation in jaw movement are more common in women. It is not clear why there is a discrepancy between incidence and prevalence rates for general populations and clinical samples, although women may be more likely to seek care for a variety of disorders, including TMD.

## PSYCHOLOGICAL AND BEHAVIORAL PROFILE

As with other chronic, painful conditions, many patients with TMD experience psychological, emotional, and behavioral sequelae of pain. Patients with TMD are more likely to suffer from depression than individuals without chronic pain (Korszun, Hinderstein, & Wong, 1996). TMD patients may report more anxiety. Activities of daily living can be markedly affected by TMD. Difficulty opening wide or chewing can result in dietary changes (e.g., increased consumption of soft foods) and changes in the way foods are eaten (e.g., smashing down a sandwich to ease biting and chewing, or in more severe cases, pureeing foods to obtain some nutrition). TMD patients may limit social activities to avoid pain produced by talking or laughing. They may take more sick days from work. Singing, kissing, and other activities involving the mouth may be avoided or limited. In short, the consequences of TMD may not be limited to the face, head, or oral region but may extend widely to other aspects of the patient's life.

The distribution of significant emotional distress is not equal across all types of TMD. Individuals with chronic pain may report considerable and debilitating psychological distress, mild difficulties, or minimal to no changes in their ability to function effectively. When these categories are applied to TMD patients, those with myofascial pain were much more likely to fall within the distressed categories than were patients diagnosed with disc displacement (Dahlström, Widmark, & Carlsson, 1997; Michelotti, Martina, Russo, & Romeo, 1998). These findings indicate that psychological problems are more likely to be present in patients diagnosed with myofascial pain than in those with disc displacement. Since epidemiological studies have shown that patients with muscle disorders outnumber those with joint-only problems, practitioners should be prepared to consider the possibility that a TMD patient, particularly one with myofascial pain, may also have a concomitant psychological disorder (Glaros, 2001).

## TYPICAL SYMPTOM PROFILE

Most cases of TMD come to the attention of clinicians when patients are in their mid-30s, and most patients range in age from early 20s to late 40s (Glaros, Glass, & Hayden, 1995). Initial symptoms can occur as early as mid-childhood. The correlation between the onset of TMD and childhood or adolescence has raised the question of whether orthodontic treatment causes TMD, but there is little convincing evidence to support this hypothesis (McNamara & Türp, 1997). Unlike many chronic pain conditions, TMD is less likely to occur after age 45. Because menopause commonly occurs in a woman's late 40s to mid-50s, the relationship between sex hormones and TMD has been raised (LeResche, Saunders, Von Korff, Barlow, & Dworkin, 1997). However, evidence in support of this hypothesis is also weak (Hatch, Rugh, Sakai, & Saunders, 2001).

The complex nature of TMD and other facial pain disorders creates difficulty in accurate and reliable diagnosis and treatment planning. The primary symptoms of TMD are pain in the TMJ and masticatory muscles, joint noises, and problems in mastication. TMD patients also complain of a variety of secondary symptoms (see Table 16.1), and many of these symptoms are associated with other disease states. For example, tinnitus can indicate an ear infection or suggest a more serious neurological condition. Secondary symptoms can be very salient in TMD sufferers, thus patients frequently see their primary care physicians for initial diagnosis and care (Glaros, Glass, & Hayden, 1995). To evaluate complaints that are ultimately diagnosed as one or more of the temporomandibular disorders, physicians use diagnostic procedures ranging from simple office examinations to MRIs, CT scans, bone scans, and spinal taps (Glaros, Glass, & Hayden, 1995). Not surprisingly, approximately 20 percent of TMD patients are told by their physicians (and their dentists) that they have no diagnosable condition or are referred elsewhere (Glaros, Glass, & Hayden, 1995).

Disease states that are present in other parts of the body may be reflected in TMD as well. For example, degenerative joint diseases such as osteoarthritis can occur in the TMJ. Similarly, medical conditions may present

**Table 16.1**   Common and Associated Symptoms of TMD

| Common Symptoms of TMD | Associated Symptoms |
| --- | --- |
| Pain in the muscles of mastication, in the preauricular area, or in the TMJ | Headache |
| | Other facial pains |
| Clicking, popping, or grating sounds in the joint | Earache |
| Difficulty opening wide | Dizziness |
| Jaw locking in the open or closed position | Tinnitus |
| Sense that occlusion (bite) is "off" | Neck, shoulder, and upper and lower back pain |

initially as TMD. For example, Raphael, Marbach, and Klausner (2000) followed a sample of individuals who originally presented with myofascial face pain. At follow-up seven years later, 23.5 percent also reported a history of fibromyalgia.

These data suggest that there is considerable overlap in the symptomatology of patients complaining of various head, neck, and facial problems. Some of these individuals may be "true" TMD patients, while others may have TMD-like symptoms that will result in other diagnoses. These statements should not be interpreted to mean that patients who present with the symptoms described in Table 16.1 can have only TMD or only some other problem. It is common for patients to present with a variety of symptoms and conditions, and a patient can certainly receive a TMD diagnosis and a non-TMD diagnosis simultaneously. The overlap in symptoms is reflected in the difficulties patients experience identifying an appropriate source of management. A study of patients at a dental school–based TMD and orofacial pain clinic demonstrated that the typical patient had sought opinions from at least three other treatment providers before presenting at the school-based clinic (Glaros, Glass, & Hayden, 1995). Patients go to physicians, dentists, chiropractic providers, physical therapists, and other health care providers for assessment and treatment.

Finally, patients can be under considerable financial pressures to seek care from a physician first, rather than a dentist. Most dental insurance plans specifically prohibit treatment for TMD, and many medical insurance plans have similar prohibitions. Thus, patients may have an incentive to seek care from a physician and to receive a diagnosis that does not allude to TMD. Medical plans may prohibit patients diagnosed with TMD from receiving financial benefits, but most medical plans treat TMD patients nonetheless, probably under a different diagnosis.

## CURRENT STANDARDS FOR ASSESSMENT AND DIFFERENTIAL DIAGNOSIS

There is general agreement that most cases of TMD involve either muscle disorders, disc displacement, degenerative changes in the TMJ, or a combination of any of these. However, many of the diagnostic schemes that have been developed suffer from a variety of limitations. These include the unknown interrater reliability of the assessment methods and, regarding final diagnoses, poor specificity, minimal biological plausibility, and failure to allow for multiple diagnoses (Glaros & Glass, 1993). Most systems also fail to assess psychological issues.

The *RDC* (Dworkin & LeResche, 1992) mentioned earlier is unique in that it requires patients to be assessed for the presence of a clinical disorder (Axis I) and for self-reported pain intensity, disability, depression, and the presence of nonspecific physical symptoms (Axis II). Studies examining the utility of this

**Table 16.2**    Screening for Suspected Temporomandibular Disorders

| Screening Questions | Screening Examination Procedures |
| --- | --- |
| Do you experience jaw pain when you move your jaw? | Palpation of the TMJ and masticatory muscles |
| Does it feel as though your jaws will "catch" or "lock" when you move your jaw? | Auscultation and observation of the joint during opening, closing, lateral, and protrusive movements |
| Do you hear noises when you move your jaw? | Measurement of opening |
| Do you currently experience headache, neck pain, or other problems in the face or head? | Intraoral examination for the presence of tooth, gingival, or other oral problems, including excessive wear from bruxism |
| Have you ever experienced injury to your jaw, head, or neck? | |

SOURCE: Adapted from guidelines published by the American Association of Orofacial Pain, http://www.aaop.org.

diagnostic scheme have shown better performance compared with other approaches (Bittencourt et al., 2001), and efforts are currently under way to evaluate the validity of this approach to the assessment of TMD patients. This section briefly summarizes some of the examination procedures used by the *RDC* and other systems to evaluate TMD. Additional information on the specific techniques used by the *RDC* to evaluate patients are available from Dworkin and LeResche (1992).

The assessment of a potential TMD patient includes a thorough history and screening (see Table 16.2), a comprehensive physical examination, and thorough behavioral and psychological assessments. Because there is considerable overlap between TMD and a variety of other medical conditions, a cursory examination may lead to an inappropriate diagnosis and incorrect treatment (Glaros & Glass, 1993).

The physical examination typically involves palpation of the TMJs and the masticatory muscles, auscultation of the joint to identify joint noises, measurement of mouth opening, and observation of opening and closing patterns. According to the *RDC* (Dworkin & LeResche, 1992), palpation of

the joint and muscles should be performed with one to two pounds of pressure, depending on the location palpated. Auscultation of the joint is usually conducted while the patient opens and closes the mouth and moves the jaw laterally and protrusively. The auscultation may reveal popping or clicking sounds on opening and closing that suggest disc displacement. Crepitus heard on auscultation as grating or grinding noises may indicate degenerative changes. Normal minimal opening is approximately 40 mm.

Additional physical assessment includes an intraoral examination to evaluate possible dental or periodontal conditions that can cause pain and, more rarely, to rule out tumors or infections that may be responsible for the patient's complaints. Excessive wear of the teeth, particularly on the occlusal (biting) surfaces, may indicate a past or current history of nocturnal teeth grinding. An examination of the ears may indicate the presence of an ear infection that can mimic TMD symptoms. Examining the general symmetry of the face, head, and jaw may provide clues to nocturnal grinding (via masseter muscle hypertrophy) and other problems (e.g., tumors or blockage of the parotid gland duct). Finally, an examination of cranial nerves and arteries will provide clues to possible neuralgias, arteritis, carotodynia, or other vascular problems.

Imaging of the TMJ can yield valuable information relative to pathological conditions that affect the condyles, disc, fossa, eminence, and the other structures of the joint complex. Several imaging techniques can be used to evaluate the TMJ, including panoramic radiographs, tomograms, magnetic resonance imaging, and arthrograms of the joint. Appropriate imaging supplements clinical examination and historical data to help aid in diagnosis and development of treatment strategies.

A series of psychological measures are collected under the guidelines of the *RDC* (Dworkin & LeResche, 1992). These include self-report measures of pain, disability, depression, and nonspecific physical conditions. Pain intensity and disability are graded from grade 0 (no TMD pain in the past six months) to grade IV (high disability, severely limiting). Depression and nonspecific physical conditions are evaluated using the Symptom Checklist–90-R Depression and Vegetative Symptom Scales (Dworkin & LeResche, 1992). Depression is rated in three groups from normal to severe based on population norms.

Normally, TMD patients do not undergo general psychological testing, but specific measures for evaluating these patients have been developed. The most successful test is the TMJ Scale, a 97-item questionnaire that requires approximately 15 to 20 minutes to complete and is scored using proprietary algorithms. The report from each testing contains 10 scales: 5 scales form the test's Physical Domain, 1 measures painful symptoms other than in the TMJ, 3 scales form the test's Psychosocial Domain, and a final Global Scale is a single predictor of the presence of a temporomandibular disorder. The test appears to have good internal consistency and construct validity (Brown & Gaudet, 1994; Levitt & McKinney, 1994).

Psychophysiological devices are available that can record opening patterns, detect joint sounds, and the like. It is not clear if these devices can adequately separate patient from nonpatient samples (i.e., have good specificity). Compared with simple visual inspection and the use of a stethoscope, their cost may not be justifiable.

## BRIEF SUMMARY OF THE LITERATURE ON BEHAVIORAL AND PSYCHOSOCIAL INTERVENTIONS

Behavioral and psychosocial interventions for TMD patients range from very simple instructions to more complex and technologically driven interventions. The behavioral and psychosocial interventions appear to be effective for pain but not disc displacement.

This section primarily focuses on individuals diagnosed with arthralgia and myofascial pain, both of which may result from parafunctional clenching. For example, Glaros and colleagues conducted a series of four studies with healthy pain-free individuals with no symptoms of TMD (Glaros, Baharloo, & Glass, 1998; Glaros & Burton, 2001; Glaros, Forbes, Shanker, & Glass, 2000; Glaros, Tabacchi, & Glass, 1998). In these studies, the participants engaged in mild to moderate clenching for as long as 20 minutes per session, for as many as eight days. These studies employed A-B-A, crossover, and randomized group assignment methodologies. During decrease training, subjects were instructed to maintain activity of the left and right temporalis and masseter muscles below a threshold selected to represent deep relaxation of the muscles. During increase training, subjects were instructed to maintain muscle activity above a threshold selected to represent tooth contact or light clenching. Electromyograph (EMG) biofeedback procedures were used to ensure that individuals

**Box 16.1**  Patient Education Information for TMD

- Your teeth will touch when you chew, swallow, or speak. Your teeth should be separated at all other times.
- If your teeth are touching, your chewing muscles are active. When the muscles are relaxed, your teeth will separate naturally.
- Do not chew gum or ice, bite your fingernails (pencils, pencil tip, erasers, etc.), bite your lips or the inside of your mouth. Keep your chewing muscles as relaxed as possible.
- Do not "pop" or "crack" your jaw.
- Use hot or cold packs to control pain. Use over-the-counter pain relievers as needed to control pain.
- Avoid hard, chewy foods and other activities that increase pain.
- Develop self-management strategies for controlling stresses.
- If you grind your teeth at night, wear a mouth guard to protect your teeth.

engaged in either increase or decrease training actually performed the task appropriately.

In all four studies, self-reported pain was significantly greater following increase training than following decrease training. Screening examinations performed by a blinded examiner showed that increase training produced symptoms of arthralgia and/or myofascial pain in approximately 25 percent of participants. Further studies using experience sampling methodology have suggested that patients diagnosed with myofascial pain have significantly higher levels of tooth contact throughout the day than people who are not patients (Glaros & Lausten, 2002; Haggerty, Glaros, & Glass, 2000).

These studies indicate that reducing parafunctional tooth contact should result in significant relief from pain. Habit reversal protocols (Bogart et al., 2002; Gramling, Neblett, Grayson, & Townsend, 1996; Kim, Glaros, & Lausten, 2002; Peterson, Dixon, Talcott, & Kelleher, 1993) reported significant reductions in pain in those receiving the protocol compared with control groups or other treatment modalities.

Indirect evidence for the efficacy of such approaches was reported in a meta-analysis of the treatments using relaxation/biofeedback for patients with TMD. Crider and Glaros (1999) reported that these techniques were effective in reducing pain compared with placebo and sham treatment conditions. Further examination of the data suggested that the degree of improvement was not related to the change in EMG activity during training. These findings suggest that teaching patients generalized relaxation skills, possibly combined with instructions to avoid tooth contact, was successful in reducing pain. Interestingly, Crider and Glaros reported that the beneficial effects from these interventions were maintained or even enhanced at follow-ups as long as two years.

It is likely that patient education and palliative home care will also benefit patients diagnosed with arthralgia or myofascial pain (see Box 16.1). Careful questioning of TMD patients will likely indicate that particular behaviors are associated with increased pain. For example, patients may benefit from avoiding hard or chewy foods that increase pain. Patients should be instructed not to "crack" or "pop" their jaws. Reductions in other oral habits may also reduce pain. Instructing patients not to chew gum, chew ice, and bite their fingernails may reduce pain as well.

Palliative home care involves little risk to patients and may reduce pain. Applications of hot or cold packs may be helpful. Use of over-the-counter analgesics may reduce pain, and mild stretching exercises may help counter muscle tightness (but probably should not be used to treat limited opening due to disc displacement without reduction). For patients who do not respond well to behavioral and psychosocial interventions, providers may consider the use of non-steroidal anti-inflammatories or tricyclic anti-depressants for the control of pain. The use of a mouth guard may also help control pain.

For patients who report significant night-time grinding, nocturnal alarms have been used successfully for short-term reduction in grinding (Cassisi, McGlynn, & Belles, 1987). These devices typically detect EMG activity associated with masseter or temporalis activity. When the activity exceeds a threshold for a specified time, an alarm sounds. On awakening, the patient is instructed to turn off the alarm and to practice relaxing the masticatory muscles. Unfortunately, removing the nocturnal alarm may cause grinding to return. A primary goal for nocturnal tooth grinders is to limit damage to the occlusal surfaces of the teeth. Such patients should therefore wear a protective mouth guard while sleeping until there is evidence that they no longer grind their teeth.

## SUMMARY

The temporomandibular disorders are a complex group of disorders. Although they share a common location in the face, jaw, and masticatory apparatus, their symptoms are quite different. Assessment of TMD must therefore be sensitive to those differences. Treatment, if it is needed, should be tailored to the patient. The selection of conservative, reversible treatment techniques will likely produce results equal to or better than more aggressive and irreversible approaches (National Institute of Dental and Craniofacial Research, n.d.). Depending on the specific symptoms, patients may benefit from some combination of home and palliative care, dental management (usually using mouth guards), behavioral techniques (emphasizing control of parafunctional activities or oral habits and cognitive-behavioral interventions for pain), and medications. Only in unusual cases should TMD patients consider surgical intervention. Considerably more research needs to be done to understand the etiologies of these disorders, and the findings from this research should lead to better, more effective treatments.

## NOTE

1. Preparation of this chapter was aided by a grant from the National Institute of Dental and Craniofacial Research (DE13563) to Alan G. Glaros.

## REFERENCES

Bittencourt, M., Mattos, C., Guerra, S., Batitucci, E., Menezes, J., & Rezende, R. (2001). Reliability comparison between two diagnostic criteria for temporomandibular disorders. *Journal of Dental Research, 80,* 186.

Bogart, R. K., Wright, E. W., Dunni, W. J., McDaniel, R. J., Hunter, C., & Peterson, A. L. (2002). Efficacy of group cognitive behavioral intervention for temporomandibular disorder (TMD) patients. *Journal of Dental Research, 81*, A-478.

Brown, D. T., & Gaudet, E. L. (1994). Outcome measurement for treated and untreated TMD patients using the TMJ scale. *Journal of Craniomandibular Practice, 12*, 216–222.

Carlsson, G. E., & LeResche, L. (1995). Epidemiology of temporomandibular disorders. In B. J. Sessle, P. S. Bryant, & R. A. Dionne (Eds.), *Progress in pain research and management: Vol. 4. Temporomandibular disorders and related pain conditions* (pp. 211–226). Seattle, WA: IASP Press.

Cassisi, J. E., McGlynn, F. D., & Belles, D. R. (1987). EMG-activated feedback alarms for the treatment of nocturnal bruxism: Current status and future directions. *Biofeedback & Self-Regulation, 12*, 13–30.

Crider, A. B., & Glaros, A. G. (1999). A meta-analysis of EMG biofeedback treatment of temporomandibular disorders. *Journal of Orofacial Pain, 13*, 29–37.

Dahlström, L., Widmark, G., & Carlsson, S. G. (1997). Cognitive-behavioral profiles among different categories of orofacial pain patients: Diagnostic and treatment implications. *European Journal of Oral Sciences, 105*, 377–383.

Duckro, P. N., Tait, R. C., Margolis, R. B., & Deshields, T. L. (1990). Prevalence of temporomandibular symptoms in a large United States metropolitan area. *Journal of Craniomandibular Practice, 8*, 131–138.

Dworkin, S. F., & LeResche, L. (1992). Research diagnostic criteria for temporomandibular disorders: Review, criteria, exams and specification, critique. *Journal of Craniomandibular Disorders, 6*, 301–355.

Fricton, J. R., & Schiffman, E. L. (1995). Epidemiology of temporomandibular disorders. In J. R. Fricton & J. R. Dubner (Eds.), *Advances in pain research and therapy: Vol. 21. Orofacial pain and temporomandibular disorders* (pp. 1–14). New York: Raven Press.

Glaros, A. G. (2001). Emotional factors in temporomandibular disorders. *Journal of the Indiana Dental Association, 79*(4), 20–23.

Glaros, A. G., Baharloo, L., & Glass, E. G. (1998). Effect of parafunctional clenching and estrogen on temporomandibular disorder pain. *Journal of Craniomandibular Practice, 16*, 78–83.

Glaros, A. G., & Burton, E. (2001). Relationship of effort in parafunctional activity to self-reported pain in temporomandibular disorder. *Journal of Dental Research, 80*, 185.

Glaros, A. G., Forbes, M., Shanker, J., & Glass, E. G. (2000). Effect of parafunctional clenching on temporomandibular disorder pain and proprioceptive awareness. *Journal of Craniomandibular Practice, 18*, 198–204.

Glaros, A. G., & Glass, E. G. (1993). Temporomandibular disorders. In R. J. Gatchel and E. B. Blanchard (Eds.), *Psychophysiological disorders* (pp. 299–356). Washington, DC: American Psychological Association.

Glaros, A. G., Glass, E. G., & Hayden, W. J. (1995). History of treatment received by TMD patients: A preliminary investigation. *Journal of Orofacial Pain, 9*, 147–151.

Glaros, A. G., Glass, E. G., & Williams, K. M. (1998). Factor analytic study of clinical examination findings in TMD patients. *Journal of Orofacial Pain, 12*, 193–202.

Glaros, A. G., & Lausten, L. (2002). Prospective assessment of parafunctional activity in temporomandibular disorder patients. *Journal of Dental Research, 81*, A-458.

Glaros, A. G., Tabacchi, K. N., & Glass, E. G. (1998). Effect of parafunctional clenching on temporomandibular disorder pain. *Journal of Orofacial Pain, 12*, 145–152.

Gramling, S. E., Neblett, J., Grayson, R., & Townsend, D. (1996). Temporomandibular disorder: Efficacy of an oral habit reversal treatment program. *Journal of Behavior Therapy & Experimental Psychiatry, 27,* 245–255.

Greene, C. S., & Laskin, D. M. (2000). Temporomandibular disorders: Moving from a dentally based to a medically based model. *Journal of Dental Research, 79,* 1736–1739.

Haggerty, C., Glaros, A. G., & Glass, E. G. (2000). Ecological momentary assessment of parafunctional clenching in temporomandibular disorder. *Journal of Dental Research, 79,* 605.

Hatch, J. P., Rugh, J. D., Sakai, S., & Saunders, M. J. (2001). Is use of exogenous estrogen associated with temporomandibular signs and symptoms? *Journal of the American Dental Association, 132*(3), 319–326.

Kim, N., Glaros, A. G., & Lausten, L. (2002). Effectiveness of habit awareness training for temporomandibular disorder pain. *Journal of Dental Research, 81,* A-458.

Korszun, A., Hinderstein, B., & Wong, M. (1996). Comorbidity of depression with chronic facial pain and temporomandibular disorders. *Oral Surgery, Oral Medicine, Oral Pathology, Oral Radiology, & Endodontics, 82,* 496–500.

LeResche, L., Saunders, K., Von Korff, M. R., Barlow, W., & Dworkin, S. F. (1997). Use of exogenous hormones and risk of temporomandibular disorder pain. *Pain, 69,* 153–160.

Levitt, S. R., & McKinney, M. W. (1994). Validating the TMJ scale in a national sample of 10,000 patients: Demographic and epidemiologic characteristics. *Journal of Orofacial Pain, 8,* 25–35.

McNamara, J. A., & Türp, J. C. (1997). Orthodontic treatment and temporomandibular disorders: Is there a relationship? Part 1: Clinical studies. *Journal of Orofacial Orthopedics, 58,* 74–89.

Michelotti, A., Martina, R., Russo, M., & Romeo, R. (1998). Personality characteristics of temporomandibular disorder patients using M.M.P.I. *Journal of Craniomandibular Disorders, 16,* 119–125.

National Institute of Dental and Craniofacial Research. (n.d.). Temporomandibular Disorders: Treatment. Retrieved April 24, 2002, from http://www.nidcr.nih.gov/health/pubs/tmd/sec6.htm

Peterson, A. L., Dixon, D. C., Talcott, G. W., & Kelleher, W. J. (1993). Habit reversal treatment of temporomandibular disorders: A pilot investigation. *Journal of Behavior Therapy & Experimental Psychiatry, 24,* 49–55.

Raphael, K. G., Marbach, J. J., & Klausner, J. (2000). Myofascial face pain: Clinical characteristics of those with regional vs. widespread pain. *Journal of the American Dental Association, 131*(7), 854–858.

Rieder, C. E., Martinoff, J. T., & Wilcox, S. A. (1983). The prevalence of mandibular dysfunction. Part I: Sex and age distribution of related signs and symptoms. *Journal of Prosthetic Dentistry, 50,* 81–88.

Rugh, J. D., & Solberg, W. K. (1985). Oral health status in the United States: Temporomandibular disorders. *Journal of Dental Education, 49,* 398–404.

# CHAPTER 17

# Asthma

PAUL LEHRER, MAHMOOD SIDDIQUE,
JONATHAN FELDMAN, AND NICHOLAS GIARDINO

**Abstract:** Asthma is a common episodic disease characterized by reversible airway obstruction caused by inflammation, bronchoconstriction, and/or mucus congestion. Although asthma exacerbations are usually triggered by allergens, airway irritants, exercise, viral infection, or exposure to cold air, they also can be triggered by stress. It is diagnosed by symptoms, pulmonary function tests, and either measures of reversibility or susceptibility to bronchoprovocation. Asthma education plays an important role in managing the disease. Patients must learn how and when to take various asthma medications, how to measure their own pulmonary function, and when to call on medical services. There is preliminary evidence that certain psychosocial stress management interventions may also be helpful in managing asthma, as may some relaxation, biofeedback, and yoga-based therapies. Evidence suggests that relaxation therapy may produce long-term benefits but short-term bronchoconstriction caused by parasympathetic rebound.

## PROFILE OF THE DISORDER

The defining characteristic of asthma is reversible airway obstruction. Although reversibility of airway obstruction is usually complete in the early stages of the disease, chronic lung inflammation can lead to "remodeling" of the airways and chronic obstructive disease (Fahy, Corry, & Boushey, 2000).[1] Aggressive medical treatment of asthma is now recommended to avoid these chronic conditions, but the effectiveness of this strategy has not been completely established. Such treatment can, however, completely eliminate current asthma symptomatology in most cases.

Asthma is very common, affecting almost one person in ten, and the prevalence of the disease is growing rapidly worldwide (Kussin & Fulkerson, 1995). It is usually an episodic disease, with periods of airway obstruction alternating with days, months, or even years of normal airway function.

For some people, asthma symptoms are limited to mild episodes of coughing and wheezing after exposure to viral infection, exercise, or cold air. In such cases, the disease can remain unrecognized for years. When asthma is mild or well regulated with medication, usually symptoms are absent and pulmonary function is normal. However, symptoms can recur during exposure to specific asthma triggers.

**Table 17.1**   Classification of Asthma Severity

| Severity Class[a] | Symptom Class | Pulmonary Function[b] |
|---|---|---|
| Mild intermittent | • Symptoms (wheeze/cough/dyspnea) ≤2 times/week<br>• Asymptomatic between exacerbations<br>• Exacerbations brief (from a few hours to a few days)<br>• Nighttime asthma symptoms ≤2 times/month<br>• Use of albuterol < twice/week (not including exercise-induced asthma) | • $FEV_1$ or PEF ≥80% predicted<br>• PEF variability <20% |
| Mild persistent | • Symptoms >2 times/week but <1 time/day<br>• Exacerbations may affect activity<br>• Nighttime asthma symptoms >2 times/month (3–4/month)<br>• Up to 4 puffs of rescue albuterol/day (not including exercise-induced asthma) | • $FEV_1$ or PEF ≥80% predicted<br>• PEF variability 20–30% |
| Moderate persistent | • Daily symptoms<br>• Daily use of inhaled short-acting albuterol<br>• Exacerbations: ≥2 times/week; may last days; affect activity<br>• Nighttime asthma symptoms >1 time/week (≥5/month)<br>• Up to 4 puffs of rescue albuterol/day (not including exercise-induced asthma) | • $FEV_1$ or PEF >60% and <80% predicted<br>• PEF variability >30% |
| Severe persistent | • Continuous symptoms<br>• Limited physical activity<br>• Frequent exacerbations<br>• Frequent nighttime asthma symptoms | • $FEV_1$ or PEF ≤60% predicted<br>• PEF variability >30% |

SOURCE: National Heart, Lung, and Blood Institute, 1997, Figure 3-4a.

a. The presence of one of the features of severity is sufficient to place a patient in that category. An individual should be assigned to the most severe grade in which any feature occurs. The characteristics noted in this table are general and can overlap because asthma is highly variable. Furthermore, an individual's classification can change over time. Patients at any level of severity can have mild, moderate, or severe exacerbations. Some patients with intermittent asthma experience severe and life-threatening exacerbations separated by long periods of normal lung function and no symptoms.

b. $FEV_1$ = forced expiratory volume in one second during a forced expiratory maneuver from maximum vital capacity; PEF = peak expiratory flow during a forced expiratory maneuver from maximum vital capacity. Percent predicted values are based on norms, classified by height, weight, age, race, and sex.

In other cases, asthma is accompanied by frequent periods of severe breathing difficulty, which can even be life threatening. Table 17.1 shows the classification of asthma symptoms, according to the most recent *Expert Panel Report* published by the National Heart, Lung, and Blood Institute (1997). As shown in the table, severity of asthma is defined both by symptoms and by measures of pulmonary function.

Asthma can be triggered by a number of events, including exposure to various allergens, viral infection, cold air, exercise, stress, and hyperventilation. Although crying, laughing, and yelling can trigger asthma episodes, it is doubtful that emotional factors play a major causative role. Accurate perception of asthma symptoms is critical for good self-care, and inability to perceive symptoms accurately is a predictor of having near-death experiences from asthma (Kikuchi et al., 1994).

Both prevalence and morbidity of asthma are related to ethnicity and socioeconomic status. In the United States, the disease is particularly prevalent among African Americans and ethnic Hispanics and, independently, among individuals with lower socioeconomic status (Centers for Disease Control and Prevention, 1998). These patterns appear to have multiple determinants, including genetic influences; differential exposure to allergens, irritants, and stress; differential access to medical care; and differences in coping resources (e.g., for avoiding allergens common in inner-city environments, such as cockroaches; for obtaining medical care; for coping with stress; etc.).

## SCREENING QUESTIONS

Initial screening for asthma will primarily involve asking about the presence of prominent asthma symptoms: coughing, chest tightness, wheezing, and difficulty breathing. These core symptoms can be accompanied by a host of other physical and psychological symptoms, including fatigue, sleeping difficulties, anxiety, panic, and irritability. Because asthma sometimes is accompanied by hyperventilation (Kinsman, Luparello, O'Banion, & Spector, 1973), a complex of hyperventilation-related symptoms may accompany asthma—primarily chest pain, feelings of unreality, headache, palpitations, tremor, and muscle tension. The symptoms usually are episodic, although they may last for anywhere from a few days to several weeks or longer. Although the symptoms often can be traced to specific asthma triggers, the patient may not always be aware of the triggers. Common asthma triggers are allergens (pollens, dust mites, cockroaches, cats, dogs, specific foods or medicines), exercise, exposure to cold dry air, smoking, air pollution, emotional stress, and respiratory infection.

After initial diagnosis, good asthma health maintenance requires the patient to know the following:

1. Personal asthma triggers and a plan to avoid or manage them.

2. Medications that physicians can prescribe and the specific uses of each. It is particularly important that the patient be able to distinguish medications that are used to obtain immediate relief from asthma symptoms (primarily albuterol) from those that are used to prevent asthma symptoms (primarily anti-inflammatory drugs, such as inhaled steroids, leukotriene inhibitors, long-acting beta-2 sympathetic stimulants, theophylline, and cromolyn). Confusing these medications can lead to poor and sometimes disastrous results.

3. How to measure personal asthma symptoms and the proper technique for using a home peak-flow meter. The patient also should calculate a "personal best" peak flow and know how to follow an "asthma action plan" when this value deteriorates to a specific level (usually below 80 percent of personal best).

## DIAGNOSTIC ASSESSMENT

Asthma is diagnosed by symptomatology, pulmonary function, and evidence of airway reactivity and/or reversibility. During an asthma flare, obstruction of the airways is present due to inflammation, mucus congestion, and/or bronchoconstriction. Symptoms of wheezing, coughing, chest tightness, and/or dyspnea (breathlessness) are often signs of asthma, although they also could reflect problems other than asthma (e.g., heart disease, other forms of lung disease, panic attack, etc.).

Presence of airway obstruction, as measured by tests of pulmonary function, is required for diagnosis. The spirometer is the device usually used for assessing pulmonary function. The patient exhales with maximum force from full vital capacity, and the device measures a number of parameters, including full vital capacity (FVC), the volume of air exhaled in the first second of this maneuver ($FEV_1$), and peak expiratory flow (PEF). Although FVC is often normal even during an asthma flare, $FEV_1$ and PEF are usually reduced, as is the ratio of $FEV_1$ to FVC. Reversibility (a defining characteristic of asthma, which distinguishes it from other chronic airway diseases) is usually measured by a bronchodilator test. Asthma is present when a clinically significant improvement in $FEV_1$ is obtained after a standard dose of bronchodilator medication (usually albuterol).

Patients whose asthma is well controlled through use of long-acting medications may have normal pulmonary function and not show a significant bronchodilator response. In such cases, a definitive diagnosis may require temporary withholding of medication and/or use of a bronchoprovocation test. This involves giving a graded dose of a known bronchoconstrictor drug, such a methacholine or histamine.

## ANATOMY AND PHYSIOLOGY

The physiology of asthma is not completely understood, although it is now defined as an inflammatory disease (National Heart, Lung, and Blood Institute, 1997). In addition to inflammation of tissues in the airways, it is usually accompanied by heightened airway irritability and constriction of airway smooth muscles. Although anyone can experience some airway reactivity to allergens, irritants, or other events that trigger bronchoconstriction, only people with asthma experience measurably long-lasting airway obstruction.

## RESEARCH ON BEHAVIORAL INTERVENTION

### Asthma Education

The most prominent behavioral intervention for asthma involves patient education. Researchers have developed a variety of multicomponent educational interventions involving a variety of approaches, including brief, written, physician-administered counseling and formal individual or group instruction materials (National Heart, Lung, and Blood Institute, 1997). Asthma education programs usually include instructing the patient about basic asthma facts and the various asthma medications, teaching techniques for using inhalers and avoiding or managing asthma triggers, devising a daily self-management plan, and completing an asthma diary for self-monitoring. Some programs also involve stress management and training in how to relate to medical practitioners (how to find a doctor, prepare for medical visits, obtain needed information, etc.) and to the medical care system (how to pay for needed medical care and where to obtain it). The goal of these programs is to eliminate asthma symptoms, avoid sudden asthma flares, minimize the need for emergency medical intervention, and generally improve quality of life. Box 17.1 presents a model asthma education program.

The most important part of an asthma education program is for each patient to develop an asthma action plan for managing acute flare-ups. To develop an adequate asthma action plan, the patient must know how to use a home peak-flow meter, his or her personal best peak flow (usually the highest value achieved during the past several weeks), and the peak-flow values and symptoms that should trigger various kinds of actions. Often the various conditions of asthma and plans for action are classified using the colors of a traffic light: a "green

---

**Box 17.1**    Recommendations for Topics in Asthma Education for Patients

Basic Facts About Asthma

- The contrast between asthmatic and normal airways
  - Hyperreactivity to irritants, cold air, or allergens
- What happens to the airways in an asthma attack
  - Inflammation
  - Constriction of the smooth muscles in the airways (bronchoconstriction)
  - Mucus congestion

Roles of Medications

- How medications work
  - Long-term control: medications that prevent symptoms, often by reducing inflammation. *Note that these medications do not produce immediate effects, and will not help in an asthma attack.*
  - Inhaled steroids
  - Long-term beta-sympathetic stimulants
  - Leukotriene inhibitors
  - Cromolyn
  - Quick relief: short-acting bronchodilator relaxes muscles around airways. *Note that these medications do produce immediate effects on asthma, but should not be heavily used for long-term prevention and control because of undesirable side effects.*
  - Beta-2 inhaled stimulants
- Stress the importance of long-term control medications and not to expect quick relief from them.

Skills

- Inhaler use: technique for taking the medication effectively
- Symptom monitoring, peak-flow monitoring, and recognizing early signs of deterioration (see Sample Asthma Action Plan, Box 17.2)

Environmental Control Measures

- Identifying and avoiding environmental precipitants or exposures

When and How to Take Rescue Actions

- Responding to changes in asthma severity (see Box 17.2)

---

SOURCE: Adapted from National Heart, Lung, and Blood Institute (1997).

---

zone" (condition is satisfactory), a "yellow zone" (caution needed, begin taking special steps), and a "red zone" (emergency action needed). A sample asthma action plan is shown in Box 17.2.

### Written Emotional Expression Exercises

People with asthma, especially children, are more likely than healthy individuals to

**Box 17.2**    Sample Asthma Action Plan

It is important in managing asthma to keep track of your symptoms, medications, and peak expiratory flow (PEF).

You can use the colors of a traffic light to help learn your asthma medications:

**GREEN** means **Go.** Use preventive (anti-inflammatory) medicine

**YELLOW** means **Caution.** Use quick-relief (short-acting bronchodilator) medicine in addition to the preventive medicine.

**RED** means **Danger!** Get help from a doctor.

**Your GREEN ZONE is**_____(80% to 100% of your personal best). Go!

Breathing is good with no cough, wheeze, or chest tightness during work, school, exercise, or play.

**Action:**

- Continue with medications listed in your daily treatment plan.

**Your YELLOW ZONE is**_____ (50% to less than 80% of your personal best). **Caution!**

Asthma symptoms are present (cough, wheeze, chest tightness).

Your peak flow number drops below_____or you notice:

- Increased need for inhaled quick-relief medicine
- Increased asthma symptoms upon awakening
- Awakening at night with asthma symptoms
- Other: _____

**Actions:**

- Take _____ puffs of _____ (quick-relief bronchodilator medicine) _____ times/day.
- Take _____ puffs of _____ (anti-inflammatory) _____ times/day.
- Begin/increase treatment with oral steroids. Take _____ mg of _____ every morning at _____ a.m. and evening at_____ p.m.
- Call your doctor (phone) _____ or emergency room _____.

**Your RED ZONE is** _____ (50% or less of your best). **Danger!**

Your peak flow number drops below _____, or you continue to get worse after increasing treatment according to the directions above.

**Actions:**

- Take _____ puffs of your quick-relief (bronchodilator) medicine_____.
  Repeat _____ times.
- Begin/increase treatment with oral steroids. Take _____ mg now.
- Call your doctor now (phone: _____ ). If you cannot contact your doctor, go directly to the emergency room (phone: _____ ).
- Other important phone numbers for transportation: _____.

AT ANY TIME, CALL YOUR DOCTOR IF:

- Asthma symptoms worsen while you are taking oral steroids, or
- Inhaled bronchodilator treatments are not lasting 4 hours, or
- Your peak flow number remains at or falls below _____ in spite of following the plan.

experience negative emotions but may be less likely to express them (Hollaender & Florin, 1983; Lehrer, Isenberg, & Hochron, 1993; Silverglade, Tosi, Wise, & D'Costa, 1994). However, empirical data as to whether and how negative emotions precipitate or exacerbate asthma attacks are mixed (Lehrer, 1998).

In one asthma study (Smyth, Soefer, Hurewitz, & Stone, 1999), participants were asked to write essays expressing their thoughts and feelings about traumatic experiences. They demonstrated clinically significant improvement in $FEV_1$ after a four-month follow-up compared with no improvement noted in control-group subjects who wrote on innocuous topics.

## Other Psychosocial Interventions

Castés et al. (1999) provided asthmatic children with a six-month program that included cognitive therapy for stress management, a self-esteem workshop, and training in relaxation and guided imagery. Improvement occurred both in clinical measures of asthma and in asthma-related immune system measures. The treatment group, but not the control group, significantly decreased their use of beta-2 stimulant medication, showed improvements in $FEV_1$, and, at the end of treatment, no longer showed a response to bronchodilators (consistent with improvement in asthma). Basal $FEV_1$ improved to normal levels in the treatment group after six months of treatment. Children in the

treatment group showed increased activity of natural killer cells, increased expression of the T-cell receptor for interleukin-2 (IL-2), and significantly decreased counts of leukocytes with low-affinity receptors for immunoglobulin E (IgE). The results suggest that, over the long term, stress management methods may have important preventive effects on asthma and may affect the basic inflammatory mechanisms that underlie this disease.

## DIRECT EFFECTS OF PSYCHOLOGICAL TREATMENTS ON THE PATHOPHYSIOLOGY OF ASTHMA

### Relaxation Training

In two reviews Lehrer et al. (1992, 2002) concluded that relaxation training often has statistically significant but small and inconsistent effects on asthma. More recent studies have yielded a similar pattern (Henry, de Rivera, Gonzalez-Martin, & Abreu, 1993; Lehrer, Hochron, Mayne, Isenberg, Carlson, et al., 1994; Lehrer, Hochron, Mayne, Isenberg, Lasoski, et al., 1997; Loew, Siegfried, Martus, Trill, & Hahn, 1996; Smyth et al., 1999; Vazquez & Buceta, 1993a, 1993b, 1993c). Differences in outcome measures, populations, and relaxation procedures across studies may explain some of the inconsistencies. Although the studies may have noted clinically significant relaxation-induced changes in pulmonary function, the changes do not occur consistently. It is possible that relaxation training may have an important effect only among people with emotional asthma triggers, or that the preexisting effects of asthma medication attenuated the effects of relaxation training in these studies.

Data from our laboratory suggest that the immediate effects of relaxation on asthma may differ from the longer-term effects (Lehrer, Hochron, Mayne, Isenberg, Carlson, et al., 1994; Lehrer, Hochron, Mayne, Isenberg, Lasoski, et al., 1997). We found that pulmonary function decreased between the beginning and end of specific relaxation sessions and that these decreases were correlated with evidence of increased parasympathetic tone. Such "parasympathetic rebound" effects are commonly seen during the practice of relaxation. A small improvement in pulmonary function was observed over six weeks of treatment, showing that the immediate effects of relaxation may differ from the longer-term effects. We have hypothesized that this improvement results from a general decrease in autonomic reactivity. Long ago, Gellhorn (1958) hypothesized that this is a general effect of relaxation methods, mediated by decreased sympathetic arousal and consequent downregulation of homeostatic parasympathetic reflexes. More recent literature confirms this hypothesis (Lehrer, 1978, 1996).

Vazquez and Buceta (1993a, 1993b, 1993c) studied the effects of an asthma education program, both alone and combined with progressive relaxation instruction. They found evidence for relaxation-induced therapeutic effects on duration of asthma attacks only among children with a history of emotional triggers. Other participants showed greater changes on this measure without relaxation instruction. At a borderline significant level, participants given relaxation training showed a greater decrease in consumption of beta-2 adrenergic stimulant (rescue) medications than those not

given relaxation training. On measures of pulmonary function, however, participants with emotional asthma triggers benefited significantly from asthma education without relaxation but not with it. The authors hypothesized that subjects receiving relaxation training put less emphasis on proper medical management of asthma. It also is possible that the parasympathetic rebound effects of relaxation interfered with effectiveness in this study.

### Biofeedback Techniques

#### EMG Biofeedback

Kotses, Harver, et al. (1991) hypothesized that changes in facial muscle tension directly produce respiratory impedance through a trigeminal-vagal reflex pathway (such that tensing these muscles produces bronchoconstriction, and relaxing them produces bronchodilation). They tested the model using frontal EMG biofeedback to increase and decrease tension in the facial muscles. Frontal EMG relaxation training decreased facial muscle tension and improved pulmonary function, while training to *increase* tension in that area had the opposite effect. EMG biofeedback training to the forearm muscles had no effects. Several recent studies from other laboratories have failed to replicate these findings, however (Lehrer, Generelli, & Hochron, 1997; Lehrer, Hochron, Carr, et al., 1996; Lehrer, Hochron, Mayne, Isenberg, Carlson, et al., 1994; Mass, Wais, Ramm, & Richter, 1992; Ritz, Dahme, & Wagner, 1998).

Another biofeedback strategy linked pulmonary function with tension in the skeletal muscles of the neck and thorax (Peper & Tibbetts, 1992). (Tension in this area often is produced by a pattern of thoracic breathing.) They used EMG biofeedback training to teach participants to relax these muscles while increasing volume and smoothness of breathing. This was done in the context of a multicomponent treatment that included desensitization to asthma sensations and training in slow diaphragmatic breathing. The latter training was carried out by a biofeedback procedure using an incentive inspirometer. At the follow-up, all subjects significantly reduced their EMG tension levels and increased their inhalation volumes. Subjects reported reductions in their asthma symptoms, medication use, emergency room visits, and breathless episodes. A small study from our laboratory did not show significant effects for this method (Lehrer, Carr, et al., 1997), but this study lacked power to determine whether some trends in the data were significant. More research on this method is warranted.

### Respiratory Resistance Biofeedback

Mass, Harden, et al. (1991) attempted to train subjects to decrease respiratory resistance by providing continuous biofeedback of this measure, using the forced oscillation method. In an uncontrolled trial, this feedback technique decreased average respiratory resistance within sessions but not between sessions (Mass, Dahme, & Richter, 1993). It did not increase $FEV_1$ (Mass, Richter, & Dahme, 1996). The researchers concluded that this type of biofeedback is not an effective technique for the treatment of bronchial asthma in adults (Mass, Richter, & Dahme, 1996).

### Respiratory Sinus Arrhythmia Biofeedback

A new biofeedback approach involves training people to increase the amplitude of respiratory sinus arrhythmia (RSA; Lehrer, Carr, et al., 1997). A manual for conducting this procedure has recently been published (Lehrer, Vaschillo, & Vaschillo, 2000). Multiple case studies from clinics in Russia support the hypothesis that RSA biofeedback training is an effective treatment for various neurotic and stress-related physical disorders (Chernigovskaya, Vaschillo, Petrash, & Rusanovskii, 1990; Chernigovskaya, Vaschillo, Rusanovskii, & Kashkarova, 1990; Pichugin, Strelakov, & Zakharevich, 1993; Vaschillo, Zingerman, Konstantinov, & Menitsky, 1983), including asthma (Lehrer, Smetankin, & Potapova, 2000).

### Yoga

Two studies of asthmatics who practiced yoga found that they experienced improvement in asthma symptoms as well as a more positive attitude, feelings of well being, and fewer symptoms of panic. One study was uncontrolled (Jain et al., 1991), while the other had a no-treatment control (Vedanthan et al., 1998). These studies suggest that yoga may have an impact on the subjective symptoms of asthma, although it is not clear whether this is also true about physiological function. However, these conclusions must remain tentative in view of the small amount of research on this topic and the wide variety of yoga methods used throughout the world.

### Hypnosis

In a controlled study of hypnosis as a treatment of asthma among children, Kohen (1995) noted improvement in asthma symptoms but not in pulmonary function compared with no treatment and waking-suggestion groups. A greater decrease in emergency room visits and missed days in school also was found in the hypnosis group. These data suggest that hypnotic interventions for asthma may improve patients' quality of life but not pulmonary function. Further evaluation of these effects is warranted. Similar findings were obtained in a later uncontrolled study among preschool children (Kohen & Wynne, 1997) for parental reports of asthma symptoms but not pulmonary function.

**Table 17.2**  Sources of Information About Asthma

| Organization | Telephone |
| --- | --- |
| American Academy of Allergy, Asthma, and Immunology | 1-800-822-2762 |
| American College of Allergy, Asthma, and Immunology *(for pamphlets or a list of board-certified doctors in your area)* | 1-800-842-7777 |
| American Lung Association | Call your local Lung Association |
| Asthma and Allergy Foundation of America | 1-800-727-8462 |
| National Allergy and Asthma Network/Mothers of Asthmatics | 1-800-878-4403 |
| National Jewish Medical and Research Center Information Service (Lung Line) | 1-800-222-5864 |

## TREATMENT PROTOCOLS

Written educational materials for patients have been published by numerous private and public agencies, including pharmaceutical companies and managed care organizations. Materials are available by telephone and from web sites of many organizations (see Table 17.2)

## CLINICAL EFFICACY AND COST-EFFECTIVENESS

Asthma education programs have been shown to be cost-effective for both children (Greineder, Loane, & Parks, 1999) and adults (Taitel, Kotses, Bernstein, Bernstein, & Creer, 1995). Studies of these programs have demonstrated improvements on measures such as frequency of asthma attacks and symptoms, medication consumption, and self-management skills (Kotses, Bernstein, et al., 1995; Wilson et al., 1996). More research, though, is needed to determine which specific components of the interventions (e.g., environmental control, peak-flow monitoring) are effective.

Relaxation methods show statistically significant improvement in asthma and may be helpful in an overall asthma management plan. The independent effects of relaxation methods, however, have not consistently been found to be clinically significant (Richter & Dahme, 1982). There is less research on the clinical effects of biofeedback methods. However, there is some evidence that biofeedback training for increasing heart rate variability may have stronger effects than do relaxation methods (Lehrer, Carr, et al., 1997). This method has much in common with methods influenced by yoga and other Eastern mind-body strategies involving slow respiration.

## SELECTION OF ALTERNATIVE TREATMENTS

Sommaruga et al. (1995) combined an asthma education program with three sessions of cognitive-behavioral therapy (CBT) focusing on areas that might interfere with proper medical management. Few significant differences on measures of anxiety, depression, and asthma morbidity (e.g., missed school or workdays) emerged between the control group receiving medical treatment alone and the CBT group. In an uncontrolled study, Park, Sawyer, and Glaun (1996) applied principles of CBT for panic disorder to asthmatic children reporting greater subjective complaints and consuming more medication than their level of pulmonary impairment warranted. In the 12 months following treatment, rate of hospitalization for asthma decreased, but other measures of clinical outcome were not analyzed. We have recently combined components of asthma education and CBT for panic disorder to develop a treatment protocol appropriate for adult asthmatics with panic disorder (Feldman, Giardino, & Lehrer, 2000), but this treatment has not yet been empirically tested. The National Heart, Lung, and Blood Institute's (1997) guidelines for asthma treatment recommend referral to mental health professionals when stress appears to interfere with medical management of asthma.

## CONCLUSION

There is evidence that psychological fac-tors can have a major impact on asthma. They may influence the ability of patients to recognixe asthma symptoms and triggers, to effectively utilize asthma medicines and medical care, and to avoid situations that my exacerbate their disease. Important factors include patients' knowledge about their disease and skill in utilizing available resources to treat it. Emotion and stress also can exacerbate asthma, both through direct psychophysiological effects on the airways and through their effects on asthma self-care behaviors, and stress management methods can be helpful for patients with emotional or stress triggers. Relaxation techniques have had limited usefulness for treating asthma, but several biofeedback techniques show promise of more potent effects.

## NOTE

1. Airway remodeling involves scarring of the airway, leading to airway narrowing that is not reversible with medication. It is thought to be caused by chronic, long-term inflammation.

## REFERENCES

Castés, M., Hagel, I., Palenque, M., Canelones, P., Corao, A., & Lynch, N. R. (1999). Immunology changes associated with clinical improvement of asthmatic children subjected to psychosocial intervention. *Brain, Behavior, and Immunity, 13,* 1–13.

Centers for Disease Control and Prevention. (1998). Surveillance for asthma—United States 1960–1995. *Morbidity & Mortality Weekly Report, 47,* 1–28.

Chernigovskaya, N. V., Vaschillo, E. G., Petrash, V. V., & Rusanovskii, V. V. (1990). Voluntary control of the heart rate as a method of correcting the functional state in neurosis. *Human Physiology, 17,* 105–111.

Chernigovskaya, N. V., Vaschillo, E. G., Rusanovskii, V. V., & Kashkarova, O. E. (1990). Instrumental autotraining of mechanisms for cardiovascular function regulation in treatment of neurotics. *The SS Korsakov's Journal of Neuropathology and Psychiatry, 90,* 24–28.

Fahy, J. V., Corry, D. B., & Boushey, H. A. (2000). Airway inflammation and remodeling in asthma. *Current Opinion in Pulmonary Medicine, 6,* 15–20.

Feldman, J. M., Giardino, N. D., & Lehrer, P. M. (2000). Asthma and panic disorder. In D. I. Mostofsky & D. H. Barlow (Eds.), *The management of stress and anxiety in medical disorders* (pp. 220–239). Needham Heights, MA: Allyn & Bacon.

Gellhorn, E. (1958). The physiological basis of neuromuscular relaxation. *Archives of Internal Medicine, 102,* 392–399.

Greineder, D. K., Loane, K. C., & Parks, P. (1999). A randomized controlled trial of a pediatric asthma outreach program. *Journal of Allergy and Clinical Immunology, 103,* 436–440.

Henry, M., de Rivera, J. L. G., Gonzalez-Martin, I. J., & Abreu, J. (1993). Improvement of respiratory function in chronic asthmatic patients with autogenic therapy. *Journal of Psychosomatic Research, 37,* 265–270.

Hollaender, J., & Florin, I. (1983). Expressed emotion and airway conductance in children with bronchial asthma. *Journal of Psychosomatic Research, 27,* 307–311.

Jain, S. C., Rai, L., Valecha, A., Jha, U. K., Bhatnagar, S. O. D., & Ram, K. (1991). Effect of yoga training in exercise tolerance in adolescents with childhood asthma. *Journal of Asthma, 28,* 437–442.

Kikuchi, Y., Okabe, S., Tamura, G., Hida, W., Homma, M., Shirato, K., et al. (1994). Chemosensitivity and perception of dyspnea in patients with a history of near-fatal asthma. *New England Journal of Medicine, 330,* 1329–1334.

Kinsman, R. A., Luparello, T., O'Banion, K., & Spector, S. (1973). Multidimensional analysis of the subjective symptomatology of asthma. *Psychosomatic Medicine, 35,* 250–267.

Kohen, D. P. (1995). Applications of relaxation/mental imagery (self-hypnosis) to the management of childhood asthma: Behavioral outcomes of a controlled study. *Hypnosis—The Journal of the European Society of Hypnosis in Psychotherapy and Psychosomatic Medicine, 22,* 132–144.

Kohen, D. P., & Wynne, E. (1997). Applying hypnosis in a preschool family asthma education program: Uses of storytelling, imagery, and relaxation. *American Journal of Clinical Hypnosis, 39,* 169–181.

Kotses, H., Bernstein, I. L., Bernstein, D. I., Reynolds, R. V. C., Korbee, L., Wigal, J. K., et al. (1995). A self-management program for adult asthma. Part I: Development and evaluation. *Journal of Allergy and Clinical Immunology, 95,* 529–540.

Kotses, H., Harver, A., Segreto, J., Glaus, K. D., Creer, T. L., & Young, G. A. (1991). Long-term effects of biofeedback-induced facial relaxation on measures of asthma severity in children. *Biofeedback & Self-Regulation, 16,* 1–21.

Kussin, P. S., & Fulkerson, W. J. (1995). The rising tide of asthma: Trends in the epidemiology of morbidity and mortality from asthma. *Respiratory Care Clinics of North America, 1,* 163–175.

Lehrer, P. M. (1978). Psychophysiological effects of progressive relaxation in anxiety neurotic patients and of progressive relaxation and alpha feedback in nonpatients. *Journal of Consulting and Clinical Psychology, 46,* 389–404.

Lehrer, P. M. (1996). Varieties of relaxation methods and their unique effects. *International Journal of Stress Management, 3,* 1–15.

Lehrer, P. M. (1998). Emotionally triggered asthma: A review of research literature and some hypotheses for self-regulation therapy. *Applied Psychophysiology and Biofeedback, 23,* 13–41.

Lehrer, P. M., Carr, R. E., Smetankine, A., Vaschillo, E., Peper, E., Porges, S., et al. (1997). Respiratory sinus arrhythmia versus neck/trapezius EMG and incentive inspirometry biofeedback for asthma: A pilot study. *Applied Psychophysiology and Biofeedback, 22,* 95–109.

Lehrer, P. M., Feldman, J., Song, H. S., & Giardino, N. (2002). Psychological aspects of asthma. *Journal of Consulting and Clinical Psychology, 70,* 691–711.

Lehrer, P. M., Generelli, P., & Hochron, S. (1997). The effect of facial and trapezius muscle tension on respiratory impedance in asthma. *Applied Psychophysiology and Biofeedback, 22,* 43–54.

Lehrer, P. M., Hochron, S., Carr, R., Edelberg, R., Hamer, R., Jackson, A., et al. (1996). Behavioral task-induced bronchodilation in asthma during active and passive tasks: A possible colinear link to psychologically induced airway changes. *Psychosomatic Medicine, 58*, 413–422.

Lehrer, P. M., Hochron, S., Mayne, T., Isenberg, S., Carlson, V., Lasoski, A. M., et al. (1994). Relaxation and music therapies for asthma among patients prestabilized on asthma medication. *Journal of Behavioral Medicine, 17*, 1–24.

Lehrer, P. M., Hochron, S., Mayne, T., Isenberg, S., Lasoski, A. M., Carlson, V., et al. (1997). Relationship between changes in EMG and respiratory sinus arrhythmia in a study of relaxation therapy for asthma. *Applied Psychophysiology and Biofeedback, 22*, 183–191.

Lehrer, P. M., Isenberg, S., & Hochron, S. M. (1993). Asthma and emotion: A review. *Journal of Asthma, 30*, 5–21.

Lehrer, P. M., Smetankin, A., & Potapova, T. (2000). Respiratory sinus arrhythmia biofeedback therapy for asthma: A report of 20 unmedicated pediatric cases using Smetankin method. *Applied Psychophysiology and Biofeedback, 25*, 193–200.

Lehrer, P. M., Vaschillo, E., & Vaschillo, B. (2000). Resonant frequency biofeedback training to increase cardiac variability: Rationale and manual for training. *Applied Psychophyisology and Biofeedback, 25*, 177–191.

Loew, T. H., Siegfried, W., Martus, P., Trill, K., & Hahn, E. G. (1996). Functional relaxation reduces acute airway obstruction in asthmatics as effectively as inhaled terbutaline. *Psychotherapy and Psychosomatics, 65*, 124–128.

Mass, R., Dahme, B., & Richter, R. (1993). Clinical evaluation of a respiratory resistance biofeedback training. *Biofeedback & Self-Regulation, 18*, 211–223.

Mass, R., Harden, H., Leplow, B., Wessel, M., Richter, R., & Dahme, B. (1991). A device for functional residual capacity controlled biofeedback of respiratory resistance. *Biomedizinische Technik, 36*, 78–85.

Mass, R., Richter, R., & Dahme, B. (1996). Biofeedback-induced voluntary reduction of respiratory resistance in severe bronchial asthma. *Behaviour Research and Therapy, 34*, 815–819.

Mass, R., Wais, R., Ramm, M., & Richter, R. (1992). Frontal muscles activity: A mediator in operant reduction of respiratory resistance? *Journal of Psychophysiology, 6*, 167–174.

National Heart, Lung, and Blood Institute. (1997). *Expert panel report 2: Guidelines for the diagnosis and management of asthma.* National Asthma Education and Prevention Program. Washington, DC: U.S. Department of Health and Human Services.

Park, S. J., Sawyer, S. M., & Glaun, D. E. (1996). Childhood asthma complicated by anxiety: An application of cognitive behavioural therapy. *Journal of Paediatrics and Child Health, 32*, 183–187.

Peper, E., & Tibbetts, V. (1992). Fifteen-month follow-up with asthmatics utilizing EMG/incentive inspirometer feedback. *Biofeedback & Self-Regulation, 17*, 143–151.

Pichugin, V. I., Strelakov, S. A., & Zakharevich, A. S. (1993). Usage of a portable device with ECG biofeedback ("cardiosignalizer") to reduce psychoemotional stress level. In A. Smetankin (Ed.), *Biofeedback: Visceral training in clinics* (pp. 149–159). St. Petersburg, Russia: Biosvyaz Corp.

Richter, R., & Dahme, B. (1982). Bronchial asthma in adults: There is little evidence for the effectiveness of behavioral therapy and relaxation. *Journal of Psychosomatic Research, 26*, 533–540.

Ritz, T., Dahme, B., & Wagner. C. (1998). Effects of static forehead and forearm muscle tension on total respiratory resistance in healthy and asthmatic participants. *Psychophysiology, 35*, 549–562.

Silverglade, L., Tosi, D. J., Wise, P. S., & D'Costa, A. (1994). Irrational beliefs and emotionality in adolescents with and without bronchial asthma. *Journal of General Psychology, 121,* 199–207.

Smyth, J. M., Soefer, M. H., Hurewitz, A., & Stone, A. A. (1999). The effect of tape-recorded training on well-being symptoms and peak expiratory flow rate in adult asthmatics: A pilot study. *Psychological Health, 14,* 487–501.

Sommaruga, M., Spanevello, A., Migliori, G. B., Neri, M., Callegari, S., & Majani, G. (1995). The effects of a cognitive behavioral intervention in asthmatic patients. *Monaldi Archives of Chest Disease, 50,* 398–402.

Taitel, M. A., Kotses, H., Bernstein, L., Bernstein, D. I., & Creer, T. L. (1995). A self-management program for adult asthma. Part II: Cost-benefit analysis. *Journal of Allergy and Clinical Immunology, 95,* 672–676.

Vaschillo, E. G., Zingerman, A. M., Konstantinov, M. A., & Menitsky, D. N. (1983). Research of the resonance characteristics for cardiovascular system. *Human Physiology, 10,* 257–265.

Vazquez, M. I., & Buceta, J. M. (1993a). Psychological treatment of asthma: Effectiveness of a self-management program with and without relaxation training. *Journal of Asthma, 30,* 171–183.

Vazquez, M. I., & Buceta, J. M. (1993b). Relaxation therapy in the treatment of bronchial asthma: Effects on basal spirometric values. *Psychotherapy & Psychosomatics, 60,* 106–112.

Vazquez, M. I., & Buceta, J. M. (1993c). Effectiveness of self-management programmes and relaxation training in the treatment of bronchial asthma: Relationships with trait anxiety and emotional attack triggers. *Journal of Psychosomatic Research, 37,* 71–81.

Vedanthan, P. K., Kesavalu, L. N., Murthy, K. C., Duvall, K., Hall, M. J., Baker S., et al. (1998). Clinical study of yoga techniques in university students with asthma: A controlled study. *Allergy and Asthma Proceedings, 19,* 3–9.

Wilson, S. R., Latini, D., Starr, N. J., Fish, L., Loes, L. M., Page, A., et al. (1996). Education of parents of infants and very young children with asthma: A developmental evaluation of the wee wheezers program. *Journal of Asthma, 33,* 239–254.

# CHAPTER 18

# Coronary Disease and Congestive Heart Disorder

## NARAS BHAT AND KUSUM BHAT

**Abstract:** Coronary artery disease and congestive heart disorder are not just "pump and pipes problems" to be fixed by wonder drugs and technical wizardry. Dynamic factors including cardiovascular and biobehavioral components determine the cardiac events and effort tolerance. Holistic cardiology treats the patient's illness behavior in addition to the anatomical heart. The three legs of the authors' new model of cardiac care include emotional tools added to the power of pills and scalpel. Reversing heart disease focuses on teaching patients to measure, monitor, and modify risk factors, including anger, depression, anxiety, and social isolation. The chapter reviews the prevailing American and European lifestyle modification protocols and outlines the authors' eclectic model, which is based on psychophysiological self-regulation and includes biofeedback monitoring of heart rate variability and structured group support. Although clinical outcome validates the biobehavioral approach, current medical economics has restricted its use. The authors suggest integrating "high-touch" behavioral modalities and "high-tech" multimedia computer training tools into mainstream medical practice.

## MEDICAL, PHYSIOLOGICAL, AND BEHAVIORAL PROFILES OF THE DISORDER

Coronary artery disease (CAD) is the most common chronic illness causing death, disability, and economic loss. In the United States, over 11 million people have CAD, and 5 million have congestive heart failure (CHF). Atherosclerotic narrowing, spasm, embolus, or blood clot of coronary arteries reduces blood and oxygen supplies to the heart muscle, causing myocardial ischemia. The process affects the bigger epicardial conductance vessels as well as microvascular intramyocardial resistance vessels. Transient ischemia can silently reduce the kinetics of heart pumping or produce anginal chest pain. If prolonged, ischemia can lead to chronic or sudden necrosis and scarring of the heart muscle. Sudden necrosis can cause cardiac arrythmia and/or sudden death. CAD manifests in one of eight clinical patterns: sudden death, CHF, cardiac arrythmia, heart attack, unstable angina, Prinzmetal's angina, angina, or silent ischemia.

CHF is the failure of the heart as a pump to meet the perfusion requirements of metabolizing tissues. Seventy-five percent of CHF is an aftermath of CAD. It afflicts 5 million people in the United States, with up to 700,000 new cases developing each year. In most cases, CHF is a progressive disorder that can be caused by many factors, all of which create continuous or excessive burdens that weaken the pumping power of the heart. Because the weakened heart cannot pump an adequate amount of oxygenated blood throughout the body, symptoms such as shortness of breath, rapid heartbeat, effort intolerance, and insomnia occur. The damaged heart also creates a buildup of fluids that causes swelling and congestion.

The malfunctioning heart in CHF causes chemical dysregulation in three domains: the sympatho-adrenal system, the renin-angiotensin system, and cytokinins. The sympathetic arousal releases an unnaturally high amount of the chemicals norepinephrine and epinephrine, leading to a vicious cycle of a weakening heart and worsening insomnia. The cells of the heart either proliferate, dilate, fibrose, or atrophy, which in turn changes the architecture of the entire heart and makes it less compliant, hypertrophied, or dilated. This process is called cardiac remodeling (Packer & Cohn, 1999). The usual management of CHF includes medications to decrease the preload (diuretics), augment cardiac muscle function (digoxin), or decrease the afterload of peripheral resistance (ACE inhibitors, beta blockers). However, recent studies have shown that there is little relation between cardiac function recorded by medical tests, including ejection fraction and the patient's effort tolerance (Consensus Trial Study Group, 1990). A newer approach to treating CHF is to view it as a dynamic, partially reversible disorder that can be improved by changing the underlying chemistry noninvasively. Diastolic heart failure, which is the failure of the heart to relax (as opposed to systolic heart failure,

the failure to contract), is partly dependent on how well the heart recuperates from the hyperaroused chemistry of the day. Sleep and stress control increase the diastolic functioning of the heart (Nixon, 1986b).

## ANATOMY AND PHYSIOLOGY OF CARDIAC DYNAMICS

Blood flow to the heart is supplied by right and left coronary arteries. Epicardial arteries are often regarded as conductance vessels, and myocardial microvasculature is regarded as a system of resistance vessels. However, the epicardial vessels are not passive conduits; they have a calcium-dependent resting tone and a catecholamine-dependent potential for spasm, even if denervation occurs after bypass surgery or transplant (Freeman & Nixon, 1985). In atherosclerotic segments of coronary arteries, endothelial dysfunction occurs, causing paradoxical or hypersensitive spasm during exercise and mental stress.

Blood flow through intramyocardial resistance vessels depends on the perfusion gradient (aortic pressure minus coronary sinus pressure or left ventricular end-diastolic pressure) and the diastolic time available for flow. Rapid heart rate during anxiety or physical stress may impose a handicap on the heart by decreasing diastolic filling and lowering coronary perfusion (Nixon, 1986b).

Conventional risk factors for coronary artery disease are grouped as (1) uncontrollable factors, such as increasing age, male sex, and hereditary predisposition; and (2) controllable factors of high blood pressure, high cholesterol, cigarette smoking, diabetes, obesity, and sedentary lifestyle. Psychosocial factors fall into five domains: hostility, chronic stress, anxiety, depression, and social isolation (Rozanski, Blumenthal, & Kaplan, 1999).

## TYPICAL SYMPTOM
## PROFILE AND ASSESSMENT

CAD typically presents with chest pain, which may radiate to the left arm or the jaw, and may be accompanied by nausea, vomiting, sweating, and shortness of breath. This symptom complex is called angina pectoris. Clinically, angina is classified according to the precipitant and duration. If it occurs only during exertion and has been stable for a long period, it is called stable angina. If pain occurs at rest, it is unstable angina. Prinzmetal's angina involves recurrent attacks due to transient spasm of coronary arteries. If the pain persists and leads to necrosis of the heart muscle, it is myocardial infarction (heart attack). Asymptomatic (silent) ischemia refers to ST segment depression in the electrocardiogram without any chest pain. CAD may weaken the heart as a pump and lead to CHF—congestion from fluid in the lungs and peripheral tissues. CHF presents as breathlessness (dyspnea), especially when lying down (orthopnea), fatigue, and effort intolerance.

The diagnosis of CAD is based on the history, physical examination, resting EKG, exercise stress test, cardiac enzymes, echocardiogram, and coronary angiogram. The EKG usually shows a depression of ST segment in angina, although in Prinzmetal's angina it could be elevated. Heart attack may be silent or present with sudden severe chest pain, irregular heartbeats, shock, or death. EKG findings of heart attack could have Q waves besides ST segment depression and inverted T waves. Necrosis of the heart muscle shows up as elevated cardiac enzymes such as CK-MB and troponin 1. An echocardiogram during angina or heart attack may show segmental wall motion abnormality. Coronary angiogram confirms the location and extent of blockage in the coronary arteries. CHF is diagnosed by patient history, the presence of edema in the feet, distension of neck veins, X-ray finding of an enlarged heart, and hemodynamic studies of reduced cardiac output and elevated ventricular diastolic pressure.

## CONVENTIONAL
## MEDICATION TREATMENT
## AND ITS SHORTCOMINGS

The conventional treatment of heart disease dwells on pills and the scalpel. Medications are given to dilate the pipes, improve the pump, and change the blood—that is, to reduce blood volume, change the cholesterol-related atherogenic chemistry, and reduce clotting potential. The surgical approach revascularizes by angioplasty, stent, atherectomy, or bypass grafts. The shortcomings of conventional treatment are epitomized by Nixon (1986b) as an "attempt to reconstruct the broken egg." Alternative treatments focus on going after the forces that broke the egg in the first place. Only 50 percent of patients with CAD have high cholesterol (Braunwald, 1997), which supports the logic of addressing other risk factors, including the psychophysiology based on dynamic factors (Nixon & Freeman, 1987).

## DYNAMIC FACTORS
## IN HEART DISEASE

Coronary arteries, like the esophagus or intestines, are dynamic, not rigid pipes. CAD is a bell-shaped curve (King & Nixon, 1988). On the upslope of the curve are people with significant artery blockage but no symptoms, on the downslope are people with significant symptoms but no fixed blockage, and in the middle are individuals with both. This means that much of CAD is due not to fixed anatomical blockage but to dynamic factors. Scientific evidence for this bell-shaped curve abounds. CAD is a marker of aging just like graying of hair. People with anginal chest pain often have the same degree of blockage as people with no chest pain at all (Mathews, 1977). Neither the number of coronary pipes clogged nor the degree of mortality or morbidity corresponds to the frequency or intensity of symptoms (James, 1983). Effort tolerance and other symptoms for a given patient can be zero to a hundred times different between a good day and a bad day (Maseri, 1980). Despite existing CAD, diagnosed or not, a person may have no symptoms for years, and then one day the symptoms appear suddenly. Pathologists studying the victims of sudden heart attack are often unable to explain the catastrophe by the degree of pipe blockage they see on autopsy. Several cases of sudden death from heart attack have had normal coronary arteries (Freeman & Nixon, 1985). Often the recurrent cardiac events are related to arteries that are not treated by angioplasty or surgery.

The dynamic factors of CAD can be cardiac and extracardiac (Freeman & Nixon, 1985). Cardiac factors come from "pipes" and "pumps." Constriction of the systemic veins acting as capacitance vessels can empty a liter or more blood into the heart and lungs, increasing the preload. Constriction of systemic resistance vessels raises the afterload pressure against which the ventricles must work. Constriction of coronary artery vasomotor tone or sudden coronary spasm can cut off circulation to the heart muscle. These pump dynamics depend on the physical and mental stress level, hyperventilation, and resulting calcium-magnesium balance.

The myocardial pump can be temporarily "stunned" (Braunwald & Kloner, 1982) or stiffened by the ischemic insult during the dynamic narrowing of coronary arteries. Stiffening can be temporarily induced by stress-induced catabolic toxicity of sympatho-adrenomedullary (S-AM) and pituitary-adrenocortical (P-AC) hormones. Repeated stunning may lead to fibrosis and permanent stiffening. Subendocardial ischemia producing stiffness can occur during stress-induced tachycardia, reducing diastolic coronary blood flow. The net effect of these cardiac dynamic factors is to reduce left ventricular compliance affecting pressure-volume relationships. Normally, a large volume of blood is accepted with minimal rise of pressure. This explains the effort intolerance and day-to-day change in symptoms based on stress arousal (Nixon, 1986a).

The extracardiac dynamic factors are dependent on the stress and coping abilities of the individual. Nixon developed his n-shaped curve to measure the relationship between stress arousal and performance. On the upslope, performance increases with effort. After the peak, more effort gives diminishing returns due to a lack of reserve energy in the body. As in beating a tired horse, the gap between intended target and reality widens. Catabolic pathways lead to vital exhaustion (Nixon, 1986b), and the brain's information channels get overloaded, affecting cognitive functions (Lipowski, 1975). The quality and quantity of sleep decreases, disturbing the body's anabolic healing power (Adam & Owaid, 1984).

## RESEARCH ON BEHAVIORAL INTERVENTION

### Anger

There have been three types of anger research. The first was that of Type A behavior. In 1974, cardiologists Friedman and Rosenman did an 8.5-year study on 3,000 men and found that Type A behavior was associated with twice the incidence of CAD. Three components in the Type A profile are time urgency, excessive competitiveness, and hostility. The National Heart, Lung, and Blood Institute proclaimed in 1981 that Type A behavior is an independent CAD risk factor.

The second kind of research showed that hostility is the toxic core of Type A behavior. A Duke University study, led by Dembroski and colleagues in 1985, looked at 12,000 men and found that the key element of Type A is hostility (Dembroski, MacDougall, Williams, Haney, & Blumenthal, 1985). The time urgency and competitiveness of Type A correlated poorly with heart disease. On the other hand, hostility was strongly correlated to CAD, as documented by angiography (Williams, 1989). In 1983, University of North Carolina research, using 25 years of follow-up, showed that the death rate among angry doctors and lawyers was five times higher than that of their counterparts who were not angry (Williams, 1989, p. 57). A report published in 1996 in the *Mayo Clinic Proceedings* stated that people with high anger measured by the Spielberger State-Trait Anger Expression Inventory had 2.5 times higher chance of reclogging their arteries after angioplasty (Goodman, Quigly, Moran, Milman, & Sherman, 1996).

The third type of anger research is that of measuring the real-time effects of anger on the heart. In 1993, a Stanford study showed that recalled anger leads to spasm of the atherosclerotic segment of the coronary artery as seen on angiogram (Boltwood, 1993). A Miami University study showed that recalled anger decreases the ejection fraction, or pumping power of the heart as seen on echocardiogram (Ironson, Taylor, Bartsokis, Dennis, & Chesney, 1992). In 1998, our study showed that the ejection fraction of the heart can be significantly improved by biofeedback-assisted anger control in heart patients (Bhat & Bhat, 1999). A study conducted at Columbia-Presbyterian Medical Center showed that anger-induced irregularity

(called heart rate variability, or HRV) happens more often during the day while a person engages in angry transactions than it does at night during sleep (Sloan, 1994). Patients in a Yale University study wore a special camera called an electronic stethoscope to measure the pumping power of the heart moment by moment (Jain, Burg, & Soufer, 1995). The study showed that during anger episodes, the ejection fraction of the heart drops and that the more such events a given person experiences, the higher the likelihood of developing cardiac events, including a heart attack.

Two kinds of heart attacks occur during stress and anger (Eliot, 1994): (1) coronary artery blockage and coagulation necrosis, which occur when the kinking spasm and clogging clot of the coronary arteries cuts off of oxygen and blood to the heart muscle; and (2) chemical burn to the heart and contraction band necrosis, in which the anger chemical, norepinephrine, increases and literally causes a chemical burn to one or more heart muscle fibers, triggering an electrical storm called ventricular fibrillation, which can result in death. Cardiologist Robert Eliot (1994) studied NASA engineers aged 28 to 35 who dropped dead when they were laid off suddenly during the Kennedy era. Autopsies showed that they did not have CAD but died of "heart burn" resulting from frustration and anger.

The antidote for anger is learned altruism. The "Mother Teresa effect" is an increase of immune power during altruism. Harvard psychologist David McLelland looked at the salivary immunoglobulin A (IgA) in two groups of medical students (McClelland & Kirshnite, 1988). The first group watched a movie of Mother Teresa ministering to the underprivileged. The second group watched a movie of violence. The Mother Teresa movie led to increased IgA, and violent movies decreased IgA. In addition, during the Mother Teresa movie, the HRV was smooth and regular, and during the violent movie the HRV was erratic and low, indicating that heart rhythm also is affected by anger. Researchers at the Institute of HeartMath duplicated the study and found that after an argument between a husband and wife, the suppression of immunoglobulin lasts for 5 to 7 hours (McCraty, Atkinson, & Tiller, 1995).

### Depression

Depression increases the CAD risk three-fold. Hopelessness (Ritcher, 1957), the magnitude of depression, and future cardiac events are closely correlated (Anda et al., 1993). Vital exhaustion has the symptom triad of fatigue, irritability, and demoralized feelings and predicts future cardiac events (Appels & Mulder, 1988). At least three detrimental psychobiological changes cluster together in depression: hypercortisolemia, impaired platelet function, and reduced HRV (Rozanski et al., 1999).

### Anxiety

Anxiety is associated with sudden cardiac death (Kawachi, Sparrow, Vokonas, & Weiss, 1994) and reduced baroreflex control of the heart (Watkin, Grossman, Krishanan, & Sherwood, 1998). Karasek, Baker, Marxer, Ahlbom, and Theorell (1981) found that job strain of high demand but low decision latitude was associated with a fourfold increase in cardiovascular deaths. Eliot (1994) found increased cardiac events in "hot reactors" who respond with heightened heart rate and blood pressure reactive to physical or mental challenge.

### Social Isolation

Lack of social network, intimacy, and instrumental support such as access to guidance and practical community services increases CAD risk at least threefold (Rozanski et al., 1999). Acculturation negatively affects CAD, as shown in Japanese Americans (Marmot & Syme, 1976) and Italian Americans (Egolf, Lasker, Wolf, & Potvin, 1992). Isolation increases blood cortisol level, heart rate, and urinary adrenaline level (Gerin, Pieper, Levy, & Pickering, 1992).

## MIND-BODY INTERVENTIONS: WHAT ARE THE CHOICES FOR HEART DISEASE?

Before a person gets heart disease, he or she has the choice of preventing it or waiting till the "crack shows you light." Once heart disease happens, the choices are to live and die with it or die from it.

When it comes to treatment, there are two levels of choices: patient's choice and doctor's choice. The patient's choice is based on whether she or he believes in "pill power" or "skill power." The doctor's choice is based on the era of medicine, as delineated by Dossey (1993), to which the doctor belongs.

- Era I: Techno-medicine or allopathic modern medicine based on tests, gadgets, surgery, and pills. This era is based on the paradigm of a mind-body split as formulated by Rene Descartes in the 17th century.
- Era II: Mind-body healing using hypnosis, meditation, imagery, and biofeedback. This era started in the 1950s.
- Era III: Transpersonal medicine based on the power of prayer, altruism, group support, and human connectedness. This era started in the 1980s.

The eclectic way to treat heart disease is to take advantage of all three eras of medicine, drawing on the power of pills to correct blood factors such as cholesterol, the power of the scalpel to open up plumbing blockages, and the power of the mind and spirit to retool the emotional imbalance.

## Nixon's Stress Control Model

Peter Nixon (1993), from London's Charing Cross Hospital, developed a model of reversing heart disease primarily by managing stress and controlling chronic hyperventilation and vigilance. The method involves regulating six elements of lifestyle that form the acronym SABRES: *S* for sleep, *A* for stress arousal, *B* for breathing, *R* for rest, *E* for effort, and *S* for self-esteem. This is pioneer work in the emotional rehabilitation of heart disease. Dean Ornish (1990), in the United States, built a model based on lifestyle changes, including low-fat diet, stress control by yoga and meditation, exercise, and group support.

## Psychophysiological Protocol

To a program of lifestyle changes, Naras Bhat (1995) added the component of anger control using biofeedback monitoring of heart rate variability. This model takes the patient from point A—a life of matter and motion—to point B—a life of matter, motion, and emotion. On the way, the individual uses measuring tools, monitoring tools, and modifying tools. The modifying tools include uprooting anger, meditation and imagery, self-disclosure, rest and activity, and mindful eating of a low-fat vegetarian diet.

The psychophysiological approach combines patient education and treatment before and after cardiac events. The program has three distinct components: books and tapes (Bhat, 1995; Ornish, 1990), weekly group meetings, and clinic visits. The weekly group class is two hours long and consists of guided meditation, discussion of one aspect of the psychophysiology of the heart, and a sharing ritual. The clinic visits use biofeedback, computers, and multimedia educational models extensively. The emotional tools include measuring, monitoring, and modifying protocols of mind-body dynamics. Five modifying

tools are used: uprooting anger, meditation and imagery, self-disclosure, rest and activity, and mindful eating. Typically, there are five structured clinic visits with specific homework assignments. The following sections summarize the treatment protocol.

*Visit 1.* Data gathering and assessment, including the following:

• Intake history to evaluate current areas of will being (level of control), ill being (medical diagnosis and symptoms), pill being (external pharmacy), well-being (healing power and belief systems), skill being (lifestyle factors), physiological signature (current pattern of physiological response to stressors using biofeedback), and emotional intelligence (EQ) scale.

• Physical diagnosis, including pulse, respiration, blood pressure, and abdominal obesity measurement.

• Chemical diagnosis, including end-tidal carbon dioxide (etCO$_2$), blood sugar, hemoglobin, insulin, cholesterol (HDL, LDL, triglycerides), lipoprotein a, homocysteine, ratio of total cholesterol to HDL, HDL subclasses, and LDL pattern A or B (Superko, 1996).

• Physiological reactivity diagnosis: Heart rate variability, muscle tension (EMG), emotional sweating (EDR), circulation level (hand temperature), breathing ratio (thoracic/abdominal), and brain wave (EEG).

• Emotional intelligence (EQ): measured by videotaped emotional learning (VEL) and emotional scales such as Beck's Anxiety and Depression Scales, Spielberger's State-Trait Anger Expression Inventory, and Stroebel's Mind-Body Intelligence Scale, Vital Exhaustion Scale, and Sleep Quality Assessment.

*Visit 2.* Review of intake data and mastery of anger control using HRV feedback.

*Visit 3*. Anxiety desensitization by interoceptive drills, relaxation tools, and monitoring meditation by EEG.

*Visit 4*. Self-disclosure training using couple's biofeedback.

*Visit 5*. Outcome measurements by repeating the scales used during the intake.

## Outcome Studies

The simple intervention of a nurse monitoring the symptoms of psychological stress after myocardial infarction produced a 50 percent reduction in mortality after one year compared with controls (Frasure-Smith & Prince, 1985). In a randomized study of 862 post-infarction patients, interventions to reduce Type A behavior reduced mortality by 50 percent (Friedman et al., 1986). Ornish et al. (1990) did a randomized study of 28 angiographically documented CAD patients who ate a vegetarian diet; practiced yoga, meditation, and exercise; and received stress management training and group support. After four years, angiography showed a 4 percent regression of blockage in the study group compared with 10 percent progression in the control group. A meta-analysis of psychosocial stress reduction in CAD patients showed a 50 percent reduction in the combined rate of mortality (Nunes, Frank, & Kornfeld, 1987). All these studies had sample sizes ranging from 200 to 1,000 compared with more than 23,000 subjects in a beta-blocker drug study (Yusuf, Peto, & Lewis, 1985).

## FUTURE DIRECTIONS FOR MIND-BODY INTERVENTION

Although the efficacy of psychosocial interventions in CAD and CHF is evidence based, there is a lack of effectiveness due to organizational, financial, and educational limitations. The medical system is well organized to focus on "putting out the fire" but not for providing fire retardant or reconstruction after the fire. Health care providers are poorly reimbursed for prevention and rehabilitation compared with acute care. Several hospitals have reduced or terminated their cardiac rehabilitation programs due to lack of funding. In addition, primary care physician training seldom includes psychosocial and alternative modalities. The Kaiser Permanente system has attempted to overcome these logistics by using nurse case managers in their MULTIFIT program (DeBusk, 1996).

One solution we find promising is to use multimedia and Internet tools to provide low-cost patient education and health care provider training. By combining high-tech and high-touch methods, the focus of treatment shifts from disease management to patient management. As Osler (1932) said, "It is important to know what kind of patient has the disease rather than what kind of disease the patient has."

## REFERENCES

Adam, K., & Owaid, I. (1984). Sleep helps healing. *British Medical Journal, 289,* 1400.

Anda, R., Williamson, D., Jones, D., Macera, C., Eaker, E., Glasman, A., & Marks, J. (1993). Depressed affect, hopelessness, and the risk of ischemic heart disease in cohort of U.S. adults. *Epidemiology, 4,* 285–294.

Appels, A., & Mulder, P. (1988). Excess fatigue as a precurser of myocardial infarction. *European Heart Journal, 9,* 758–764.

Bhat, N. (1995). *How to reverse and prevent heart disease and cancer.* San Francisco: New Edition.

Bhat, N., & Bhat, K. (1999). Anger control using biofeedback: A clinical model for heart patients. *Biofeedback, 27*(4), 15–17.

Boltwood, E. (1993). Anger report predicts coronary artery vasomotor response to mental stress in atherosclerotic segments. *American Journal of Cardiology, 72,* 1361–1365.

Braunwald, E. (1997). Cardiovascular medicine at the turn of the millennium: Triumphs, concerns, and opportunities. *New England Journal of Medicine, 337,* 1360–1369.

Braunwald, E., & Kloner, R. A. (1982). The stunned myocardium: Prolonged, postischemic ventricular dysfunction. *Circulation, 66*(6), 1146.

Consensus Trial Study Group. (1990). Hormones regulating cardiovascular function in patients with severe congestive heart failure and their relation to mortality. *Circulation, 82,* 1730–1736.

DeBusk, R. (1996). MULTIFIT: A new approach to risk factor modification. *Cardiology Clinics of North America, 14*(1), 143–157.

Dembroski, T., MacDougall, J. M., Williams, R. B., Haney, T. L., & Blumenthal, J. A. (1985). Components of type A, hostility, and anger-in: Relationship to angiographic findings. *Psychosomatic Medicine, 47*(3), 219–231.

Dossey, L. (1993). *Healing words.* New York: HarperSanFrancisco.

Egolf, G., Lasker, J., Wolf, S., & Potvin, L. (1992). The Roseto effect: A 50-year comparison of mortality rates. *American Journal of Public Health, 82,* 1089–1092.

Eliot, R. (1994). *From stress to strength.* New York: Bantam Books.

Frasure-Smith, N., & Prince, R. (1985). The ischemic heart disease life stress monitoring program: Impact on mortality. *Psychosomatic Medicine, 47,* 431.

Freeman, L. J., & Nixon, P. (1985). Dynamic causes of angina pectoris. *American Heart Journal, 110*(5), 1087–1092.

Friedman, M., & Rosenman, R. H. (1974). *Type A behavior and your heart.* London: Wildwood House.

Friedman, M., Thoreson, C. E., Gill, J. J., Ulmer, D., Powell, L. H., & Price, V. A. (1986). Alteration of type A behavior and its effect on cardiac recurrences in post-myocardial infarction patients: Summary results of the Recurrent Coronary Prevention Project. *American Heart Journal, 112,* 653.

Gerin, W., Pieper, C., Levy, R., & Pickering, T. G. (1992). Social support in social interaction, a moderator of cardiovascular reactivity. *Psychosomatic Medicine, 54,* 324–336.

Goodman, M., Quigly, M. A., Moran, G., Milman, H., & Sherman, M. (1996). Hostility predicts restenosis after percutaneous transluminal coronary angioplasty. *Mayo Clinic Proceedings, 71,* 729–734.

Ironson, G., Taylor, C. B., Bartsokis, T., Dennis, C., & Chesney, M. (1992). Effects of anger on left ventricular ejection fraction in coronary artery disease. *American Journal of Cardiology, 70,* 281–285.

Jain, D., Burg, M., & Soufer, R. (1995). Prognostic implications of mental stress induced silent ventricular dysfunction in patients with stable anginal pectoris. *American Journal of Cardiology, 76,* 30–35.

James, T. (1983). Chance and sudden death. *Journal of the American College of Cardiology, 1,* 164–183.

Karasek, R., Baker, D., Marxer, F., Ahlbom, A., & Theorell, T. (1981). Job decision latitude, job demands, and cardiovascular disease: A prospective study of Swedish men. *American Journal of Public Health, 71,* 694–705.

Kawachi, I., Sparrow, D., Vokonas, P. S., & Weiss, S. T. (1994). Symptoms of anxiety and coronary artery disease: The normative aging study. *Circulation, 90,* 2225–2229.

King, J., & Nixon, P. (1988). A system of cardiac rehabilitation: Psychophysiological basis of practice. *British Journal of Occupational Therapy, 51*(11), 378–384.

Lipowski, Z. (1975). Sensory and information input overload: Behavioral effects. *Comprehensive Psychiatry, 16,* 199–202.

Marmot, M., & Syme, S. L. (1976). Acculturation and coronary heart disease in Japanese Americans. *American Journal of Epidemiology, 104,* 225–247.

Maseri, A. (1980). Pathogenetic mechanism of angina pectoris. *British Heart Journal, 43*(6), 648–660.

Mathews, M. (1977). *Angina pectoris.* Edinburgh, Scotland: Churchill Livingstone.

McClelland, D., & Kirshnite, C. (1988). The effects of motivational arousal through films on salivary immunoglobulin A. *Psychological Health, 2,* 31–52.

McCraty, R., Atkinson, M., & Tiller, W. A. (1995). The effect of emotions on short-term heart rate variability using power spectrum analysis. *American Journal of Cardiology, 76*(14), 1089–1093.

National Heart, Lung, and Blood Institute. (1981). Coronary prone behavior and coronary heart disease: A critical review. *Circulation, 63,* 199–215.

Nixon, P. (1986a, Spring). Consensus meeting: Coronary artery bypass surgery—Is it enough? *Quality of Life and Cardiovascular Care,* 125–132.

Nixon, P. (1986b). Exhaustion: Cardiac rehabilitation's starting point. *Physiotherapy, 72*(5), 224.

Nixon, P. (1993). The broken heart—Counteraction by SABRES. *Journal of the Royal Society of Medicine, 86,* 468–471.

Nixon, P., & Freeman, L. J. (1987). What is the meaning of angina pectoris today? *American Heart Journal, 114*(6), 1542–1546.

Nunes, E., Frank, K. A., & Kornfeld, D. S. (1987). Psychologic treatment for the type A behavior pattern and coronary artery disease: A meta-analysis of the literature. *Psychosomatic Medicine, 48,* 159–173.

Ornish, D. (1990). *Dean Ornish's program for reversing heart disease.* New York: Ballantine Books.

Ornish, D., Brown, S. E., Scherwitz, L. W., Billings, J. H., Armstrong, W. T., Ports, T. A., et al. (1990). Can lifestyle changes reverse coronary artery disease? *Lancet, 336,* 129–133.

Osler, W. (1932). *Aequanimitas.* New York: McGraw-Hill.

Packer, M., & Cohn, N. (1999). Consensus recommendations for management of chronic heart failure. *American Journal of Cardiology, 83,* 2A–8A.

Ritcher, C. (1957). On the phenomenon of sudden death in animals and man. *Psychosomatic Medicine, 19,* 190–198.

Rozanski, A., Blumenthal, J. A., & Kaplan, J. (1999). Impact of psychosocial factors on the pathogenesis of cardiovascular disease and implications for therapy. *Circulation, 99,* 2192–2217.

Sloan, R. (1994). Cardiac autonomic control and hostility in healthy subjects. *American Journal of Cardiology, 74,* 298–300.

Superko, R. (1996). Lipid disorders contributing to coronary artery disease: An update. *Current Problems in Cardiology, 21,* 736–780.

Watkin, L., Grossman, P., Krishanan, R., & Sherwood, A. (1998). Anxiety and vagal control of heart attack. *Psychosomatic Medicine, 60,* 498–502.

Williams, R. (1989). *The trusting heart.* New York: Random House.

Yusuf, S., Peto, R., & Lewis, J. (1985). Beta blockage during and after myocardial infarction: An overview of randomized trials. *Progress in Cardiovascular Diseases, 27,* 335–371.

# CHAPTER 19

# Back Pain: Musculoskeletal Pain Syndrome

## GABRIEL E. SELLA

**Abstract:** Back pain is a common disorder that produces lingering suffering and impairment and requires extensive and expensive medical intervention. The chapter reviews the anatomy and physiology of the human back, highlighting the role of upright bipedal posture in back pain. The author advocates a thorough medical and kinesiological evaluation, including surface electromyography (SEMG) assessment of muscular activation and dynamics. He proposes a multidisciplinary treatment model comprising guided relaxation, SEMG biofeedback, hypnosis, cognitive therapy, psychotherapy, and selective use of alternative therapies such as neurofeedback.

## PROFILES OF BACK PAIN

### Medical Profile

Back pain is one of the most common symptomatic complaints in medical practice, especially within the pain specialty. Statistics show that the yearly expenditure on back pain and related issues in the United States is in the range of $80 billion to $90 billion per year (Bigos & Battie, 1987). Most back pain presentations are acute and resolve within one to three months of treatment. Fewer than 5 percent of patients become chronic back pain sufferers. The situation is considered chronic if the pain does not resolve within six months.

Most back pain suffering is functional and of myofascial etiology. Less than 10 percent of back pain is of structural origin, including disc herniation, root compression, tendonal or ligamental ruptures or derangements, vertebral structure fracture, and arthrosis (Cailliet, 1993).

### Pathophysiological Profile

The bipedal position acquired by human beings in the course of evolution has had a great influence on the function of the back and trunk (Hollingshead, 1976; Maigne, 1996). Table 19.1 illustrates that the human back is an incomplete evolutionary hybrid. After at least one million years of human existence, it is still better suited for quadripedal stance and motion. Most of the functional etiology of back pain could, in one way or another, be the result of incompatibility of the vertebromuscular anatomy and the requirements of the bipedal position and function.

**Table 19.1**   Functional Changes of the Trunk and Back from the Quadripedal to the Bipedal Position

| Cranium and Vertebral Column | Quadripedal Position | Bipedal Position |
|---|---|---|
| Head | • Position on neck usually extended for movement or surveillance of environment, flexed for feeding. | • Position on neck mainly neutral, but head weighs heavily on the entire column. |
| Neck | • Vertebral position mainly horizontal, with strong posterior muscles needed to sustain the head.<br>• Disc pressure mainly vertical, with head weight pressure sustained mainly by the ligaments and muscles. | • Vertebral position vertical with weaker muscles sustaining the head.<br>• Disc pressure horizontal with high head pressure on discs against gravity. |
| Upper back and thorax | • Muscles adapted for ambulation sustained well by the bony structures of the upper thoracic column, shoulder girdle, and upper rib cage. | • Muscles adapted for the ballistic motion of the upper limbs.<br>• Weight of upper limbs and shoulders increases the gravitational pressure on the vertebral column and associated structures. |
| Mid- and low back | • Used mainly for lateral motion.<br>• Disc pressure mainly vertical. | • Used for bending and rotation in addition to flexion and extension.<br>• Disc pressure horizontal and maximal at region of L4 or L5 to S1 (the region of most herniations). |
| Low back and hip | • Sacroiliac complex in horizontal position, able to sustain contents, such as a fetus, vertically, weighing on the abdominal muscles against gravity. | • Sacroiliac complex in vertical position, able to sustain contents, such as fetus, horizontally, weighing against the pelvic floor |
| Vertebral ligaments | • Anterior longitudinal ligament structurally larger and stronger than the posterior longitudinal ligament.<br>• Good adaptation to horizontal pressure of the column against gravity. | • Same anatomy, poor adaptation for ligamental support in the vertical position.<br>• Posterior ligament overused because of frequent back flexion, functional in human activities. |
| Discs | • Structure well adapted for vertical pressure (sustained well below by the anterior longitudinal ligament) with little pressure against gravity from superior structures. | • Structure poorly adapted for horizontal pressure, increasing against gravity from C1 to L5 or S1.<br>• "Weakest area" against herniation in the lateral aspects, around the root exits. |
| Paravertebral muscles | • Function mainly in the horizontal position, well adapted for running, bending, and sustaining the limb muscles for jumping, such as from branch to branch. | • Function mainly in the vertical position, equivocally adapted to sustain the vertebral column in standing, running, and sustaining ballistic motion of the upper limbs. |

**Table 19.1**    *Continued*

| *Cranium and Vertebral Column* | *Quadripedal Position* | *Bipedal Position* |
|---|---|---|
| Trunk muscles | • Well adapted to quadripedal stance and motion. | • Functionally adaptable to the bipedal stance and motion.<br>• More easily injured because of excess requirements in terms of the (1) ballistic and weight-carrying requirements of the upper limbs and (2) postural, gait, and ambulation requirements of the lower limbs. |
| Nerve roots | • Exits and course relatively free of muscle or other pressure. | • Exits more amenable to disc protrusion, herniation, compression, or muscle pressure (e.g., piriformis pressure on the sciatic nerve). |

In clinical practice, the most common back pain presentation is of myofascial origin. In this condition, the affected muscle and fascia are usually the subject of an acute acceleration, commonly resulting from a sudden and unexpected motion (Travell & Simons, 1983). A typical example would be that of a whiplash injury. Consequent to the injury, there is a localized inflammation resulting from fiber or fascial damage. Consequent to the inflammation, there may be scarring, frequently in the form clinically recognized as tender or trigger points. The generalized, inflammation-type pain may become more specific and recognizable as myofascial-type pain (Braddom, 1996; Pope, Anderson, Frymoyer, & Chaffin, 1991).

The myofascial unit may contract in a "splinting activity," and the resulting localized contraction may disrupt the functional and structural integrity of a whole muscle. Moreover, there is subsequent disruption of the primary myotatic or functional unit, which can affect additional adjacent functional units (Travell & Simons, 1983).

Muscles and myotatic units function in contralateral pairs. In the case of the back,

structural and functional myotatic balance is paramount to the standing and sitting positions, ambulation, gait, and posture. To understand back pain, it is relevant to understand the anatomy, kinesiology, and kinesiopathology of the myofascial mantle of the trunk (Travell & Simons, 1983). Back pain is a disruption of the equilibrium of at least one component and affects the whole structure. In the bipedal position, the trunk muscles have to function in a balanced and well-supporting manner while contending with (1) the gravitational pull, (2) the weight and positional change of the heavy head on the relatively weaker neck, (3) the ballistic and weight-carrying requirements of the upper limbs, and (4) the stance, gait, posture, and ambulation requirements of the lower limbs. Any disruption of equilibrium due to myofascial injury will be reflected in back or trunk dysfunction, including pain.

## Psychophysiological and Psychological Profiles

Once myotatic/myofascial dysfunction is under way, the transmission of pain also brings into play a number of additional psychological and neurophysiological mechanisms. Melzack and Wall (1988) developed the gate theory, later updated as the neuromatrix theory, which highlights the role of a number of excitatory and inhibitory mechanisms in the final experience of pain. Between the periphery and the brain, the original pain signal can be magnified, minimized, and changed in quality to form the final pain experience. Neurochemical, cognitive, affective, and interpersonal factors influence the final pain experience and the degree of suffering. Nelson (1999) reviews current theories of pain transmission. He emphasizes that once established, a neurosignature of pain—a pattern of nerve impulses associated with pain—can be evoked repeatedly by new sensory inputs and by a variety of psychological and psychophysiological triggers.

### Behavioral Profile

The trunk muscles comprise neck muscles (e.g., sternocleidomastoid, or SCM), upper-back muscles (e.g., trapezius), midback muscles (e.g., latissimus dorsi), paraspinal muscles, and thoracic muscles (e.g., pectoralis major and minor). They serve mainly a postural and support function, helping to maintain the body and trunk erect or in the sitting position, and are paramount to flexing, extending, rotating, and bending. Some trunk muscles also assist in respiration. Muscles that derive from the branchial arches serve "double duty," postural support and emotional expression.

Emotions such as anxiety and joy are conveyed by these muscles through different patterns of breathing. The branchial-derived muscles of the neck and upper back show emotions such as sadness or pride through the posture. The paraspinal muscles, especially those of the lumbosacral area, convey arrogance or submission through changes in back posture. Altogether, the trunk muscles

convey a body language of power or sexual expression. This expressive function of the body further implicates itself in the previously mentioned neuromatrix of pain transmission. Functional bracing of the musculature under emotional stress interacts with emotionally based activation of the limbic brain and autonomic nervous systems to increase the magnitude of the pain experience and color the affective tone of that experience.

## TYPICAL SYMPTOM PROFILE AND DIAGNOSTIC ASSESSMENT

The presence and magnitude of several common features define the individual patient's muscular pain syndrome.

1. The intensity and frequency of pain in specific trunk locations.

2. The presence of tender or trigger points and pain radiating from those points.

3. The presence of radicular- or neuritic-related pain on the trunk.

4. The effects of pain on sleep, urination, defecation, and sexual intercourse.

5. The effects of pain on the ability to exercise, especially in terms of the trunk range of motion.

6. Any changes in pain pattern, intensity, or frequency related to changes in the level of emotional tension.

The diagnostic criteria for muscular pain syndrome include (1) the absence of neurological involvement (ruling out disc disease or herniation or the compression of nerve roots at any particular vertebral level); (2) the absence of neurological involvement in terms of radicular or neuritic radiation to well-defined dermatomes; and (3) the absence of organ disease that radiates pain to the trunk dermatomes.

The diagnostic examination identifies specific myofascial involvement, including

---

**Box 19.1** Screening for Chronic Back Pain

Health professionals who suspect the presence of a back pain disorder should gather information on the following as a brief screen:

1. History of the back pain: etiology in terms of trauma, repetitive motion, or other occupational disease; concomitance with other organ or system disease, states of tension, etc.
2. Location of the pain in a specific trunk region, such as thorax, upper back, mid-back, low back or hip, abdomen, pelvis, or in a combination of regions.
3. Intensity and frequency of the trunk pain on a semiquantitative scale.
4. Difficulties with performance of trunk or back range of motion in the course of activities of daily living or vocational tasks.
5. Effect of tension of emotional origin on the intensity and frequency of the pain and the converse—i.e., the effect of the trunk pain on the emotional state or intensity of tension.
6. Effect of the trunk pain on family and social relationships.
7. Effect of the pain on financial status.

---

(1) the presence of primary or secondary trigger points and myofascial pain radiation in well-defined or maverick patterns; and (2) varying degrees of effects of muscular dysfunction on vegetative functions and the converse (e.g., emotional tension can increase the activity of accessory muscles of respiration, such as the SCM and trapezius, causing overall fatigue and development of spasm, tender points, and pain in those muscles).

Assessing a patient who suffers from back pain begins with a complete history of injury, pain, and any medical and therapeutic interventions (see Box 19.1). Traditional medical testing and psychological testing relevant to chronic back pain are both important to assessment (see Boxes 19.2 and 19.3).

Criteria for behavioral assessment include the presence of pain and related symptoms in the absence of organic manifestations or history of trauma. Behavioral assessment identifies a possible need for a combination of treatments, including psychotherapy, physical or occupational therapy, and

pharmacotherapy for trunk pain and related symptoms. Behavioral assessment also identifies the role of emotional tension in the etiology of pain.

Differential diagnosis in chronic back pain includes screening for systemic diseases that can produce trunk pain, weakness, and other symptoms. In the primary or metastatic state, cancer can produce pain and weakness. Endocrine disease (e.g., hyper- or hypothyroidism) can cause muscular weakness, tension, and fatigue. Muscular weakness and fatigue are also associated with adrenal disease (e.g., Cushing's syndrome). Metabolic diseases such as renal or liver disease can change the electrolyte balance and produce muscular weakness, tremor, and fatigue.

Myofascial pain syndrome, secondary to trauma or to other etiology, often produces localized and/or radiating muscle pain and dysfunction. Neurological disease invariably produces muscle weakness, functional imbalance, pain, and fatigue. Psychophysiological states, including fibromyalgia and chronic fatigue, cause pain, weakness, and fatigue

---

**Box 19.2**     Medical Testing in the Assessment of Chronic Back Pain

1. X rays of vertebral column, thoracic cage, and pelvic bones to rule out fractures or arthrosis.
2. Bone scan to rule out occult disease, such as cancer, trauma, and rheumatic conditions.
3. MRI or CT scan to rule out disc disease or fracture conditions not visible on simple X rays.
4. CT scan or myelogram done in conditions of neurologic disease to rule out severe nerve compression (necessary before disc or other surgery).
5. Laboratory testing, including biochemistry and muscular enzymes to rule out muscular disease.
6. Laboratory testing aimed at end-organ disease that may affect the myofascial mantle.

---

**Box 19.3**     Common Reasons for Psychological Testing in the Assessment of Chronic Back Pain

1. Preoperative screening to rule out personality traits which would point to a negative functional outcome of surgery in terms of poor medical compliance, ineffective pain reduction, and poor prognosis for return to a normal lifestyle.
2. The need for understanding of emotional states, especially depression and anxiety, that may modulate the intensity or frequency of trunk symptoms, especially pain.
3. Special testing related to specific conditions, such as psychological testing of personality, mood, and cognitive traits in conditions such as dyspareunia with pelvic muscle pain.

---

(see Chapter 23 on fibromyalgia and Chapter 24 on chronic fatigue syndrome).

## ANATOMY, PHYSIOLOGY, AND PATHOLOGY

Bony functional anatomy relies on the intact structure and structural relationships of the vertebrae, facets and related structures, discs, and ligaments. Any disruption in the equilibrium of these structures will automatically result in vertebromuscular imbalance and resulting dysfunction, including gait and postural disequilibria and pain. Muscular anatomy and myofascial mantle connections must be intact to provide natural equilibrium in stance and gait. Although the trunk muscles are interconnected by the fascial mantle and function as a unit, it is relevant to understand the trunk as a three-dimensional entity. The anterior aspect is formed by the anterior thoracic muscles and the abdominal muscles. The inferior aspect is formed by the pelvic muscles, connected fascially and through the bones to the anterior muscles and to the posterior or hip muscles. The lateral musculature creates a bridge between the anterior and posterior aspects and serves in motions such as bending and rotating, in respiratory functions, and in structural support to the anterior and posterior muscles. The posterior muscles can be divided into two groups: (1) the paravertebral (paraspinal) muscles, which are connected directly and only to the vertebrae, and (2) the superficial group, which connects the thoracolumbar region to the hip and to the neck and shoulder on the other (e.g., the latissimus dorsi).

There are two components of innervation to the trunk muscles: (1) sensory and motor neurons, including pain fibers, of the central nervous system, and (2) the sympathetic and parasympathetic fibers of the autonomic nervous system. The intactness of bilateral neural stimulation is paramount to the equilibrium of the back musculature function.

The neural input serves several functions, the most common of which is postural, in terms of maintenance of gait and support for the activity of the ballistic muscles of the limbs. A related function is specific to the maintenance of the head and neck in neutral position and the hip and lower limbs in stance and ambulatory functions. Disruption of neural innervation naturally biases the equilibrium in favor of the intact component and renders postural equilibrium impossible.

When conduction of the autonomic nervous system is disrupted, vegetative dysfunction (e.g., incontinence) and changes in the tone of muscles that become dysfunctional (e.g., pelvic floor pain) can result.

The pathology of back pain comprises myofascial, neurological, endocrine, and traumatic factors.

- Primary trigger points can elicit the formation of secondary trigger points.
- Protective guarding and other defensive movements can become more dysfunctional in time, leading to possible brain engram changes and chronic muscular dysfunctions.
- Root compression and nerve compression lead to muscular weakness, pain, and fatigue.

- Metabolic disease or cancer directly produce pain and dysfunction.
- Physical trauma can affect any organ in the trunk region.

## RESEARCH ON BEHAVIORAL INTERVENTIONS

SEMG is an electrophysiological modality. From the vantage point of the skin, SEMG assesses the electric potentials generated by skeletal muscles during rest or activity. It is a dual assessment modality for the electric potentials either in the amplitude domain (the summation of action potentials during any moment in time) or in the frequency domain (the summation of action potentials at any given frequency in time). SEMG is commonly used to assess muscular electric potentials in health and disease. It is used just as commonly in its neuromuscular reeducation or biofeedback role to retrain and normalize control of skeletal muscles found to express abnormal patterns of electrical potentials during rest or activity.

SEMG has been the subject of several studies (Ahern, Follick, Council, Laser-Wolston, & Litchman, 1988; Biederman, Inglis, & Monga, 1989; Dolce & Raczynski, 1985; Nicolaisen & Jorgensen, 1985; Nouwen, VanAkkerveeken, & Versloot, 1987; Robinson, Cassisi, O'Connor, MacMillan, 1992; Roy, DeLuca, Emley, & Buijs, 1995; Seidel, Beyer, & Brauer, 1987; Sihvonen, Partanen, & Hanninen, 1998; Wolf & Basmajian, 1977; Wolf, Basmajian, Russe, & Kutner, 1979). Although the studies have been very useful for the field, large sample studies on the subject of behavioral investigation and protocols for treatment are needed, especially in the area of chronic back and trunk pain. Ideally, there should be multicenter, double-blind, prospective studies in the area of behavioral/biofeedback investigation and treatment modalities.

Using SEMG, the author tested 6,400 muscles, and the data derived from this study form the bases of several books and articles (Sella, 1997, 1998a, 1998b, 1999a, 1999b, 1999c, 2000a, 2000b, 2000c, 2000d, 2000e, 2000f). Part of the study focused on the muscular activity of several muscles through the trunk range of motion (Sella, 1999b, 1999c, 2000c, 2000d, 2000e, 2000f). Data are presented in this chapter on statistical SEMG activity and resting potentials patterns, based on comparisons between muscles of asymptomatic individuals and those of patients with myofascial pain syndrome.

Table 19.2 presents the largest normative database created to date on the subject of the SEMG of the segmental range of motion of the back and trunk. It comprises 1,098 muscles tested through activity and rest for seven segments of the trunk and back. The activity and resting averages (μV RMS) and the normalization (percent) to the average group value are presented for 19 muscles. The data are used as reference value for the SEMG testing of symptomatic and asymptomatic muscles of 102 individuals with myofascial pain syndrome (MPS).

Table 19.3 shows that for asymptomatic muscles at rest, the ratio of resting values to reference values is about 60 percent. For symptomatic muscles at rest, the ratio of the resting values to the reference (asymptomatic) values is about 180 percent. The data for the muscular activity of the asymptomatic muscles are roughly 70 percent of those of the reference values. The activity value of symptomatic muscles is roughly 200 percent higher than that of the reference (asymptomatic) values.

Hence, the data from Table 19.3 demonstrate that individuals with back complaints diagnosed with MPS have resting values approximately 180 percent higher and activity values 200 percent higher than asymptomatic individuals. Thus SEMG investigation provides a clear diagnostic differentiation of symptomatic versus asymptomatic muscles in the condition of MPS. Data from symptomatic muscles in a variety of diagnoses of conditions presenting with back pain are awaited at the clinical and epidemiological levels.

## TREATMENT PROTOCOLS

### Classical Medical Protocols

Physical and occupational therapy protocols typically involve one to three months of exercise, three times a week, aimed at functional musculoskeletal rehabilitation. The primary goal of active physical therapy is to restore agility, range of motion, strength, and endurance. Passive physical therapy aims to reduce pain and inflammation through neurostimulation, transcutaneous electrical nerve stimulation (TENS), ultrasound, and similar procedures. Trigger point injections are frequently followed by range-of-motion and stretching exercises. Medical therapies largely consist of medication for analgesia and muscular relaxation. Chiropractic or osteopathic therapies include specialized massage and other passive manual manipulations of the spine and musculature. Neurosurgical procedures, which are rarely needed, reduce nerve or root complexion and subsequent muscular dysfunction.

### Alternative Medicine Protocols

Because of the relative lack of success of most of the classical medical protocols, the last few years have seen the increased development and popular approval of "alternative" treatments. These include acupuncture, moxibustion, and herbal remedies.

### Behavioral Protocols

The behavioral protocols include biofeedback, hypnosis, psychotherapy (including

Table 19.2    SEMG of 19 Trunk Muscles, Database Values (μV RMS) and Ranking

| Muscle | Number | Flexing | Extending | Rotating | Bending | Squatting | Average ± Standard Deviation | Normalization (percent) | Resting Average | Normalization (percent) |
|---|---|---|---|---|---|---|---|---|---|---|
| Levator scapulae | 10 | 10.1 | 18.1 | 13.3 | 6.2 | 11.2 | 11.2 ± .7 | 196 | 6.9 | 283 |
| Upper trapezius | 51 | 11.4 | 10.5 | 8 | 7.2 | 10.5 | 9 ± .48 | 157 | 4.1 | 168 |
| L1 paraspinal | 155 | 11.3 | 3.3 | 10.2 | 5.6 | 9.6 | 8 ± .43 | 140 | 2.58 | 106 |
| L3 paraspinal | 39 | 14.1 | 3.4 | 9 | 4.8 | 9.3 | 7.8 ± .33 | 136 | 2.2 | 90 |
| T8 paraspinal | 39 | 7.8 | 6.1 | 9.6 | 5.6 | 9.6 | 7.7 ± .5 | 135 | 3.31 | 136 |
| L5 paraspinal | 304 | 10.1 | 3.6 | 8.9 | 6.7 | 7.8 | 7.6 ± .41 | 133 | 2.01 | 82 |
| Quadratus lumborum | 110 | 6.4 | 3.1 | 8.2 | 5 | 6.2 | 6 ± .42 | 105 | 2.49 | 102 |
| Latissimus dorsi | 28 | 7.4 | 4.3 | 3.9 | 5.3 | 6.7 | 5.2 ± .25 | 91 | 2.12 | 87 |
| Internal oblique | 23 | 3.3 | 8 | 3.8 | 5.3 | 5.7 | 5 ± .24 | 87 | 1.26 | 52 |
| Gluteus maximus | 70 | 6.2 | 3.4 | 4.5 | 5.6 | 5.2 | 5 ± .26 | 87 | 1.84 | 75 |
| Transversus abdominis | 23 | 2 | 11.3 | 5.7 | 4.4 | 3.1 | 5 ± .28 | 87 | 2.11 | 86 |
| T1 paraspinal | 70 | 6.2 | 4 | 4.8 | 4.2 | 5.1 | 4.7 ± .25 | 82 | 2.39 | 98 |
| Intercostalis VII | 18 | 1.4 | 3.6 | 5.9 | 6.2 | 1.5 | 4.4 ± .31 | 77 | 1.12 | 46 |
| External oblique | 40 | 3.4 | 3.7 | 4.2 | 4.6 | 4.3 | 4.1 ± .24 | 71 | 1.81 | 74 |
| Gluteus medius | 28 | 3.5 | 5.7 | 4.1 | 4 | 3.5 | 4.1 ± .63 | 71 | 1.8 | 74 |
| Pectoralis major | 28 | 2.4 | 4.7 | 3.5 | 4 | 5.5 | 3.9 ± .26 | 68 | 1.48 | 61 |
| T7 paraspinal | 12 | 9.7 | 2.1 | 3.7 | 1.4 | 3.5 | 3.5 ± 3 | 61 | 3.3 | 135 |
| Rhomboid major | 12 | 3.9 | 2.9 | 2.8 | 3.3 | 3.1 | 3.2 ± .09 | 56 | 2.3 | 94 |
| Rectus abdominis | 38 | 2.7 | 4.9 | 2.6 | 3 | 3.5 | 3.2 ± .19 | 56 | 1.2 | 49 |
| Total | 1,098 | 6.5 | 5.6 | 6.1 | 4.4 | 6 | 5.7 ± .3 | 100 | 2.44 | 100 |

**Table 19.3**  SEMG Testing for Musculoskeletal Pain Syndrome: Asymptomatic and Symptomatic Muscle Tonus (µV) and Ratio to Reference Values

| Muscles | Number | Resting Asymptomatic Tonus | Ratio (percent) | Resting Symptomatic Tonus | Ratio (percent) | Activity Asymptomatic Tonus | Ratio (percent) | Activity Symptomatic Tonus | Ratio (percent) |
|---|---|---|---|---|---|---|---|---|---|
| | | | | **Paraspinal** | | | | | |
| Reference T1 | 6 | 2.39 | 41 | | 145.2 | 4.7 | 42.3 | | 151.3 |
| T1 | | 0.98 | | 3.47 | | 1.99 | | 7.11 | |
| Reference T7 | 1 | 3.3 | 37.6 | | 50.3 | 3.5 | 90.6 | | 130.6 |
| T7 | | 1.24 | | 1.66 | | 3.17 | | 4.57 | |
| Reference T8 | 3 | 3.3 | 78.2 | | 161.8 | 7.7 | 103.9 | | 226.8 |
| T8 | | 2.58 | | 5.34 | | 8 | | 17.46 | |
| Reference L1 | 23 | 2.58 | 72.9 | | 151.2 | 8 | 68 | | 161.9 |
| L1 | | 1.88 | | 3.9 | | 5.44 | | 12.95 | |
| Reference L5 | 22 | 2.01 | 84.6 | | 268.7 | 7.6 | 68.4 | | 184.2 |
| L5 | | 1.7 | | 5.4 | | 5.2 | | 14 | |
| **Average ratio (percent)** | | | 62.8 | | 155.4 | | 74.6 | | 170.9 |
| **Total number** | 55 | | | | | | | | |
| | | | | **Midback and hip** | | | | | |
| Reference quadratus lumborum | 21 | 2.49 | 61.8 | | 135.3 | 6 | 75.2 | | 219.5 |
| Quadratus lumborum | | 1.54 | | 3.37 | | 4.51 | | 13.17 | |

| Muscles | Number | Resting Asymptomatic | | Resting Symptomatic | | Activity Asymptomatic | | Activity Symptomatic | |
|---|---|---|---|---|---|---|---|---|---|
| | | *Tonus* | *Ratio (percent)* | *Tonus* | *Ratio (percent)* | *Tonus* | *Ratio (percent)* | *Tonus* | *Ratio (percent)* |
| Reference gluteus maximus | 9 | 1.84 | 71.7 | | 178.3 | 5 | 86 | | 141.6 |
| Gluteus maximus | | 1.32 | | 3.28 | | 4.3 | | 7.1 | |
| **Average ratio (percent)** | | | **66.8** | | **156.8** | | **80.6** | | **180.6** |
| **Total number** | **30** | | | | | | | | |
| | | | | *Upper back and thoracic* | | | | | |
| Reference upper trapezius | 6 | 4.1 | 84.6 | | 185.4 | 9 | 63.6 | | 292.7 |
| Upper trapezius | | 3.47 | | 7.6 | | 5.72 | | 26.34 | |
| Reference levator scapulae | 5 | 6.9 | 38.8 | | 342.6 | 11.2 | 32.1 | | 224.3 |
| Levator scapulae | | 2.68 | | 23.64 | | 3.6 | | 25.12 | |
| Reference rhomboid major | 1 | 2.3 | 66.1 | | 136.1 | 3.2 | 97.8 | | N/A |
| Rhomboid major | | 1.52 | | 3.13 | | 3.13 | | N/A | |
| **Average ratio (percent)** | | | **63.2** | | **221.4** | | **64.5** | | **258.5** |
| **Total number** | **12** | | | | | | | | |
| **Overall average muscles ratio** | | | **64.3** | | **177.9** | | **73.2** | | **203.3** |

Note: Tonus = Electric potential of muscular tonus in μV RMS; ratio = of value to reference value.

cognitive therapy), and combinations of classical medical treatment and psychophysiological modalities. Several biofeedback modalities are useful in training general relaxation (see Chapter 8 on biofeedback and Chapter 10 on relaxation strategies). General relaxation in turn serves to reduce sympathetic innervations of the muscles, via the muscle spindles, reducing excess activation. General relaxation also reduces pain transmission and renders pain more tolerable for the individual. The use of SEMG biofeedback directly serves to reduce chronic lingering muscle tensions, reduce co-contraction in adjacent and distant muscle groups, and reduce asymmetries in muscle tension and activation. Cognitive therapy and hypnosis alter the subjective perception of pain by changing the individual's interpretations and attributions about pain and by helping the individual focus on something other than pain. Psychotherapy serves to moderate depression and anxiety, both of which exacerbate pain, and redirect the individual's behavior and attention into adaptive coping behaviors and psychosocial activities.

## Neurofeedback

Neurofeedback, or EEG biofeedback, also has many applications to chronic pain. A number of small studies and anecdotal reports describe the use of alpha-theta slow-wave training, to reduce overall cortical activation, or to reduce focal areas of hyper-activation, producing a reduction in the intensity of pain (Byers, 1998, pp. 141–149).

In addition, Rosenfeld (1998) has trained specific brain responses (somatosensory-evoked potentials) in rats and humans and demonstrated specific changes in the perception of pain. Further research is needed to refine protocols and demonstrate the efficacy of neurofeedback for pain.

## OUTCOME STUDIES

### Clinical Efficacy

Most back pain suffering lasts between one and two months. It is more likely that these data refer to pain of functional origin, such as simple sprain or strain. Treatment in the form of medication (muscle relaxants, nonsteroidal analgesics and anti-inflammatories) in combination with active and passive physical therapy usually suffices for pain and spasm relief. Five percent of back pain sufferers become chronic—that is, experience symptoms that last for more than three to six months. A small number of these persons have disc-related pathology and end up with discectomies. The general results are good in only 50 percent of these cases. Most chronic back pain sufferers have a number of psychological issues affecting their pain, including depression resulting directly from the pain as well as the socioeconomic difficulties related to lack of work.

A number of chronic patients develop MPS. In the best scenario, MPS symptoms can be relieved within three to six months, which allows the back pain sufferer to return to a normal lifestyle. All too often, however, problems involving insurance and workers compensation cause delays in treatment. Anxiety and depression combined with economic and family problems can slow the process of healing and prevent the individual from returning to a normal lifestyle. Until society addresses this problem seriously, back pain will cost society and the citizen enormous amounts of money that would be better used for treatment and vocational rehabilitation. Unfortunately outcome studies of chronic back pain suffering are not yet available, because there are no funds available to look into what society does not want to see.

When behavioral interventions are implemented along with classical medical treatment, back pain or trunk pain suffering can be relieved better than with either modality alone. The SEMG biofeedback component, applied properly to specific suffering muscles and not to ill-defined regions, helps teach the patient the control and self-reliance necessary to relearn and apply normal motions rather than consistently employing dysfunctional muscular activities during motion or rest. There is no other modality that can teach patients "anew" how to perform muscular movements in a normal fashion and to control resting in such a way that muscles can really rest.

## Cost-Effectiveness of Recommended Interventions

Combining classical medical and physical therapy with SEMG biofeedback is practical and cost-effective for the following reasons:

1. The combined treatment is more intensive and shorter, usually lasting only three months.

2. Only with the addition of SEMG biofeedback can the patient learn how to move or relax affected muscles and thus achieve self-control.

3. Muscular dysfunction and pain (in that order) are reduced as the patient learns the relationship between improving muscular function and lessening pain.

4. Medical and legal proof of improvement is gained when the patient is motivated to improve the level of dysfunction, lack of improvement is obvious in unmotivated patients, who should be placed into another program.

Patients who are not motivated to follow the SEMG biofeedback program and seek narcotic analgesics instead require a program of psychological counseling.

## THE SELECTION OF ALTERNATIVE TREATMENTS FOR BACK PAIN

As discussed in the previous sections, back pain needs to be considered within the topic of trunk pain. Trunk pain may result from a number of etiologies. Therefore, treatment should be directed to the specific etiology and diagnosis. In behavioral medicine, as in traditional medicine, there is a benign neglect of the fact that back pain of musculoskeletal origin needs to be investigated and treated comprehensively. The treatment should include self-control and self-understanding methodologies, especially including SEMG biofeedback in conjunction with psychological counseling (mainly cognitive psychotherapy) in cases of chronic back pain.

The use of behavioral or biofeedback therapy without a thorough medical investigation or the use of medical treatment without concomitant SEMG muscular testing and SEMG biofeedback treatment offers only drawbacks and demonstrates the lack of bridging between the two treatment paradigms. The patient is the loser, and society as a whole pays the price for the lack of communication and collaboration between the two bona fide fields.

In some cases, other alternative therapies, single or in combination, may be useful to relieve the pain, although no long-term studies have been done. As scientists, we need to keep our eyes open to new developments and use them in a focused manner whenever warranted.

# REFERENCES

Ahern, D. K., Follick, M. J., Council, J. R., Laser-Wolston, N., & Litchman, H. (1988). Comparison of lumbar paravertebral EMG patterns in chronic low back pain patients and non-patient controls. *Pain, 34,* 153–160.

Biederman, H. J., Inglis, J., & Monga, T. N. (1989). Differential treatment responses on somatic pain indicators after EMG biofeedback training in back pain patients. *International Journal of Psychosomatics, 36,* 53–57.

Bigos, S. J., & Battie, M. C. (1987). Surveillance of back problems in industry. In N. M. Hadler (Ed.), *Clinical concepts in regional musculoskeletal illness* (pp. 99–315). New York: Grune & Stratton.

Braddom, R. L. (Ed.). (1996). *Physical medicine and rehabilitation.* Philadelphia: W. B. Saunders.

Byers, A. P. (Ed.) (1998). *The Byers neurotherapy reference library* (2nd ed.). Wheat Ridge, CO: Association for Applied Psychophysiology and Biofeedback.

Cailliet, R. (1993). *Pain: Mechanism and management. R. Cailliet Pain Series.* Philadelphia: Davis.

Dolce, J. J., & Raczynski, J. M. (1985). Neuromuscular activity and electromyography in painful backs: Psychological & biomechanical models in assessment and treatment. *Psychological Bulletin, 97,* 502–520.

Hollingshead, W. H. (1976). *Functional anatomy of the limbs and back.* Philadelphia: W. B. Saunders.

Maigne, R. (1996). *Diagnosis and treatment of pain of vertebral origin.* Baltimore: Williams & Wilkins.

Melzack, R., & Wall, P. D. (1988). *The challenge of pain.* New York: Penguin.

Nelson, D. V. (1999). Understanding chronic pain: Whither biofeedback? *Biofeedback, 27(3),* 4–15.

Nicolaisen, T., & Jorgensen, K. (1985). Trunk strength, back muscle endurance and low-back trouble. *Scandinavian Journal of Rehabilitative Medicine, 17,* 121–127.

Nouwen, A., VanAkkerveeken, P. F., & Versloot, J. M. (1987). Patterns of muscular activity during movement in patients with chronic low back pain. *Spine, 12(8),* 777–782.

Pope, M., Anderson, G., Frymoyer, J., & Chaffin, D. (Eds.). (1991). *Occupational low back pain assessment, treatment and prevention.* St. Louis, MO: Mosby.

Robinson, M. E., Cassisi, J. E., O'Connor, P. D., & MacMillan, M. (1992). Lumbar SEMG during isotonic exercise. Chronic low back pain patients vs. controls. *Journal of Spinal Disorders, 5,* 1.

Rosenfeld, P. J. (1998). Neurotherapy for pain management. In A. P. Byers (Ed.), *The Byers neurotherapy reference library* (2nd ed., pp. ix). Wheat Ridge, CO: Association for Applied Psychophysiology and Biofeedback.

Roy, S. H., DeLuca, C. J., Emley, M., & Buijs, R. J. C. (1995). Spectral EMG assessment of back muscles in patients with low back pain undergoing rehabilitation. *Spine, 20(1),* 38–48.

Seidel, H., Beyer, H. & Brauer, D. (1987). Electromyographic evaluation of back muscle fatigue with repeated sustained contraction of different strengths. *European Journal of Applied Physiology, 56,* 592–602.

Sella, G. E. (1997). Gender patterns of muscular utilization: The S-EMG analysis of the elbow range of motion. *Disability: The International Journal of the American Academy of Disability Evaluating Physicians, 6(3),* 1–24.

Sella, G. E. (1998a). Surface EMG (S-EMG) analysis of the shoulder range of motion. *Disability: The International Journal of the American Academy of Disability Evaluating Physicians, 7(2),* 171–181.

Sella, G. E. (1998b). Muscular activity of the shoulder range of motion: Surface EMG (S-EMG) analysis. *Europa MedicoPhysica, 34*(4), 19–36.

Sella, G. E. (1999a). S-EMG of the hip ROM protocol: A study of consistency and repeatability/reliability of electrical activity of nineteen muscles. *Europa MedicoPhysica, 35*(2), 83–92.

Sella, G. E. (1999b). *Neuro-muscular testing with S-EMG* (2nd ed.). Martins Ferry, OH: GENMED Publishing.

Sella, G. E. (1999c). *Muscles in motion: Surface EMG analysis of the human body range of motion* (3rd ed.). Martins Ferry, OH: GENMED Publishing.

Sella, G. E. (2000a). Dynamic S-EMG: A methodology for the establishment of normative database in trunk muscles of asymptomatic individuals [Abstract]. *Back Pain and Disability Unraveling Puzzle*, New York University Medical Center, November 30–December 2, 2000.

Sella, G. E. (2000b, December). Surface electromyography testing: Sensitivity, specificity, positive and negative predictive values. *Europa MedicoPhysica, 36*(4), 183–190.

Sella, G. E. (2000c). *Guidelines for neuro-muscular re-education with S-EMG biofeedback.* Martins Ferry, OH: GENMED Publishing.

Sella, G. E. (2000d). *Graphics of motion: The electromyography of muscular dynamics.* Martins Ferry, OH: GENMED Publishing.

Sella, G. E. (2000e). *Muscular dynamics: Electromyography assessment of energy and motion.* Martins Ferry, OH: GENMED Publishing.

Sella, G. E. (2000f). Internal consistency, reproducibility and reliability of S-EMG testing. *Europa MedicoPhysica, 36*(1), 31–38.

Sihvonen, T., Partanen, J., & Hanninen, O. (1998). Averaged (RMS) surface EMG in testing back function. *Electromyography and Clinical Neurophysiology, 28*, 335–339.

Travell, J., & Simons, D. (1983). *Myofascial pain and dysfunction: A trigger point manual* (Vols. I & II). Baltimore: Williams & Wilkins.

Wolf, S. L., & Basmajian, J. V. (1977). Assessment of paraspinal electromyographic activity in normal subjects and in chronic back pain patients using a muscle biofeedback device. In E. Asmussen & K. Jorgensen (Eds.), *Biomechanics VI-B* (pp. 319–324). Baltimore: University Park Press.

Wolf, S. L., Basmajian, J. V., Russe, C., & Kutner, M. (1979). Normative data on low back mobility and activity levels. *American Journal of Physical Medicine, 58*, 217–229.

# CHAPTER 20

# The Metabolic Syndrome: Obesity, Type 2 Diabetes, Hypertension, and Hyperlipidemia

ANGELE McGRADY, RAYMOND BOUREY, AND BARBARA BAILEY

**Abstract:** The metabolic syndrome should be approached as an entity because diabetes, hypertension, hyperlipidemia, and obesity share common etiological, physiological, and psychological factors. The practitioner treating patients with this syndrome should consider that inactivity and overeating, superimposed on genetic predisposition, form a cascade of metabolic events leading to overt disease. Psychological and social factors have an impact on etiology and maintenance of the disorder. Medical, psychophysiological therapies, and lifestyle modifications are best combined to achieve positive outcomes.

## INTRODUCTION TO THE METABOLIC SYNDROME

An epidemic rages at a staggering pace, for the first time unrelated to infectious or toxic agents. The comorbid conditions of abdominal obesity, type 2 diabetes, hypertension, and hyperlipidemia have their roots in evolutionarily and genetically determined inactivity and hedonistic appetites. Once present, the components of this deadly quartet, now termed the metabolic syndrome, confer significant risk for cardiovascular and cerebrovascular disease (Bouchard, 1995; Pi-Sunyer, Laferrere, Aronne, & Bray, 1999; Zimmet, McCarty, & de Courten, 1997).

The apparent behavioral basis of the metabolic syndrome makes it, on the surface, well suited to nonpharmacological intervention. However, two factors make it difficult to design programs that are acceptable to patients: (1) Fatigue and lassitude are the only overt symptoms, and (2) successful treatment depends on patient compliance. Therefore, many practitioners avoid nonpharmacological approaches.

We have chosen to focus on the metabolic syndrome (including type 2 diabetes) at the expense of its less common metabolic relatives. Primary care of patients with type 1 diabetes (formerly called insulin-dependent diabetes mellitus) or gestational diabetes is best assigned to subspecialists in diabetology with support by a team of nurse-educators, dietitians, exercise physiologists, social workers, and psychologists. Issues facing medical caregivers of these patients are beyond the scope of this chapter.

## TYPE 2 DIABETES MELLITUS

### Definition and Diagnosis

Diabetes mellitus is a state characterized by hyperglycemia. Seemingly simple, the diagnosis of diabetes is confounded by the definition of hyperglycemia and the variability of human physiology. The level of blood glucose that defines diabetes has been debated and modified through three major consensus efforts in the last 25 years (Expert Committee, 1997). Significant hyperglycemia predicts pathology, but even minimal elevations in blood glucose have been associated with pancreatic islet dysfunction (Bourey et al., 1993) and vascular disease (Barrett-Connor, Wingard, Criqui, & Suarez, 1984; Haffner, 1998; Mykkanen, Laakso, Penttila, & Pyorala, 1991; Stamler et al., 1979; Yeap, Russo, Fraser, Wittert, & Horowitz, 1996).

Type 2 diabetes is associated with insulin resistance and defective insulin secretion. Although previously referred to as noninsulin-dependent diabetes mellitus, most patients require insulin within five years of diagnosis. The term *adult-onset diabetes* implies another characteristic of this disease that is no longer pathognomonic. Not only do more than 10 percent of adult-onset diabetics demonstrate a typical autoimmune-mediated response similar to type 1 at onset of the disease (Tuomi, Carlsson, et al., 1999; Tuomi, Group, et al., 1993), but type 2 diabetes is occurring more frequently in children and adolescents (Ledermann, 1995; Lehto et al., 1997).

Table 20.1 shows the diagnostic criteria for type 2 diabetes recently adopted by the American Diabetes Association (2001).

### Prevalence

The Centers for Disease Control and Prevention (1998) estimate that about 6 percent of the population, or 15.7 million people, have diabetes, with 800,000 new cases diagnosed each year. Prevalence increases with age, obesity, hypertension, and hyperlipidemia. Type 2 diabetes tends to run in families, but research has yet to produce a common gene for susceptibility. The phenotype seems dependent on a particular environment and lifestyle, so diabetes does not usually occur in the absence of a sedentary lifestyle and easily available food. Perhaps the most striking example is that of the Pima Indians of Arizona. This group exhibits a prevalence of diabetes in middle-aged persons of 54 percent (men) and 37 percent (women) compared with their poorer relatives who scratch out an agrarian existence in the Sierra Madre Mountains of Mexico and carry only 6 percent and 11 percent prevalence, respectively (Ravussin, Valencia, Esparza, Bennett, & Schulz, 1994). Therefore, type 2 diabetes appears to arise as a consequence of behavioral patterns superimposed on a permissive genetic state and should be considered both preventable and, at least in its early stages, treatable by behavioral therapies.

## ESSENTIAL HYPERTENSION

### Definition and Diagnosis

A person suffering from hypertension is defined as having a "systolic blood pressure of 140 mm Hg or greater, diastolic blood pressure of 90 mm Hg or greater, or taking antihypertensive medication" (Joint National Committee, 1997). These seemingly arbitrary values were decided through several national consensus conferences weighing the data correlating blood pressure with the risk of end-organ damage over time. Thus the

**Table 20.1** Criteria for Diagnosis of Type 2 Diabetes

| State | Glucose Concentration [mg/dL (mM)] | | |
|---|---|---|---|
| | Whole blood Venous | Capillary | Plasma Venous |
| Fasting | >110 (6.1) | >110 (6.1) | >126 (11.1) |
| 2 hours postglucose load | >180 (10.0) | >200 (11.1) | >200 (11.1) |

presence of comorbid disorders influences the criterion blood pressure. Since cardiovascular disease is a major problem in persons with diabetes, the American Diabetes Association (2000b) blood pressure treatment goal for adults is less than 130/85 mm Hg.

Most hypertension runs in families and occurs without obvious etiology so is termed *essential hypertension (EHT)*, and indeed the name may be quite appropriate. Mechanisms to generate high blood pressure may confer evolutionary advantage in the face of either salt deprivation or massive blood loss and trauma (Neel, Weder, & Julius, 1998). The resultant high blood pressure may truly have been "essential" to survival and distinguishes EHT from the more uncommon hormonal causes of high blood pressure.

### Prevalence

Approximately 50 million Americans have sustained, elevated blood pressure (Burt et al., 1995). Although hypertension occurs in all races, special attention has been directed to the increased prevalence in African American men who demonstrate an earlier onset and more rapid rate of development of stage 3 hypertension (Joint National Committee, 1997).

### HYPERLIPIDEMIA

### Definition and Diagnosis

Until recently, population statistics were used to define normal cholesterol content as in the 250 to 300 mg/dL range. It is now recognized that those levels will, over the course of a lifetime, result in cholesterol accumulation in deposits in unwanted places like arterial walls. So, the term *desirable* cholesterol level has largely replaced the word (and the statistical concept of) *normal*. Hyperlipidemia is now defined as blood lipid levels that are not desirable. High total serum cholesterol is defined as levels greater than 240 mg/dL, which corresponds to the 80th percentile of the U.S. population (Expert Panel, 1993). The term *hyperlipidemia* subsumes all blood lipids, including cholesterol-carrying subtypes and triglycerides. Current recommendations derive from data on the association of calculated low-density lipoprotein (LDL) with heart disease. Table 20.2 summarizes the dietary and drug therapy of hyperlipidemia. Considering that the calculation of LDL also involves total cholesterol as well as high-density lipoprotein (HDL) and triglycerides, a simple definition of *hyperlipidemia* escapes us.

The definition of hyperlipidemia requiring pharmacotherapy has been tailored for groups with other associated risk factors for heart disease, such as family history of coronary heart disease, tobacco use, hypertension, and diabetes mellitus (Expert Panel, 1993). Once hyperlipidemia is identified, a search should proceed for possible exacerbating conditions. These include diabetes, hypothyroidism, and excessive alcohol use, as well as common medications such as estrogens and beta blockers. For individuals with diabetes, recommended levels are LDL

Table 20.2    Therapy of Hyperlipidemia

|  | Initiation Level | LDL Goal |
|---|---|---|
| *Dietary Therapy* | | |
| Without CHD and with fewer than 2 risk factors | ≥160 mg/dL | <160 mg/dL |
| Without CHD and with 2 or more risk factors | ≥130 mg/dL | <130 mg/dL |
| With CHD | >100 mg/dL | ≤100 mg/dL |
| *Drug Treatment* | *Consideration Level* | *LDL Goal* |
| Without CHD and with fewer than 2 risk factors | ≥190 mg/dL[a] | <160 mg/dL |
| Without CHD and with 2 or more risk factors | ≥160 mg/dL | <130 mg/dL |
| With CHD | ≥130 mg/dL[b] | ≤100 mg/dL |

SOURCE: Expert Panel (1993).

CHD = coronary heart disease.

a  In men under 35 years of age and premenopausal women with LDL cholesterol levels of 190–219 mg/dL, drug therapy should be delayed except in high-risk patients such as those with diabetes.

b  In CHD patients with LDL-cholesterol levels 100-129 mg/dL, the physician should exercise clinical judgment in deciding whether to initiate drug treatment.

cholesterol below 100 mg/dL, HDL cholesterol below 45 mg/dL, and triglycerides below 200 mg/dL (American Diabetes Association, 2000a).

## Prevalence

Due to ongoing changes in definition, true prevalence data for hyperlipidemia is difficult to obtain. If *hypercholesterolemia* is defined by values greater than 240 mg/dL, then about 20 percent of the adult population of the United States is afflicted (Expert Panel, 1993).

## LONG-TERM COMPLICATIONS OF THE METABOLIC SYNDROME

A striking association exists among the disorders of the metabolic syndrome in risk factors, etiology, and complications. The primary long-term effect of the syndrome is acceleration of atherosclerosis and increased incidence of cerebrovascular and cardiovascular events, including stroke and myocardial

infarction. Diabetes ravages the body through the effects of chronic hyperglycemia and associated glycosylation products that have an "aging" effect, causing deterioration of the vascular endothelium, the glomeruli, neural networks, and immune system. Progressive, irreversible damage to the pancreas results in further hyperglycemia and eventually insulin deficiency. Diabetes is the leading cause of new blindness, heart disease death, end-stage renal disease, and lower extremity amputations (Centers for Disease Control and Prevention, 1998). Patients with diabetes are 1.5 times more likely to be hospitalized and on average remain hospitalized for 1.7 more days than people who are not diabetic (Diabetes Research Working Group, 1999). The primary sites (and consequences) of damage attributed to hypertension are the arteries, (stroke or myocardial infarction), the heart (congestive heart failure), and the kidneys (proteinuria and failure). Hyperlipidemia is also associated with pathological sequelae, notably, coronary heart disease (Barrett-Connor et al., 1984; Groop, 2000).

**Table 20.3**  Sample Screening Questions for Diabetes

| Questions | Relevance |
|---|---|
| Do you have a family history of diabetes? | People with type 2 diabetes typically have other relatives with the disease. The genetic predisposition to diabetes increases from 25% if one parent has the disease to 50%–75% if both parents have it. |
| Are you over 45 years old? | Type 2 diabetes is typically diagnosed after age 40. The ADA recommends people over age 45 have a fasting plasma glucose test (no food intake for at least 8 hours). If it is normal (<126 mg/dL), then rescreen every 3 years. |
| Do you have polydipsia, polyphagia, and polyuria? | These are the 3 classic symptoms of diabetes. If a patient has these and a random plasma glucose level >200 mg/dL, then a diagnosis of diabetes can be made. |
| Are you at your desired body weight? | Obesity is a key risk factor for diabetes. Obesity is defined as >20% over desired body wt. or body mass index >27 kg/m². |
| What is your race or ethnic background? | Incidence of diabetes is more common in certain ethnic groups such as African Americans, Hispanics, American Indians, Asian Americans, and Pacific Islanders. |
| Have you ever been told that you had "borderline" diabetes or that your blood sugar was elevated? | Impaired glucose tolerance has often been referred to as borderline diabetes. These patients have had an elevated blood sugar but not high enough to meet diagnostic criteria. These patients are at high risk for developing overt diabetes if lifestyle changes are not implemented. |
| Do you have high blood pressure? | EHT can contribute to the chronic complications of diabetes (e.g., nephropathy, cardiovascular and neurovascular disease). |
| Do you have an elevated HDL and/or triglyceride level? | Low risk patients have: LDL <100 mg/dL, HDL >45 mg/dL, and triglycerides <200 mg/dL. |
| (Women) Do you have a history of gestational diabetes or babies weighing over 9 lbs at birth? | About 4% of women experience glucose intolerance during pregnancy. They are at high risk for developing diabetes after delivery. At 6 weeks postpartum, a 75-gram oral glucose tolerance test should be done. If normal, reevaluate every 3 years. |
| Are you taking steroids, thiazides, diuretics, estrogen, Dilantin, or nicotinic acid? | These drugs can cause impaired glucose tolerance and hyperglycemia. |

SOURCE: Adapted from the American Diabetes Association (2000a, 2000b).

## SCREENING

Because about 8 million people have undiagnosed diabetes (Centers for Disease Control and Prevention, 1998), screening patients for the disease is very important. Sample screening questions are listed in Table 20.3.

---

Box 20.1    Components of the Metabolic Syndrome

- Central obesity (visceral fat accumulation)
- Hypertension
- Hyperlipidemia: high LDL, low HDL, high triglycerides
- Insulin resistance
- Decreased thermogenic response
- Sex steroid abnormalities
- Hyperresponsive hypothalamic pituitary axis
- Low insulin-like growth factor (IGF-I)
- Depression
- Adrenal incidentalomata
- Fibrinolysis plasminogen activator inhibitor (PAI-1)
- Endothelial dysfunction
- Sakkinen
- Elevated resting heart rate
- Fatty liver

---

## PATHOPHYSIOLOGICAL AND PATHOPSYCHOLOGICAL MECHANISMS

The metabolic syndrome has evolved through the years to include several related problems, which are summarized in Box 20.1. The high incidence of obesity, diabetes, hypertension, and hyperlipidemia in the general population of Western societies strongly supports the notion of a common genetic and physiological backdrop, which might have, in the past, conferred an evolutionary advantage. Therefore, the hypothesis suggesting that the phenotype of the metabolic syndrome represents a morbid collision between genes essential to premodern survival and modern affluence has remained popular (Groop, 2000; Neel et al., 1998).

The psychophysiological mechanisms underlying the metabolic syndrome are increased appetite, poor food choices, and a behavioral tendency to inactivity. Low socioeconomic status is associated with an unhealthy lifestyle, poor eating habits, and lack of exercise. In a study of healthy women, 63 percent of the association between obesity and low socioeconomic status could be explained by reproductive history, maladaptive dietary habits, and a composite of psychological factors comprising self-esteem and job strain (Wamala, Wolk, & Orth-Gomer, 1997). In the Whitehall study of people with and without diabetes, heart disease was higher in the lowest socioeconomic group, and mortality among diabetic people in the lowest socioeconomic group was twice as high as that of diabetic persons in the highest socioeconomic group (Chaturvedi, Jarrett, Shipley, & Fuller, 1998). Urban adults with low socioeconomic status also demonstrated an increased risk for cardiovascular disease (Winkleby, Kraemer, Ahn, & Varady, 1998). In blacks, the presence of three or more risk factors was associated with low income and education, substantiating the influence of poverty, fewer food choices, and lack of knowledge about healthy living habits (Diez-Roux, Northridge, Morabia, Bassett, & Shea, 1999).

The impact of stressful life events on physiology is particularly relevant to the metabolic syndrome. Perceived stress accompanied by a defeatist attitude leads to activation of the hypothalamic-pituitary-adrenal (HPA) axis, and high cortisol levels antagonize the actions of insulin. For example, people who have experienced very stressful events (e.g., the death of a partner and moving from a cherished family home) are more likely to test positive for diabetes during screening. The stress-induced alteration of endocrine function must affect the pancreatic beta cells for a sufficient time to produce the prediabetic condition; short-term exposure is without serious consequences (Mooy, De Vries, Grootenhuis, Bouter, & Heine, 2000). In a study of 302 diabetic patients assessed for mood, stressful life events, body size, and mood state, body mass index was associated with stress, and negative mood correlated with waist/hip ratio (Bell, Summerson, Spangler, & Konen, 1998). Behavioral factors, such as preference for fats and sweets, are clearly related to increasing risk of obesity (Devlin, Yanovski, & Wilson, 2000).

Psychological factors have been correlated with increased risk for EHT and cardiovascular disease (Dimsdale, 1997; Forrest, Becker, Kuller, Wolfson, & Orchard, 2000; Jonas, Franks, & Ingram, 1997). For example, a long-term study of 3,310 originally normotensive persons tracked for up to 22 years found that negative affect was associated with higher risk for hypertension. Compared with Caucasian women, black African Americans women showed a larger increase in relative risk per unit of negative affect (Jonas & Lando, 2000).

The thrifty-gene hypothesis was proposed (Neel, 1962; Neel et al., 1998; Sharma, 1998; Wendorf & Goldfine, 1991) to explain the presence of genes that conferred an evolutionary selection advantage to our hunter-gatherer ancestors. The genotype fostered increased fat synthesis and storage during periods of high food availability, thereby providing adaptation to periods of low food availability. The idea of a single gene underlying the development of the metabolic syndrome was abandoned because the term *syndrome* implies a collection of phenotypes that appear to be tied together by a common physiology.

Besides genetic influences, the environment of Western society promotes obesity through hedonistic appetite and sloth. These attributes are shared by much of the adult animal kingdom, facilitating accumulation of stored energy as fat for periods without food, such as migration or hibernation. The seasonal control of fat stores in animals is associated with hyperinsulinemia, insulin resistance, and glucose intolerance, strikingly similar to the basis of the metabolic syndrome in humans. One particularly stunning finding in animals, such as hamsters, is that they can increase fat stores and weight without increasing caloric intake. How many patients have tried to tell us that? When seasonally lean, animals' peak insulin levels seem to shift to a period of low lipogenic responsiveness.

Much of the research to elucidate the physiological mechanisms of the metabolic syndrome has centered on the central nervous system and the neurons of the hypothalamus and suprachiasmatic regions that control food intake and thermogenesis. Nuclei controlling sleep, appetite, metabolic rate, and arousal are proximate and interrelated. Some major neurotransmitters and peptides involved in appetite and metabolism include neuropeptide Y (NPY), thyrotropin-releasing hormone, corticotropin-releasing hormone (CRH), urocortin, and orexin, among others. The similarity between Cushing's syndrome and the metabolic syndrome suggests that disruption of the CRH and the HPA axes is a major contributor to the development of obesity, diabetes, hypertension, and hyperlipidemia. CRH inhibits gonadotropin-releasing hormone, somato-statin, and NPY while increasing orexigenic effects through glucocorticoids, fat appetite, and increased carbohydrate consumption (Cavagnini, Croci, Putignano, Petroni, & Invitti, 2000; Pasquali & Vicennati, 2000).

The autonomic nervous system represents another regulator of metabolism under normal and stress conditions. For instance, stress-induced increases in noradrenergic activity result in increased hepatic gluconeo-genesis, adipose lipolysis, insulin resistance, and feeding behavior. Insulin resistance is present in persons with EHT who are of normal weight but have impaired endothelium-dependent vasodilation (Kotchen, 1996).

Normally, insulin attenuates the vasoconstrictive effects of reflex sympathetic activity, but persons with EHT lack this modulatory effect (Lembo, Iaccarino, Rendina, Volpe, & Trimarco, 1994). Even though insulin activates the sympathetic nervous system in healthy subjects, resulting in elevated heart rate, blood pressure remains unchanged because of vasodilation, particularly in skeletal muscle (Hulthén, Endre, Mattiasson, & Berglund, 1995). Hyperinsulinemia produces a net increase in muscle sympathetic activity and norepinephrine release (Sowers, 1997). Sympathetic hyperactivity and parasympathetic underactivity remain central to the etiology and maintenance of sustained EHT (Brook & Julius, 2000).

## ANXIETY, DEPRESSION, AND THE METABOLIC SYNDROME

Anxiety and depression predict later EHT in whites aged 45 to 64 years and in blacks aged 25 to 64 years, based on a study of 2,992 normotensive individuals who were followed for 7 to 16 years. Possible pathways include sympathetic arousal, increased blood pressure reactivity, neurotransmitter dysregu-lation, and more frequent high-risk behaviors

(Jonas et al., 1997). In diabetes, stable psychosocial factors, such as marriage and higher educational level, were associated with better glycemic control. Sustained high blood glucose resulting from chronic stress is mediated by the stress hormones in contrast to briefer neural effects on blood glucose (Peyrot, McMurry, & Kruger, 1999). Stressful life events are associated with increased variability in blood glucose, increased glycohemoglobin values, and the necessity of adding insulin to oral medicine (Mooy et al., 2000; Surwit & Schneider, 1993). When 151 persons with type 2 diabetes were evaluated for psychosocial effects on progression of disease, significant correlations were found among depression, poor social support, low socioeconomic status, and the presence of diabetic complications (Miyaoka, Miyaoka, Motomiya, Kitamura, & Asai, 1997).

In patients with type 1 and type 2 diabetes, 71 percent had at least one psychiatric illness in their lifetime; mood and anxiety disorders were the most common. Glycohemoglobin values were significantly higher in those who had recently been emotionally ill compared with the patients who had never been ill (Lustman, Griffith, & Clouse, 1988). The self-care of depressed persons is often disrupted and is manifested by poor diet, lack of exercise, less frequent monitoring of glucose levels, and delayed medication (Goodall & Halford, 1991). Clinical depression has a worse course in persons with diabetes, resulting in an independent morbidity (Gavard, Lustman, & Clouse, 1993).

## INTERVENTIONS FOR THE METABOLIC SYNDROME

The primary goal for prevention and treatment of the metabolic syndrome is a physiological state of homeostasis that is not associated with the development of cerebrovascular or

---

**Box 20.2**    Preventing Essential Hypertension

- Quit smoking
- Lose weight
- Restrict sodium intake below 100 mmol per day.
- Limit alcohol intake to 1–2 drinks per day.
- Get 30–45 minutes of aerobic activity on most days.
- Maintain adequate potassium intake (90 mmol per day).
- Maintain adequate intakes of calcium and magnesium.

SOURCE: Joint National Committee (1997).

---

cardiovascular disease within the natural lifetime of the individual. Fighting years of evolutionary pressure has proved expectedly hard and unacceptable to Western societies, though encouraging success in treatment has been accomplished on a small scale in some isolated studies (De Lorgeril et al., 1996; Stephenson, 2000). Risk factors may be modified by behavioral change, including exercise and change in eating habits. For example, a program of moderate intensity aerobic activity was found to reduce the risk for development of type 2 diabetes in adults (Hu et al., 1999). Stress management interventions can teach individuals to decrease the impact of stressful situations and thereby lower risk for development and worsening of the metabolic syndrome. For behavioral therapy to be effective, patients must realize the seriousness of the disorder and commit themselves to change. Box 20.2 lists the lifestyle changes that can help prevent essential hypertension; Box 20.3 describes EHT treatment goals, which are based on patient risk.

The biopsychosocial model proposes that psychological and psychosocial factors play a critical role in fostering acceptance and commitment to change. Psychosocial factors may affect blood glucose independently of adherence (self-care) by increasing liver production of glucose in response to stress hormones (Peyrot et al., 1999). Using an empowerment framework in patient education means teaching skills, giving information, and designing plans based on the patient's own goals and capabilities (Bo, Cavallo-Perin, & Gentile, 1999). Behavior change depends on the patients' feelings of empowerment in their abilities to care for themselves. In addition, providers' can enhance patients' motivation for autonomy by helping to set goals and supporting efforts at self-management (Glasgow & Anderson, 1999).

People with diabetes need the skills to make good decisions and act appropriately in their own behalf, despite societal pressures (Anderson et al., 1995). In the elderly, there are special considerations to ensure understanding of the regimen and facilitate adherence. The dietitian and the diabetes educator play important roles in helping the elderly manage their diabetes (Fonseca & Wall, 1995). Glasgow, Fisher, et al. (1999) diagrammed a pyramid of psychosocial factors with culture at its base and personal coping at the apex. Influences on the person with diabetes range from the interpersonal and informal or subtle to more formal, institutional factors. Practitioners treating persons with the metabolic syndrome must recognize the myriad of influences affecting the choices that people make, identify the gaps in knowledge or skills and the barriers to change before designing appropriate interventions.

**Box 20.3**    Goals of Therapy

- Control blood pressure to the following:
  - Below 140/90 mm Hg for patients with uncomplicated hypertension; set a lower goal for those with target organ damage or clinical cardiovascular disease.
  - Below 130/85 mm Hg for patients with diabetes.
  - Below 125/75 mm Hg for patients with renal insufficiency with proteinuria greater than 1 gram per 24 hours.
- Begin with lifestyle modifications (see Box 20.2) for all patients. Be supportive!
- Add pharmacological therapy if blood pressure remains uncontrolled.
- Start with a diuretic or beta blocker unless there are compelling indications to use other agents. Use low dose and titrate upward. Consider low-dose combinations.
- If no response, try a drug from another class or add a second agent from a different class (diuretic if not already used).
- Educate patient and family about psychosocial factors
- Maintain good communication with patient.
- Discuss how to integrate treatment into daily activities.
- Keep care inexpensive and simple.
- Favor once-daily dosing and long-acting formulations.
- Use combination tablets, when needed.
- Consider using generic formulas or larger tablets that can be divided to decrease costs.
- Consider using nurse case management.

SOURCE: Joint National Committee (1997).

Questionnaires have been used to define the internal and external barriers to modification of diet and exercise in persons with diabetes. Internal barriers include being too busy or too lazy. External barriers include lack of transportation or financial resources. Those who identified external barriers were more likely to make changes than those who identified internal barriers (Ziebland, Thorogood, Yudkin, Jones, & Coulter, 1997). Once the obstacles to adherence and the specific situations associated with poor adherence are identified, it is important to teach patients ways of coping with these obstacles (Schlundt, Rea, Kline, & Pichert, 1994).

## STANDARDS OF CARE

Standards of medical care for people with diabetes were recently revised (American Diabetes Association, 2001). The standards delineate the goals of treatment for type 1 and type 2 diabetes and specific components of a medical history, physical exam, laboratory tests, and management plan that should be performed at the initial and ongoing office visits. Table 20.4 shows the necessary contents of a complete medical history for patients with diabetes. Tables 20.5 and 20.6 list the components of the physical examination and laboratory evaluation, respectively, for patients with diabetes.

**Table 20.4**    Components of the Medical History for Diabetes

| *Initial Visit* | *Ongoing Visits* |
|---|---|
| 1. Symptoms, laboratory results related to diagnosis | 1. Frequency, causes, and severity of hypo- and hyperglycemia |
| 2. Nutritional assessment, weight history | 2. Blood glucose monitoring |
| 3. Previous and present treatment plan<br>a. Medications (prescription and over-the-counter)<br>b. Medical nutrition therapy<br>c. Self-management training<br>d. Blood glucose monitoring results and use of data | 3. Patient regimen adjustments<br>4. Adherence problems<br>5. Lifestyle changes<br>6. Symptoms of complications<br>7. Other medical illnesses |
| 4. Current treatment program | 8. Medications (prescription and over-the-counter) |
| 5. Exercise history | |
| 6. Acute complications (hypoglycemia, hyperglycemia, ketoacidosis) | 9. Psychosocial issues, stresses |
| 7. History of infections: dental, urinary, skin, lower extremity | 10. Tobacco and alcohol use |
| 8. Chronic complications of diabetes: eye, renal, peripheral vascular disease, gastrointestinal, nervous system | |
| 9. Medication history (prescription and over-the-counter) | |
| 10. Family history: essential hypertension, diabetes, hyperlipidemia, cardiovascular disease, stroke | |
| 11. Coronary heart disease risk factors: smoking, essential hypertension, hyperlipidemia, family history, obesity | |
| 12. Psychosocial/economic/lifestyle factors | |
| 13. Tobacco and alcohol use | |

Forms, kept in the medical record, remind providers about physical exams and laboratory tests, and facilitate documentation of care (see Figure 20.1). Regular use of the forms signals a need for a change in management and thereby helps health care providers identify trends in blood glucose that may predict increasing severity of the disease. If symptoms of mood or anxiety disorders are noted, the patient should be evaluated and either medical management or cognitive-behavioral therapy initiated.

Evaluation of the efficacy of the management plan is necessary before changes in regimen are proposed. Table 20.7 summarizes factors to be considered in assessing the management plan before the initial visit with a new physician (initial visit) and during visits for established patients (ongoing visits).

**Table 20.5** Components of the Physical Examination for Diabetes

| Initial Visit | Ongoing Visits |
|---|---|
| 1. Height and weight | 1. Every regular diabetes visit<br> a. Weight<br> b. Blood pressure<br> c. Previous abnormalities on the physical exam |
| 2. Blood pressure | 2. Annual examinations<br> a. Physical<br> b. Eyes with dilated pupils<br> c. Feet (more often in patients with high-risk conditions such as Charcot foot) |
| 3. Examinations:<br> a. Ophthalmoscopic<br> b. Cardiac<br> c. Thyroid<br> d. Pulses<br> e. Feet<br> f. Skin<br> g. Neurological<br> h. Oral cavity | |
| 4. Sexual maturation (if prepubertal) | |

**Table 20.6** Components of the Laboratory Evaluation for Diabetes

| Initial Visit | Ongoing Visits |
|---|---|
| 1. Fasting plasma glucose (optional) | 1. Glycosylated hemoglobin<br> a. Quarterly if treatment changes or patient is not meeting goals<br> b. Twice per year if stable |
| 2. Glycosylated hemoglobin | 2. Fasting plasma glucose (optional) |
| 3. Fasting lipid profile | 3. Fasting lipid profile annually, unless low risk |
| 4. Serum creatinine | 4. Microalbumin measurement annually (indicated) |
| 5. Urinalysis | |
| 6. Urine culture (if indicated) | |
| 7. Electrocardiogram (adults) | |

Use of medications in primary prevention of cardiovascular disease (i.e., patients with no identified atherosclerotic process) typically involves the use of water-soluble hydroxy-methyl-glutaryl-coenzyme A (HMG-CoA) reductase inhibitors. These drugs are not metabolized by the liver, do not cross the blood-brain barrier, and are supported by the West of Scotland study (Shepherd et al., 1995). Most recently,

## Diabetes Care Flow Sheet

| | INTERVAL | GOALS | visit date / / | visit date / / | visit date / / | visit date / / | visit date / / | visit date / / | visit date / / | visit date / / |
|---|---|---|---|---|---|---|---|---|---|---|
| WT. | Q visit | IBW= | lbs/kg | lbs/kg | lbs/kg | lbs/kg | lbs/kg | lbs/kg | lbs/kg | lbs/kg |
| ?Diet | " | | ☐yes ☐no | ☐yes ☐no | ☐yes ☐no | ☐yes ☐no | ☐yes ☐no | ☐yes ☐no | ☐yes ☐no | ☐yes ☐no |
| ?Exercise | " | | ☐yes ☐no | ☐yes ☐no | ☐yes ☐no | ☐yes ☐no | ☐yes ☐no | ☐yes ☐no | ☐yes ☐no | ☐yes ☐no |
| ?SMBG | " | | ☐yes ☐no | ☐yes ☐no | ☐yes ☐no | ☐yes ☐no | ☐yes ☐no | ☐yes ☐no | ☐yes ☐no | ☐yes ☐no |
| $HbA_{1c}$ | Q 3-6 mos. | <7% | | | | | | | | |
| BP | Q visit | <135/80 | | | | | | | | |
| ?Smoking | | | ☐no ☐yes | ☐no ☐yes | ☐no ☐yes | ☐no ☐yes | ☐no ☐yes | ☐no ☐yes | ☐no ☐yes | ☐no ☐yes |
| ASA | | | ☐yes ☐no | ☐yes ☐no | ☐yes ☐no | ☐yes ☐no | ☐yes ☐no | ☐yes ☐no | ☐yes ☐no | ☐yes ☐no |
| Cholesterol | Q 1 yr | <200 | | | | | | | | |
| HDL | " | >45(m) >55(w) | | | | | | | | |
| LDL | " | <100 | | | | | | | | |
| TG | " | <200 | | | | | | | | |
| BUN Cr | " | | | | | | | | | |
| microalbumin | " | <30 ug/mg Cr | | | | | | | | |
| or 24 h U albumin | | <30 mg/day | | | | | | | | |
| Cr Cl | | | | | | | | | | |
| Fundus exam | Q 1 yr | | ☐NL ☐BDR ☐PDR | ☐NL ☐BDR ☐PDR | ☐NL ☐BDR ☐PDR | ☐NL ☐BDR ☐PDR | ☐NL ☐BDR ☐PDR | ☐NL ☐BDR ☐PDR | ☐NL ☐BDR ☐PDR | ☐NL ☐BDR ☐PDR |
| most recent retinal exam | Q 1 yr | | Dr. ___ | Dr. ___ | Dr. ___ | Dr. ___ | Dr. ___ | Dr. ___ | Dr. ___ | Dr. ___ |
| Foot exam | Q visit | | PULSES ☐nl ☐abnl SENSAT ☐nl ☐abnl ULCER ☐no ☐yes | PULSES ☐nl ☐abnl SENSAT ☐nl ☐abnl ULCER ☐no ☐yes | PULSES ☐nl ☐abnl SENSAT ☐nl ☐abnl ULCER ☐no ☐yes | PULSES ☐nl ☐abnl SENSAT ☐nl ☐abnl ULCER ☐no ☐yes | PULSES ☐nl ☐abnl SENSAT ☐nl ☐abnl ULCER ☐no ☐yes | PULSES ☐nl ☐abnl SENSAT ☐nl ☐abnl ULCER ☐no ☐yes | PULSES ☐nl ☐abnl SENSAT ☐nl ☐abnl ULCER ☐no ☐yes | PULSES ☐nl ☐abnl SENSAT ☐nl ☐abnl ULCER ☐no ☐yes |
| most recent pod eval | | | Dr. ___ | Dr. ___ | Dr. ___ | Dr. ___ | Dr. ___ | Dr. ___ | Dr. ___ | Dr. ___ |

**Figure 20.1**  Diabetes Care Flow Sheet

Note: Wallet-size cards are available from the American Diabetes Association (call 1-800-ADA-ORDER or go to http://store.diabetes.org) for clients to record test results.

pravastatin has been found to offer some protection against the development of diabetes (Freeman et al., 2001).

## BEHAVIORAL AND COMPLEMENTARY THERAPIES

### Diabetes Mellitus

A collaborative problem-solving behavioral approach can improve dialogue between the provider and the patient. First, define the problem in the context of the patient's culture and ability to understand. Then develop an action plan and set realistic goals on a time line. Explore the available medications and behavior-change strategies. Track the patient's progress on a regular basis, reinforce positive change, and make adjustments in the plan based on patient feedback. No single plan can be expected to cover many years of illness, so modifications are to be expected (Glasgow, Fisher, et al., 1999).

In depressed patients, both antidepressants and cognitive-behavioral therapy (CBT) should be considered. The antidepressants have variable effects on blood glucose, depending on whether tricyclics or selective serotonin reuptake inhibitors (SSRIs) are used. The former are associated with hyperglycemia, while the SSRIs have more of a hypoglycemic effect (Goodnick, Henry, & Buki, 1995; Potter VanLoon et al., 1992). CBT has been useful in depressed persons

**Table 20.7**    Evaluation of the Diabetes Management Plan

| *Initial Visit* | *Ongoing Visits* |
| --- | --- |
| 1. Short- and long-term goals of management | 1. Short- and long-term goals of management |
| 2. Medications (prescription and over-the-counter) | 2. Medications (prescription and over-the-counter) |
| 3. Medical nutrition therapy | 3. Adequacy of glycemic control |
| 4. Lifestyle changes | 4. Frequency/severity of hypoglycemia |
| 5. Self-management education | 5. Blood glucose monitoring results |
| 6. Monitoring: glucose test results | 6. Complications: eye, renal, skin, feet, etc. |
| 7. Referral to specialists if needed | 7. Control of dyslipidemia |
| 8. Agreement on continuing support/follow-up with other health care providers such as dietitian, nurse educator, exercise specialist, counselor | 8. Blood pressure |
| 9. Pneumococcal and influenza vaccines | 9. Body weight |
| | 10. Medical nutrition therapy |
| | 11. Exercise regimen |
| | 12. Adherence to self-management training |
| | 13. Referral to specialists; annual eye exam |
| | 14. Psychosocial adjustment and issues |
| | 15. Knowledge and skills regarding diabetes self-management |
| | 16. Smoking cessation (if indicated) |
| | 17. Annual influenza vaccine |

with type 2 diabetes, as shown in a study of 42 people with scores higher than 14 on the Beck Depression Inventory. Patients in the CBT group showed greater improvement in depressive symptoms and were more likely to go into remission compared with patients in the control group. Failures in the CBT group were those with lower compliance to self-monitoring of blood glucose and more complications (Lustman, Freedland, Griffith, & Clouse, 1998). CBT also was associated with lessening of diabetes-related anxiety in adolescents with type 2 diabetes (Hains, Davies, Parton, Totka, & Amoroso-Camarata, 2000).

Mind-body therapies used to treat persons with diabetes have shown variable results. Thirty-two patients with type 2 diabetes completed a study in which EMG feedback and progressive relaxation training were provided. In the group as a whole, relaxation training was no more effective than intensive conventional treatment. However, patients in the relaxation group who evidenced high trait anxiety levels showed improved glucose tolerance and decreased plasma cortisol (Lane, McCaskill, Ross, Feinglos, & Surwit, 1993). In another study, anxiety, tension, and skin conductance decreased with relaxation, indicating that the subjects had learned the relaxation response, but no changes in blood glucose were documented (Jablon, Naliboff, Gilmore, & Rosenthal, 1997).

In type 1 diabetes, several studies suggested positive effects of biofeedback-assisted relaxation therapy on blood glucose (McGrady, Bailey, & Good, 1991; McGrady, Graham, & Bailey, 1996). In contrast, patients who showed symptoms of depression were not able to lower blood glucose after a similar behavioral treatment regimen (McGrady & Horner, 1999). A small study of 15 adolescents with type 1 diabetes found that stress management (cognitive restructuring and problem solving) decreased anxiety levels and improved coping abilities but did not change blood glucose (Hains et al., 2000). At this time, the differential effects of relaxation therapy in type 1 and type 2 diabetes require further study.

Thermal biofeedback-assisted relaxation has been useful for people with diabetes-related circulation problems. Forty subjects with diabetes were given biofeedback training to increase toe temperature and blood volume pulse; results showed improvements in circulation in the feet, which could decrease complications of diabetes (Rice and Schindler, 1992).

Yoga reduced blood glucose and decreased the need for oral hypoglycemic drugs in a group of 149 people with type 2 diabetes who practiced yoga for 40 days. Yoga training consisted of one and one-half hours a day of relaxation, breathing training, and postures while patients were hospitalized. Two thirds of the patients demonstrated a fair to good response in blood glucose (Jain, Uppal, Bhatnagar, & Talukdar, 1993).

## Essential Hypertension

Two stress management education approaches, transcendental meditation and progressive muscle relaxation, were compared with lifestyle modification education in 100 adult African Americans with mild EHT. Transcendental meditation decreased systolic blood pressure by 10.7 mm Hg and diastolic blood pressure by 6.4 mm Hg, and the relaxation group decreased systolic blood pressure by 4.7 mm Hg and diastolic blood pressure by 3.3 mm Hg. Only small changes were observed in the education group. These results compare favorably with other non-pharmacological therapies of EHT such as sodium reduction and exercise (Schneider et al., 1995).

The effects of transcendental meditation on total peripheral resistance were analyzed in 32 healthy long-term practitioners of the technique compared with a group of controls. Systolic blood pressure and total peripheral resistance decreased and correlated with decreased cortisol and sympathetic activity (Barnes, Treiber, Turner, Davis, & Strong, 1999). Elderly blacks taught the transcendental meditation technique were able to decrease blood pressure more than the education and progressive muscle relaxation groups (Alexander et al., 1996).

Exercise, weight management, and the two combined were compared with wait-list control in 133 sedentary, overweight, unmedicated persons with high normal blood pressure, stage 1 and 2 EHT. Patients in the treatment groups decreased systolic and diastolic blood pressure as well as TPR, while cardiac output increased. The weight management group demonstrated lower fasting and postprandial blood glucose. The best effects were those found in the group that received the combination of exercise and weight management (Blumenthal et al., 2000). A program of weight loss and low sodium diet was tested in older obese persons with EHT, while the reduced sodium diet was also given to elderly persons with EHT who were not obese. Both interventions were effective for up to 36 months (Whelton et al., 1998).

Several types of feedback—direct blood pressure feedback as well as EMG, thermal, skin conductance, and heart rate variability biofeedback—have been tested in persons with EHT. Direct blood pressure feedback was used without relaxation therapy in early studies by Engel, Glasgow, and Gaarder (1983). The experimental group showed a decrease in systolic blood pressure of 7.3 mm Hg compared with 4.4 mm Hg in the control group. Glasgow, Engel, and D'Lugoff (1989) proposed that feedback and relaxation therapy should be offered in a specific sequence and not initially combined. Blood pressure feedback followed by relaxation training with daily home practice was suggested to be the most effective in lowering blood pressure. Direct blood pressure feedback, using a device that measures blood pressure from the finger, has also been applied to white-coat hypertension, a type of hypertension identified when an individual manifests elevated blood pressure in the doctor's office or clinic but maintains normal blood pressure at home. After a two-week monitoring period, subjects participated in four sessions of biofeedback. Significant decreases in systolic and diastolic blood pressure were recorded in addition to decreased blood pressure responses to mental stress challenge (Nakao, Nomura, Shimosawa, Fujita, & Kuboki, 2000).

Forehead EMG biofeedback with adjunctive relaxation has been studied extensively in EHT. An early study of 22 trained subjects and 16 controls showed statistically significant decreases in both systolic (11.2 mm Hg) and diastolic (5.7 mm Hg) blood pressure (McGrady, Yonker, Tan, Fine, & Woerner, 1981). Jurek, Higgins, and McGrady (1992) combined EMG feedback and diuretic medication to produce an additive effect. Goebel, Viol, and Orebaugh (1993) also reported small but consistent decreases in blood pressure and antihypertensive medication compared to a believable control group.

The application of thermal biofeedback to EHT is reviewed in Blanchard (1990). An advantage in lowering blood pressure was observed in those patients trained to increase the temperature of their hands compared to the group receiving progressive relaxation (Blanchard et al., 1986). Over a three-year period, 108 individuals participated in a study of autogenic training with thermal feedback taught in a group setting. Home practice was recommended. The experimental group showed significant decreases in systolic and diastolic blood pressure, increases in finger temperature, and decreases in trait anxiety and plasma aldosterone (McGrady, 1994).

Persons with ambulatory blood pressure of at least 140/90 mm Hg participated in 10 hours of stress management ($n = 27$) or were wait listed ($n = 33$) until after the control period. The intervention was customized to patients' psychological risk factors. Blood decreased in the immediate treatment group (6.1 mm Hg systolic and 4.3 mm Hg diastolic). Similar reductions were observed in the wait-list group eventually treated. The extent of the systolic blood pressure decrease was related to reduced psychological stress and change in anger coping styles. Starting levels of blood pressure were strongly related with degree of change (Linden, Lenz, & Con, 2001).

Stress management plus exercise was compared with exercise alone in patients with heart disease. At the end of treatment, patients in the combined treatment group decreased their global distress score and blood pressure reactivity to psychological challenge, the latter particularly important for lowering risk (Turner, Linden, van der Wal, & Schamberger, 1995). An important meta-analysis of trials of relaxation-based therapies showed that the starting blood pressure is predictive for the amount of decrease in blood pressure. When adjustments are made for differing starting blood pressure, the best nondrug treatments were as efficacious as several drug regimens (Linden & Chambers, 1994).

One study compared respiratory sinus arrhythmia (RSA) feedback with thermal biofeedback in EHT. Both types of feedback were effective in lowering blood pressure, despite differences in mediating mechanisms. It was suggested that RSA feedback lowers blood pressure through an increase in parasympathetic function, while both EMG and thermal feedback are effective due to a decrease in sympathetic function (Herbs, 1994).

Efforts to define the long-term maintenance of decreased blood pressure in persons with EHT trained with biofeedback-assisted relaxation have proven to be complicated. The natural progression of hypertension and changes in medication must be factored into the analysis of long-term biofeedback effects. Nonetheless, some patients are able to maintain lower blood pressure years after the end of therapy (Blanchard et al., 1986; Leserman et al., 1989; McGrady, Nadsady, & Schumann-Brzezinski, 1991).

## Hyperlipidemia

Detailed descriptions of weight management programs are beyond the scope of this chapter, but the primary care practitioner treating the metabolic syndrome should be aware of the significant influence of psychological factors in obesity. In addition to the medical adverse effects of long-term overweight are the psychological concomitants. In a society where a large body results in negative attitudes and overt hostility directed toward the overweight person, it becomes clear that treatment must consider the multifaceted nature of the problem. Approaches to therapy need to include behavioral and social components (Faith, Fontaine, Cheskin, & Allison, 2000).

Behavioral programs comprising exercise, better eating habits, and psychological support are considered to be ideal (Devlin et al.,

2000). However, most people trying to lose weight do not use the recommended combination of weight management and physical activity. Conclusions based on a survey of 100,000 adults were that at least one third of the men and women who were attempting to lose or maintain weight were engaged in one or the other, but not both (Serdula et al., 1999). Diet without exercise does not lower LDL levels in men or women with high-risk lipoprotein levels (Stefanick, Mackey, Sheehan, Ellsworth, Haskell, & Wood, 1998).

## PREDICTION OF TREATMENT RESPONSE

A success rate of 50 percent to 65 percent based on a criterion decrease in blood pressure of 5 mm Hg mean arterial pressure in studies of biofeedback in EHT fostered interest in trying to determine if blood pressure response could be predicted. In a study of 40 individuals with EHT, 23 were classified as successful while 10 failed. Treatment was most successful for patients with the highest levels of anxiety, muscle tension, urinary cortisol, and heart rate and the coolest hand temperatures. In addition, high normal stimulated plasma renin activity predicted success in contrast to low renin activity (McGrady & Higgins, 1989; McGrady, Utz, Woerner, Bernal, & Higgins, 1986; Weaver & McGrady, 1995).

There have been variable results in studies of patients with diabetes concerning which patient characteristics might predict better response. External barriers to adherence seemed easier to overcome than feelings of deprivation (Schlundt et al., 1994). Depression has been suggested to interfere with a positive response to biofeedback-assisted relaxation (McGrady & Horner, 1999); and poorer adherence to self-monitoring of blood glucose predicted a poorer response to cognitive-behavioral therapy for depression

(Lustman et al., 1998). In contrast, patients with a sense of empowerment and self-confidence were better able to manage their diabetes regimen (Howorka et al., 2000).

## CONCLUSION

The metabolic syndrome should be approached as an entity in a combined medical and behavioral framework. Successful treatment of any of the major elements may result in improvement of the others. Understanding of the psychosocial factors contributing to etiology and worsening of the syndrome is critical for the health care provider. Additional research testing psychophysiological therapy on blood glucose, blood pressure, and the lipid profile is urgently needed.

## REFERENCES

Alexander, C. N., Schneider, R. H., Staggers, F., Sheppard, W., Clayborne, B. M., Rainforth, M., et al. (1996). Trial of stress reduction for hypertension in older African Americans. *Hypertension, 28,* 228–237.

American Diabetes Association. (2000a) Report of the expert committee on the Diagnosis and Classification of Diabetes Mellitus. *Diabetes Care, 23*(Suppl. 1), S4–S19.

American Diabetes Association. (2000b). Screening for type 2 diabetes Position Statement. *Diabetes Care, 23*(Suppl. 1), S20–S23.

American Diabetes Association. (2001). American Diabetes Association clinical practice recommendations 2001. *Diabetes Care, 24*(Suppl. 1), S1–S133.

Anderson, R. M., Funnell, M. M., Butler, P. M., Arnold, M. S., Fitzgerald, J. T., & Feste, C. C. (1995). Patient empowerment. *Diabetes Care, 18,* 943–949.

Barnes, V. A., Treiber, F. A., Turner, J. R., Davis, H., & Strong, W. B. (1999). Acute effects of transcendental meditation on hemodynamic functioning in middle-aged adults. *Psychosomatic Medicine, 61,* 525–531.

Barrett-Connor, E., Wingard, D. L., Criqui, M. H., & Suarez, L. (1984). Is borderline fasting hyperglycemia a risk factor for cardiovascular death? *Journal of Chronic Disease, 37,* 773–779.

Bell, R. A., Summerson, J. H., Spangler, J. G., & Konen, J. C. (1998). Body fat, fat distribution, and psychosocial factors among patients with type 2 diabetes mellitus. *Behavioral Medicine, 24,* 138–143.

Blanchard, E. B., (1990). Biofeedback treatments of essential hypertension. *Biofeedback & Self-Regulation, 15*(3), 209–228.

Blanchard, E. B., McCoy, G. C., Musso, A., Gerardi, M. A., Pallmeyer, T. P., Gerardi, R. J., et al. (1986). A controlled comparison of thermal biofeedback and relaxation training in the treatment of essential hypertension: I. Short-term and long-term outcome. *Behavior Therapy, 17,* 563–579.

Blumenthal, J. A., Sherwood, A., Gullette, E. C., Babyak, M., Waugh, R., Georgiades, A., et al. (2000). Exercise and weight loss reduce blood pressure in men and women with mild hypertension: Effects on cardiovascular, metabolic, and hemodynamic functioning. *Archives of Internal Medicine, 160,* 1947–1958.

Bo, S., Cavallo-Perin, P., & Gentile, L. (1999). Prevalence of patients reaching the targets of good control in normal clinical practice. *Diabetes Care,* 22(12), 2092.

Bouchard, C. (1995). Genetics and the metabolic syndrome. *International Journal of Obesity and Related Metabolic Disorders, 19*(Suppl. 1), S52–S59.

Bourey, R. E., Kohrt, W. M., Kirwan, J. P., Staten, M. A., King, D. S., & Holloszy, J. O. (1993). Relationship between glucose tolerance and glucose-stimulated insulin response in 65-year-olds. *Journal of Gerontology, 48,* M122–M127.

Brook, R. D., & Julius, S. (2000). Autonomic imbalance, hypertension and cardiovascular risk. *American Journal of Hypertension, 13,* 1125–1225.

Burt, V. L., Culter, J. A., Higgins, M., Horan, M. J., Labarthe, D., Whelton, P., et al. (1995). Trends in the prevalence, awareness, treatment, and control of hypertension in the adult US population. Data from the health examination surveys, 1960 to 1991. *Hypertension, 26,* 60–69.

Cavagnini, F., Croci, M., Putignano, P., Petroni, M. L., & Invitti, C. (2000). Glucocorticoids and neuroendocrine function. *International Journal of Obesity Related Metabolic Disorders, 24*(Suppl. 2), S77–S79.

Centers for Disease Control and Prevention. (1998). *National diabetes fact sheet: National estimates and general information on diabetes in the United States* (rev. ed.). Atlanta, GA: U.S. Department of Health and Human Services.

Chaturvedi, N., Jarrett, J., Shipley, M. J., & Fuller, J. H. (1998). Socioeconomic gradient in morbidity and mortality in people with diabetes: Cohort study findings form the Whitehall study and the WHO multinational study of vascular disease in diabetes. *British Medical Journal, 316,* 100–105.

De Lorgeril, M., Salen, P., Martin, J. L., Mamelle, N., Monjaud, I., Touboul, P., et al. (1996). Effect of a Mediterranean type of diet on the rate of cardiovascular complications in patients with coronary artery disease. Insights into the cardioprotective effect of certain nutriments. *Journal of the American College of Cardiology 28,* 1103–1108.

Devlin, M. J., Yanovski, S. Z., & Wilson, G. T. (2000). Obesity: What mental health professionals need to know. *American Journal of Psychiatry, 157,* 854–866.

Diabetes Research Working Group. (1999). *Conquering diabetes: A strategic plan for the 21st century* (NIH Publication No. 99-4398). Washington, DC: National Institutes of Health.

Diez-Roux, A. V., Northridge, M. E., Morabia, A., Bassett, M. T., & Shea, S. (1999). Prevalence and social correlates of cardiovascular disease risk factors in Harlem. *American Journal of Public Health, 89*(3), 302–308.

Dimsdale, J. E., (1997). Symptoms of anxiety and depression as precursors to hypertension. *Journal of the American Medical Association, 277,* 574–575.

Engel, B. T., Glasgow, M. S., & Gaarder, K. R. (1983). Behavioral treatment of high blood pressure: II. Follow-up results and treatment recommendations. *Psychosomatic Medicine, 45*(1), 23–29.

Expert Committee. (1997). Report of the Expert Committee on the diagnosis and classification of diabetes mellitus. *Diabetes Care, 20,* 1183–1197.

Expert Panel on Detection, Evaluation, and Treatment of High Blood Cholesterol in Adults (Adult Treatment Panel II). (1993). Summary of the second report of the National Cholesterol Education Program (NCEP). *Journal of the American Medical Association, 269,* 3015–3023.

Faith, M. S., Fontaine, K. R., Cheskin, L. J., & Allison, D. B. (2000). Behavioral approaches to the problems of obesity. *Behavior Modification, 24*(4), 459–493.

Fonseca, V., & Wall, J. (1995). Diet and diabetes in the elderly. *Clinics in Geriatric Medicine, 11,* 613–624.

Forrest, K. Y. Z., Becker, D. J., Kuller, L. H., Wolfson, S. K., & Orchard, T. J. (2000). Are predictors of coronary heart disease and lower-extremity arterial disease in type I diabetes the same? A prospective study. *Atherosclerosis, 148,* 159–169.

Freeman, D. J., Norrie, J., Sattar, N., Neely, R. D., Cobbe, S. M., Ford, I., et al. (2001). Pravastatin and the development of diabetes mellitus: Evidence for a protective treatment effect in the West of Scotland Coronary Prevention Study. *Circulation, 103,* 357–362.

Gavard, J. A., Lustman, P. J., & Clouse, R. E. (1993). Prevalence of depression in adults with diabetes. *Diabetes Care, 16,* 1167–1178.

Glasgow, M. S., Engel, B. T., & D'Lugoff, B. C. (1989). A controlled study of a standardized behavioral stepped treatment for hypertension. *Psychosomatic Medicine, 51,* 10–26.

Glasgow, R. E., & Anderson, R. M. (1999). In diabetes care, moving from compliance to adherence is not enough. *Diabetes Care, 22*(12), 2090–2091.

Glasgow, R. E., Fisher, E. B., Anderson, B. J., LaGreca, A., Marrero, D., Johnson, S. B., et al. (1999). Behavioral science in diabetes. *Diabetes Care, 22,* 832–843.

Goebel, M., Viol, G. W., & Orebaugh, C. (1993). An incremental model to isolate specific effects of behavioral treatments in essential hypertension. *Biofeedback & Self-Regulation, 18*(4), 255–280.

Goodall, T.A. , & Halford, W. K. (1991). Self-management of diabetes mellitus: A critical review. *Health Psychology, 10,* 1–8.

Goodnick, P. J., Henry, J. H., & Buki, V. M. (1995). Treatment of depression in patients with diabetes mellitus. *Journal of Clinical Psychiatry, 56,* 128–136.

Groop, L. (2000). Genetics of the metabolic syndrome. *British Journal of Nutrition, 83*(Suppl. 1), S39–S48.

Haffner, S. M. (1998). The importance of hyperglycemia in the nonfasting state to the development of cardiovascular disease. *Endocrine Reviews 19,* 583–592.

Hains, A. A., Davies, W. H., Parton, E., Totka J., & Amoroso-Camarata, J. (2000). A stress management intervention for adolescents with type 2 diabetes. *The Diabetes Educator, 26,* 417–424.

Herbs, D. (1994). The effects of heart rate pattern biofeedback versus skin temperature biofeedback for the treatment of essential hypertension. Unpublished doctoral dissertation, California School of Professional Psychology, San Diego.

Howorka, K., Pumpria, J., Wagner-Nosiska, D., Grillmayr, H., Schlusche, C., & Schabmann, A. (2000). Empowering diabetes out-patients with structured education: Short-term and long-term effects of functional insulin treatment on perceived control over diabetes. *Journal of Psychosomatic Research, 48,* 37–44.

Hu, F. B., Sigal, R. J., Rich-Edwards, J. W., Colditz, G. A., Solomon, C. G., Willett, W. C., Speizer, F. E., & Manson, J. E. (1999). Walking compared with vigorous physical activity and risk of type 2 diabetes in women. *Journal of the American Medical Association, 282,* 1433–1439.

Hulthén, U. L., Endre, T., Mattiasson, I., & Berglund, G. (1995). Insulin and forearm vasodilation in hypertension-prone men. *Hypertension, 25,* 214–218.

Jablon, S. L., Naliboff, B. D., Gilmore, S. L., & Rosenthal, M. J. (1997). Effects of relaxation training on glucose tolerance and diabetic control in type II diabetes. *Applied Psychophysiology and Biofeedback, 22,* 155–69.

Jain, S. C., Uppal, A., Bhatnagar, S. O. D., & Talukdar, B. (1993). A study of response pattern of non-insulin dependent diabetics to yoga therapy. *Diabetes Research and Clinical Practice, 19,* 69–74.

Joint National Committee. (1997). The sixth report of the Joint National Committee on prevention, detection, evaluation and treatment of high blood pressure. *Archives of Internal Medicine, 157,* 2413–2446.

Jonas, B. S., Franks, P., & Ingram, D. D. (1997). Are symptoms of anxiety and depression risk factors for hypertension? *Archives of Family Medicine, 6,* 43–49.

Jonas, B. S., & Lando, J. F. (2000). Negative affect as a prospective risk factor for hypertension. *Psychosomatic Medicine, 62,* 188–196.

Jurek, I. E., Higgins, J. T., Jr., & McGrady, A. (1992). Interaction of biofeedback-assisted relaxation and diuretic in treatment of essential hypertension. *Biofeedback & Self-Regulation, 17*(2), 125–141.

Kotchen, T. A. (1996). Attenuation of hypertension by insulin-sensitizing agents. *Hypertension, 28,* 219–223.

Lane, J. D., McCaskill, C. C., Ross, S. L., Feinglos, M. N., & Surwit, R. S. (1993). Relaxation training for NIDDM. *Diabetes Care, 16,* 1087–1094.

Ledermann, H. M. (1995). Maturity-onset diabetes of the young (MODY) at least ten times more common in Europe than previously assumed? *Diabetologia, 38,* 1482.

Lehto, M., Tuomi, T., Mahtani, M. M., Widen, E., Forsblom, C., Sarelin, L., et al. (1997). Characterization of the MODY3 phenotype. Early-onset diabetes caused by an insulin secretion defect. *Journal of Clinical Investigation, 99,* 582–591.

Lembo, G., Iaccarino, G., Rendina, V., Volpe, M., & Trimarco, B. (1994). Insulin blunts sympathetic vasoconstriction through the 2-adrenergic pathway in humans. *Hypertension, 24,* 429–438.

Leserman, J., Stuart, E. M., Mamish, M. E., Deckro, J. P., Beckman, R. J., Friedman, R., et al. (1989). Nonpharmacologic intervention for hypertension: Long-term follow-up. *Journal of Cardiopulmonary Rehabilitation, 9,* 316–324.

Linden, W., & Chambers, L. A. (1994). Clinical effectiveness of non-drug therapies for hypertension: A meta-analysis. *Annals of Behavioral Medicine, 16,* 35–45.

Linden, W., Lenz, J. W., Con, A. H. (2001). Individualized stress management for primary hypertension: A randomized trial. *Archives of Internal Medicine, 161,* 1071–1080.

Lustman, P. J., Freedland, K. E., Griffith, L. S., & Clouse, R. E. (1998). Predicting response to cognitive behavior therapy of depression in type 2 diabetes. *General Hospital Psychiatry, 20,* 302–306.

Lustman, P. J., Griffith, L. S., & Clouse, R. E. (1988). Depression in adults with diabetes. *Diabetes Care, 11,* 605–612.

McGrady, A. V. (1994). Effects of group relaxation training and thermal biofeedback on blood pressure and related psychophysiological variables in essential hypertension. *Biofeedback & Self-Regulation, 19*(1), 51–66.

McGrady, A. V., Bailey, B. K., & Good, M. P. (1991). Controlled study of biofeedback-assisted relaxation in type 1 diabetes. *Diabetes Care, 14,* 360–365.

McGrady, A. V., Graham, G., & Bailey, B. (1996). Biofeedback-assisted relaxation in insulin dependent diabetes: A replication and extension study. *Annals of Behavioral Medicine, 22*(3), 155–169.

McGrady, A. V., & Higgins, J. T., Jr. (1989). Prediction of response to biofeedback-assisted relaxation in hypertensives: Development of a hypertensive predictor profile (HYPP). *Psychosomatic Medicine, 51,* 277–284.

McGrady, A. V., & Horner, J. (1999). Role of mood in outcome of biofeedback-assisted relaxation therapy in insulin dependent diabetes mellitus. *Applied Psychophysiology and Biofeedback, 24,* 79–88.

McGrady, A. V., Nadsady, P. A., & Schumann-Brzezinski, C. (1991). Sustained effects of biofeedback-assisted relaxation therapy in essential hypertension. *Biofeedback & Self-Regulation, 16*(4), 399–413.

McGrady, A. V., Utz, S. W., Woerner, M., Bernal, G. A. A., & Higgins, J. T. (1986). Predictors of success in hypertensives treated with biofeedback-assisted relaxation. *Biofeedback & Self-Regulation, 11*(23), 95–103.

McGrady, A. V., Yonker, R., Tan, S. Y., Fine, T. H., & Woerner, M. (1981). The effects of biofeedback-assisted relaxation training on blood pressure and selected biochemical parameters in patients with essential hypertension. *Biofeedback & Self-Regulation, 6*(3), 343–353.

Miyaoka, Y., Miyaoka, H., Motomiya, T., Kitamura, S., & Asai, M. (1997). Impact of sociodemographic and diabetes-related characteristics on depressive state among non-insulin-dependent diabetic patients. *Psychiatry and Clinical Neurosciences, 51,* 203–206.

Mooy, J. M., De Vries, H., Grootenhuis, P. A., Bouter, L. M., & Heine, R. J. (2000). Major stressful life events in relation to prevalence of undetected type 2 diabetes. *Diabetes Care, 23,* 197–201.

Mykkanen, L., Laakso, M., Penttila, I., & Pyorala, K. (1991). Aysmptomatic hyperglycemia and cardiovascular risk factors in the elderly. *Atherosclerosis, 88,* 153–161.

Nakao, M., Nomura, S., Shimosawa, T., Fujita, T., & Kuboki, T. (2000). Blood pressure biofeedback treatment of white-coat hypertension. *Journal of Psychosomatic Research , 48,* 161–169.

Neel, J. V. (1962). Diabetes mellitus: A "thrifty" genotype rendered detrimental by "progress"? *American Journal of Human Genetics, 14,* 353–362.

Neel, J. V., Weder, A. B., & Julius, S. (1998). Type II diabetes, essential hypertension, and obesity as "syndromes of impaired genetic homeostasis": The "thrifty genotype" hypothesis enters the 21st century. *Perspective of Biologic Medicine, 42,* 44–74.

Pasquali, R., & Vicennati, V. (2000). Activity of the hypothalamic-pituitary-adrenal axis in different obesity phenotypes. *International Journal of Obesity Related Metabolic Disorders, 24*(Suppl. 2), S47–S49.

Peyrot, M., McMurry, J. F., & Kruger, D. F. (1999). A biopsychosocial model of glycemic control in diabetes: Stress, coping and regimen adherence. *Journal of Health and Social Behavior, 40,* 141–158.

Pi-Sunyer, F. X., Laferrere, B., Aronne, L. J., & Bray, G. A. (1999). Therapeutic controversy: Obesity—A modern day epidemic. *Journal of Clinical Endocrinology Metabolism, 84,* 3–12.

Potter VanLoon, B. J. P., Radder, J. K., Frolich, M., Krans, H. M., Zwinderman, A. H., & Meinders, A. E. (1992). Fluoxetine increases in insulin action in obese nondiabetic and in obese non-insulin-dependent diabetic individuals. *International Journal of Obesity, 16,* 79–85.

Ravussin, E., Valencia, M. E., Esparza, J., Bennett, P. H., & Schulz, L. O. (1994). Effects of a traditional lifestyle on obesity in Pima Indians. *Diabetes Care, 17,* 1067–1074.

Rice, B. I., & Schindler, J. V. (1992). Effect of thermal biofeedback-assisted relaxation training on blood circulation in the lower extremities of a population with diabetes. *Diabetes Care, 15,* 853–858.

Schlundt, D. G., Rea, M. R., Kline, S. S., & Pichert, J. W. (1994). Situational obstacles to dietary adherence for adults with diabetes. *Journal of the American Dietetic Association, 94,* 877–878.

Schneider, R. H., Staggers, F., Alexander, C. N., Sheppard, W., Rainforth, M., Kondwani, K., et al. (1995). A randomized controlled trial of stress reduction for hypertension in older African Americans. *Hypertension, 26,* 820–827.

Serdula, M. K., Mokdad, A. H., Williamson, D. F., Galuska, D. A., Mendlein, J. M., & Heath, G. W. (1999). Prevalence of attempting weight loss and strategies for controlling weight. *Journal of American Medical Association, 282,* 1353–1358.

Sharma, A. M. (1998). The thrifty-genotype hypothesis and its implications for the study of complex genetic disorders in man. *Journal of Molecular Medicine, 76,* 568–571.

Shepherd, J., Cobbe, S. M., Ford, I., Isles, C. G., Lorimer, A. R., Macfarlane, P. W., et al. (1995). Prevention of coronary heart disease with pravastatin in men with hypercholesterolemia. West of Scotland Coronary Prevention Study Group. *New England Journal of Medicine, 333,* 1301–1307.

Sowers, J. R. (1997). Insulin and insulin-like growth factor in normal and pathological cardiovascular physiology. *Hypertension, 29,* 691–699.

Stamler, R., Stamler, J., Dyer, A., Cooper, R., Collette, P., Berkson, D. M., et al. (1979). Asymptomatic hyperglycemia and cardiovascular diseases in three Chicago epidemiologic studies. *Diabetes Care, 2,* 142–143.

Stefanick, M. L., Mackey, S., Sheehan, M., Ellsworth, N., Haskell, W. L., & Wood, P. D (1998). Effects of diet and exercise in men and postmenopausal women with low levels of HDL cholesterol and high levels of LDL cholesterol. *New England Journal of Medicine, 339,* 12–20.

Stephenson, J. (2000). Health agencies update: A DASH of heart help. *Journal of the American Medical Association, 284,* 1371.

Surwit, R. S., & Schneider, M. S. (1993). Role of stress in the etiology and treatment of diabetes mellitus. *Psychosomatic Medicine, 4,* 380–393.

Tuomi, T., Carlsson, A., Li, H., Isomaa, B., Miettinen, A., Nilsson, A., et al. (1999). Clinical and genetic characteristics of type 2 diabetes with and without GAD antibodies. *Diabetes, 48,* 150–157.

Tuomi, T., Group, L. C., Zimmet, P. A., Rowley, M. J., Knowles, W., & MacKay, I. R. (1993). Antibodies to glutamic acid decarboxylase reveal latent autoimmune diabetes mellitus in adults with a non-insulin dependent onset of disease. *Diabetes, 42,* 359–362.

Turner, L., Linden, W., van der Wal, R., & Schamberger, W. (1995). Stress management for patients with heart disease: A pilot study. *Heart Lung, 24,* 145–53.

Wamala, S. P., Wolk, A., & Orth-Gomer, K. (1997). Determinants of obesity in relation to socioeconomic status among middle-aged Swedish women. *Preventive Medicine, 26*(5), 734–744.

Weaver, M. T., & McGrady, A. (1995). A provisional model to predict blood pressure response to biofeedback-assisted relaxation. *Biofeedback & Self-Regulation, 20*(3), 229–240.

Wendorf, M., & Goldfine, I. D. (1991). Archaeology of NIDDM. Excavation of the "thrifty" genotype. *Diabetes, 40,* 161–165.

Whelton, P. K., Appel, L. J., Espeland, M. A., Applegate, W. B., Ettinger, W. H., Kostis, J. B., et al. (1998). Sodium reduction and weight loss in the treatment of hypertension in older persons: a randomized controlled trial of nonpharmacological interventions in the elderly (TONE). *Journal of the American Medical Association, 279*(11), 839–846.

Winkleby, M. A., Kraemer, H. C., Ahn, D. K., & Varady, A. N. (1998). Ethnic and socioeconomic differences in cardiovascular disease risk factors. *Journal of the American Medical Association, 280,* 356–362.

Yeap, B. B., Russo, A., Fraser, R. J., Wittert, G. A., & Horowitz, M. (1996). Hyperglycemia affects cardiovascular autonomic nerve function in normal subjects. *Diabetes Care, 19,* 880–882.

Ziebland, S., Thorogood, M., Yudkin, P., Jones, L., & Coulter, A. (1997). Lack of willpower or lack of wherewithal? "Internal" and "external" barriers of changing diet and exercise in a three-year follow-up of participants in a health check. *Social Science & Medicine, 46*(4–5), 461–467.

Zimmet, P. Z., McCarty, D. J., & de Courten, M. P.(1997). The global epidemiology of non-insulin-dependent diabetes mellitus and the metabolic syndrome. *Journal of Diabetes Complications, 11,* 60–68.

CHAPTER 21

# Functional Bowel
# and Anorectal Disorders

OLAFUR S. PALSSON AND ROBERT W. COLLINS

**Abstract:** Functional bowel and anorectal disorders collectively affect at least half of the U.S. population and are often treated in primary care settings. A significant proportion of patients with these problems fail to gain adequate relief from conventional medical management, which predominantly consists of education, reassurance, and pharmacological interventions targeting individual symptoms. Empirically validated mind-body treatment alternatives with high success rates exist for incontinence, constipation, and irritable bowel syndrome. Patients with these three disorders, as well as patients with lower gastrointestinal tract symptoms in general who have failed conventional management or who exhibit a clear relationship between psychosocial issues and their gastrointestinal problems, should be routinely considered for behavioral and psychophysiological treatment.

## MEDICAL, PHYSIOLOGICAL, AND BEHAVIORAL PROFILES OF THE DISORDERS

Functional bowel and anorectal disorders are a subset of the functional gastrointestinal (GI) disorders (Drossman, Corazziari, Talley, Thompson, & Whitehead, 2000). They are common in the general population and are often encountered in primary care clinics. Although they rarely pose a threat to patients' lives, they are associated with reduced quality of life, impaired life functioning, and increased medical expenses to patients and society. They are often chronic and sometimes severe. Behavioral and psychophysiological treatments often constitute an important part of successful management of these disorders.

Five specific functional disorders of the bowel (irritable bowel syndrome, functional abdominal bloating, functional constipation, functional diarrhea, and functional abdominal pain syndrome) and three functional anorectal disorders (functional fecal incontinence, functional anorectal pain, and pelvic floor dyssynergia) are currently recognized. Collectively, these disorders plague at least half the U.S. population: A detailed 1993 U.S.-population-based survey (Drossman, Li, et al., 1993) of 5,430 individuals found 44 percent of respondents had functional bowel disorders and 26 percent had functional anorectal disorders, with significant overlap between these categories. These disorders are generally more prevalent in women than in men, and women seek health care for these problems more readily than males (Thompson et al., 2000; Whitehead, Wald, Diamant, et al., 2000).

By virtue of their classification as functional disorders, both these disorders presumably do *not* involve biological or structural pathology, and abnormal physiological functioning is central to their nature. The first assumption has generally been borne out by research, but the evidence has been mixed in regard to the latter. Abnormalities in physiological functioning are sufficiently predominant and well defined in some of these disorders to serve as diagnostic criteria for the disorder. In pelvic floor dyssynergia, for example, paradoxical muscle tension during elimination is used to diagnose the condition.

In other disorders, evidence has been reliably detected in group-based studies of abnormal physiological responses or patterns. However, the abnormal physiological responses are not evident in all (or nearly all) patients and therefore are not diagnostically useful. This is the case for irritable bowel syndrome, in which excessive physiological response to intestinal stimulation, hypermotility, and heightened intestinal pain sensitivity are seen in a substantial proportion of patients in many studies, but not in nearly all individuals (Whitehead, 1996; Whitehead & Palsson, 1998). In still other disorders in this category, such as functional abdominal pain (Kingham, Bown, Colson, & Clark, 1984), there is little evidence or data on abnormal physiological findings.

Research on psychological functioning in patients with functional bowel and anorectal disorders has generally found patients to show high psychological distress compared with healthy controls and other medical patients (Drossman, 1999; Jarrett et al., 1998). Anxiety, depression, and somatization test scores are commonly significantly

elevated (Whitehead, 1996). Many patients (in some studies the majority of patients assessed) meet the formal criteria for comorbid affective (mood) disorders—a diagnosis sometimes identified as a negative prognostic indicator for behavioral treatment approaches (Drossman, 1999; Dykes, Smilgin Humphreys, & Bass, 2001; Nehra, Bruce, Rath-Harvey, Pemberton, & Camilleri, 2000; Whorwell, Prior, & Colgan, 1987). Neuroticism, a personality trait associated with excess negative affect over time and threat perception, has repeatedly been found to be elevated in these disorders (Whitehead, 1996). Other psychological personality profile disturbances have also been found to characterize some of these disorders (Heymen, Wexner, & Gulledge, 1993).

Psychological and social factors associated with childhood bowel and anorectal disorders are very poorly understood compared with those associated with adult disorders. It is hard to say whether it is the parent, the child, both, or an overly busy, two-working-parents or divorced-parents culture ("War of the Diapers," 1999) that is contributing most to toileting delays and other childhood elimination problems.

Adult patients with functional bowel and anorectal disorders often report high life stress and past traumatic life experiences (Drossman, Corazziari, et al., 2000; Whitehead, 1996). In particular, a history of sexual abuse is reported by as many as 40 percent to 50 percent of these patients, more than is reported by patients with any other medical disorder (Drossman, 1995; Leroi, Berkelmans, Denis, Hemond, & Devroede, 1995; Leroi, Bernier, et al., 1995).

Psychological distress contributes significantly to the severity of functional bowel and anorectal symptoms (Drossman, 1999; Drossman, Whitehead, et al., 2000; Jarrett et al., 1998). It is at present unclear, however, whether the impact of psychological functioning on symptoms occurs through physiological effects or through amplifying somatization and illness behavior. Empirical research has shown only a modest or no relationship between the magnitude of physiological abnormalities and that of psychological distress (Whitehead, 1996).

Not only do psychological factors contribute to the manifestation of functional bowel and anorectal disorders, but these disorders often have severe negative impacts on the psychological well-being and social and occupational functioning of patients. Fecal incontinence, which occurs in about 2 percent of children (by definition after age four) and mostly (about 95 percent) takes the form of a constipated, overflow incontinence, can become a source of very great conflict within the family and in child care settings beyond the home (American Gastroenterological Association, 1999; Collins, 1980; Whitehead, Wald, & Norton, 2001). Adults who continue to be incontinent or who develop incontinence (approximately 2 percent overall) will likely suffer just as greatly, fear leaving home, and miss out on being active and having a normal life (Whitehead, Wald, & Norton, 2001). The overall incidence of fecal incontinence approaches 15 percent after the age of 50 and finally becomes a major factor in nursing home placements for the elderly, where it approaches 50 percent among the residents (Jorge & Wexner, 1993; Whitehead, Wald, & Norton, 2001). Irritable bowel syndrome, which affects 10 percent to 20 percent of the general population and most commonly begins in early adulthood, is one of the leading causes of work absenteeism in the United States and can severely disrupt normal social and intimate relationship functioning.

## TYPICAL SYMPTOM PROFILE AND ASSESSMENT

Until the early 1990s, functional bowel and anorectal disorders were generally loosely and inconsistently diagnosed. An international effort in gastroenterology began in 1988 to develop consensus criteria for these and other functional GI disorders. The product of that effort was the establishment of specific consensus criteria for functional GI disorders, the so-called Rome criteria, which have gradually won broad acceptance in the field, both in research and clinical practice. The current version of these criteria is the Rome II criteria published in 2000 (Drossman, Corazziari, et al., 2000). The bowel and anorectal disorder criteria are summarized in Table 21.1.

A definite diagnosis typically requires both *inclusion* of a set of characteristic symptoms of one of the disorders and the *exclusion* of likely competing biological or structural explanations for the patient's symptoms. In addition to physical examination, one or more tests may be appropriate for the latter purpose. Depending on the nature of the symptoms and the health risk profile of the patient, these may be endoscopy or radiological studies, anal manometry, blood samples, stool tests to rule out infection or parasites, or breath hydrogen tests. Constipation and incontinence, in particular, warrant a thorough diagnostic evaluation to search for possible structural and physiological causes. An authoritative set of guidelines may be found in the "Consensus Conference Report: Treatment Options for Fecal Incontinence" (Whitehead, Wald, & Norton, 2001).

Mental health professionals working with these patients should collaborate with physicians and be well acquainted with the common tests and assessment procedures to ensure that other, and often more dangerous, conditions involving pathophysiology are properly ruled out. They should not undertake treatment until this has been done, as identification of biological pathology might otherwise be delayed or obscured. They

**Table 21.1**   Summary of Diagnostic Requirements for Bowel and Functional Anorectal Disorders

| Bowel Disorders | Description |
| --- | --- |
| Irritable bowel syndrome | 12+ weeks in the past year of abdominal discomfort or pain relieved by defecation, associated with altered stool frequency, and/or associated with altered stool form |
| Functional abdominal bloating | 12+ weeks in the past year of abdominal discomfort, bloating, or visible distension |
| Functional constipation | 12+ weeks in the past year including two or more of the following: Straining >1/4 of defecations Lumpy or hard stools >1/4 of defecations Sensation of incomplete evacuation >1/4 of defecations Sensations of anorectal blockage >1/4 of defecations Manual maneuvers to facilitate >1/4 of defecations <3 defecations per week |
| Functional diarrhea | 12+ weeks in the past year of loose or watery stools >3/4 of the time without abdominal pain |
| Functional abdominal pain syndrome | 6+ months of continuous or nearly continuous abdominal pain that impairs daily life functioning and has little or no relationship with physiological events such as eating |

| Functional Anorectal Disorders | Description |
| --- | --- |
| Functional fecal incontinence | 1+ month of recurrent uncontrolled fecal passage associated with fecal impaction, diarrhea, or nocturnal anal sphincter dysfunction in a patient who is developmentally at least four years old |
| Functional anorectal pain | |
| Levator ani syndrome | 12+ weeks total in the last year of chronic or recurrent rectal pain lasting 20 minutes or longer |
| Proctalgia fugax | Recurrent but intermittent brief (seconds to a few minutes) episodes of anal or lower rectal pain |
| Pelvic floor dyssynergia (previously anismus) | Patient meets criteria for functional constipation, but there is incomplete evacuation and physiological (manometry or EMG) or radiological evidence for inappropriate contraction or lack of pelvic floor relaxation during defecation attempts |

SOURCE: Drossman, Corazziari, et al. (2000).

should also be sensitive to the need for further evaluation if treatment has been ineffective. Whitehead, Wald, and Norton (2001), for example, recommend that patients who fail to respond to treatment for fecal incontinence in a well-informed primary care setting within a reasonable time (e.g., four to eight weeks) should be referred for further evaluation.

There are numerous factors to attend to in the clinical assessment interview of patients with lower GI functional complaints, and many of these will influence treatment decisions. Some of the factors are matters that good clinicians attend to in general behavioral medicine practice, such as the history of the presenting problems and a general medical, psychiatric, and social history. Because a host of pharmacological agents influence gastrointestinal functioning, special attention also needs to be paid to use of prescription, over-the-counter, and recreational drugs, and use of tobacco, caffeine, alcohol, and herbal supplements. Dietary habits should also be examined, as fiber intake, specific food sensitivities, and lactose intolerance may have a contributory role in symptoms. Current life stress, symptoms of anxiety and depression, and any relationship of these with the presenting symptoms are always important considerations.

## CONVENTIONAL MEDICAL TREATMENTS AND THEIR SHORTCOMINGS

Due to the fact that anxiety, heightened somatic focus, and worry about potential harm from these functional GI problems are more common than not, patient education, reassurance, and establishment of a good therapeutic relationship are considered standard and important components of good conventional medical management (Drossman, 1999).

Beyond those general therapeutic measures, which are sufficient to ameliorate the symptoms of some patients, conventional medical treatment typically is largely limited to pharmacological interventions for individual symptoms. Such symptomatic treatment varies greatly in success, depending on the disorder, individual patients, and symptoms targeted (Drossman, Corazziari, et al., 2000).

Treatment of the pain that is central to irritable bowel syndrome, and functional abdominal and anorectal pain has met with limited success. Common analgesics are largely ineffective for that purpose, as they are designed to target peripheral pain rather than pain in the gastrointestinal tract. Concerns about addiction potential and overdosing limit the use of narcotics. Antidepressant medications, on the other hand, have been found to act as "central analgesics" (Thompson et al., 2000) and can reduce abdominal discomfort, which can interfere with daily activity, and have an impact on the depression of patients who have significant vegetative depressive symptoms (e.g., sleep, appetite, or libido impairment).

Anxiolytic medication is often used to treat the prevalent anxiety of functional GI patients, but the value of these drugs for gastrointestinal disorders remains to be proven, and their sedative effects and addiction potential limit their utility (Thompson et al., 2000).

Bran and other sources of fiber, such as whole-grain foods or fiber bulk laxatives, have long been recommended to patients for management of constipation. Fiber supplementation has the advantages of being benign, inexpensive, and readily available to all patients. In sufficient doses (optimally at least 30 grams per day), fiber added to the diet can improve constipation, hard stools, and straining. Some patients report improvement in diarrhea and pain as well. It should be noted, however, that some patients either receive no benefit or experience significant worsening of their bowel symptoms from increased fiber intake. Furthermore, up to half of patients may fail to comply due to flatulence, distention, or abdominal discomfort. Among those who continue treatment, however, improvement is seen in up to 80 percent of cases (Thompson et al., 2000).

Laxatives other than fiber are commonly available and widely used by patients. Although they can help constipation, they are often inappropriately and excessively used in the general population (Heaton & Cripps, 1993) and by patients with functional bowel disorders, and chronic use can do more harm than good.

Dietary approaches to the management of the functional bowel and anorectal disorders have often been tried. There have been some reports of success with elimination diets in controlling diarrhea, but these remain largely unproven (Thompson et al., 2000).

Antidiarrheal medications often help to control functional diarrhea and diarrhea associated with irritable bowel syndrome, but the common antidiarrheal drugs frequently have troublesome side effects (Whitehead, Wald, Diamant, et al., 2000).

Surgical interventions are generally not called for in the treatment of functional bowel and anorectal disorders but are sometimes used to relieve constipation associated with severe colonic inertia. Although constipation improves in at least half of these patients after surgery, serious and lasting side effects such as diarrhea or incontinence are common (Pfeiffer, Agachan, & Wexner, 1996).

Conventional management of childhood fecal incontinence and constipation is problematic and deserves a special mention here. The predominant method for treating childhood encopresis has been habit training that is highly reliant on oral laxatives, which has resulted in long-term remission rates of only around 60 percent in extensive reviews (Felt et al., 1999; Lowery, Srour, Whitehead, & Schuster, 1985; Whitehead, Wald, & Norton, 2001). This approach can require months of treatment, and most parents and pediatricians use harsh stimulant vegetable laxatives and problematic mineral oils. Presenters at the 1999 Consensus Conference on Fecal Incontinence advised against the use of such harsh agents. A very clear bias emerged among pediatric authors and practitioners in the 1970s and 1980s for using oral laxatives to the exclusion of more

immediately acting suppositories or enemas (Levine, 1982; Levine & Bakow, 1976).

Cultural concerns over sexual connotations of using the anal route may prevent the more benign, and often more helpful, use of suppositories and enemas and may inappropriately discourage adequate examination of children with anorectal disorders. Gold, Levine, Weinstein, Kessler, and Pettei (1999) found that 77 percent of 128 children referred for chronic constipation had not had a rectal examination, a basic and critical medical procedure for diagnosis before referral. Fifty-four percent of these children were found to have fecal impaction. Fifty-two percent of the children in this study had received stimulant laxative therapy, and 71 percent of that subset had not had prior digital rectal examination. While abuse of children can be a valid concern, a legitimate and important medical procedure such as a rectal exam must not be ignored.

In summary, conventional medical management of functional bowel and anorectal disorders consists of education, reassurance, and drug therapy, sometimes supplemented by diet adjustment and increased fiber intake. Such management helps the majority of patients. However, 25 percent to 40 percent of patients (Felt, et al., 1999; Lowery, et al., 1985; Whitehead, Wald, & Norton, 2001; Whorwell, Prior, & Colgan, 1987) will continue to suffer from chronic, and sometimes debilitating, symptoms without any lasting relief from standard medical management.

These treatment refractory patients, as well as those with prominent chronic psychological distress or clear association between stress and GI symptoms, are proper candidates for psychological and psychophysiological interventions. Furthermore, some mind-body treatment approaches, detailed in the next section, have shown such high and reliable success rates in research that they rival or outperform standard medical treatment and might be considered as the first choice for treating incontinence, pelvic floor dyssynergia, and irritable bowel syndrome.

## BEHAVIORAL AND PSYCHOPHYSIOLOGICAL INTERVENTIONS

Broad-ranging psychological and psychophysiological interventions have been tested for functional bowel and anorectal disorders.

*Biofeedback* is the therapeutic modality that most directly addresses the essence of functional GI disorders, because it aims to directly normalize the abnormalities in physiological functioning that are thought to underlie symptom production. Biofeedback has been demonstrated to be effective in the treatment of pelvic floor dyssynergia (Enck, 1993; Rao, Enck & Loenig-Baucke, 1997) and fecal incontinence (Enck, 1993) in adults and children and has been used as a component in multimodal treatment of irritable bowel syndrome (Schwartz, Taylor, Scharff, & Blanchard, 1990).

Cognitive and cognitive-behavioral therapies identify maladaptive thoughts and perceptual biases that exacerbate or trigger symptoms or cause excess emotional distress. The treatment aims at giving patients control over both their symptoms and the impact of the symptoms on their lives. This approach has been demonstrated to be effective in the treatment of irritable bowel syndrome (Toner et al., 1998).

Behavioral interventions aim at (1) changing specific behaviors directly related to symptoms, such as voiding behavior, that can influence bowel functioning directly, or (2) correcting maladaptive behavioral responses that produce psychological distress (Corney, Stanton, Newell, Clare, & Fairclough, 1991). These interventions have been used successfully in habit training for

fecal incontinence (Lowery et al., 1985) and are often a complementary component to other approaches to treatment.

Hypnotherapy has been mostly used in the treatment of irritable bowel syndrome, where a therapeutic approach centering on gut-directed imagery and physiological relaxation has been found to help many patients (Gonsalkorale et al., 1999; Whorwell, Prior, & Colgan, 1987).

Psychodynamic and interpersonal therapy approaches have been used only in a limited way in reported work on functional bowel and anorectal disorders and are reported to have a beneficial impact on symptoms of irritable bowel syndrome (Guthrie, Creed, Dawson, & Tomenson, 1991; Svedlund, 1983). These treatments aim at ameliorating the effect that difficulties in interpersonal relationships have on the symptoms and well-being of patients.

Stress management training, such as progressive muscle relaxation or autogenic training, makes good sense in light of the ubiquitous findings of heightened distress in patients with these disorders. Stress management training has been found to reduce the symptoms of irritable bowel syndrome (Blanchard, Greene, Scharff, & Schwarz-McMorris, 1993; Lynch & Zamble, 1989; Shaw et al., 1991) and is often combined with another specific psychological intervention, such as cognitive therapy, hypnosis, or biofeedback. The rationale for this approach is to neutralize the sympathetic arousal that may amplify or trigger gastrointestinal symptoms, as well as to improve patients' well-being. Biofeedback (typically thermal or EMG biofeedback training) has also been used for general relaxation.

The cognitive and cognitive-behavioral treatment modalities are often combined in various ways in the treatment of functional bowel and anorectal disorders. For example, a treatment package for irritable bowel syndrome consisting of progressive muscle relaxation, thermal biofeedback, cognitive therapy and education has been empirically tested and found to be effective in the treatment of irritable bowel syndrome (Schwartz et al., 1990), although there is no evidence that it is more effective than simpler single-modality treatments in treating this disorder.

Initially, some patients have negative reactions to the suggestion of psychological treatment for their functional GI problems because they take it to imply that the physician thinks their problems "all in their heads." Physicians should therefore introduce psychological treatment to patients as complementary to ongoing medical care. It may be necessary to explain that such therapy reduces the psychological impact of the functional disorder, helps relieve stress that exacerbates the symptoms, and does not imply that the patient suffers exclusively from a psychological disorder. Some patients who are unreceptive to psychological treatment, even after careful explanation of the rationale for such intervention, are more accepting of biofeedback training, which is more readily identified as a treatment of the body than the mind.

### Effective Protocols and Interventions

As previously noted, standard medical management helps the symptoms of many patients with functional bowel and anorectal disorders. It is common, therefore, to refer patients to mind-body treatments only when conventional management fails. However, empirically validated mind-body treatments with high success rates should be routinely considered in addition to, or sometimes in place of, standard medical approaches (especially drug therapy or surgery), as they are largely without harmful side effects and give patients a sense of control over their own health. To be considered empirically validated, a mind-body therapy should minimally meet the following four criteria:

1. It is more effective than conventional management.

2. Several formal empirical studies have been published by multiple research teams, showing consistently high success rate.

3. Well-described and replicable treatment protocols exist.

4. Follow-up studies for one year or longer have been done, with treatment gains substantially maintained.

In addition, placebo-controlled studies and comparisons with standard management are highly desirable to establish the superiority of the treatments in question over nonspecific interventions or routine medical care.

The following mind-body treatments presently meet all four criteria in the treatment of functional disorders of the bowel and anorectum.

*Biofeedback for Fecal Incontinence.* Many uncontrolled studies have been conducted, and the vast majority of these support the efficacy of this treatment. A systematic review (Enck, 1993) has suggested that three fourths of patients achieve clinically significant improvement using this approach.

*Biofeedback for Pelvic Floor Dyssynergia.* Biofeedback offers a reliably effective treatment for pelvic floor dyssynergia. Because the treatment has no side effects and is more effective than alternatives, it is considered a first line of treatment for pelvic floor dyssynergia. Systematic reviews (Enck, 1993; Rao et al., 1997) and several large series of patients (Patanar et al., 1997) suggest that at least two thirds of patients benefit from this approach. The treatment aims at teaching patients to relax the external anal sphincter during defecation attempts.

*Hypnosis Treatment for Irritable Bowel Syndrome.* Hypnosis treatment for irritable bowel syndrome has been reported to be successful in more than a dozen studies. It has been tested in a randomized placebo-controlled trial (Whorwell, Prior, & Faragher, 1984), and a large case series (205 patients) has been reported (Gonsalkorale et al., 1999). Improvement is typically seen in 80 percent or more of patients treated with a course of 7 to 12 sessions; remarkably, this high success rate is also seen in studies involving only patients with severe problems who have failed conventional management (Palsson, Turner, & Johnson, 2000; Whorwell, Prior, & Colgan, 1987; Whorwell, Prior, & Faragher, 1984). Fully standardized protocols have been tested (Palsson, Burnett, Meyer, & Whitehead, 1997; Palsson, Turner, & Johnson, 2000) and are available to clinicians with proper training and experience in clinical hypnosis.

*Cognitive-Behavioral Therapy for Irritable Bowel Syndrome.* The success rate of this treatment is as high as 80 percent, and the efficacy of this therapy has been established in several studies (Greene & Blanchard, 1994; Payne & Blanchard, 1995; Toner et al., 1998; Van Dulmen, Fennis, & Bleijenberg, 1996), including controlled trials (Payne & Blanchard, 1995). The treatment can be conducted in structured format, and scripts are available for handling common therapy situations (Toner et al., 1998).

Unfortunately, no empirically validated psychological or mind-body treatment protocols currently exist for functional abdominal bloating, functional diarrhea, and functional abdominal or anorectal pain.

### Long-Term Outcome Studies

Functional bowel and anorectal disorders are generally chronic in nature, although many have an intermittent course, and spontaneous recovery sometimes occurs. Many studies of behavioral and psychophysiological

interventions for functional GI disorders only include three to six months of follow-up. Several studies, however, have demonstrated that the clinical improvement effected by these treatments can last at least one to four years. Examples include the following:

- Gains from hypnosis treatment for irritable bowel syndrome have proven to be well maintained at one-year and two-year follow-up (Whorwell, Prior, & Colgan, 1987; Palsson, Turner, & Johnson, 2000).

- A follow-up (Chiotakakou-Faliakou, Kamm, Roy, Storrie, & Turner, 1998) of 100 adults treated with biofeedback for constipation refractory to conventional treatment showed that 57 percent of patients improved after two years.

- Habit training for fecal incontinence in children showed the therapeutic gain to be well maintained at three-year follow-up, with 61 percent of patients experiencing excellent results after that time (Lowery et al., 1985).

- A four-year follow-up of patients with multicomponent treatment involving progressive muscle relaxation, thermal biofeedback, cognitive therapy, and education found that the majority of patients still showed at least a 50 percent reduction in primary symptom scores for irritable bowel syndrome (Schwartz et al., 1990).

Such long-term benefits from mind-body therapies for functional bowel and anorectal disorders support the cost-effectiveness of these treatments and the value of considering these approaches in the management of functional GI disorders.

### FUTURE DIRECTIONS

### The Need for Further Research

With the exception of biofeedback studies, the bulk of research on mind-body therapies for functional bowel and anorectal disorders has focused on irritable bowel syndrome. Psychological and psychophysiological therapies for other disorders need to be developed and empirically tested.

Investigations of better alternatives to the current conventional treatment of functional lower GI disorders in children have especially been neglected. Promising alternatives have repeatedly been identified, but adequate efforts have not been made to produce the research data necessary for systematic empirical validation of these alternatives.

Psychologist Logan Wright (1973, 1975), for example, introduced a procedure a quarter of a century ago that rapidly overcame anismus and guaranteed daily defecation using the anal route. His procedure dramatically reduced the average number of soilings from 17.14 in the first week to 2.16 for week two and 0.50 for week four. This dramatic and rapid response is much better than that observed with the oral route.

Another example of a promising treatment alternative for children is provided in the *Clean Kid Manual* (Collins, 2002). This manual is currently used by several pediatricians across the country in treating their patients, and parents are ordering the manual directly after many months of frustration with the traditional pediatric method.

## Broadening the Standard Medical Approach to Functional Lower GI Disorders

The realities of today's dominant health care environment are that primary care clinicians are the principal caretakers of patients with functional bowel and anorectal disorders. Conventional management of these disorders could become more effective by integrating successful elements of mind-body therapies into standard medical care. Structured procedures for primary care clinicians that incorporate both the psychological, physiological, and biomedical aspects of these problems could be developed and taught in medical settings. Judging from what has been found effective for functional GI disorders to date, relaxation, cognitive restructuring, education, and empathy would likely be important elements in such comprehensive biopsychosocial interventions.

Additionally, physicians who manage the health care of functional GI patients should form close collaborations with behavioral clinicians with expertise in the psychological and psychophysiologicial therapies that have been empirically validated for these problems.

## REFERENCES

American Gastroenterological Association, Clinical Practice and Practice Economics Committee. (1999). *Gastroenterology, 116*(3), 735–760.

Blanchard, E. B., Greene, B., Scharff, L., & Schwarz-McMorris, S. P. (1993). Relaxation training as a treatment for irritable bowel syndrome. *Biofeedback & Self-Regulation, 3*, 125–132.

Chiotakakou-Faliakou, E., Kamm, M. A., Roy, A. J., Storrie, J. B., & Turner, I. C. (1998). Biofeedback provides long-term benefit for patients with intractable, slow and normal transit constipation. *Gut, 42*(4), 517–521.

Collins, R. W. (1980). *Enuresis and encopresis.* In R. H. Woody (Ed.), *Encyclopedia of clinical assessment* (pp. 286–294). San Francisco: Jossey-Bass.

Collins, R. W. (2002, March 20). *The clean kid manual* [Excerpts]. Retrieved from http://www.soilingsolutions.com/html/clean_excerpts.htm

Corney, R. H., Stanton, R., Newell, R., Clare, A., & Fairclough, P. (1991). Behavioural psychotherapy as a treatment for irritable bowel syndrome. *Journal of Psychosomatic Research, 35,* 461–469.

Drossman, D. A. (1995). Sexual and physical abuse and gastrointestinal illness. *Scandinavian Journal of Gastroenterology, 208*(4, Suppl.), 90–96.

Drossman, D. A. (1999). Do psychosocial factors define symptom severity and patient status in irritable bowel syndrome? *American Journal of Medicine, 107*(5, Suppl. A), 41S–50S.

Drossman, D. A., Corazziari, E., Talley, N. J., Thompson, W. G., & Whitehead, W. E. (Eds.). (2000). *Rome II: The functional gastrointestinal disorders* (2nd ed.). McLean, VA: Degnon Associates.

Drossman, D. A., Li, Z., Andruzzi, E., Temple, R. D., Talley, N. J., Thompson, W. G., et al. (1993). U.S. householder survey of functional gastrointestinal disorders. Prevalence, sociodemography, and health impact. *Digestive Diseases and Sciences, 38*(9), 1569–1580.

Drossman, D. A., Whitehead, W. E., Toner, B. B., Diamant, N., Hu, Y. J., Bangdiwala, S. I., et al. (2000). What determines severity among patients with painful functional bowel disorders? *American Journal of Gastroenterology, 95*(4), 974–980.

Dykes, S., Smilgin-Humphreys, S., & Bass, C. (2001). Chronic idiopathic constipation: A psychological enquiry. *European Journal of Gastroenterology and Hepatology, 13*(1), 39–44.

Enck, P. (1993). Biofeedback training in disordered defecation: A critical review. *Digestive Diseases & Sciences, 38,* 1953–1960.

Felt, B., Wise, C. G., Olson, A., Kochhar, P., Marcus, S., & Coran, A. (1999). Guideline for the management of pediatric idiopathic constipation and soiling. *Archives of Pediatrics and Adolescent Medicine, 153*(4), 380–385.

Gold, D. M., Levine, J., Weinstein, T. A., Kessler, B. H., & Pettei, M. J. (1999). Frequency of digital rectal examination in children with chronic constipation. *Archives of Pediatric and Adolescent Medicine, 153*(4), 377–379.

Gonsalkorale, W.M., Cooper, P., Cruikshanks, P., Miller, V., Randles, J., Whelan, V., et al. (1999). Hypnotherapy for severe irritable bowel syndrome: Gender differences in response? *Gastroenterology, 116,* A999.

Greene, B., & Blanchard, E. B. (1994). Cognitive therapy for irritable bowel syndrome. *Journal of Consulting and Clinical Psychology, 62,* 576–582.

Guthrie, E., Creed, F., Dawson, D., & Tomenson, B. (1991). A controlled trial of psychological treatment for the irritable bowel syndrome. *Gastroenterology, 100,* 450–457.

Heaton, K. W., & Cripps, H. A. (1993). Straining at stool and laxative taking in an English population. *Digestive Diseases & Sciences, 38,* 1004–1008.

Heymen, S., Wexner, S. D., & Gulledge, A. D. (1993). MMPI assessment of patients with functional bowel disorders. *Diseases of the Colon and Rectum, 36*(6), 593–596.

Jarrett, M., Heitkemper, M., Cain, K. C., Tuftin, M., Walker, E. A., Bond, E. F., et al. (1998). The relationship between psychological distress and gastrointestinal symptoms in women with irritable bowel syndrome. *Nursing Research, 47*(3), 154–161.

Jorge, J. M., & Wexner, S. D. (1993). Etiology and management of fecal incontinence. *Diseases of the Colon and Rectum, 36*(1), 77–97.

Kingham, J. G., Bown, R., Colson, R., & Clark, M. L. (1984). Jejunal motility in patients with functional abdominal pain. *Gut, 25*(4), 375–380.

Leroi, A. M., Berkelmans, I., Denis, P., Hemond, M., & Devroede, G. (1995). Anismus as a marker of sexual abuse. *Digestive Diseases and Sciences, 40,* 1411–1416.

Leroi, A. M., Bernier, C., Watier, A., Hemond, M., Goupil, G., Black, R., et al. (1995). Prevalence of sexual abuse among patients with functional disorders of the lower gastrointestinal tract. *International Journal of Colorectal Disease, 10*(4), 200–206.

Levine, M. D. (1982). Encopresis: Its potentiation, evaluation, and alleviation. *Pediatric Clinics of North America, 29*(2), 315–330.

Levine, M. D., & Bakow, H. (1976). Children with encopresis: A study of treatment outcome. *Pediatrics, 58*(6), 845–852.

Lowery, S. P., Srour, J. W., Whitehead, W. E., & Schuster, M. M. (1985). Habit training as treatment of encopresis secondary to chronic constipation. *Journal of Pediatric Gastroenterology and Nutrition, 4*(3), 397–401.

Lynch, P. M., & Zamble, E. (1989). A controlled behavioral treatment study of irritable bowel syndrome. *Behavior Therapy, 20,* 509–524.

Nehra, V., Bruce, B. K., Rath-Harvey, D. M., Pemberton, J. H., & Camilleri, M. (2000). Psychological disorders in patients with evacuation disorders and constipation in a tertiary practice. *American Journal of Gastroenterology, 95*(7), 1755–1758.

Palsson, O. S., Burnett, C. K., Meyer, K., & Whitehead, W. E. (1997). Hypnosis treatment for irritable bowel syndrome. Effects on symptoms, pain threshold and muscle tone. *Gastroenterology, 112,* A803.

Palsson, O. S., Turner, M. J., & Johnson, D. A. (2000). Hypnotherapy for irritable bowel syndrome: Symptom improvement and autonomic nervous system effects. *Gastroenterology, 118*(4), A174.

Patanar, S. K., Ferrara, A., Levy, J. R., Larach, S. W., Williamson, P. R., & Perozo, S. E. (1997). Biofeedback in colorectal practice: A multi-center, statewide, three-year experience. *Diseases of the Colon and Rectum, 40,* 827–831.

Payne, A., & Blanchard, E. B. (1995). A controlled comparison of cognitive therapy and self-help support groups in the treatment of irritable bowel syndrome. *Journal of Consulting and Clinical Psychology, 63*(5), 779–786.

Pfeiffer, J., Agachan, F., & Wexner, S. D. (1996). Surgery for constipation: A review. *Diseases of the Colon and Rectum, 39*(4), 444–460.

Rao, S. S., Enck, P., & Loenig-Baucke, V. (1997). Biofeedback therapy for defecation disorders. *Digestive Diseases, 15*(Suppl. 1), 78–92.

Schwartz, S. P., Taylor, A. E., Scharff, L., & Blanchard, E. B. (1990). Behaviorally treated irritable bowel syndrome patients: A four-year follow-up. *Behavior Research and Therapy, 28*(4), 331–335.

Shaw, G., Srivastava, E. D., Sadlier, M., Swann, P., James, J. Y., & Rhodes, J. (1991). Stress management for irritable bowel syndrome: A controlled trial. *Digestion, 50,* 36–42.

Svedlund, J. (1983). Psychotherapy in irritable bowel syndrome: A controlled outcome study. *Acta Psychiatrica Scandinavica, 67*(Suppl.), 1–86.

Thompson, W. G., Longstreth, G., Drossman, D. A., Heaton, K., Irvine, E. J., & Muller-Lisner, S. (2000). C. Functional bowel disorders, and D. Functional abdominal pain. In D. A. Drossman, E. Corazziari, N. J. Talley, W. G. Thompson, & W. E. Whitehead (Eds.), *Rome II: The functional gastrointestinal disorders* (2nd ed., pp. 351–432). McLean, VA: Degnon Associates.

Toner, B. B., Segal, Z. V., Emmott, S., Myran, D., Ali, A., DiGasbarro, I., et al. (1998). Cognitive-behavioral group therapy for patients with irritable bowel syndrome. *International Journal of Group Psychotherapy, 48*(2), 215–243.

Van Dulmen, A. M., Fennis, J. F., & Bleijenberg, G. (1996). Cognitive-behavioral group therapy for irritable bowel syndrome: Effects and long-term follow-up. *Psychosomatic Medicine, 58*(5), 508–514.

War of the diapers. (1999, January 25). *Time,* p. 64.

Whitehead, W. E. (1996). Psychosocial aspects of functional gastrointestinal disorders. *Gastroenterology Clinics of North America*, 25(1), 21–34.

Whitehead, W. E., & Palsson, O. S. (1998). Is rectal sensitivity a biological marker for irritable bowel syndrome: Psychological influences on pain perception in irritable bowel syndrome. *Gastroenterology*, *115*(5), 1263–1271.

Whitehead, W. E., Wald, A., Diamant, N. E., Enck, P., Pemberton, J. H., & Rao, S. S. (2000). Functional disorders of the anus and rectum. In D. A. Drossman, W. Corazziari, N. J. Talley, W. G. Thompson, & W. E. Whitehead (Eds.), *Rome II: The functional gastrointestinal disorders* (2nd ed., pp. 483–532). McLean, VA: Degnon Associates.

Whitehead, W. E., Wald, A., & Norton, N. J. (2001). Consensus conference report: Treatment options for fecal incontinence. *Diseases of the Colon and Rectum*, 44(1), 131–144.

Whorwell, P. J., Prior, A. & Colgan, S. M. (1987). Hypnotherapy in severe irritable bowel syndrome: Further experience. *Gut*, 28(4), 423–425.

Whorwell, P. J., Prior, A., & Faragher, E. B. (1984). Controlled trial of hypnotherapy in the treatment of severe refractory irritable-bowel syndrome. *Lancet*, 2, 1232–1234.

Wright, L. (1973). Handling the encopretic child. *Professional Psychology*, *4*(5), 137–144.

Wright, L. (1975). Outcome of a standardized program for treating psychogenic encopresis. *Professional Psychology*, 6(11), 453–456.

# CHAPTER 22

# Urinary Incontinence

## OLAFUR S. PALSSON

**Abstract:** Urinary incontinence is a major clinical problem that affects a large proportion of adults, primarily women and the elderly. With careful diagnosis and appropriate therapy, current methods can help 80 percent of patients with urinary incontinence. Standard treatment approaches include pelvic floor exercises, bladder training, medications, and surgery. Behavioral and psychophysiological methods have successfully addressed the most common types of urinary incontinence.

## MEDICAL, PHYSIOLOGICAL, AND BEHAVIORAL PROFILES OF THE DISORDERS

Urinary incontinence (UI), or involuntary loss of urine, is a major clinical problem that affects approximately half of all adult women to some degree (Harrison & Memel, 1994) and is approximately 10 times more common in women than in men (MacLennan, Taylor, Wilson, & Wilson, 2000). Among women, UI is more prevalent after menopause and among the elderly (Brown et al., 1999; Harrison & Memel, 1994; MacLennan et al., 2000). Even in women in the age range from 20 to 49, however, UI incidence has been reported to be as high as 47 percent (Harrison & Memel, 1994). Many cases of UI are mild. However, 17 million adults (Khoury, 2001) suffer from significant UI problems that reduce their quality of life and are associated with substantial disability, dependency, and emotional toll. The direct annual costs of managing UI in the United States were estimated in 1995 to be $26.3 billion (Wagner & Hu, 1998).

Urinary incontinence occurs for numerous reasons. It can have neurological, structural/anatomical, physiological, psychophysiological, mental, behavioral, and even situational causes, and it is not uncommon for more than one of these factors to synergistically produce the problem. This chapter cannot accommodate detailed discussion of the broad spectrum of reasons for incontinence problems but does address the characteristics of the major types and outline effective treatment options.

The urinary bladder is a reservoir with a wall that contains interlaced bundles of smooth muscles. The muscular wall, called the detrusor, relaxes to allow storage of the urine produced by the kidneys. When it receives appropriate signals from the brain, it contracts to produce emptying (urination or micturition). Stretch sensors in the bladder wall send information via the spine to the brain, enabling the brain to monitor the degree of fullness in the bladder. Normal filling and emptying of the bladder are largely under the control of the autonomic nervous system (ANS), based on information from the stretch sensors. When there is little fluid in the bladder, the sympathetic branch of the ANS is stimulated, which causes the smooth muscles of the detrusor to relax and stretch so the bladder can accommodate more fluid. Simultaneously, the parasympathetic branch of the ANS is inhibited, which keeps the internal sphincter contracted, holding the urine securely in the bladder.

When the bladder volume reaches approximately 300 cc, the brain normally recognizes fullness. When bladder emptying is desired, the brain stimulates the parasympathetic nerves to the bladder and inhibits sympathetic nerve activity. This results in contraction of the detrusor smooth muscles and relaxation of the internal bladder sphincter, allowing urine to escape. The wall contraction continues during that process, pushing the urine out to overcome resistance in the urethra. Once the bladder is empty, parasympathetic inhibition and sympathetic stimulation resume, allowing filling to begin again. The external bladder sphincter usually plays little role in continence but can help to block urination briefly when needed, both in deliberate withholding and to prevent urine loss during transient pressure increases in the abdomen, such as during coughing, sneezing, or laughing.

Factors that increase risk for incontinence include diabetes mellitus, large body mass index, bearing children (with the risk increasing after each birth), and increasing age (MacLennan et al., 2000; Persson, Wolner-Hanssen, & Rydhstroem, 2000). Regarding the last factor, it is important to recognize that normal aging does not cause UI. However, aging results in biological changes

(such as pelvic muscle atrophy, reduced sensation, and decreased bladder size) and accumulating events (such as urinary tract infections, fecal impaction, obstetric trauma, prostate problems, immobility) that make incontinence more likely to occur.

## TYPICAL SYMPTOM PROFILES

Most cases of UI fall into one of four categories:

1. *Urge incontinence, or detrusor overactivity* (also called uninhibited or overactive bladder, detrusor instability, or detrusor hyperreflexia), is marked by a recurrent, sudden urge to urinate and frequent voiding. The symptoms are produced by inappropriate early contractions of the muscles in the bladder wall due to defective ANS inhibition or by excessive afferent sensory stimulation from the bladder. This can result from several diseases and physiological changes and becomes more likely with aging. Urge incontinence is not associated with any consistent pathophysiological evidence detectable by tests or physical exam; therefore, diagnosis is primarily based on history.

2. *Overflow incontinence* is characterized by markedly reduced urinary stream, incomplete or unsuccessful voiding, and frequent or continuous dribbling of urine. The causes are either a bladder with lessened or absent contractile ability (hypotonic or atonic bladder) or obstruction in the urine outflow. Either cause produces higher than normal bladder volumes with pressure that exceeds the resistance of the urethra, causing dribbling, whereas the obstruction or muscle dysfunction causes voiding difficulty. In men, bladder outlet obstruction is usually due to prostate enlargement. Physical examination of urge incontinence patients often reveals a distended bladder and in men, prostate

enlargement. Measurement of urine volume after voiding can show excess residual volume, and urodynamic testing can demonstrate decreased urinary flow rates.

3. *Stress incontinence, or outlet incompetence,* is characterized by loss of small amounts of urine when pressure in the abdominal area increases, such as when coughing and sneezing or during exercise. It is commonly caused by weakening or laxity of the striated pelvic floor muscles responsible for keeping the urethra closed when intra-abdominal pressure rises. Common reasons for stress incontinence in women include pelvic muscle laxity after childbirth and atrophy of muscles after menopause. Stress incontinence can also result from weakness of the bladder sphincters. In men, stress incontinence is generally limited to those who have suffered damage to the internal sphincter due to urological procedures.

4. *Functional incontinence* is unwanted voiding (not reaching a bathroom) caused by some external factor in individuals who have a normal urinary system and would otherwise be continent. Factors that may cause this include the effects of medications, physical problems impairing the ability to reach a bathroom when needed, or cognitive impairment such as dementia or delirium. Functional incontinence generally is not associated with any significant findings on physical examination or urodynamic testing and needs to be determined based on assessment of the patient's medications, cognitive and physical abilities, and the situations surrounding incontinence episodes.

In addition to these four types, incontinence can result from various physical trauma, such as pelvic floor trauma related to childbirth or fistulas. Finally, some patients have both urge and stress incontinence, which is designated as *mixed incontinence.*

## ASSESSMENT AND DIAGNOSIS

In assessment and diagnosis of UI, the clinical interview is perhaps the single most important method. Factors to determine in the interview include the history; frequency, circumstances, and quantity of urine loss (see Box 22.1); bowel habits (which can affect UI); past medical history; current medications (many medications influence urine production and modulate voiding); fluid and caffeine intake; and effect of the problem on the patient's life (Culligan & Heit, 2000; Tries & Eisman, 1995). Physical examination is a standard component of the assessment of UI and may reveal physical causes of incontinence such as fecal impaction, prostate enlargement, and the enlarged bladder of overflow incontinence. Urodynamic testing can be helpful—especially in assessing urge or stress incontinence (Abrams, Blaivas, Stanton, & Andersen, 1988)—and sometimes laboratory tests or radiological studies are called for when symptoms or history indicate their use. Often, however, a thorough clinical interview and a physical exam are sufficient to establish definite diagnosis and initiate treatment (Culligan & Heit, 2000).

## CONVENTIONAL MEDICAL TREATMENTS

Urinary incontinence is in most cases a highly treatable condition. It is estimated that if adequately diagnosed and managed, 80 percent of cases can be markedly improved (Burkhart, 2000). Therapeutic efforts should generally begin with conservative treatment options (Khoury, 2001; National Institutes of Health, 1988) such as pelvic floor exercises. Stress and urge incontinence, the most common types of UI (Culligan & Heit, 2000), are also the ones that most readily lend themselves to conservative and noninvasive

---

**Box 22.1**     Key Questions for Determining the Type and Severity of Urinary Incontinence

**DETERMINING TYPE**

*Stress Incontinence*

- Do you leak urine when you cough, laugh, lift something or sneeze? How often?

*Urge Incontinence*

- Do you ever leak urine when you have a strong urge on the way to the bathroom? How often?
- How frequently do you empty your bladder during the day?
- How many times do you get up to urinate after going to sleep? Is it the urge to urinate that wakes you?
- Do you ever leak urine during sex?

*Overflow Incontinence*

- Does it hurt when you urinate?
- Do you ever feel that you are unable to completely empty your bladder?

**DETERMINING SEVERITY**

- Do you wear pads that protect you from leaking urine? How often do you have to change them?
- Do you ever find urine on your pads or clothes and were unaware of when the leakage occurred?

---

Adapted with permission from Culligan and Heit (2000).

---

treatment. Physicians have a variety of effective therapy options at their disposal.

*Medications.* Estrogen replacement therapy, administered either orally or topically in the vagina in the form of an estrogen ring or estrogen cream, helps many women with stress and urge incontinence, as estrogen thickens the urethral mucosa (Bhatia, Bergman, & Karram, 1989). Tolterodine and extended-release oxybutynin chloride have become first-line pharmacological treatment agents for urge incontinence and have favorable side-effect profiles (Culligan & Heit, 2000). Alpha-adrenergic drugs, which increase resting urethral tone, improve stress incontinence in 20 percent to 60 percent of patients (Fantl, 1996). Tricyclic antidepressants are also used to treat urge incontinence.

*Pelvic Floor Exercises.* Kegel exercises (Kegel, 1948) are therapeutic pelvic floor exercises that aim at increasing muscle strength and contraction reflexes to sudden rise in intra-abdominal pressure. Gaining awareness of the pelvic floor muscle contractions is also an important component of these exercises. Typically, repeated series of 5- to 10-second contractions, followed by an equal period of relaxation contractions, should be performed daily. Kegel exercises are primary useful for stress incontinence, can yield improvements for up to 83 percent of patients (Ceresoli et al., 1993; Hahn, Milsom, Fall, & Ekelund, 1993), and seem to work best for younger women and those with milder symptoms (Bishop, Dougherty, Mooney, Gimotty, & Williams, 1992; Elia & Bergman, 1993).

*Vaginal Weights.* Also called vaginal cones, these devices are carried in the vagina for 15 minutes twice a day, providing powerful sensory feedback that makes the pelvic floor contract around the cone and retain it. As the pelvic floor muscles become stronger, the weight of the cones is gradually increased. In controlled studies, cones have been at least as effective as routine pelvic floor exercises and require less teaching time (Haken, Benness, Cardozo, & Cutner, 1991; Norton & Baker, 1990), but they are often used in combination with Kegel-type exercises.

*Electrical Stimulation of the Pelvic Floor.* This treatment can help both stress and urge incontinence. Urge incontinence is treated by short-term maximal stimulation (Eriksen, 1989) whereas stress incontinence is typically treated by lower intensity long-term stimulation (Hahn, Sommer, & Fall, 1991). Electrical stimulation has been used less in

the United States than in Europe, perhaps due to difficulties in obtaining third-party reimbursement. That may change quickly, however, as the Health Care Financing Administration (2000b) recently approved Medicare coverage of this treatment based on favorable research evidence.

*Pessaries.* These mechanical support devices are carried in the vagina and are among the oldest of all medical devices. They are often useful in managing stress incontinence (Viera & Larkins-Pettigrew, 2000).

*Surgical Procedures.* The most common procedures are retropubic urethropexies and suburethral slings. They are good options for patients who do not respond to conservative management and have severe symptoms of genuine stress incontinence, with reported long-term success rates at 80 percent and higher (Leach et al., 1997; Ulmsten, Henriksson, Johnson, & Varhos, 1996). Incontinence due to structural problems of various kinds is also often successfully addressed by surgery.

## BEHAVIORAL AND PSYCHOPHYSIOLOGICAL INTERVENTIONS

Behavioral and psychophysiological approaches can contribute substantially to effective management of stress, urge, and mixed incontinence and most commonly consist of bladder training and biofeedback.

The term *bladder training* encompasses both timed voiding or habit training (voiding on a fixed schedule) and prompted voiding (where the patient is asked at regular intervals about the need to void). Bladder training regimens are popular, widely used, and often effective with UI patients in nursing homes to treat urge incontinence. In one study, they have also been reported to help stress incontinence (Fantl, Wyman, McClish, et al., 1991). Patient education and positive reinforcement are important components of such training (Fantl, Wyman, Harkins, & Hadley, 1990).

Biofeedback, often requiring no more than four to six sessions, has proven effective in several studies (e.g., Burgio, Whitehead, & Engel, 1985; Burns, Pranikoff, Nochasjski, Desotelle, & Harwood, 1990; Burton, Pearce, Burgio, Engel, & Whitehead, 1988; Ceresoli et al., 1993; Glavind, Nohr, & Walter, 1996; Susset, Galea, & Read, 1990), with significant therapeutic effects on both urge and stress incontinence. UI biofeedback uses feedback from electromyographic and pressure sensors to correct incontinence-related physiological activity. Because of the complexity of the voiding process and the various reasons for problems, several measuring channels should be used (Tries & Eisman, 1995). The training aims at reinforcing bladder inhibition, strengthening pelvic muscle tone and contractions, or maintaining stable bladder pressure while contracting pelvic floor muscles. Although clearly effective, it is unclear whether biofeedback has distinct advantages over other methods. Several studies have typically failed to demonstrate clear outcome differences of biofeedback and comparison methods (Burns et al., 1990; Burton et al., 1988; Ceresoli et al., 1993). However, Glavind et al. (1996) found biofeedback to lead to more improvement than pelvic floor exercises alone in a study of 40 women (91 percent versus 22 percent on an objective test at three-month follow-up). Many research protocols and clinical treatment programs use biofeedback in combination with pelvic floor exercises and/or bladder training. Apart from biofeedback effects alone, biofeedback instruments can also be used to significantly enhance teaching of pelvic floor exercises (Burgio, Robinson, & Engel, 1986).

## EFFECTIVE PROTOCOLS AND INTERVENTIONS

The many ways in which interventions are combined in the treatment of urinary incontinence make it hard to assess which single interventions are effective and how much different components add to the outcome. Surgery, biofeedback, bladder training, and pelvic floor exercises, however, have been demonstrated individually to have an 80 percent or better success rate in select UI patient groups. Some examples of such effective interventions are described in the following paragraphs.

Retropubic urethropexies and suburethral slings are surgical procedures that have reportedly corrected genuine stress incontinence successfully in 80 percent to 96 percent of cases (Leach et al., 1997; Ulmsten et al., 1996). However, since surgery, unlike other inventions, can sometimes result in serious and lasting side effects, other options should be explored first.

In a study of 15 women with stress and urge incontinence, Susset et al. (1990) reported that 87 percent of patients improved on an objective measure (pad weights) and 80 percent of patients reported 100 percent symptom improvement from intravaginal pressure biofeedback combined with use of home training devices.

Jarvis and Millar (1980) conducted a randomized and controlled trial of inpatient bladder training with 60 women. After treatment, 83 percent were continent and symptom free compared with 23 percent of controls.

In a comparison of pelvic floor exercises alone or combined with biofeedback, Ceresoli et al. (1993) found that 82 percent of patients using the exercises alone and 89 percent also receiving biofeedback had at least 60 percent improvement in urinary loss (group differences were not statistically significant).

## LONG-TERM OUTCOME STUDIES

Follow-up in studies of behavioral and psychophysiological treatments, as well as other conservative management methods, has unfortunately been limited in most cases to a period of less than a year after treatment. Empirical literature on the long-term success of conservative management methods for urinary incontinence is therefore almost nonexistent, and what little there is tends to rely on small samples or the effects of heterogenous interventions. However, there are indications that some conservative approaches such as bladder training and pelvic floor exercises have beneficial effects lasting a number of years (Hahn, Milsom, et al., 1993; Lagro-Janssen & van Weel, 1998; Weinberger, Goodman, & Carnes, 1999). Surgical interventions for stress incontinence show excellent long-term outcomes beyond 48 months with an 80 percent or better success rate. (Leach et al., 1997; Richter et al., 2001; Ulmsten et al., 1996)

## FUTURE DIRECTIONS

New and promising treatments for urinary incontinence, such as extracorporeal magnetic innervation (Galloway et al., 1999), new medications, and minimally invasive surgical solutions, keep emerging and are likely to add to the arsenal of currently effective treatments for UI. Behavioral and psychophysiological methods have been amply demonstrated to be useful in the treatment of UI, but further research work remains in the field to refine and demonstrate which protocols and combinations are most effective—especially for biofeedback, which is practiced in a bewildering number of ways. Long-term outcome studies of significant size are sorely needed for all of the conservative management methods.

Lack of reimbursement has hindered many UI patients from benefiting from some of the benign and effective treatment alternatives. The mounting body of research evidence on these methods is gradually removing such obstacles, and much wider access to options other than medications and surgery is foreseeable. For example, based on review of the research and clinician expert testimonies, the Health Care Financing Administration (2000a, 2000b) has recently established a national policy mandating coverage for electrical stimulation and biofeedback for Medicare beneficiaries with UI, when certain conditions are met.

## REFERENCES

Abrams, P., Blaivas, J. G., Stanton, S. L., & Andersen, J. T. (1988). The standardisation of terminology of lower urinary tract function. The International Continence Society Committee on Standardisation of Terminology. *Scandinavian Journal of Urology and Nephrology, 114*(Suppl.), 519.

Bhatia, N. N., Bergman, A., & Karram, M. M. (1989). Effects of estrogen on urethral function in women with urinary incontinence. *American Journal of Obstetrics and Gynecology, 160*, 176–181.

Bishop, K. R., Dougherty, M., Mooney, R., Gimotty, P., & Williams, B. (1992). Effects of age, parity, and adherence on pelvic muscle response to exercise. *Journal of Obstetrical and Gynecological Neonatal Nursing, 21*, 401–406.

Brown, J. S., Grady, D., Ouslander, J. G., Herzog, A. R., Varner, R. E., & Posner, S. F. (1999). Prevalence of urinary incontinence and associated risk factors in post-menopausal women. Heart & Estrogen/Progestin Replacement Study (HERS) Research Group. *Obstetrics and Gynecology, 94,* 66–70.

Burgio, K. L., Robinson, J. C., & Engel, B. T. (1986). The role of biofeedback in Kegel exercise training for stress urinary incontinence. *American Journal of Obstetrics and Gynecology, 154*(1), 58–64.

Burgio, K. L., Whitehead, W. E, & Engel, B. T. (1985). Urinary incontinence in the elderly. Bladder-sphincter biofeedback and toileting skills training. *Annals of Internal Medicine 103*(4), 507–515.

Burkhart, K. S. (2000). Urinary incontinence in women: Assessment and management in the primary care setting. *Nurse Practitioners Forum, 11*(4), 192–204.

Burns, P. A., Pranikoff, K., Nochasjski, T., Desotelle, P., & Harwood, M. K. (1990). Treatment of stress incontinence with pelvic floor exercises and biofeedback. *Journal of the American Geriatric Society, 38,* 341–344.

Burton, J. R., Pearce, K. L., Burgio, K. L., Engel, B. T., & Whitehead, W. E. (1988). Behavioral training for urinary incontinence in elderly ambulatory patients. *Journal of the American Geriatric Society, 36,* 693–698.

Ceresoli, A., Zanetti, G., Seveso, M., Bustros, J., Montanari, E., Guarneri, A., et al. (1993). Perineal biofeedback versus pelvic floor training in the treatment of urinary incontinence. *Archivio Italiano di Urologia, Andrologia, 65*(5), 559–560.

Culligan, P. J., & Heit, M. (2000). Urinary incontinence in women: Evaluation and management. *American Family Physician, 62,* 2433–44, 2447, 2452.

Elia, G., & Bergman, A. (1993). Pelvic muscle exercises: When do they work? *Obstetrics and Gynecology, 81,* 283–286.

Eriksen, B. C. (1989). Maximal electrostimulation of the pelvic floor in female idiopathic detrusor instability and urge incontinence. *Neurourology and Urodynamics, 8,* 219–230.

Fantl, J. A. (1996). *Urinary incontinence in adults: Acute and chronic management/urinary incontinence in adults. Guideline panel update* (Clinical Practice Guideline No. 2, AHCPR Publication No. 96–0682). Rockville, MD: U.S. Department of Health and Human Services, Agency for Health Care Policy and Research.

Fantl, J. A., Wyman, J. F., Harkins, S. W., & Hadley, E. C. (1990). Bladder training in the management of lower urinary tract dysfunction in women. A review. *Journal of the American Geriatric Society, 38,* 329–332.

Fantl, J. A., Wyman, J. F., McClish, D. K., Harkins, S. W., Elswick, R. K., Taylor, J. R., et al. (1991). Efficacy of bladder training in older women with urinary incontinence. *Journal of the American Medical Association, 265,* 609–613.

Galloway, N. T., El-Galley, R. E., Sand, P. K., Appell, R. A., Russell, H. W., & Carlan, S. J. (1999). Extracorporeal magnetic innervation therapy for stress urinary incontinence. *Urology, 53,* 1108–1111.

Glavind, K., Nohr, S. B., & Walter, S. (1996). Biofeedback and physiotherapy versus physiotherapy alone in the treatment of genuine stress urinary incontinence. *International Urogynecology, 7,* 339–343.

Hahn, I., Milsom, I., Fall, M., & Ekelund, P. (1993). Long-term results of pelvic floor training in female stress urinary incontinence. *British Journal of Urology, 72,* 421–427.

Hahn, I., Sommer, S., & Fall, M. (1991). A comparative study of pelvic floor training and electrical stimulation for the treatment of genuine female stress urinary incontinence. *Neurourology and Urodynamics, 10,* 545–554.

Haken, J., Benness, C., Cardozo, L., & Cutner, A. (1991). A randomised trial of vaginal cones and pelvic floor exercises in the management of genuine stress incontinence. *Neurourology and Urodynamics, 10,* 393–394.

Harrison, G. L., & Memel, D. S. (1994). Urinary incontinence in women: Its prevalence and its management in a health promotion clinic. *British Journal of General Practice, 44,* 149–152.

Health Care Financing Administration. (2000a, October 5). *Pelvic floor electrical stimulation for treatment of urinary incontinence* (Decision Memorandum No. CAG-0021N). Retrieved May 17, 2002, from http://www.hcfa.gov/coverage/8b3-w4.htm

Health Care Financing Administration. (2000b, October 6). *Biofeedback for treatment of urinary incontinence* (Decision Memorandum No. CAG-0020N). Retrieved May 17, 2002, from http://www.hcfa.gov/coverage/8b3-x4.htm

Jarvis, G. J., & Millar, D. R. (1980). Controlled trial of bladder drill for detrusor instability. *British Medical Journal, 281,* 1322–1323.

Kegel, A. H. (1948). Progressive resistance exercise in the functional restoration of the perineal muscles. *American Journal of Obstetrics and Gynecology, 56,* 238–249.

Khoury, J. M. (2001). Urinary incontinence. No need to be wet and upset. *North Carolina Medical Journal, 62*(2), 74–77.

Lagro-Janssen, T., & van Weel, C. (1998). Long-term effect of treatment of female incontinence in general practice. *British Journal of General Practice, 48*(436), 1735–1738.

Leach, G. E., Dmochowski, R. R., Appell, R. A., Blaivas, J. G., Hadley, H. R., Luber, K. M., et al. (1997). Female stress urinary incontinence clinical guidelines: Panel summary report on surgical management of female stress urinary incontinence. The American Urological Association. *Journal of Urology, 158,* 875–880.

MacLennan, A. H., Taylor, A. W., Wilson, D. H., & Wilson, D. (2000). *British Journal of Obstetrics and Gyneacology, 107*(12), 1460–1470.

National Institutes of Health. (1988). Urinary incontinence in adults. *NIH Consensus Statement, 7*(5), 1–32.

Norton, P., & Baker, J. (1990). Randomized prospective trial of vaginal cones vs. Kegel exercises in postpartum primiparous women. *Neurourology and Urodynamics, 9,* 434–435.

Persson, J., Wolner-Hanssen, P., & Rydhstroem, H. (2000). Obstetric risk factors for stress urinary incontinence: A population-based study. *Obstetrics and Gynecolology, 96*(3), 440–445.

Richter, H. E., Varner, R. E., Sanders, E., Holley, R. L., Northen, A., & Cliver, S. P. (2001). Effects of pubovaginal sling procedure on patients with urethral hypermobility and intrinsic sphincteric deficiency: Would they do it again? *American Journal of Obstetrics and Gynecology, 184*(2), 14–19.

Susset, J. G., Galea, G., & Read, L. (1990). Biofeedback therapy for female incontinence due to low urethral resistance. *Journal of Urology, 143,* 1205–1208.

Tries, J., & Eisman, E. (1995). Urinary incontinence: Evaluation and biofeedback training. In M. Schwartz and Associates (Eds.), *Biofeedback: A practitioner's guide* (pp. 597–632). New York: Guilford.

Ulmsten, U., Henriksson, L., Johnson, P., & Varhos, G. (1996). An ambulatory surgical procedure under local anesthesia for treatment of female urinary incontinence. *International Urogynecologic Journal of Pelvic Floor Dysfunction, 7,* 81–86.

Viera, A. J., & Larkins-Pettigrew, M. (2000). Practical use of the pessary. *American Family Physician, 61,* 2719–2726, 2729.

Wagner, T. H., & Hu, T. W. (1998). Economic costs of urinary incontinence [Editorial]. *International Urogynecological Journal of Pelvic Floor Dysfunction, 9*, 127–128.

Weinberger, M. W., Goodman, B. M., & Carnes, M. (1999). Long-term efficacy of nonsurgical urinary incontinence treatment in elderly women. *Journals of Gerontology, Series A: Biological Sciences and Medical Sciences, 54*(3), M117–M121.

# CHAPTER 23

# *Fibromyalgia*

## C. C. STUART DONALDSON AND GABRIEL E. SELLA

**Abstract:** Fibromyalgia is a disorder marked by widespread pain and "tender points" throughout the body, accompanied by sleep disturbance, cognitive deficits, reduced energy, and a variety of other symptoms. The authors overview current knowledge about fibromyalgia and advocate a central, systemic origin for this disorder. The chapter provides screening questions, diagnostic guidelines, and a summary of a treatment approach integrating medication, relaxation therapies, physical therapy, biofeedback, and neurofeedback.

## PROFILE OF THE DISORDER

The American College of Rheumatology (ACR) criterion for the diagnosis of fibromyalgia is that of widespread pain throughout the body involving at least 11 of 18 tender points. These points are displayed throughout the body, including the neck, shoulders, chest, back, arms, hips, and knees (see Wolfe, Smythe, et al., 1990, for specific details). In addition, sleep disturbances, poor immediate recall, poor concentration, and a decreased ability to multitask are reported. Symptoms such as irritable bowel syndrome, headaches, and temporomandibular joint pain are also reported.

The demographics of this population indicate that it is predominantly female (more than 80 percent) and primarily prevalent between the ages of 40 and 64, with the average age of onset being 47.8 years (White, Speechley, Harth, & Ostbye, 1999). Wolfe, Ross, Anderson, Russell, and Hebert (1995) suggest that many of the elderly population who are diagnosed with arthritis may actually be suffering from fibromyalgia, thus increasing the incidence rate for the 60-to-79 age range. The onset appears to be associated with a number of different factors, including trauma to the neck (Buskila, Neumann, Vaisberg, Alkalay, & Wolfe, 1997), low-back pain (Older et al., 1998), virus (Goldenberg, Mossey, & Schmid, 1995), stress (Donaldson, Sella, & Mueller, 1998), and a combination of these factors. This appears to be a long-lasting dysfunction, with the average length of time in pain reported as 78.7 months (Goldenberg et al., 1995).

AUTHORS' NOTE: The authors wish to acknowledge with thanks the following people for their help in generating and preparing ideas for this work. In no particular order: Dr. H. Mueller, Myosymmetries, Edmonton, Alberta; Mary Donaldson, M.Ed.; and Leslie Snelling, B.A., Myosymmetries, Calgary, Alberta.

Despite extensive research and investigation, fibromyalgia represents one of the more difficult challenges facing the health care practitioner. It is estimated that between 2 percent and 3.3 percent of the total population of North America suffer from this dysfunction (White et al., 1999; Wolfe, Ross, et al., 1995), yet the etiology and consequently the treatment of this dysfunction remains poorly understood. Numerous theories abound as to the etiology, including biochemical (Bennett, Clark, Campbell, & Burckhardt, 1992; Griep, Boersma, & de Kloet, 1993; Russell, Michalek, Vipaio, Fletcher, & Wall, 1989; Russell, Orr, et al., 1994; Yunus, Dailey, Aldag, Masi, & Jobe, 1992), psychological (Older et al., 1998; Yunus, Ahles, Aldag, & Masi, 1991), and sleep related (alpha intrusion; Moldofsky, Scarisbrick, England, & Smythe, 1975).

The widespread nature of the pain suggests a systemic process involved with the dysfunction. However, extensive investigations for blood markers suggesting a rheumatological disorder are promising but have not been conclusive. There is a growing body of evidence that suggests the presence of biochemical abnormalities in the fibromyalgia etiology. The suggested imbalances include a generalized deficiency of serotonin (Russell, Michalek, et al., 1989), low levels of serum tryptophan and other amino acids (Yunus, Dailey, et al., 1992), increased levels of substance P (Russell, Orr, et al., 1994), and low serum levels of the insulin-like growth factor IGF-1 (Bennett et al., 1992). In addition, there is evidence of an enhanced pituitary release of adrenocorticotropic hormones (ACTHs) and a low response of this hormone to neuroendocrine tests (Griep et al., 1993).

Another avenue explored in an effort to explain this generalized pain phenomenon is that of sleep deprivation. Sleep comprises four stages distinguished by the percentage of low-frequency, slow-wave brain activity and two cycles characterized by either REM (rapid eye movement) or non-REM sleep. As the stages progress, there is more delta activity and thus "deeper" sleep. It is during slow-wave sleep that the restorative processes are thought to occur and substances such as serotonin and IGF-1 come into play.

A study by Moldofsky et al. (1975) demonstrated a disruption of non-REM slow-wave sleep in "fibrositis" subjects and the ability to replicate fibromyalgia symptoms in healthy subjects by depriving them of stage 4 sleep. Moldofsky et al. suggest that this disruption may be attributable to a disturbance in serotonin metabolism. In addition, a study by Bennett et al. (1992) suggested that a lack of slow-wave sleep disrupts the release of growth hormone–1 (GH-1). However, both these findings have been disputed by other studies (Older et al., 1998), and thus the delta-alpha sleep dysregulation theory remains debatable.

## SCREENING QUESTIONS

The primary purpose of the screening questions is to provide a differential diagnosis. Most current screening procedures examine for rheumatology factors, which are discussed in detail later in the chapter. What is often missed is an adequate work-up of muscle activity primarily for the purpose of differentiating fibromyalgia from myofascial pain syndromes. A recent paper suggested that 38 percent of referrals for fibromyalgia were myofascial pain syndromes (Donaldson, Sella, & Mueller, 1998). Table 23.1 lists some of the more common differences between the two conditions.

## CHRONIC BENIGN PAIN AND FIBROMYALGIA

Fibromyalgia falls into the area of chronic benign pain as defined by the International

**Table 23.1** Comparison of Various Features of Fibromyalgia Syndrome and Myofascial Pain Syndrome Based on Clinical Samples

| Features | Fibromyalgia Syndrome | Myofascial Pain Syndrome |
|---|---|---|
| Musculoskeletal pain | Widespread | Regional/occasionally widespread |
| Tender points | Multiple, widespread | Regional |
| Referred pain | Minimal | Follows well-defined patterns |
| Taut band | Similar to normal controls | Similar to normal controls |
| Twitch response | Probably similar to normal controls | Similar to normal controls |
| Fatigue | Dominates | Variable with activity |
| Poor sleep | Dominates | Variable with pain |
| Headaches | Common | Common |
| Irritable bowel | Common | Rare |

Association for the Study of Pain (Mersky & Bogduk, 1994). Chronic benign pain is defined as pain of a non-life-threatening nature that lasts for more than six months. Numerous authors (e.g., Birbaumer, Flor, Lutzenberger, & Elbert, 1995; Coderre, Katz, Vaccarino, & Melzack, 1993; Flor & Turk, 1996) have recently investigated chronic pain as a neurological phenomenon. The preliminary results of these works indicate that the central nervous system (CNS), including the dorsal horn and the cortex, may react to the pain and then be involved with the maintenance of chronic pain. Donaldson, Sella, and Mueller (1998) and Mueller, Donaldson, Nelson, and Layman (2001) applied this thinking to fibromyalgia, suggesting that the disorder may involve CNS and peripheral neurological dysfunctions.

## ANATOMY AND PHYSIOLOGY: THE NEURAL PLASTICITY MODEL

Before proceeding with a discussion of the proposed neural mechanisms involved with fibromyalgia, a discussion of the concepts of neural sensitization, or plasticity, is necessary. Neural sensitization, or plasticity (hereafter referred to as plasticity), refers to the process whereby the CNS or the peripheral nervous system (1) grows in size, (2) alters

the areas of innervation (Flor et al., 1993), or (3) becomes more responsive to the pain signal (Coderre et al., 1993) due to repeated exposure to the pain signal. Similar in manner to the way neural pathways become more efficient in transmitting a neural signal during learning (e.g., learning to play the piano), the neurological system becomes more efficient at transmitting the pain signal. Coderre et al. go on to state,

> In some cases peripheral tissue damage or nerve injury leads to a pathological state characterized by one or more of the following: pain in the absence of a noxious stimulus, increased duration of response to brief stimulation, reduced pain threshold, increased responsiveness to suprathreshold stimulation, and spread of pain and hyperalgesia to uninjured tissue. (p. 259)

## DIAGNOSTIC ASSESSMENT

Application of the concept of neural plasticity to fibromyalgia suggests that pathological changes should be seen in both the peripheral and central nervous systems. The application of surface electromyographic (SEMG) and EEG neurotherapy assessment techniques enable clinicians to identify these changes.

Before proceeding with the SEMG assessment, it is important that a comprehensive medical evaluation of fibromyalgia symptoms be conducted. In every case, the intensity and frequency of symptoms may differ. A listing of all symptoms should include (1) presence of each symptom, (2) span of presence, (3) intensity, (4) frequency, (5) worsening in either intensity or frequency in the presence or absence of treatment and environmental factors, (6) improvement in either intensity or frequency of symptoms in the presence or absence of treatment and environmental factors, (7) listing of different treatments and symptomatic response in time, and (8) overall symptomatic change from the beginning of the appearance of symptoms to the time of the evaluation or reevaluation.

The medical evaluation needs to be comprehensive and should rule out systemic disease and somatoform disorders to determine the absence of either before considering the diagnosis of fibromyalgia or related conditions. The essential points of the evaluation, with special focus on fibromyalgia, myofascial pain syndrome, and other muscular painful conditions, are as follows:

1. History of the condition, including a description of the primary etiology of the condition (e.g., acute posttraumatic, chronic, postrepetitive motion injury, etc.). The time span from the original initiation of the pain symptoms to the time of the evaluation has to be described in detail, especially regarding the investigation, diagnostic process, treatment, and success rate of the rehabilitation.

2. Review of systems, with special regard to any injury or condition that might contribute to the maintenance or enhancement of the muscular type pain, fatigue, and concomitant symptoms of depression, anxiety, and especially sleep disorder.

3. Physical examination, with special focus on every system in terms of conditions that might contribute actively to the maintenance of the fibromyalgia or related symptoms. Such examination needs to include a comprehensive questionnaire, especially involving the pain and emotional symptoms, history thereof, and treatment up to the point of the evaluation.

4. Objective evaluation of the muscular pain components in terms of SEMG of all the affected muscles as well as muscles known to cocontract with the symptomatic muscles, goniometry to assess any changes in the joints' range of motion, dynamometry to assess loss of strength, dolorimetry to assess the pain perception pattern, and other tests as necessary (White et al., 1999).

5. Neuropsychological tests related to the emotional component of the pain, including anxiety and depression.

6. Sleep studies when there is sleep disturbance, especially associated with lack of dreaming, early awakening, and sensation of sleepiness during the day.

Once the medical investigation is completed, an SEMG evaluation can be conducted. Surface electromyography, through the examination of the electrical activity of the muscles, indirectly allows for examination of the nervous system. Primarily, this is seen in three phenomena: (1) increased resting level of muscle activity, (2) muscle co-contractions, and (3) muscle imbalances.

Increased muscle activity at rest means that muscles that should be electrically quiet at rest (recovering from the contractions and allowing blood flow to remove the lactic acid) are not. They remain hyperactive, causing fatigue and pain. Unpublished data indicate that the resting levels of fibromyalgia sufferers are approximately 11 percent greater (lower) than the resting levels of nonpain sufferers as reported by various authors (e.g., Donaldson & Donaldson, 1990; Sella, 1999). A co-contraction is defined as an increase in electrical activity of a muscle from resting level when another muscle in another part of the body is contracting performing a movement. For example, Donaldson, Snelling, MacInnis, Sella, and Mueller (in press) demonstrated that fibromyalgia sufferers lying supine on a table, during rotation of the head, increase the activity of the wrist extensors (forearm tender point), gluteus minimus (buttocks tender point), and vastus medialis (knee tender point). This phenomenon was seen in 40 out of 40 individuals carefully screened and diagnosed with fibromyalgia. Muscle imbalances are documented during movement and at rest. The electrical activity of a muscle on one side of the body is compared to that of its contralateral partner (i.e., the same muscle on the right side). Fibromyalgia sufferers show differences in various muscle pairs doing the same movement, which Donaldson, Sella, and Mueller (1998) demonstrated correlated quite strongly (80 percent) with trigger-point activity in the upper trapezius. Sella (1999) found high specificity (77 percent) and sensitivity (63 percent) values for muscle imbalance measures when comparing painful to nonpainful muscles.

It is postulated that the increased muscle activity, for whatever reason, is the cause of the generalized pain as seen in fibromyalgia sufferers and could represent the cause of the development of tender points and trigger points. This, of course, remains to be proven.

Examination of the activity of the CNS, particularly the brain-wave activity, shows changes in cortical activity. Particularly, the changes involve an increase in slow brain-wave activity (delta, theta, and the lower frequencies of alpha) throughout the frontal cortex for fibromyalgia sufferers. Donaldson, Sella, and Mueller (1998) and Mueller et al. (2001) reported that increased frontal slow-wave activity was seen in all fibromyalgia sufferers. Successful rehabilitation of this phenomenon was associated with a reduction of symptoms. Other authors (Billiot, Budzynski, & Andrasik,

1997) reported this phenomenon with chronic fatigue syndrome. It is not known what this increased slow-wave phenomena represents. Increased slow-wave activity has been found in individuals suffering from various types of viral infections (Westmoreland, 1993) and in individuals exposed to toxic chemicals (Van Sweden, 1993).

In summary, the neurological system appears to react to the constant stimulation of the pain signal, producing changes in both the peripheral nervous system and the CNS. These changes may be used as markers for understanding and treating fibromyalgia.

## TREATMENT PROTOCOLS

The treatment of fibromyalgia follows directly from the assessment. First, a comprehensive evaluation of fibromyalgia symptoms is necessary in every case, though the intensity and frequency of symptoms may differ. A listing of all symptoms by (1) presence, (2) span of presence, (3) intensity, (4) frequency, (5) worsening in either intensity or frequency in the presence or absence of treatment and environmental factors, (6) improvement in either intensity or frequency in the presence or absence of treatment and environmental factors, (7) listing of different treatments and symptomatic response in time, and (8) overall symptomatic change from the beginning of the appearance of symptoms to the time of the evaluation or reevaluation.

The pain component cannot be treated specifically with just one type of medication. Different analgesic classes may prove useful in reducing pain intensity and/or frequency for a determined period. Combined classes of medicines may prove more useful (e.g., Tramadol and Vicoprofen) in that they may reduce pain by "attacking" different receptors. Opiates may be reserved for complicated cases, which have shown a poor response to pain treatment with other classes of analgesics. All pain medications must be prescribed and taken under clear guidelines and control. Recently Teitelbaum (personal communication, December 29, 1999) indicated that in a double-blind study, the application of a combination of medications and naturopathic substances significantly reduced fibromyalgia symptoms. The readers need to be cautioned that this work is preliminary and needs further review.

The anxiety/depression component may be controlled with adequate doses of anxiolytic/antidepressant agents. Different medications may be used in the same individual over time if the response is less than adequate. The response to medication may differ according to the intensity of the anxiety/depression symptoms over time.

Sleep inadequacy may be treated partially with antidepressant medication. It may be relevant to consider nutritional supplements such as tryptophan and/or melatonin before adding a specific sleep medication, especially of the benzodiazepine group.

### Behavioral Intervention

Alleviation of the pain with nonpharmacological techniques is promising. Basmajian and De Luca (1985) identified four possible neurological mechanisms that can be involved in the disruption of motor control: (1) centrally mediated reciprocal inhibition, (2) centrally mediated coactivation, (3) peripherally mediated reciprocal inhibition, and (4) peripherally mediated coactivation. As one or several of these mechanisms may be involved with fibromyalgia, a multifaceted strategy is recommended, consisting of (1) trying to calm the system with relaxation training techniques; (2) altering the muscle (peripheral) activity using different SEMG techniques, physical therapy, and massage therapy; and (3) altering CNS activity using EEG neurotherapy techniques. (These methods are discussed in more detail later in the chapter.) The basic premise is to reduce the sources of pain in the periphery and reduce CNS dysfunction while not irritating or reinforcing the pain pathways.

There are several different methods to reduce muscle imbalances and cocontractions. The use of the Donaldson Protocol© for the restoration of muscle balance fits here, as this treatment is designed to gently reduce the muscle imbalances without irritating the system. Briefly, the Donaldson Protocol includes (1) comparing the activity of the same muscle on each side of the body doing the same movement, and (2) uptraining the side that is lower in activity while keeping the hyper (higher) side lower than the up-training side. Response to treatment is usually immediate, with the hyperactive side decreasing in activity, consequently decreasing pain. For more details on this protocol, see Donaldson and Donaldson (1990). Other SEMG techniques that serve to quiet the muscle activity (such as relaxation training) also fit here and are useful.

The increased frontal slow-wave activity of the CNS may be altered using neurofeedback techniques. There are a number of techniques, including traditional procedures such as theta-beta therapy, fixed-frequency light therapy, and variable-frequency light therapy, known as FNS® (Ochs, 1996a, 1996b). FNS is a form of neurotherapy that involves monitoring scalp potentials between 1 and 40 Hz and returning a feedback signal related to them in the form of a profoundly low power energy field, the characteristics of which are not yet well understood. Each of these techniques is designed to reduce the increased frontal slow-wave activity as seen in the fibromyalgia sufferer. However, research in this area is lacking, with no double-blind studies reported in the literature. Reports of improvement are primarily anecdotal in nature or single case studies.

## Alternative Treatments

Relaxation training of any type serves to reduce the generalized arousal of the system. Hypnosis, self-hypnosis, autogenics, and visualization techniques can all be used, depending on individual tastes and needs. Progressive muscle relaxation has the advantage of reducing the muscle's resting levels but runs the risk of irritating any existing muscle imbalances and co-contractions so should be applied carefully. Surface EMG techniques can be used to monitor and control the muscle activity.

Numerous forms of physical therapy (e.g., Feldenkreis, Sahrmann muscle work, and cranial sacral therapy) are also available. These particular techniques are recommended because they involve gentle manipulation of the muscles and joints while not irritating the nervous system. Ice and heat applied with massage therapy also work well. Transcutaneous nerve stimulation and other variations of it are not recommended, as the long-term effect is poor. Some of the newer microcurrent techniques (e.g., Alpha Stim®) appear to have promise, but further research is needed.

## OUTCOME STUDIES

A more recent trend in the literature is to view the treatment of fibromyalgia from a multidisciplinary approach. The overall effectiveness of combining treatment modalities focused on both the central and peripheral nervous systems in alleviating the complex psychological and somatic complaints associated with fibromyalgia is demonstrated by a recent clinical outcomes study by Donaldson, Sella, and Mueller (1998) and Mueller et al. (2001). Both these retrospective studies demonstrated that a multidisciplinary approach to the treatment of fibromyalgia shows a high success rate with positive long-term results.

Donaldson, Sella, and Mueller (1998) studied 252 consecutive referrals to a chronic pain treatment center over a period of one year. All subjects were physician referred, with 157 meeting the criteria for fibromyalgia as defined by the American College of Rheumatology (Wolfe, Smythe, et al., 1990). All subjects received a four-point evaluation that included (1) trigger-point evaluation, (2) SEMG evaluation, (3) physiotherapy evaluation, and (4) an EEG evaluation as designed by Ochs (1996a, 1996b). This evaluation was then repeated posttreatment, whenever possible. All subjects received a comprehensive treatment program that included (1) trigger-point therapy, (2) physiotherapy, (3) SEMG neuromuscular retraining as outlined in Donaldson, Sella, and Mueller (1998), and (4) EEG neurotherapy as designed by Ochs (1996a, 1996b).

These subjects were on average 44.2 years old (range 14 to 85), 80 percent female, in pain for an average of seven years, with a total score of 29.3 on the McGill Pain Questionnaire. Surface EMG evaluation showed significant muscle dysfunctions primarily affecting the upper trapezius (47.2 percent of the sample) and other muscles in the neck. The EEG evaluation indicated the presence of elevated theta activity 28.1 percent of the time, alpha activity 14.3 percent of the time, and theta/alpha activity 17.3 percent of the time. This dominance was evident at 8 of 13 sites examined, including FP, F3, Fz, C3, Cz, C4, and Pz.

A combined therapy program of SEMG biofeedback, massage therapy, physiotherapy, and EEG neurotherapy showed, after one year, that out of 44 who had completed treatment, 4 reported increased symptoms, 10 reported virtually a 100 percent decrease in symptoms, and the remaining 30 all improved to varying degrees. There was a marked pattern to the improvement; with the cognitive dysfunctions clearing up in two to three weeks, the pain decreasing and becoming localized in two to three months, and the sleep improving in approximately three months. Long-term follow-up of the subjects that improved showed they maintained the improvement over a further one-year follow-up.

Mueller et al. (2001) reported on a series of 30 consecutive fibromyalgia referrals, treated using a multidisciplinary approach. Although there was some individual variation, patients were generally treated three to five times per week with EEG-Driven Stimulation (EDS was a precursor to FNS) exclusively until changes in their cognitive and emotional states and improvement in their sleep was reported. Once this shift became apparent (mean of $16 \pm 6$ weeks), the number of EDS sessions per week was reduced, and weekly sessions of physical therapies were added. Physical therapies included some combination of trigger-point massage, myofascial and positional release, stretch and spray, SEMG-assisted neuromuscular retraining, prescribed muscle stretching, and strengthening exercises, depending on each patient's needs. As a group, these patients averaged 37.3 ($\pm$15.6) hours of EDS and 14.7 ($\pm$8.0) hours of physical therapies over the course of approximately three to four months of treatment.

Significant decreases in average levels of cortical delta (1 to 4 Hz), theta (4 to 8 Hz), and alpha (8 to 12 Hz) activity as measured in pre- and posttreatment brain maps (31.3 percent, 28.9 percent, and 18.7 percent reductions, respectively) were noted. Concurrently significant differences (pre- to posttreatment) were obtained on the Symptom Check List–90-R (Derogatis, 1994), the Fibromyalgia Impact Questionnaire (Burckhardt, Clark, & Bennett, 1991), and repeated patient self-reports of selected key symptoms using a visual analog scale (VAS). Patients rated themselves as an average of 62.2 percent ($\pm$21.6 percent) improved overall at the time of their follow-up an average of 8.2 ($\pm$4.3) months after treatment was terminated. Similarly, patients

reported a significant reduction in number of positive tender points from 15 ($\pm$2) at intake to 8 ($\pm$3) at discharge.

The data just presented and clinical data generated by Donaldson and at various clinics throughout North America are consistent in that they suggest that change in the CNS activity is necessary before change in the remainder of the symptomatology may occur. These findings point to a centrally mediated control mechanism as a key component to change. Presently, it is not known if just treating the CNS will result in long-term symptom reduction. Treating the peripheral musculature and peripheral nervous system is still needed to ensure long-term and/or permanent change.

## CONCLUSION

Fibromyalgia represents a complex and puzzling problem for the health care professional. The ACR criteria for diagnosis of this dysfunction is based on the presence of 11 of 18 tender points occurring throughout the body, emphasizing the diffuse nature of the pain component to this problem. In addition, various cognitive, emotional, and other health problems (e.g., headaches) are reported, and sleep problems are well documented. Further compounding the problem is the variety of reported causes of this dysfunction. It is difficult to make sense of how trauma, virus, stress, and neck pain all can produce the same dysfunction!

To make some sense of these seemingly unrelated problems, much investigation has occurred involving biochemical markers in the blood, brain, and other systems in the body. These results are not clear or have not been replicated. Recently, researchers have begun examining the role of the brain in chronic benign pain and, in particular, fibromyalgia. Presently, this work is very preliminary and needs further investigation.

Today there is no easy answer—no silver bullet—in the treatment of fibromyalgia. Current research that is showing some success with this problem is multifaceted in nature, treating the problem with several therapies. While there is hope for the future, let us remain critical in the present and "do no harm."

## REFERENCES

Basmajian, J., & De Luca, C. (1985). *Muscles alive: Their functions revealed by electromyography* (5th ed.). Baltimore: Williams & Wilkins.

Bennett, R., Clark, S., Campbell, S., & Burckhardt, C. (1992). Low levels of somatomedin C in patients with the fibromyalgia syndrome: A possible link between sleep and muscle pain. *Arthritis and Rheumatism, 35*(10), 1113–1116.

Billiot, K., Budzynski, T., & Andrasik, F. (1997). EEG patterns and chronic fatigue syndrome. *Journal of Neurotherapy, 2*(2), 20–30.

Birbaumer, N., Flor, H., Lutzenberger, W., & Elbert, T. (1995). The corticalization of chronic pain. *Advances in Pain Research and Therapy, 22*, 331–343.

Burckhardt, C., Clark, R., & Bennett, R. (1991). The fibromyalgia impact questionnaire: Development and validation. *Journal of Rheumatology, 18*, 728–733.

Buskila, D., Neumann, L., Vaisberg, G., Alkalay, D., & Wolfe, F. (1997). Increased rates of fibromyalgia following cervical spine injury. *Arthritis and Rheumatism, 40*(3), 446–452.

Coderre, T., Katz, J., Vaccarino, A., & Melzack, R. (1993). Contribution of central neuroplasticity to pathological pain: Review of clinical and experimental evidence. *Pain, 52*, 259–285.

Derogatis, L. (1994). *SCL-90-R: Administration, scoring and procedures manual* (3rd ed.). Minneapolis, MN: National Computer Systems.

Donaldson, C. C. S., & Donaldson, M. (1990). Multichannel EMG assessment and treatment techniques. In J. R. Cram (Ed.), *Clinical EMG for Surface Recordings* (Vol. 2, pp. 143–173). Nevada City, CA: Clinical Resources.

Donaldson, C. C. S., Sella, G., & Mueller, H. (1998). Fibromyalgia: A retrospective study of 252 consecutive referrals. *Canadian Journal of Clinical Medicine, 5*(6), 116–127.

Donaldson, C. C. S., Snelling, L. S., MacInnis, A. L., Sella, G. E., & Mueller, H. H. (in press). Diffuse muscular coactivation (DMC) as a potential source of pain in fibromyalgia—Part 1. *Neurorehabilitation, 17*(1).

Flor, H., Birbaumer, N., Furst, M., Lutzenberger, W., Elbert, T., & Braun, C. (1993). Evidence of enhanced peripheral and central responses to painful stimulation in chronic pain. *Psychophysiology, 30*, 9.

Flor, H., & Turk, D. (1996). Integrating central and peripheral mechanisms in chronic muscular pain. *Pain Forum, 5*(1), 74–76.

Goldenberg, D., Mossey, C., & Schmid, C. (1995). A model to assess severity and impact of fibromyalgia. *Journal of Rheumatology, 22*(12), 2313–2318.

Griep, E., Boersma, J., & de Kloet, R. (1993). Altered reactivity of the hypothalamic-pituitary-adrenal axis of the primary fibromyalgia syndrome. *Journal of Rheumatology, 20*(3), 469–474.

Mersky, H., & Bogduk, N. (Eds.). (1994). *Classification of chronic pain: Descriptions of chronic pain syndromes and definitions of pain terms* (2nd ed.). Seattle, WA: International Association for the Study of Pain.

Moldofsky, H., Scarisbrick, P., England, R., & Smythe, H. (1975). Musculoskeletal symptoms and non-REM sleep disturbance in patients with "fibrositis syndrome" and healthy subjects. *Psychosomatic Medicine, 37,* 341–351.

Mueller, H., Donaldson, C. C. S., Nelson, D., & Layman, M. (2001). Treatment of fibromyalgia incorporating EEG-driven stimulation: A clinical outcomes study. *Journal of Clinical Psychology 57*(7), 933–952.

Ochs, L. (1996a). *FNS: Background: Operating manual* (Flexyx Publication No. 1). Walnut Creek, CA: Flexyx Publications.

Ochs, L. (1996b). *FNS: Operating manual* (Flexyx Publication No. 2). Walnut Creek, CA: Flexyx Publications.

Older, S., Battafarano, D., Danning, C., Ward, J., Grady, E., Derman, S., et al. (1998). The effects of delta wave sleep interruption on pain thresholds and fibromyalgia-like symptoms in healthy subjects; correlations with insulin-like growth factor I. *Journal of Rheumatology, 25*(6), 1180–1186.

Russell, I., Michalek, J., Vipaio, G., Fletcher, E., & Wall, K. (1989). Serum amino acids in fibrositis/fibromyalgia syndrome. *Journal of Rheumatology, 19,* 158–163.

Russell, I., Orr, M., Littman, B., Vipraio, G., Alboukrek, D., Michalek, J., et al. (1994). Elevated cerebrospinal fluid levels of substance P in patients with the fibromyalgia syndrome. *Arthritis and Rheumatism, 37*(11), 1593–1601.

Sella, G. E. (1999). Surface EMG testing: Sensitivity, specificity, positive and negative predictive values. *Europa MedicoPhysics, 36*(4), 183–190.

Van Sweden, B. (1993). Toxic encephalopathies. In E. Niedermeyer & F. Da Silva (Eds.), *Electromyography: Basic principles, clinical applications, and related fields* (pp. 643–651). Baltimore: Williams & Wilkins.

Westmorland, B. (1993). The EEG in cerebral inflammatory processes. In E. Niedermeyer & F. Da Silva (Eds.), *Electromyography: Basic principles, clinical applications, and related fields* (pp. 291–304). Baltimore: Williams & Wilkins.

White, K., Speechley, M., Harth, M., & Ostbye, T. (1999). The London fibromyalgia epidemiology study: The prevalence of fibromyalgia syndrome in London, Ontario. *Journal of Rheumatology, 26*(7), 1570–1576.

Wolfe, F., Ross, K., Anderson, J., Russell, I., & Hebert, L. (1995). The prevalence and characteristics of fibromyalgia in the general population. *Arthritis and Rheumatism, 38*(1), 19–28.

Wolfe, F., Smythe, H. A., Yunus, M. B., Bennett, R. M., Bombardiare, C., Goldenberg, D. L., et al. (1990). The American College of Rheumatology 1990 criteria for the classification of fibromyalgia: Report of the multicenter criteria committee. *Arthritis and Rheumatism, 33,* 160–172.

Yunus, M., Ahles, T., Aldag, J., & Masi, A. T. (1991). Relationship of clinical features with psychological status in primary fibromyalgia. *Arthritis and Rheumatism, 34*(1), 15–21.

Yunus, M., Dailey, J., Aldag, J., Masi, A. T., & Jobe, P. (1992). Plasma tryptophan and other amino acids in primary fibromyalgia: A controlled study. *Journal of Rheumatology, 19,* 90–94.

# CHAPTER 24

# Chronic Fatigue Syndrome

CHARLES W. LAPP

**Abstract:** Chronic fatigue syndrome is a disorder characterized by debilitating fatigue, recurrent flulike symptoms, and neurocognitive symptoms such as difficulties with memory, concentration, comprehension, recall, calculation, and expression. A sleep disorder is not uncommon. All these symptoms are aggravated by even minimal physical exertion or emotional stress, and relapses can occur spontaneously. Although there is no curative treatment, rest and symptomatic therapies can palliate the symptoms. The cause of this disorder is unknown, but it is not thought to be infectious. Emerging evidence strongly indicates that its etiology may be associated with disturbances at the neuroendocrinological interface (Habib, Gold, & Chrousos, 2001).

## CLINICAL PRESENTATION

Fatigue is an extremely common symptom and one of the most frequent complaints reported by individuals seeking primary care. In a study performed at the General Medical Clinic at Harvard's Brigham and Women's Hospitals, approximately 25 percent of patients listed chronic fatigue as a major complaint (Buchwald, Sullivan, & Komaroff, 1987). Only a small percentage of that population, however, will have prolonged fatigue significant enough to affect lifestyle and the ability to work. It is this subset of more severely and persistently fatigued persons that currently defines chronic fatigue syndrome.

### Differentiating Chronic Fatigue from Chronic Fatigue Syndrome

What is the difference between everyday chronic fatigue and chronic fatigue syndrome (CFS)? Three characteristics define the syndrome: (1) The fatigue is persistent and debilitating enough to cause significant changes in lifestyle and work; (2) the fatigue is accompanied by recurrent flulike symptoms such as achiness, joint discomfort, feverishness, generalized malaise, sore throat, and lymph node tenderness; and (3) significant neurocognitive difficulties are present, including problems with short-term memory, concentration, and processing. In addition, CFS is frequently accompanied by a sleep disorder; irritable bowel and bladder; vascular headaches; sensitivities to chemicals, odors, and fumes; temporomandibular disorders; and widespread muscle pain. Fibromyalgia has been diagnosed in over 70 percent of CFS cases, suggesting that these "overlap syndromes" are very closely related or share a common pathogenesis (see Chapter 23 on fibromyalgia). Table 24.1 summarizes the common symptoms of chronic fatigue syndrome.

**Table 24.1**  Symptoms of Chronic Fatigue Syndrome

| Symptom | Patients with the CFS Reporting Symptom (percent) | |
| --- | --- | --- |
| | Study 1[a] | Study 2[b] |
| Easy fatigability | 100 | 100 |
| Difficulty concentrating | 90 | 79 |
| Headache | 90 | 81 |
| Sore throat | 85 | 73 |
| Tender lymph nodes | 80 | 71 |
| Muscle aches | 80 | 83 |
| Joint aches | 75 | 67 |
| Feverishness | 75 | 43 |
| Difficulty sleeping | 70 | 66 |
| Psychiatric problems | 65 | 67–70 |
| Allergies | 55 | – |
| Abdominal cramps | 40 | 45 |
| Weight loss | 20 | 13 |
| Rash | 10 | 30 |
| Rapid pulse | 10 | – |
| Weight gain | 5 | 24 |
| Chest pain | 5 | – |
| Night sweats | 5 | – |
| Diarrhea | 33 | – |
| Cough | 54 | – |
| Bedridden | 6 | – |
| Shut in | 17 | – |
| Part-time work | 28 | – |
| Fulfill all responsibilities | 48 | – |
| Abrupt flu-like onset | 65 | – |

a. Straus (1988)
b. Buchwald, Cheney, et al. (1992)

## Etiology

The majority of CFS cases occur abruptly, frequently following an acute viral illness. This fact, when coupled with a history of "epidemics," has led many to think that CFS is infectious. However, no epidemiological data exist to support this contention. Alternatively, CFS could be triggered by environmental factors, abnormalities of the immune or neuroendocrine systems, or other putative mechanisms that all lead to the same final pathway. In a minority of subjects, the onset is gradual over months to years, and no obvious event can be identified.

## Epidemiology

The first reports of CFS involved relatively small numbers of assertive young white women, so the disorder was derogatorily referred to as "yuppie flu." Epidemiological studies soon showed that CFS was present in men, minorities, and all age groups. Large surveillance studies by the Centers for Disease Control and Prevention (2000) have established that women are three to seven times more likely than men to contract CFS and that the disorder affects all segments of society, including rich and poor, educated and uneducated. The largest and most comprehensive community-based study was published by Jason, Richman, Rademaker, et al. (1999). This study established a prevalence of 200 to 800 cases per 100,000, depending on age, gender, and ethnicity, making CFS more prevalent than multiple sclerosis, systemic lupus (Komaroff, 2000a), and HIV infection (Centers for Disease Control, 2002).

## Pathophysiology

The cause of CFS is currently unknown, but research has uncovered several physiological abnormalities that might be clues. Immunologically, CFS patients show a pattern of immune activation with discreet and predictable evidence of T-cell activation, increased populations of CD8 cytotoxic/suppressor cells, poor natural killer-cell function, and immune complexes (Buchwald, Cheney, et al., 1992). Neurologically, hyperintense T2-weighted signals are seen in the majority of MRIs (Schwartz et al., 1994), regional cerebral blood is reduced on SPECT scan (Ichise et al., 1992; Schwartz et al., 1994), and autonomic dysfunction can be demonstrated in a majority of subjects by tilt-table testing (Bou-Houlaigah, Rowe, Kan, & Calkins, 1995; Freeman & Komaroff, 1997; Lapp, 1996; Schondorf, Benoit, Wein, & Phaneuf, 1999). Elegant neuroendocrine studies reveal dysfunction of the hypothalamic-pituitary-gonadal-adrenal axis leading to reduced corticotropin-releasing hormone responsiveness, growth hormone deficiency, low 24-hour cortisol production, and hyporesponsiveness to adrenocorticotrophic hormone (Bennett, Clark, & Walczyk, 1998; Demitrack et al., 1991). These findings are precisely opposite those seen in major depression, adding credence to the conclusion that depression is not a cause of CFS. As will be discussed shortly, such observations are also consistent with

the rapidly evolving understanding of dysfunctional characteristics of the body's stress system (Habib et al., 2001).

Investigators have reported that autonomic dysfunction, or *dysautonomia,* is demonstrable in up to 96 percent of persons with CFS (Bou-Houlaigah et al., 1995). The most dramatic manifestation of this is an abnormal vasodepressor reaction—neurally mediated hypotension or vasovagal syncope—in response to upright posture (Wilke, Fouad-Tarazi, Cash, & Calabrese, 1998). Others have reported postural orthostatic tachycardia syndrome (Schondorf & Low, 1993), symptomatic orthostatic tachycardia syndrome (Lapp, 1996), and milder forms of orthostatic intolerance. It is hypothesized that the orthostatic intolerance causes symptoms by lowering systemic blood pressure and cerebral perfusion (Komaroff, 2000b), but dysautonomia may also explain palpitations, sweats, temperature intolerance, dysphagia, irritable bowel or gut dysmotility, polyuria, and other CFS symptoms. The problem may be exacerbated by low blood and plasma volume reported in persons with CFS (Streeten & Bell, 1998). Thus patients feel worse the more they are upright, while the supine position is most comfortable.

## TYPICAL SIGNS AND DIAGNOSTIC CRITERIA

### Physical Examination

The physical examination is typically normal or nonspecific, but there are subtleties to look for. Early in the course of illness, the patient may have a low-grade temperature, less than 100.5 °F degrees orally. The blood pressure tends to be low, probably due to low blood volume and autonomic abnormalities (Bou-Houlaigah et al., 1995; Streeten & Bell, 1998). Swollen or tender lymph nodes are common in the neck and axillae. Most CFS patients will have fibromyalgia with classical tender points, sacroiliac tenderness, and allodynia.

## Laboratory and Radiological Findings

Routine laboratory tests are usually unrevealing in CFS. Nevertheless, clues sometimes appear, such as a low sedimentation rate, atypical lymphocytosis (which occurs in more than 2 percent of cases), or a low-level antinuclear antibody titer (Bates et al., 1995; Buchwald & Komaroff, 1991).

Radiologically, hyperintense T2-weighted lesions may appear on cranial MRI in over 80 percent of patients (Buchwald, Cheney, et al., 1992), and reduced cerebral blood flow in temporal and midbrain areas may be seen on the SPECT scan (Ichise et al., 1992; Schwartz et al., 1994).

## Defining the Disorder

Without a gold standard, specific laboratory tests, or any pathognomonic physical finding, a disorder can only be diagnosed by a clinical case definition. Such was the case in 1988, when a panel of the Centers for Disease Control and Prevention defined a heterogeneous group of patients with persistent fatigue, cognitive dysfunction, and flu-like symptoms. They published a working case definition and called this novel disorder *chronic fatigue syndrome*, which emphasized both the persistence of the illness and the most prevalent symptoms (Holmes et al., 1988). In 1994, the case definition was revised to clarify some semantic vagaries and exclude most physical findings (Fukuda et al., 1994). These criteria are now accepted worldwide and are known as the International Case Definition Criteria for CFS. These criteria were adopted to define a heterogeneous group for research purposes

only, but in the absence of any accepted clinical criteria, the International Case Definition Criteria are commonly used to diagnose CFS in the medical office (see Box 24.1).

Conditions that exclude a diagnosis of CFS are active medical conditions known to cause fatigue, melancholic depressive illness or psychosis, bipolar depression, morbid obesity, eating disorders, and alcohol or substance abuse.

## TRADITIONAL MANAGEMENT OF CHRONIC FATIGUE SYNDROME: THE STEPWISE APPROACH TO TREATMENT

Disorders for which there are no known causes and no known cures are treated expectantly with supportive and symptomatic therapies. An approach that serves CFS patients well is a stepwise approach that begins with reassurance and education and includes exercise, diet, and treatment of specific symptoms.

## Reassurance and Education

Because of the nature of the disorder, many persons with CFS have seen many providers in an attempt to find out what is causing their myriad symptoms. Patients are often rebuked or discounted by uncaring, uninformed physicians who do not recognize the classical symptoms of CFS. Thus many patients need to be reassured that they have a recognized disorder and that there is hope for improvement. Most are relieved just to hear that they are neither crazy nor dying. It is helpful to briefly review the pathophysiology of CFS with patients so they can appreciate the origin of their symptoms and understand why routine tests have been unrevealing. Next, the clinician should set realistic expectations and goals for the patient, making it clear that there is no known cure

---

**Box 24.1**  1994 International Case Definition Criteria for Chronic Fatigue Syndrome

Chronic fatigue syndrome is a syndrome characterized by fatigue that is:

- Medically unexplained
- New in onset
- Of at least 6 months duration
- Not the result of ongoing exertion or relieved by rest, and
- Causes a substantial reduction in previous levels of occupational, educational, social, or personal activities

In addition, there must be four or more of the following symptoms:

- Impaired memory or concentration
- Postexertional malaise lasting more than 24 hours
- Unrefreshing sleep
- Myalgias
- Migratory multijoint pain without swelling, heat, or redness (arthralgia)
- Headaches of a new type, pattern, or severity
- Recurrent nonsuppurative pharyngitis
- Cervical or axillary lymph node tenderness

CFS is excluded for the purposes of research, however, by other currently active medical conditions that are known to cause significant fatigue, major depressive or psychotic illnesses (including bipolar disorder and schizophrenia), dementia, morbid obesity (BMI $\geq$ 45), current eating disorders, and alcohol or substance abuse.

---

SOURCE: Fukuda et al. (1994).

---

for chronic fatigue syndrome but that treatment can improve many symptoms. A majority of persons with CFS return to near normal activity, but this process may take years. The physician should assure the patient of continued care and suggest that psychological counseling may help to cope with such a long-term illness.

### Activity

The next step is to encourage regular activity. Prolonged bed rest should be avoided due to problems with physical deconditioning. The patient should be advised to balance light activity with frequent rest periods. Although patients will resist exercise at first for fear of triggering a relapse, they can be coached to do interval exercise safely. Two to five minutes of activity (walking, biking, swimming, light weights, aerobics, etc.) at a self-selected pace should be alternated with 5 minutes of rest, and then repeated as tolerated. With interval exercise, all but the sickest patients can achieve several minutes of activity daily.

### Nutrition

The next priority is to optimize the patient's health with good nutrition, vitamins, and supplements. A prudent carbohydrate-based diet with lots of fruits and vegetables, potato, rice, pasta, and light meats (chicken, turkey, and scaly fish) seems tolerated best in CFS, while heavy meals with red meat and fried or greasy foods are more difficult to digest, cause slow peristalsis, and are innately fatiguing. Patients with irritable bowel symptoms and diarrhea may benefit from a diet low in dairy and gluten (wheat) products. Empirically, many patients do not tolerate refined sugar, excess caffeine, and alcohol.

## Symptomatic Therapies

The next step in traditional patient management is to address specific symptoms.

*Sleep.* Sleep is probably the most important symptom to address because without adequate sleep, anyone would be irritable, moody, achy, and miserable. Sedatives or hypnotics of lesser or greater potency may be necessary, with vigilant awareness of the potential development of habituation or tolerance. Relaxation therapies can also be helpful (see Chapter 28 for further behavioral strategies to enhance sleep).

*Pain.* Pain may arise from muscles, joints, or headaches. The usual cautions in using analgesic medications have to be observed, although the risk of habituation to narcotics is remarkably low in persons with chronic, nonmalignant pain, and pain relief should not be withheld for fear of "addiction" unless, of course, the patient has a past history of drug or alcohol abuse (Portenoy, 1990).

*Central activation (reduction of fatigue and cognitive dysfunction).* Fatigue and cognitive dysfunction are the two most common concerns in CFS patients. Fatigue can be managed by resting frequently, but additional cognitive dysfunction ("brain fog") makes the illness dreadful, leading to discouragement, frustration, depressed mood, and anxiousness. Some of these feelings may be attributed

to reduced serotonin levels in the blood and cerebrospinal fluid (Russell et al., 1992). Accordingly, serotonin agonists, such as the tricyclic antidepressants and selective serotonin reuptake inhibitors, are frequently prescribed. The increase in serotonin not only improves mood but also improves sleep quality and motivation. Agents with norepinephrine agonism (for example, amitriptyline and venlafaxine) have the added benefit of raising the pain threshold.

*Drugs.* Recently, amphetamine-like drugs have been used to activate the central nervous system. While the exact mechanism of action is undefined, this class of drug may work by (1) direct stimulation, (2) improving the attentional deficits typical of CFS, (3) reducing daytime somnolence, (4) enhancing the antidepressant drugs, or (5) raising the blood pressure. Long-acting stimulants such as phentermine or sustained-release Dexedrine are convenient for once-a-day use, but methylphenidate is equally effective. Modafinil was introduced specifically for the treatment of daytime hypersomnolence but has been shown effective in treating the fatigue associated with multiple sclerosis and fibromyalgia (Rammohan et al., 2002), as well as chronic fatigue syndrome.

Orthostatic intolerance is treated with volume expansion, beta blockade, and alpha agonism.

## BEHAVIORAL AND NEUROPSYCHIATRIC ASPECTS OF CFS: A NEW PARADIGM FOR DISEASE

For the past century, the dominant medical paradigm has been that illness or disease is defined by a physical injury, infection, or some other specific, etiologic factor. There is now a large and growing body of evidence that CFS is not a disease of "simple causation" but a disorder that involves profound and multiple physiological changes that result in the symptomatology that characterizes the condition. The autonomic dysfunction referred to earlier (Bou-Houlaigah et al., 1995) is likely to be a reflection of chronic hypoactivation of the stress system as described by Habib et al. (2001). Thus a gradually increasing understanding of the intimate and interactive relationships between the neurological, endocrine, and immunological systems is leading us toward defining a new disease paradigm.

## Depression and Chronic Fatigue Syndrome

Many physicians and lay people still believe that CFS is due to depression alone. This misunderstanding is perpetuated by uninformed practitioners who either equate "fatigue" with depression or who have achieved some success treating persons secondarily depressed by debilitating CFS. Scientific evidence, however, shows that depression is physiologically and clinically quite different from CFS (Bakheit, Behan, Dinan, Gray, & O'Keane, 1992; Bou-Houlaigah et al., 1995; Demitrack et al., 1991; Farrar, Locke, & Kantrowitz, 1995; Mountz et al., 1995; Schondorf et al., 1999). Table 24.2 summarizes the differences between major depression and CFS.

## EFFECTIVE ALTERNATIVE AND BEHAVIORAL TREATMENT INTERVENTIONS

### Alternative Therapies

Many persons with CFS turn to complementary and alternative therapies as a consequence of poor general and informational support from their physicians and the absence of effective allopathic treatments (Ax, Gregg, & Jones, 1997). A recent surveillance study

by the Centers for Disease Control and Prevention (Nisenbaum, Reyes, Jones, & Reeves, 2001) identified various forms of treatment used to treat chronic fatigue. Seventy-nine percent used traditional medical therapies, but a majority also relied on vitamins (79 percent), exercise (64 percent), dietary changes (54 percent). In addition, 36 percent reported using herbal remedies, acupuncture, or homeopathy.

Good scientific studies of complementary and alternative therapies in CFS are few. The strongest body of support seems to be for acupuncture, which is advocated mostly for the management of chronic pain. Some results have been equivocal because of design, sample size, and difficulties in blinding both operators and subjects. The National Institutes of Health promulgated a comprehensive consensus statement in 1997, concluding that acupuncture showed good efficacy as an adjunctive treatment for fibromyalgia and myofascial pain as well as more traditional pain syndromes such as postoperative and postdental pain, osteoarthritis, low-back pain, and carpal tunnel syndrome.

### Meditation, Hypnosis, Biofeedback, and Neurofeedback

Stress may exacerbate CFS and fibromyalgia, so it is not surprising that a number of papers support mind-body interventions, including muscle biofeedback, hypnosis, and relaxation training, for stress reduction in CFS (National Institutes of Health, 1997). Kaplan demonstrated the positive impact that meditation and visual imagery can have on fibromyalgia patients (Kaplan, Goldenberg, & Galvin-Nadeau, 1993). Likewise, muscle biofeedback, hypnosis, and relaxation training are widely recommended for stress reduction in CFS.

Electroencephalograph (EEG) biofeedback (also called neurofeedback) has been used by our group and others (James &

**Table 24.2** Differences Between Major Depression and Chronic Fatigue Syndrome

| Feature | Major Depression | CFS |
|---|---|---|
| Fatigue | 28% of cases | 100% of cases |
| Postexertional malaise | 19% of cases | 79–87% of cases |
| Sleep disorder | Early awakening, light sleep | Early onset of REM |
| | | Alpha-intrusion |
| | | Myoclonus, restless legs |
| Exercise | Helps | Intolerant |
| HPG axis | Excess cortisol | Low cortisol output |
| | Hyper-response to ACTH | Poor response to ACTH, CRH |
| | No response to buspirone | Hyperprolactinemia with |
| | | buspirone challenge |
| SPECT scan | Cortical abnormalities | Low CBF in thalamus, caudate, |
| | | and temporal lobes |
| Mood | Hopeless, helpless | Proactive and vocal |
| | Vegetative | Tend to overexert |
| Onset | Insidious | Abrupt |
| Incidence | Sporadic | Clusters and epidemics occur |
| Response to therapy | Usually positive | Usually unresponsive |

SOURCES: Bakheit et al. (1992); Demitrack et al. (1991); Farrar, Locke & Kantrowitz (1995); Jason, Richman, Friedberg, et al. (1997); Jorge & Goodnick (1997); Mountz et al. (1995).
NOTE: HPGA = hypothalamic-pituitary-gonadal axis, CBF = cerebral blood flow, REM = rapid eye movement

Folen, 1996). Neurofeedback can facilitate relaxation effects, or it can increase cortical activation and sharpen attention, depending on the training protocol. Hence neurofeedback can improve sleep and quality of life as well as produce measurable improvements in cognitive and functional abilities. The drawback to this therapy, however, is the large number of visits required for success. The number of skilled neurofeedback practitioners is small but growing (see Chapter 9 for an introduction to neurofeedback and Chapter 23 for a discussion of the application of neurofeedback to fibromyalgia).

### Cognitive-Behavioral Therapy

Cognitive-behavioral therapy (CBT) is a biopsychosocial approach to CFS management. Cognitive therapy assumes that somatic symptoms are perpetuated by errant illness beliefs and maladaptive coping. That is, certain cognitions and behaviors may perpetuate symptoms and impairments. Cognitive therapists believe that abnormal emotions and physiology are perpetuated by "catastrophic interpretations" that lead to excessive emotion and beliefs that somatic symptoms are beyond the control of the individual. Intensive cognitive-behavioral treatment, administered by skilled therapists, is directive and emphasizes self-help, education, correction of inaccurate beliefs, and the application of appropriate coping skills (See Chapter 12 for an overview of CBT.)

Numerous studies have applied CBT to chronic fatigue syndrome. Recent studies in the United Kingdom (Deale, Chalder, Marks, & Wessley, 1997; Sharpe et al., 1996) have demonstrated a reasonable improvement (return to work or school activity or a 10-point increase in the Karnofsky score) for approximately 70 percent of those who completed the program. This suggests that when both cognitive and behavioral components are addressed by expert therapists, CBT can be an effective long-term treatment for CFS (Price & Couper, 2000).

As encouraging as this research may sound, there are numerous problems with

CBT. First, CBT requires a therapist with special skills and a firm knowledge of chronic fatigue syndrome. Second, group therapy has not been shown to be effective, so treatment must be one-on-one and relatively long term (Price & Couper, 2000). Third, as earlier studies demonstrated, even skilled therapists may be unsuccessful. Fourth, CBT has only been studied in moderately ill persons who may not represent the majority of patients with CFS. CBT may not be as helpful either in mild community-based cases or in the extremely debilitated patient who is home or bed bound. Last, and most important, the CBT model tends to denigrate the medical/biological realities of CFS, which is contradictory to most patients' perspectives. Thus referrals for CBT must be carefully worded to acknowledge the medical aspects of the disorder while emphasizing the relative improvements possible through cognitive and behavioral change. Educating patients in a mind-body integrative view of CFS facilitates their acceptance of referrals for CBT and other behavioral interventions (see Chapter 2 for a description of the Trojan horse role induction, a strategy to optimize the referral of medical patients for mind-body services).

## Aerobic Activity

Although several studies have suggested short-term benefits from aerobic exercise in patients with fibromyalgia (McCain, 1986; Wigers, Stiles, & Vogel, 1996), this is one area where CFS is clinically different from fibromyalgia. Persons with CFS typically have an exacerbation of pain, cognitive difficulties, and flulike feelings with exercise and are thus advised to start with a low level of activity, take frequent rest intervals, and increase their physical activity very slowly. Although no studies satisfactorily demonstrate long-term benefits from exercise in CFS, several studies clearly show an increase postexercise in cognitive dysfunction,

neurohormonal abnormalities, excess cytokine production, and reduced cerebral blood flow in CFS (Blackwood, MacHale, Power, Goodwin, & Lawrie, 1998; Cheney, Lapp, & Davidson, 1992; LaManca et al., 1998; Ottenweller, Sisto, McCarty, & Natelson, 2001; Peterson et al., 1994).

In addition, numerous research studies have established that patients with CFS have reproducible abnormalities on cardiopulmonary exercise testing, including a high resting heart rate, reduced capacity to perform aerobic work, an early onset of the anaerobic threshold, and defects in the neuroendocrine response to exercise (Cheney et al., 1992; DeBecker, Roeykens, McGregor, & DeMeirleir, 2001). Clinically, CFS patients often show exacerbations of their symptoms with exertion and can trigger prolonged relapses with overexertion (Lapp, 1997). Thus not only do persons with CFS have a limited functional capacity, but exceeding that capacity may be disastrous to their health and well-being. The goal, then, is to find a middle ground between too little activity (i.e., deconditioning or isolation) and too much activity (i.e., flare or relapse). Low-level interval aerobic activity has been most successful in the author's experience, as recently confirmed by Clapp et al. (1999). Clapp's subjects walked on a treadmill at a self-selected comfortable pace for 10 discontinuous repetitions of 3 minutes of exercise separated by 3 minutes of recovery. Thirty minutes of interval exercise did not exacerbate any symptoms, although subjects felt beforehand that they could not exercise continuously for 30 minutes without triggering a flare. Personal experience and reports from several rehabilitation programs support that persons with CFS can tolerate exercise well if it is low level, aerobic, and interval.

## Physical Therapies

The least data seems to be available for the physical therapies, although many patients report improvement from the use of cool to hot packs, various forms of massage, neuromuscular release, cranial sacral therapy (particularly for cervicogenic pain and headache), and manipulation (or chiropracty).

## Dietary and Vitamin Supplements

Scientific studies of diet and vitamin supplementation in CFS are lacking, but the premise of optimizing health is a reasonable one and seemingly supported by literature on related conditions. The neurocognitive symptoms of $B_{12}$ deficiency in the elderly, for example, are similar to those seen in CFS (Beck, 1998), and hypomagnesemia is well known to cause fatigue and muscle weakness. Research has documented abnormalities in $B_{12}$ metabolism (Regland et al., 1998), decreased intracellular potassium (Burnet, 1998; Burnet, Yeap, Chatterton, & Gaffney, 1996), and hypomagnesemia (Cox, Campbell, & Dowson, 1991); therefore, many clinicians recommend supplementation with these vitamins. Folate and multivitamins are recommended when high doses of $B_{12}$ are employed (Lapp, 1999) to avoid subacute combined degeneration and competition of $B_{12}$ with other B vitamins. Uncontrolled studies of dietary supplements have purported to show improvement in overall symptoms and vitality using multiple-symptom questionnaires and visual analogue scales for outcome measurements (Rigden, 1998). Empirically, many clinicians report the benefit of a prudent diet that is low in fat, presumably because red meats and greasy foods exacerbate the autonomic-related gut motility disorder and irritable bowel symptoms so common in persons with CFS.

Herbal supplements have been used by many clinicians and patients alike in an effort to counteract some of the known biochemical and neurocognitive abnormalities found in CFS. Herbal approaches include treatment with ubiquinone (coenzyme Q) and nicotinamide-adenine dinucleotide (NAD) to improve mitochondrial function and adenosine triphosphate (ATP) production; *Gingko biloba* to improve cerebral blood flow and cognition; dehydroepiandrosterone (DHEA) to supplement the lower levels of this hormone caused by mild adrenocortical suppression; and melatonin, kava kava, and valerian used individually or in combination to combat sleep disruption. There is some evidence that oxidation radicals may be increased in CFS (Manuel y Keenoy, Moorkens, Vertommen, & DeLeeuw, 2001), so many holistic practitioners recommend treatment with vitamin C, vitamin E, glutathione, *N*-acetylcysteine, garlic, or one of the proanthocyanidins. Supplements and herbal remedies may pose health risks to some patients and can interfere with traditional therapies. Such remedies should be taken, therefore, only with the full knowledge and agreement of the attending physician.

## Unusual and Extreme Therapies

The desperation of this illness drives many patients to try extreme measures for relief, but there are no satisfactory controlled studies that support the use of chelation, intravenous treatments, enemas, reflexology, desensitization, peroxide, or oxygen inhalation therapy for the treatment of CFS. While many patients report improvement with magnet therapy, again there are no satisfactory randomized, placebo-controlled trials, and even strong supporters of this therapy cannot provide a reasonable physiological explanation as to how magnetic fields might help.

## CONCLUSION: LONG-TERM MANAGEMENT OF CFS

Our most important message for clinical practice is that research supports a combination of therapies as most effective in the long-term management of CFS (Buckelew et al., 1998; Clapp, et al., 1999; Eaton, 1996). Although many treatments have been effective in the short term, it appears that a combination of traditional medical therapy, interval aerobic exercise, relaxation therapy, biofeedback, cognitive-behavioral therapy, and general educational support is typically necessary for the best long-term results in chronic fatigue syndrome.

## REFERENCES

Ax, S., Gregg, V. H., & Jones, D. (1997). Chronic fatigue syndrome: Sufferers' evaluation of medical support. *Journal of the Royal Society of Medicine, 90*(5), 250–254.

Bakheit, A. M., Behan, P. O., Dinan, T. G., Gray, C. E., & O'Keane, V. (1992). Possible upregulation of hypothalamic 5-hydroxytryptamine receptors in patients with postviral fatigue syndrome. *British Medical Journal, 304*(6833), 1010–1012.

Bates, D. W., Buchwald, D., Lee, J., Kith, P., Doolittle, T., Rutherford, C., et al. (1995). Clinical laboratory tests in patients with chronic fatigue syndrome. *Archives of Internal Medicine, 155*(1), 97–103.

Beck, W. S. (1998). Cobalamin and the nervous system. *New England Journal of Medicine, 318*(26), 1752–1754.

Bennett, R., Clark, S. C., & Walczyk, J. (1998). A randomized, double-blind, placebo-controlled study of growth hormone in the treatment of fibromyalgia. *American Journal of Medicine, 104*(3), 227–231.

Blackwood, S. K., MacHale, S. M., Power, M. J., Goodwin, G. M., & Lawrie, S. M. (1998). Effects of exercise on cognitive and motor function in chronic fatigue syndrome and depression. *Journal of Neurology, Neurosurgery, and Psychiatry, 65*(4), 541–546.

Bou-Houlaigah, I., Rowe, P. C., Kan, J., & Calkins, H. (1995). The relationship between neurally mediated hypotension and the chronic fatigue syndrome. *Journal of the American Medical Association, 274*, 961–967

Buchwald D., Cheney, P. R., Peterson, D. L., Berch, H., Wormsley, S. B., Geiger, A., et al. (1992). A chronic illness characterized by fatigue, neurologic and immunologic disorders and active HHV6 infection. *Annals of Internal Medicine, 116*, 106–113

Buchwald, D. S., & Komaroff, A. L. (1991). Review of laboratory findings for patients with chronic fatigue syndrome. *Review of Infectious Diseases, 13*(Suppl. 1), S12–S28.

Buchwald, D. S., Sullivan, J. L., & Komaroff, A. L. (1987). Frequency of "chronic active Epstein-Barr virus infection" in a general medical practice. *Journal of the American Medical Association, 257*(17), 2303–2307.

Buckelew, S. P., Conway, R., Parker, J., Deuser, W. E., Read, J., Witty, T. E., et al. (1998). Biofeedback/relaxation training and exercise interventions for fibromyalgia. *Arthritis Care and Research, 11*(3), 196–209.

Burnet, R. B. (1998). Total body potassium in CFS. In T. K. Roberts (Ed.), *Proceedings of the international conference on the clinical and scientific basis of chronic fatigue syndrome* (p. 31). Sydney, Australia: T. K. Roberts.

Burnet, R. B., Yeap, B. B., Chatterton, B. E., & Gaffney, R. D. (1996). Chronic fatigue syndrome: Is total body potassium important? *Medical Journal of Australia, 164*(6), 314–318.

Centers for Disease Control and Prevention. (2000, September 7). National Center for Infectious Diseases chronic fatigue syndrome Web site. Retrieved May 8, 2002, from http://www.cdc.gov/ncidod/diseases/cfs

Centers for Disease Control and Prevention. (2002, February 2). National Center for HIV, STD and TB Prevention Web site. Retrieved May 22, 2002, from http://www.cdc.gov/hiv/stats.htm

Cheney, P. R., Lapp, C. W., & Davidson, M. (1992, October). *Bicycle ergometry with gas analysis and neuroendocrine response to exercise in CFS.* Paper presented at the International CFS/CFIDS/ME Research Conference, Albany, NY.

Clapp, L. L., Richardson, M. T., Smith, J. F., Wang, M., Clapp, A. J., et al. (1999). Acute effects of thirty minutes of light-intensity, intermittent exercise on patients with chronic fatigue syndrome. *Physical Therapy, 79*(8), 749–756.

Cox, I. M., Campbell, M. J., & Dowson, D. (1991). Red blood cell magnesium and chronic fatigue syndrome. *Lancet, 337*(8744), 757–760.

Deale, A., Chalder, T., Marks, I., & Wessley, S. (1997). Cognitive behavior therapy for the chronic fatigue syndrome: A randomized controlled trial. *American Journal of Psychiatry, 15*(3), 408–414.

DeBecker, P., Roeykens, J., McGregor, N., & DeMeirleir, K. (2001, January). *Measuring the exercise capacity in female CFS patients.* Paper presented at the American Association for Chronic Fatigue Syndrome Fifth International Research and Clinical Conference, Seattle, WA.

Demitrack, M. A., Dale, J. K., Straus, S. E., Laue, L., Listwak, S., Kruesi, M. J., et al. (1991). Evidence for impaired activation of the hypothalamic-pituitary-adrenal axis in patients with chronic fatigue syndrome. *Journal of Clinical Endocrinology and Metabolism, 73*(6), 1224–1234.

Eaton, K. K. (1996). Cognitive behaviour therapy for the chronic fatigue syndrome. Use of an interdisciplinary approach. *British Medical Journal, 312*(7038), 1097–1098.

Farrar, D. J., Locke, S. E., & Kantrowitz, F. G. (1995). Chronic fatigue syndrome. *Behavioural Medicine, 21*(1), 5–16.

Freeman, R., & Komaroff, A. L. (1997). Does chronic fatigue syndrome involve the autonomic nervous system? *American Journal of Medicine, 104*, 957–964

Fukuda, K., Straus, S. E., Hickie, I., Sharpe, M. C., Dobbins, J. G., Komaroff, A. L., et al. (1994). The chronic fatigue syndrome: A comprehensive approach to its definition and study. *Annals of Internal Medicine, 121*, 953–959.

Habib, K. E., Gold, P. W., Chrousos, G. P. (2001). Neuroendocrinology of stress. *Endocrinology and Metabolism Clinics of North America, 30*(3), 695–728.

Holmes, G. P., Kaplan, J. E., Gantz, N. M., Komaroff, L. A., Schonberger, L. B., & Straus, S. E. (1988). Chronic fatigue syndrome: A working case definition. *Annals of Internal Medicine, 108*(3), 387–389.

Ichise, M., Salit, I. E., Abbey, S. E., Chung, D. G., Gray, B., Kirsh, J. C., et al. (1992). Assessment of regional cerebral perfusion by 99Tc-HMPAO SPECT in chronic fatigue syndrome. *Nuclear Medicine Communications, 13*(10), 767–772.

James, L. C., & Folen, R. A. (1996). EEG biofeedback as a treatment for chronic fatigue syndrome. *Behavioural Medicine, 22*(2), 77–81.

Jason, L. A., Richman, J. A., Friedberg, F., Wagner, L., Taylor, R., & Jordan, K. M. (1997). Politics, science, and the emergence of a new disease: The case of chronic fatigue syndrome. *American Psychologist, 52*(9), 973–983.

Jason, L. A., Richman, J. A., Rademaker, A. W., Jordan, K. M., Plioplys, A. V., Taylor, R. R., et al. (1999). A community based study of chronic fatigue syndrome. *Archives of Internal Medicine, 159*, 2129–2137.

Jorge, C. M., & Goodnick, P. J. (1997). Chronic fatigue syndrome and depression: Biological differentiation and treatment. *Psychiatric Annals, 27*(5), 365–371.

Kaplan, K. H., Goldenberg, D. L., & Galvin-Nadeau, M. (1993). The impact of a meditation-based stress reduction program on fibromyalgia. *General Hospital Psychology, 15*(5), 284–289.

Komaroff, A. L. (2000a). The biology of chronic fatigue syndrome. *American Journal of Medicine, 108*, 169–171.

Komaroff, A. L. (2000b). The physical basis of CFS. *CFS Research Review, 1*(2), 1–3, 11.

LaManca, J. J., Sisto, S. A., DeLuca, J., Johnson, S. K., Lange, G., Pareja, J., et al. (1998). Influence of exhaustive treadmill exercise on cognitive functioning in chronic fatigue syndrome. *American Journal of Medicine, 105*(Suppl. 3A), 59S–65S.

Lapp, C. W. (1996, October). *Neurally mediated hypotension and symptomatic orthostatic tachycardia in CFS.* Paper presented at the AACFS Clinical & Research Conference, San Francisco.

Lapp, C. W. (1997). Exercise limits in chronic fatigue syndrome. *American Journal of Medicine, 103*(1), 83–84.

Lapp, C. W. (1999). Using cobalamin for the management of CFS. *CFIDS Chronicle, 12*(6), 14–17.

Manuel y Keenoy, B., Moorkens, G., Vertommen, J., & DeLeeuw, I. (2001). Antioxidant status and lipoprotein peroxidation in chronic fatigue syndrome. *Life Science, 68*(17), 2037–2049.

McCain, G. (1986). Role of physical fitness in the fibrositis/fibromyalgia syndrome. *American Journal of Medicine, 81*(3A), 73–77.

Mountz, J. M., Bradley, L. A., Modell, J. G., Alexander, R. W., Triana-Alexander, M., Aaron, L. A., et al. (1995). Fibromyalgia in women. Abnormalities of regional cerebral blood flow in the thalamus and the caudate nucleus are associated with low pain threshold levels. *Arthritis and Rheumatism, 38*(7), 926–938.

National Institutes of Health. (1997, November). *NIH Consensus Statement on Acupuncture, 15*(5), 1–34.

Nisenbaum, R., Reyes, M., Jones, A., & Reeves, W. C. (2001, February). Course of illness among patients with chronic fatigue syndrome in Witchita, Kansas. Paper presented at the American Association for Chronic Fatigue Syndrome Fifth International Research and Clinical Conference, Seattle, WA.

Ottenweller, J. E., Sisto, S. A., McCarty, R. C., & Natelson, B. H. (2001). Hormonal responses to exercise in chronic fatigue syndrome. *Neuropsychobiology, 43*(1), 34–41.

Peterson, P. K., Sirr, S. A., Grammith, F. C., Schenck, C. H., Pheley, A. M., Hu, S., et al. (1994). Effects of mild exercise on cytokines and cerebral blood flow in chronic fatigue syndrome patients. *Clinical Diagnostic Laboratory Immunology, 1*(2), 222–226.

Portenoy, R. K. (1990). Chronic opioid therapy in non-malignant pain. *Journal of Pain Symptom Management, 5*(Suppl. 1), S46–S62.

Price, J. R., & Couper, J. (2000). Cognitive behavioral therapy for adults with chronic fatigue syndrome. *Cochrane Database Systematic Review, 2*, CD001027.

Rammohan, K. W., Rosenberg, J. H., Pollak, C. P., Lynn, D. J., Blumenfeld, A., & Nagaraja, H. N. (2002, February). Efficacy and safety of modafinil (Provigil) for the treatment of fatigue in multiple sclerosis. *Journal of Neurology, Neurosurgery & Psychiatry, 72*(2), 150.

Regland, B., Andersson, L., Abrahamsson, J., Bagby, J., Dryehag, L. E., Germgard, T., et al. (1998). One-carbon metabolism and CFS. In T. K. Roberts (Ed.), *Proceedings of the international conference on the clinical and scientific basis of chronic fatigue syndrome* (p. 142). Sydney, Australia: T. K. Roberts.

Rigden, S. (1998). *Functional medicine adjunctive nutritional support for chronic fatigue syndrome.* Gig Harbor, WA: HealthComm International.

Russell, I. J., Michalek, J. E., Vipraio, G. A., Fletcher, E. M., Javors, M. A., & Bowden, C. A. (1992). Platelet 3H-imipramine uptake receptor density and serum serotonin levels in patients with fibromyalgia/fibrositis syndrome. *Journal of Rheumatology, 19*(1), 104–109.

Schondorf, R., Benoit, J., Wein, T., & Phaneuf, D. (1999). Orthostatic intolerance in the chronic fatigue syndrome. *Journal of the Autonomic Nervous System, 75*, 192–201

Schondorf, R., & Low, P. A. (1993). Idiopathic postural orthostatic tachycardia syndrome: An attenuated form of acute pandysautonomia? *Neurology, 43*(1), 132–137.

Schwartz, R. B., Garada, B. M., Komaroff, A. L., Tice, H. M., Gleit, M., Jolesz, F. A., et al. (1994). Detection of intracranial abnormalities in patients with chronic fatigue syndrome: comparison of MR imaging and SPECT. *American Journal of Roentgenology, 162*(4), 935–941.

Sharpe, M., Hawton, K., Simkin, S., Surawy, C., Hackman, A., Klimes, I., et al. (1996). Cognitive behavior therapy for the chronic fatigue syndrome: A randomized controlled trial. *British Medical Journal, 312*(7022), 22–26.

Straus, S. (1988). The chronic mononucleosis syndrome. *Journal of Infectious Diseases, 157*(3), 405–412.

Streeten, D., & Bell, D. S. (1998). Circulating blood volume in chronic fatigue syndrome. *Journal of Chronic Fatigue Syndrome, 4*(1), 3–11.

Wigers, S. H., Stiles, T. C., & Vogel, P. A. (1996). Effects of aerobic exercise versus stress management treatment in fibromyalgia. A 4.5 year prospective study. *Scandinavian Journal of Rheumatology, 25*(2), 77–86.

Wilke, W. S., Fouad-Tarazi, F. M., Cash, J. M., & Calabrese, L. H. (1998). The connection between CFS and neurally mediated hypotension. *Cleveland Clinic Journal of Medicine, 65*(5), 261–266.

# CHAPTER 25

# Attention Deficit Hyperactivity Disorder

JOEL F. LUBAR

**Abstract:** Attention deficit hyperactivity disorder is a lifelong disorder with a genetic basis and lingering effects into adult years. The author describes the profile of attention deficit hyperactivity disorder and its basis in neurophysiology. He provides guidelines for assessment using clinical interviews, behavior checklists, continuous performance tests, and baseline electroencephalograph (EEG) measurements. He proposes a protocol of EEG biofeedback training (neurofeedback) to alter cerebral activity and correct the neural dysfunction underlying attention problems. He recommends a comprehensive treatment program integrating academic training and neurofeedback. The author cites the growing number of outcome studies replicating his original research and documenting the effectiveness of neurofeedback for attention disorders. The research indicates that neurofeedback produces positive long-term modifications in cortical activity and cognitive function.

## MEDICAL, PHYSIOLOGICAL, AND BEHAVIORAL PROFILES OF THE DISORDER

Attention deficit hyperactivity disorder (ADD/HD), as currently characterized in the *Diagnostic and Statistical Manual of Mental Disorders (DSM-IV)*, consists of three main forms: inattentive, hyperactive-impulsive, and combined (American Psychiatric Association, 1994). These terms replace older classifications such as *hyperkinetic disorder of childhood,* a term popular in the 1970s, and *minimal brain dysfunction syndrome,* popular from 1940 to 1960 (Whalen & Henker, 1991). The disorder is regarded as neurologically based, primarily involving

dysfunction in the prefrontal lobes and in the associated dopaminergic and, to some extent, noradrenergic systems of the brain (J. F. Lubar & J. O. Lubar, 1999).

Research over the last five decades has begun to crystallize our understanding of the prefrontal lobe in much more detail. Fuster (1997) has cited considerable evidence indicating that the frontal lobe can be thought of as three interconnected systems. First, the lateral prefrontal cortex is extremely important for planning and organizing behavior. It is involved in the formulation and execution of different behavioral schemas. Barkley (1997) refers to this function as reconstitution. It involves the ability to reformulate new plans and new schemes of action when previous ones have not been effective. Clearly individuals with attention deficit hyperactivity disorder have significant difficulties in planning, organizing, understanding consequences of behavior, and reformulating behavioral plans when things have not worked in the past, which often leads to "giving up." The dorsal lateral prefrontal cortex is extremely important for working or recent memory function and for holding information during periods of delay or interference.

The second portion of the frontal lobe is the anterior cingulate and medial prefrontal cortex. These areas have been referred to as regions of "executive attention" by Posner and Raichle (1997) and involve planning in terms of carrying out a task that involves integration of sensory information leading to motor responses. An example would be the intention to begin a project such as homework.

The third system is primarily involved in inhibitory control and involves the orbital-frontal cortex (more on the right side than the left side) and portions of the medial cortex. These areas project heavily through the amygdala and other limbic structures and ultimately down to the hypothalamus, with outputs to the autonomic nervous system as well as brain-stem motor nuclei.

Deficits in inhibitory control are very often seen in individuals with the hyperactive form of attention deficit disorder. These individuals often exhibit inappropriate social behavior and behaviors associated with oppositional defiant disorder, conduct disorders, and, for the more severe cases, antisocial personality disorder.

Taken together, the three components of frontal lobe function clearly underlie the importance of the frontal lobe as the organizing structure in the brain for all the systems and lower systems in terms of sensory integration, motor outflow, and autonomic organization. Halstead (1947) characterized the frontal lobes very well in his phrase the "organs of civilization"—that is, the portion of the brain that differentiates complex human behavior, planning, judgment, and social behaviors and is not as developed in less complex species. What is characterized as attention deficit today was previously characterized as a "deficit in moral behavior associated with wanton destructiveness" (Still, 1902), which summarizes in part the constellation of problems seen in some individuals with attention deficit disorder or with prefrontal lobe injury.

There is considerable evidence from the work of Kenneth Blum and colleagues (Miller & Blum, 1995; Nobel, Blum, Ritchie, Montgomery, & Sheridan, 1991) that there are specific genetic alleles associated with metabolism of dopamine that are abnormal in nearly 50 percent of individuals that experience ADD/HD, particularly the hyperactive form. Another important recent finding is that ADD/HD is a lifelong, pervasive disorder that does not diminish in adolescence or adulthood but undergoes a transformation. Many people who experienced the hyperactive type of attention deficit disorder as children experience the inattentive or combined form as adolescents and adults. On the other hand, children with the inattentive form are likely to continue to experience that form. Estimates of the proportion of individuals who experienced ADD/HD as children and continued to experience it as adolescents and adults have ranged as high as 90 percent. Findings by Zametkin et al. (1990) employing PET technology and Amen and Carmichael (1997) using SPECT imaging confirm the pervasiveness of this disorder from childhood through late adulthood.

Behaviorally, ADD/HD is characterized by inattentiveness, inability to stay focused on tasks that are perceived as boring or irrelevant to the individual, difficulty in meeting deadlines, generalized difficulty in concentration, focusing and task completion of homework or assignments in class, poor

---

**Box 25.1    Screening Questions for ADD/HD**

1. Do you find it difficult to keep your mind on tasks?
2. Are you easily distracted from what you are doing?
3. Do you frequently fail to complete tasks you have begun?
4. Are you frequently disorganized, losing things, forgetting plans, or neglecting details?
5. Are you restless, overactive, and fidgety?
6. Do you do things impulsively, without thinking about the consequences?

If the individual or a family member responds positively to more than one of these screening questions, a more complete assessment should be conducted.

---

performance academically for reasons not associated with learning disabilities or mental retardation. In the case of the hyperactive or combined component, there is also restlessness, excessive activity, and often inappropriate behavior in social situations. Health professionals who suspect that a patient has an attention problem should ask the questions shown in Box 25.1 as a brief screen for ADD/HD.

## TYPICAL SYMPTOM PROFILE AND ASSESSMENT

ADD/HD rarely occurs in isolation but is often associated with a variety of comorbidities, including obsessive-compulsive disorder, oppositional-defiant disorder, conduct disorder, and in extreme cases, antisocial personality disorder and learning disabilities. For this reason, it is important to determine the relative contribution of each of these combinations of comorbidities with the central core of symptoms related to attention deficit disorder. There is considerable and increasing evidence that individuals with ADD/HD show a different pattern of EEG activity than nonclinical controls. Studies by Mann, Lubar, Zimmerman, Miller, and Muenchen (1992) showed that individuals experiencing the inattentive form of ADD/HD have more

slow activity in the theta and low alpha range in the frontal portion of the cortex and decreased high-frequency activity in the beta range in the posterior portion of the cortex. This is particularly evident during academic challenges such as reading and drawing tasks. Studies by Riccio, Hynd, Cohen, and Gonzalez (1993) at the University of Georgia also reported decreased frontal lobe activation in these individuals. A recent multicenter study involved the contributions of eight clinics and a total of more than 480 cases both with and without attention deficit disorder (Monastra et al., 1999). This study showed that individuals with ADD/HD between the ages of 6 and 30 differed significantly from nonclinical controls in the measure of the percentage of theta power divided by the percentage of beta power recorded at the vertex location on the scalp. These differences were highly significant and correlated very well with behavioral, psychometric, and continuous performance measures. A second paper involved 469 additional cases aged 6 to 20 (Monastra, Lubar, & Linden, 2001). This study, using the theta/beta ratio and Cz (vertex) location, obtained reliabilities greater than 0.90 with rating scale and continuous performance measures. Groups with ADD/HD could be differentiated from nonclinical controls with at least 90 percent accuracy by EEG measures.

---

**Box 25.2**    Components in the Assessment of ADD/HD

1. Clinical interview
   a. Educational and work history
   b. Family and social history
   c. Review of *DSM-IV* criteria
2. Behavior checklists completed by patient, family, and/or teacher
   a. Hawthorne Attention Deficit Disorders Evaluation Scale
   b. Conners Parent and Teacher Rating Scales
   c. Brown Attention Deficit Disorders Scale
3. Computerized continuous performance tests
   a. Test of Variables of Attention (TOVA)
   b. Conners Continuous Performance Test (CPT)
   c. Intermediate Visual and Auditory (IVA) Continuous Performance Test
4. Neurometric/EEG measures
   a. Multichannel quantitative EEG
   b. Single-site theta-beta ratios

---

As shown in Box 25.2, the comprehensive assessment of ADD/HD employs behavior rating scales such as the ADDES (Attention Deficit Disorders Evaluation Scale) by McCarney (1989), as well as those employed by Barkley (1990), Conners (1990), and others. Additional measures that correlate highly with the diagnosis of ADD/HD are based on performance on continuous performance tests such as the Intermediate Visual and Auditory (IVA) Continuous Performance Test or the Test of Variables of Attention (TOVA) diagnostic systems. Continuous performance tests essentially involve the presentation of two stimuli, through either the auditory or visual channels. The subject is required to respond to one of the two stimuli. Performance is measured by errors of omission, commission, impulsivity, and variability. Errors of omission involve the individual not responding when the appropriate stimulus is presented. Omission errors are indicative of inattention and may be associated with daydreaming or "disappearing" during the task. Errors of commission involve responding to the negative stimulus rather than withholding a response. Commission errors are associated in hyperactivity with impulsivity and are markers of prefrontal lobe dysfunction. Measures of response time and response variability are also highly correlated with the diagnosis of ADD/HD.

Taken together, a careful family history, performance on a continuous performance test, the EEG measures, and behavior rating scales, when all highly correlated, provide an accurate diagnosis of attention deficit hyperactivity disorder. The same measures may also provide some insight as to whether there may be underlying depression, oppositional defiant disorder, anxiety, or other comorbidities. The poorest measure is response to stimulant medication. The reason for this is that most individuals, whether they experience ADD/HD or not, respond positively to stimulant medication with decreased restlessness or increased focus and concentration. Therefore, stimulant medications do not provide a differential diagnosis for this disorder.

## CONVENTIONAL MEDICATION TREATMENT AND ITS SHORTCOMINGS

The conventional treatment for ADD/HD relies heavily on stimulant medications such as methylphenidate (Ritalin), supplemented under ideal conditions by educational accommodations, family counseling, and behavior modification to compensate for lack of focus and personal disorganization. When successful, stimulant medications reduce restless hyperactivity, increase attention to task, and decrease distractibility and impulsiveness (Barkley, 1990; Resnick, 2000). Most family members and health professionals report improvement in the inattentive individual's ability to plan and follow through with tasks.

There are significant problems, however, with relying exclusively on medications. Stimulant medications can inhibit growth rates of young persons, interfere with sleep, and trigger increased moodiness and irritability (National Institutes of Health, 2000; Pagliaro & Pagliaro, 1999, pp. 359–365). Some children and adults show inadequate response to medication, with only marginal reduction in hyperactivity and distractibility (Hallowell & Ratey, 1994). More serious (but fortunately infrequent) side effects include elevated blood pressure and heart rhythms, seizures, Tourette's syndrome, and changes in blood chemistry (Pagliaro & Pagliaro, 1999). Many individuals require frequent dosing (every 3 to 4 hours) on standard stimulant medications and experience a fading of attention and/or an increase in irritability as each dosage of the medication fades. Physicians frequently prescribe a combination of antidepressant medications with stimulants to level the individual's mood during the "stimulant fade" period, but antidepressants carry their own list of adverse effects. Several slow-release versions of the

stimulants have been approved, such as Concerta (methylphenidate HCl), but not all individuals show the same benefit from the slow-release medications, and some show more sleep disturbance on the longer-acting products. Only minimal research is available on the longer-term use of stimulants and on the use of higher doses of stimulant medication (National Institutes of Health, 2000).

Patient compliance is also a problem with exclusive reliance on pharmacotherapy for ADD/HD. Many parents are distrustful of any medication-oriented approach, and antipsychiatric newspaper articles and political action groups have sensitized parents against "drugging your child" (Sudderth & Kandel, 1997). The stimulants are controlled substances used on the street as "speed" or "uppers," raising parental concerns. The individual's own resistance is also frequently a limiting factor in the effectiveness of medication-oriented therapies. Patient education can increase compliance with medication, but both children and adults frequently show intermittent or constant resistance. Many youngsters resist taking the stimulant medications, which they frequently label as "hyper pills" and associate with emotionally disturbed or mentally impaired classmates. The need to go to the school office midday to take a second dose of the standard stimulant medication increases the stigma of these medications. It is also a major challenge for an individual whose primary problem is inattention and disorganization to remember to take medicines on a consistent schedule day after day, year after year. I have repeatedly observed that the long-term track record for remaining on stimulant medications from childhood into adulthood is all too low.

Patients and parents frequently express preferences for alternative therapies. Many of the alternative therapies, however, including nutritional modifications, have failed to show adequate magnitudes of effect to replace the use of stimulant and antidepressant medications (Resnick, 2000). The remainder of this chapter discusses neurofeedback as an alternative therapy that is producing substantial benefit for the majority of children and adults who complete a course of treatment.

## BEHAVIORAL AND PSYCHOPHYSIOLOGICAL INTERVENTIONS: NEUROFEEDBACK

Roughly 1,200 practitioners in the United States and many in Asia, Australia, Canada, Europe, Israel, and South America currently use EEG biofeedback (neurofeedback) to help overcome symptoms of ADD/HD. This approach has grown rapidly because studies have shown it to be extremely effective not only for symptomatic relief but also for altering the underlying cerebral dysfunction associated with the disorder by changing EEG activity and perhaps the underlying neurometabolic abnormalities. The first controlled study of neurofeedback intervention was published by Lubar and Shouse (1976) with a single case. Additional cases published by Shouse and Lubar (1979) were blind crossover studies with independent evaluations in classroom settings. These studies showed that training children to increase the sensorimotor rhythm (SMR)—a brain rhythm associated with inhibition of motor outflow from the motor cortex—and to inhibit 4-to-8-Hz theta activity associated with inattention showed significant improvements in the classroom. This original series of studies involved an ABA crossover design so that during part of the study, the conditions were reversed, leading to worsening of symptoms, and then reversed again to the original condition, leading to an improvement in symptoms both at home and in classroom settings. The study ended with the slow withdrawal of

medication and maintenance of the positive results that were obtained during the feedback training. In 1984, J. O. Lubar and J. F. Lubar published case studies showing the effectiveness of neurofeedback training. Later, a controlled study (Lubar, Swartwood, Swartwood, & O'Donnell, 1995) correlated the improvement on TOVA scores with decreased slow activity in the EEG over the course of neurofeedback training. There was an improvement in TOVA scores and increased scores on the WISC-R measure of IQ. The full-scale IQ improvement was approximately 12 points.

Several groups have replicated this research, including Linden, Habib, and Radojevic (1996) and, most recently, Thompson and Thompson (1998), whose study included 111 subjects—98 children and 13 adults—ranging from 5 to 63 years old. Tansey (1991) showed changes in WISC-R scores following EEG biofeedback training. Rossiter and La Vaque (1995) showed that EEG biofeedback training was at least as effective as psychostimulants for individuals with ADD/HD. Altogether, approximately 45 published studies employing neurofeedback have replicated the original work (Lubar & Shouse, 1976) and extended it to larger populations, including those with several subtypes of attention deficit disorder. Several studies also replicated that original work in individuals with comorbid attention deficit disorder and learning disabilities. In addition, numerous presentations at meetings of professional societies have described replications of the original findings.

It is important, however, to emphasize that the use of neurofeedback by itself is not an appropriate complete treatment. I use cognitive strategies that combine neurofeedback with academic training (see Box 25.3). I have used this model since the 1970s, and several other groups employ the same model.

---

**Box 25.3**    Patient and Family Education

Intervention with the individual with attention problems is more effective when patients and their families are educated about the nature of attention problems and about behavioral strategies to compensate for impaired attention. Patients and families should be given the following information:

1. Attention deficits are real neurologically based disorders, which significantly impair academic learning, social learning, and vocational functioning.
2. Attention deficits can cause problems beyond the classroom, including physical clumsiness, frequent accidents, poor time management, and careless mistakes on the job.
3. Failure to address attention problems commonly results in lifelong patterns of underachievement, low self-esteem, and impaired social functioning.
4. Neither lecturing nor punishing the individual with an attention problem will correct the inattention or personal disorganization.
5. Attention deficits rarely disappear after adolescence, and many adults require continued intervention.
6. Many individuals will continue to show some impairment in attention even after the best medical, behavioral, and psychophysiological interventions.
7. Behavioral methods can assist the individual to organize tasks, manage time, and otherwise compensate for inattention and disorganization.

---

Although studies involving neurofeedback alone also show positive results, these are more appropriate in validating research protocols as opposed to clinical interventions.

## EFFECTIVE PROTOCOLS AND INTERVENTIONS

The protocol that Lubar and Shouse (1976) developed originally involved training an increase in SMR (12 to 15 Hz) over the motor cortex and at the same time inhibiting slow activity in the range of 4 to 8 Hz for children and 6 to 10 Hz for adolescents and adults. Determining the best locations for training requires referential or bipolar measurements from individual locations on the scalp or a multichannel quantitative EEG involving 19 electrodes and examining locations that show the greatest amount of slow activity compared with fast activity measured through theta/beta or alpha/beta ratios. Recently, Chabot, Orgill, Crawford, Harris, and Serfontein (1999) described at least half a dozen subtypes of ADD/HD based on quantitative EEG measurements in over 400 cases. Some of these subtypes involved excessive frontal beta activity rather than deficient beta activity in posterior locations. These subtypes may be associated with individuals that experience a combination of attention deficit disorder and alcoholism. The reasons for this are findings by John, Prichep, Friedman, and Easton (1988) and Peniston and Kulkosky (1990) indicating that in alcoholics there is excessive beta activity and deficit alpha and theta activity. However, in individuals that have both attention deficit disorder and addictive disorders, a pattern appears to be emerging consisting of a bimodal distribution of excessive slow activity and excessive fast activity simultaneously with deficit activity in the middle frequencies (alpha). The treatment protocols for this subtype would involve decreasing frontal beta activity while inhibiting slow activity and increasing activity in the high alpha or SMR range. Because there is considerable evidence in the neurological literature that most forms of attention deficit hyperactivity disorder involve frontal lobe dysfunction, protocols are being developed that are directed at changing activity in the prefrontal regions. These protocols must take into account that the prefrontal region is difficult to work with because of eye movement artifact. The protocols may involve either decreasing excessive slow activity in the inattentive form or decreasing excessive fast activity in aggressive subtypes and in subtypes associated with addictive disorders.

It is now clear that the traditional neurofeedback approach of simply decreasing central slowing and increasing beta activity has progressed to looking at the quantitative EEG in more detail and employing protocols which are designed to normalize specific abnormalities regardless of where they occur in cerebral cortical locations. Most clinics that employ EEG biofeedback for ADD/HD claim that their success rates—as measured by psychometric changes, continuous performance tests, rating scales, and changes in EEG measures—range anywhere from 60 percent to 90 percent. Even higher degrees of success might be obtained by employing specific protocols for individuals in some of the more unusual subtypes of ADD/HD.

## LONG-TERM OUTCOME STUDIES

A very important criterion that needs to be applied to outcome studies in this area is whether the treatment effects are long lasting or not. A study of 52 cases followed up to 10 years after treatment, using the Connors scale as an index for attention, showed that the improvement with neurofeedback treatment appeared to be stable and long lasting (Lubar, 1995). Since many researchers and clinicians have entered this field recently, it is imperative that they continue to follow their patients as long as possible to determine whether the effects are more or less permanent. Occasionally, booster sessions are needed for some cases, but it has been my experience following patients up to 14 years posttreatment that once they learn the techniques and incorporate the changes that occur into their daily living, they do far better than they did previously. Overall, the groups that are employing this technique claim that they are able to reduce medication needs by anywhere from 40 percent to 80 percent. This does not imply that neurofeedback is a substitute for medication but that it is a powerful adjunctive technique that, in many cases, reduces individuals' dependence on medication. This is particularly true for those that experience the inattentive form of attention deficit disorder rather than the hyperactive or hyperactive-impulsive forms.

## FUTURE DIRECTIONS

For neurofeedback to become a mainstream treatment for ADD/HD, it must move from small clinical studies to larger multicenter studies. At the current time, multicenter studies are being initiated as well as studies in school systems to determine whether neurofeedback can be integrated directly with the curriculum. The most frequent criticism of using biofeedback to treat ADD/HD was that the published studies primarily involved small numbers of patients with a lack of randomized group selection. Often there is a confounding of results because neurofeedback is combined with other approaches such as behavior therapy, psychotherapy, medication, and parenting skills. However, some of the studies have employed only neurofeedback approaches. Basically, the majority of recent neurofeedback studies have been observational studies submitted by clinicians working in clinical settings, as opposed to controlled research in laboratory settings. Recently, however, the *New England Journal of Medicine* has published two important papers (Benson & Hartz, 2000; Concato, Shah, & Horowitz, 2000) that show that the results of observational studies are very similar to those obtained in controlled clinical trials with random assignment. These papers deal with large meta-analyses of medical interventions and provide the first and clearest evidence that observational studies not employing random assignment, double-blind approaches and ABA crossover designs may be just as valuable as the more traditional "court of science" approach. Clearly, both kinds of studies are necessary at this point. The

controlled studies with random assignment of individuals into different groups to compare outcome are important to show, as clearly as possible, the strength of neurofeedback in and of itself. In the clinical context, however, it is preferable to combine neurofeedback with other approaches.

Managed care and insurance carriers are beginning to recognize neurofeedback as a viable intervention and are beginning to cover the cost of neurofeedback training for many of their clients. There is a growing realization that neurofeedback is aimed at the underlying neurological and neurochemical basis for the disorder rather than at the symptoms, and it appears from the data collected so far that the effects are long lasting. The growth curve of neurofeedback for the evaluation and treatment of ADD/HD is still in its early stages, but rapid, continued development of this technology can be expected over the next decade.

## REFERENCES

Amen, D. G., & Carmichael, B. D. (1997). High resolution brain SPECT imaging in ADHD. *Annals of Clinical Psychiatry, 9,* 81–86.

American Psychiatric Association. (1994). *Diagnostic and statistical manual of mental disorders* (4th ed., *DSM-IV*). Washington, DC: Author.

Barkley, R. A. (1990). *Attention deficit hyperactivity disorder: A handbook for diagnosis and treatment.* New York: Guilford.

Barkley, R. A. (1997). Behavioral inhibition, sustained attention, and executive functions: Constructing a unifying theory of ADHD. *Psychological Bulletin, 121,* 65–94.

Benson, K., & Hartz, A. J. (2000). A comparison of observational studies and randomized controlled trials. *New England Journal of Medicine, 342*(25), 1878–1886.

Chabot, R. J., Orgill, A. A., Crawford, G., Harris, M. J., & Serfontein, G. (1999). Behavioral and electrophysiological predictors of treatment response to stimulants in children with attention disorders. *Journal of Child Neurology, 14*(6), 343–351.

Concato, J., Shah, N., & Horowitz, R. (2000). Randomized controlled trials, observational studies, and the hierarchy of research designs. *New England Journal of Medicine, 342*(25), 1887–1892.

Conners, C. K. (1990). *Conners' rating scales manual.* North Tonawanda, NY: MHS.

Fuster, J. M. (1997). *The prefrontal cortex: Anatomy, physiology, and neuropsychology of the frontal lobe* (3rd ed.). Philadelphia: Lippincott-Raven.

Hallowell, E. M., & Ratey, J. J. (1994). *Driven to distraction: Recognizing and coping with attention deficit disorder from childhood through adulthood.* New York: Touchstone.

Halstead, W. C. (1947). *Brain and intelligence: A quantitative study of the frontal lobes.* Chicago: University of Chicago Press.

Intermediate Visual and Auditory Continuous Performance Test (IVA). Available through BrainTrain, 727 Twin Ridge Lane, Richmond, VA 23235.

John, E. R., Prichep, L. S., Friedman, J., & Easton, P. (1988). Neurometrics: Computer-assisted differential diagnosis of brain dysfunctions. *Science, 293,* 162–169.

Linden, M., Habib, T., & Radojevic, V. (1996). A controlled study of EEG biofeedback effects on cognitive and behavioral measures with attention-deficit disorder and learning disabled children. *Biofeedback & Self-Regulation, 21,* 35–49.

Lubar, J. F. (1995). Neurofeedback for the management of attention deficit hyperactivity disorders. In M. S. Schwartz (Ed.), *Biofeedback: A practitioner's guide* (2nd ed., pp. 493–522). New York: Guilford.

Lubar, J. F., & Lubar, J. O. (1999). Neurofeedback assessment and treatment for attention deficit/hyperactivity disorders (ADD/HD). In J. R. Evans & A. Abarbanel (Eds.), *Introduction to quantitative EEG and neurotherapy* (pp. 103–143). New York: Academic Press.

Lubar, J. F., & Shouse, M. N. (1976). EEG and behavioral changes in a hyperkinetic child concurrent with training of the sensorimotor rhythm (SMR): A preliminary report. *Biofeedback & Self-Regulation, 3,* 293–306.

Lubar, J. F., Swartwood, M. O., Swartwood, J. N., & O'Donnell, P. (1995). Evaluation of the effectiveness of EEG neurofeedback training for ADHD in a clinical setting as measured by changes in TOVA scores, behavioral ratings, and WISC-R performance. *Biofeedback & Self-Regulation, 20,* 83–99.

Lubar, J. O., & Lubar, J. F. (1984). Electroencephalographic biofeedback of SMR and beta for treatment of attention deficit disorders in a clinical setting. *Biofeedback & Self-Regulation, 9,* 1–23.

Mann, C. A., Lubar, J. F., Zimmerman, A. W., Miller, B. A., & Muenchen, R. A. (1992). Quantitative analysis of EEG in boys with attention deficit/hyperactivity disorder (ADHD). A controlled study with clinical implications. *Pediatric Neurology, 8,* 30–36.

McCarney, S. B. (1989). *The attention deficit disorders evaluation scale* (Home version, technical manual). Columbia, MO: Hawthorne Educational Services.

Miller, D. K., & Blum, K. (1995). *Overload: Attention deficit disorder and the addictive brain.* Kansas City, MO: Andrews & McMeel.

Monastra, V. J., Lubar, J. F., & Linden, M. K. (2001). The development of a quantitative electroencephalographic scanning process for attention deficit-hyperactivity disorder: Reliability and validity studies. *Neuropsychology, 15*(1), 136–144.

Monastra, V. J., Lubar, J. F., Linden, M., VanDeusen, P., Green, G., Wing, W., Phillips, A., & Fenger, T. N. (1999). Assessing attention deficit hyperactivity disorder via quantitative electroencephalography: An initial validation study. *Neuropsychology, 13*(3), 424–433.

National Institutes of Health. (2000). National Institutes of Health consensus development conference statement: Diagnosis and treatment of attention-deficit hyperactivity disorder (ADHD). *Journal of the American Academy of Child and Adolescent Psychiatry, 39,* 182–193.

Nobel, E., Blum, K., Ritchie, T., Montgomery, A., & Sheridan, P. (1991). Allelic association of the D2 dopamine receptor gene with receptor-binding characteristics in alcoholism. *Archives of General Psychiatry, 48,* 648–654.

Pagliaro, L. A., & Pagliaro, A. M. (1999). *Psychologists' neuropsychotropic drug reference*. Philadelphia, PA: Taylor & Frances.

Peniston, E. G., & Kulkosky, P. J. (1990). Alcoholic personality and alpha-theta brainwave training. *Medical Psychotherapy, 3,* 37–55.

Posner, M. I., & Raichle, M. E. (1997). *Images of the mind*. New York: W. H. Freeman.

Resnick, R. J. (2000). *The hidden disorder: A clinician's guide to attention deficit hyperactivity disorder in adults*. Washington, DC: American Psychological Association.

Riccio, C. A., Hynd, G. W., Cohen, M. J., & Gonzalez, J. J. (1993). Neurological basis of attention deficit hyperactivity disorder. *Exceptional Children, 60*(2), 118–124.

Rossiter, T. R., & La Vaque, T. J. (1995). A comparison of EEG biofeedback and psychostimulants in treating attention deficit hyperactivity disorders. *Journal of Neurotherapy, 1,* 48–59.

Shouse, M. N., & Lubar, J. F. (1979). Sensorimotor rhythm (SMR) operant conditioning and methylphenidate in the treatment of hyperkinesis. *Biofeedback & Self-Regulation, 4,* 299–311.

Still, G. F. (1902). The Coulstonian lectures on some abnormal psychological conditions in children. *Lancet, 1,* 1008–1012, 1163–1168.

Sudderth, D. B., & Kandel, J. (1997). *Adult ADHD: The complete handbook*. Rocklin, CA: Prima Health.

Tansey, M. (1991). Wechsler (WISC-R) changes following treatment of learning disabilities via EEG biofeedback training in a private setting. *Australian Journal of Psychology, 43,* 147–153.

Test of Variables of Attention (TOVA). Available from Universal Attention Disorders Inc., 4281 Katella Avenue, #215, Los Alamitos, CA 90720.

Thompson, L., & Thompson, M. (1998). Neurofeedback combined with training in metacognitive strategies: Effectiveness in students with ADD. *Applied Psychophysiology and Biofeedback, 23*(4), 243–263.

Whalen, C. K., & Henker, B. (1991). Therapies for hyperactive children: Comparisons, combinations, and compromises. *Journal of Consulting and Clinical Psychology, 59,* 126–137.

Zametkin, A. J., Nordahl, T., Gross, M., King, A. C., Semple, W. E., Rumsey, J., et al. (1990). Cerebral glucose metabolism in adults with hyperactivity of childhood onset. *New England Journal of Medicine, 323,* 1361–1366.

# CHAPTER 26

# Anxiety Disorders

DONALD MOSS

**Abstract:** This chapter introduces anxiety disorders and suggests screening, education, and therapy for anxiety in primary care. The author reviews a comprehensive range of assessment tools, including medical, psychiatric, cognitive, behavioral, physiological, and neurometric assessment. The conventional treatment of anxiety disorders calls for anxiolytic and antidepressant medication combined with cognitive-behavioral therapy. Mind-body interventions include relaxation therapies, breathing retraining, biofeedback, and neurofeedback.

## PSYCHOLOGICAL AND DEMOGRAPHIC PROFILE OF ANXIETY DISORDERS

Everyday life is filled with worries and fears, some transient and others lingering. Health professionals designate anxieties, worries, and fears as anxiety disorders when they become so intense and frequent as to disrupt everyday life. Anxiety disorders are among the most common mental health problems that health professionals in primary care and mental health clinics encounter (Kessler et al., 1994). The Epidemiological Catchment Area Survey suggests that in the course of a lifetime, approximately 15 percent of the population suffers a diagnosable anxiety disorder (Regier, Narrow, & Rae, 1990).

Anxiety disorders affect all social and age groups within the population, but several groups face higher risk. Anxiety disorders are twice as common in women (9.7 percent incidence in a one-month period) as in men (4.7 percent in a one-month period). Population groups most vulnerable to anxiety disorders include individuals 25 to 44 years old, females, separated and divorced individuals, and those with low socioeconomic status (Regier, Narrow, & Rae, 1990). The average age of onset for any anxiety disorder is 16.4 years and even earlier for some disorders. The average age of onset for social phobia is 11.6 years (Regier, Rae, Narrow, Kaelber, & Schatzberg, 1998). Early onset of an anxiety disorder has lingering consequences, with heightened risk for later major depression and addictive disorders (Regier, Rae, et al., 1998).

## A COMPREHENSIVE BIOCHEMICAL, PSYCHOPHYSIOLOGICAL, COGNITIVE, AND BEHAVIORAL MODEL OF ANXIETY DISORDERS

The current understanding of anxiety disorders emphasizes the overall interaction of

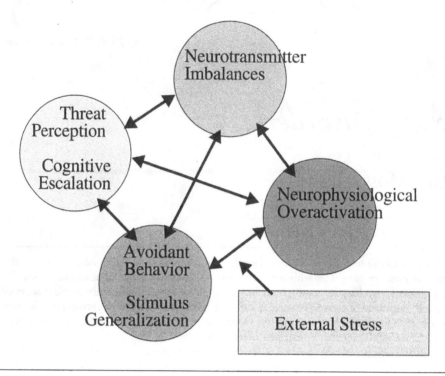

**Figure 26.1** Comprehensive Model of Anxiety

biochemical vulnerability, physiological activation, cognitive fears, behavioral avoidance patterns, and a stressful environment (see Figure 26.1). As Peter Lang and S. J. Rachman observed, distinct aspects of anxiety do not covary reliably (Rachman, 1982, 1999). They are loosely coupled, or discordant. An individual can overcome avoidance behavior yet remain cognitively afraid and neurophysiologically activated. Similarly, an individual can relax his or her body yet continue to label a situation as a threat. This is critical because treatment should target each aspect of anxiety distinctly, as the patient's presentation demands.

### Biochemical Vulnerability

Biological psychiatry has identified a number of neurotransmitters implicated in anxiety disorders. The unavailability of serotonin in the synaptic cleft, the gap between

neurons, appears to play a role in obsessive-compulsive disorder and at least an accessory role in the rest of the anxiety disorders. Serotonin serves as a "chemical messenger" across the synapse. Both anxiety and depressive symptoms decrease when medication blocks the uptake of serotonin into receptors on the neuronal dendrites and increases the availability of serotonin.

There are also probable abnormalities at gamma-aminobutyric acid (GABA) receptors in anxiety disorders. GABA is an inhibitory neurotransmitter that reduces efferent and afferent activity to and from the limbic brain (the emotional brain, including the amygdala and the hippocampus). When GABA levels are low, there is a heightening of subjective distress, including both anxiety and depression. The benzodiazepine medications, widely used in anxiety disorders, modulate the activity of GABA in the brain (Bernstein, 1995; Nutt & Malizia, 2001).

## Neurophysiological Activation: General

Anxiety disorders most often manifest in the form of a bewildering array of physical symptoms, including tense musculature, hyperventilation, rapid heart rate, chest pain and tightness, sweating and trembling, dizziness, racing thoughts, difficulty getting one's breath, nausea, abdominal discomfort, hot flashes, chills, and other somatic symptoms. When an individual feels the presence of threat, whether objective or perceived, the hypothalamic-pituitary-adrenal axis mobilizes the body for emergency action. Current research shows interaction among neurotransmitter systems, neuroendocrinological processes, and neuroanatomical structures in mediating stress responses, normal anxiety, and the anxiety disorders (Antai-Otong, 2000).

## Respiratory Psychophysiology

"The mind and breathing are interdependent and regular respiration produces a serene mind." (Yue Yanggui, *Questions and Answers of Meisha*, cited by Xiangcai, 2000, p. 7)

The physiology of respiration plays a central role in anxiety disorders (Fried, 1990, 1993; Timmons & Ley, 1994). Rapid breathing (hyperventilation) "blows off" carbon dioxide ($CO_2$) and reduces $CO_2$ in the air stream as well as in arterial blood. This lowered level of $CO_2$, called hypocapnia, induces cerebral vasoconstriction and hypoxia and increases sympathetic nervous system (SNS) arousal and later fatigue. Hypocapnia causes a rise in blood pH, which is counteracted by renal excretion of bicarbonate ion. The resulting changes in alkali systems and in extracellular and intracellular chemistry produce many of the symptoms of hypocapnia (Nixon, 1994; von Scheele & von Scheele, 1999). The symptoms of hypocapnia (Fried, 1990, pp. 88–91) show up in almost all physiological systems:

1. Cardiovascular: palpitations, tachycardia, precordial pain, cutaneous vasoconstriction.

2. Neurological—central: dizziness, disturbance of consciousness and vision.

3. Neurological—peripheral: paresthesia, tetany.

4. Respiratory: shortness of breath, wheezing, chest tightness.

5. Gastrointestinal: globus, dysphagia, epigastric pain, aerophagy.

6. Musculoskeletal: muscle pain, tremors, tetany.

7. Psychic: tension, anxiety.

8. General: fatigue, weakness, exhaustion, sleep disturbance, nightmares.

These symptoms are central to the presentation of panic disorder and the phobias and overlap extensively with the symptomatic presentation of generalized anxiety disorder and social phobia. Recent research in Sweden by von Scheele and von Scheele (personal communication, November 19, 2001) raises the possibility that hypercapnia may play a similar role in the etiology of symptoms, but further research is necessary to clarify the significance of excesses in carbon dioxide.

There has been controversy about the role of respiration in anxiety disorders, as earlier studies sometimes failed to support the role of hyperventilation in inducing panic disorder (Gorman et al., 1984; Papp, Klein, & Gorman, 1993). However, in a series of elegant empirical studies, often using ambulatory monitoring of breathing and $CO_2$ levels while individuals were exposed to flight and driving situations, Roth and colleagues verified the presence of various forms of irregular respiration and responses to respiration in anxiety patients. On taking a deep breath, patients with generalized anxiety disorder showed more heart rate acceleration than controls (Roth, Wilhelm, & Trabert, 1998). Before and after taking that deep breath, respiratory $CO_2$ was lower in those with generalized anxiety disorder and lowest in patients with panic disorder compared with that of normal controls.

In another study during an air flight, phobics paused more during inspiration than controls (Wilhelm & Roth, 1998a). Phobics showed more autonomic instability during flight, including skin conductance fluctuations and an absence of synchrony between respiration and heart rate. Both patients with panic disorder and those with social phobia felt more anxious during voluntary hyperventilation in another study, and those with panic disorder recovered more slowly than normal controls after hyperventilation (Wilhelm, Gerlach, & Roth, 2001). Wilhelm and Roth (1998b) also reported that phobics showed a greater elevation of heart rate on entering a plane than controls, suggesting the role of anticipatory anxiety and its impact on the cardiovascular system. Other teams have also recently demonstrated the role of hyperventilation. Nardi, Valenca, Nascimento, Mezzasalma, and Zin (2001) showed that 61.5 percent of panic disorder patients, 22.7 percent of social phobics, and only 4 percent of controls had a panic attack after voluntary hyperventilation. Abelson, Weg, Nesse, and Curtis (2001) found striking irregularities in the respiration of panic disorder patients and showed that cognitive manipulation could modify the respiratory pattern.

## Neurocortical Activation Patterns

The human brain, especially the neocortex, is a critical structure in higher mental processes such as thinking, attention, and perception. Electrocortical patterns in the human cortex shape the current state of mind and the manner of attunement to the surrounding experiential world. The state of mind when the brain is dominated by fast electrical waves in the frequency range of 20 to 28 Hz is more likely to be worrisome, fearful, and suspicious, whereas a dominant pattern of slow waves in the range of 8 to 12 Hz is likely to produce a relaxed, calm state of mind. Other cortical patterns are also commonly identified in anxiety states, including a paradoxical suppression of slow-wave activity (Sattlberger & Thomas, 2000; Thomas & Sattlberger, 1997) and an overactivation on the cortical midline overlying the anterior cingulate gyrus driving obsessional thinking. Researchers and practitioners differ in exactly how they designate frequency bands. However, Table 26.1 shows a typical designation of frequency bands and a subjective description of the typical subject's experiencing when each band dominates the electroencephalograph (EEG).

Subcortical brain structures also play a critical role in the emotions, including anxiety. The emotional brain (or limbic brain) includes three subcortical structures—the thalamus, the amygdala, and the hippocampus—which are functionally organized into an emotional system integrated with the right prefrontal cortex (LeDoux, 1996). Other subcortical structures have been identified as critical in specific anxiety disorders, including the caudate nucleus and the anterior cingulate gyrus in obsessive-compulsive disorder, and the locus ceruleus in posttraumatic stress disorder. Early life events, especially successful mother-child infant bonding, are critical in the integration of subcortical emotional systems with cortical control centers. Problems in early bonding result in weaknesses in limbic-cortical circuits and a resultant emotional dysregulation (Schore, 1994). Individuals with emotional dysregulation remain emotionally reactive and labile and show extreme swings in anxiety and mood as adults.

**Table 26.1**   Commonly Used Designations of Cortical Frequency Ranges

| Frequency Range (Hz)[a] | Label | Subjective State |
|---|---|---|
| 2–4 | Delta | Sleep states |
| 4–7 | Theta | Daydreaming, imagery |
| 8–12 | Alpha | Awake, receptive, meditative |
| 12–20 | Low beta | Activated, focused |
| | | Special subset of beta range with focused thinking |
| 20-28 | High beta | Hypervigilance, anxiety, panic |

a. Researchers differ in precise cutting points for these frequency ranges.

## Physiology and Cognition: The Escalation of Anxiety

Psychophysiological research on anxiety disorders shows a variety of symptom patterns, depending on the specific anxiety disorder and the individual. In many cases basal heart rate, autonomic functions, and metabolism are elevated continuously, with further elevation during times of heightened anxiety or panic. These physical accompaniments of anxiety frighten the anxious individual, and the person's fear about "what is wrong in my body" in turn plays a role in further escalating the anxiety. Clark's (1986) classic formulation of panic disorder is that the subject makes a "catastrophic interpretation" of certain bodily sensations, such as elevated heart rate, and hence begins to panic (see also Rachman, 1996). Typical catastrophic fears in panic are that "I am dying" (from a heart attack, cancer, or some terrible undiagnosed disease), "I am going crazy," "I am losing my mind," or "I am losing control." Cognitive therapies aim to eliminate or reduce this subjective escalation of the anxiety response. The physical manifestations of anxiety may confuse medical caregivers and lead to costly testing and treatments, often with little benefit for the individual.

The cognitive approach to anxiety highlights the critical role of distorted thoughts and distorted cognitive schemas in the onset of anxiety (Beck & Emery, 1985; Salkovskis, 1996; Wells, 1997). The obsessive-compulsive individual, for example, perceives the world as a dangerous place full of germs and sources of contamination. The individual adopts various safety behaviors to address this perception of danger, believing that "By constant cleaning and avoiding contact with filth, I can survive." The cognitive therapist challenges the distorted schema of danger and invites the individual to engage in experiments that can disprove the fears.

## Avoidance Behavior and Stimulus Generalization

The obsessive-compulsive example just described highlights the role of avoidance behaviors and their interdependence with core fears and cognitive distortions. The phobic, for example, adopts the cognitive schema that "Several places carry special danger for me. By going there I could lose my mind, die, or lose complete control." Then the phobic engages in the defensive behavior of avoiding such places and situations, hoping to remain safe. The behavioral avoidance pattern maintains the perception of threat, as the individual never enters the situation and never has the opportunity to master or disprove the fear.

In addition, behavioral approaches emphasize the "classical conditioning" effect of stimulus generalization. Once a fear of a particular stimulus is established, fear begins to attach as well to adjacent situations and to stimuli that occur in the presence of the original feared object. An individual may first experience a panic attack in a crowded supermarket and gradually come to fear entering other stores, other public places, riding to the store, riding anywhere, and eventually even leaving the home. Behavioral therapies rest heavily on exposure therapies, such as systematic desensitization, which overcome the avoidance patterns and the generalized fears that support the avoidance.

## SCREENING FOR ANXIETY DISORDERS

Anxiety disorders are largely treatable, yet when they progress untreated, they cause dramatic suffering and often disability. The single most important intervention for the health professional regarding anxiety disorders is to identify the individual with anxiety early in the course of the disorder.

### Anxiety Disorders in Medical Settings

Patients with anxiety disorders present in high numbers in emergency rooms and primary health care clinics, yet often anxiety disorders and other mental health problems remain undetected. Even when mental health disorders are recognized, a larger number of patients receive treatment in general medical settings than from mental health specialists (Cummings, Cummings, & Johnson, 1997; Narrow, Regier, Rae, Manderscheid, & Locke, 1993). Current health maintenance organizations have instituted practices, including gatekeeping requirements and larger co-pays for mental health than for medical services, which reinforce the long-standing reluctance of the general public to accept referral for mental health specialty services (Narrow et al., 1993). Cardiac clinics, gastrointestinal clinics, oncology clinics,

geriatric medicine practices, and other medical specialty clinics all see large numbers of anxiety disorders presenting as medical disorders. Patients with chronic anxiety disorders have a documented higher incidence of developing medical illnesses, including atherosclerosis and cerebrovascular, ischemic heart, gastrointestinal, hypertensive, and respiratory diseases (Bowen, Senthilselvan, & Barale, 2000). Conversely, many specific medical disorders create increased risk for anxiety and other mental health disorders. Children with asthma, for example, report more anxiety symptoms than do children with diabetes; those asthmatic children with psychiatric symptoms also show poorer self-esteem and lower social competence (Vila et al., 1999). Adults with asthma suffer similar elevated prevalence rates for anxiety disorders (Jonas, Wagener, Lando, & Feldman, 1999).

### Diagnostic Categories

Anxiety disorders are classified according to objective diagnostic criteria, following the *Diagnostic and Statistical Manual of Mental Disorders* (or *DSM-IV*), the diagnostic manual of the American Psychiatric Association (1994). The *DSM-IV* classifies anxiety problems into panic disorder, the phobias, generalized anxiety disorder, obsessive-compulsive disorder, posttraumatic stress disorder, acute stress disorders, and "adjustment disorder with anxious features." Pharmacotherapies, cognitive therapies, and behavioral therapies have become more effective as research has allowed the development of treatment plans sensitive to differences among diagnostic groupings (Moss, 2001; Moss, 2002). Obsessive-compulsive disorder, for example, responds better to the selective serotonin reuptake inhibitors (SSRIs) and to specific cognitive-behavioral interventions, such as "exposure and response prevention." Precise diagnostic assessment goes farther than specifying a *DSM-IV* diagnosis. Identification of

**Table 26.2**     Medical Illnesses and Factors Causing Anxiety-Like Symptoms

| System | Specific Disorder | Symptoms |
|---|---|---|
| Cardiovascular | Angina, myocardial infarction, arrhythmias, hypertension | Tachycardia, palpitations, ischemia, chest pain |
| Gastrointestinal | Peptic ulcer, Crohn's disease | Abdominal pain, diarrhea, upset stomach |
| Hematological | Anemia | Fatigue, shortness of breath, palpitations |
| Metabolic | Cushing's syndrome, hyper- and hypothyroidism, hypoglycemia, menopause, porphyria | Insomnia, irritability, fatigability tremulousness, restlessness, faintness, palpitations |
| Neurological | Encephalopathies, seizure disorders | Headache, dizziness, light-headedness, paresthesias |
| Respiratory | Asthma | Shortness of breath, suffocation, fears |

a faulty cognitive schema underlying anxiety serves as a basis for more strategic cognitive therapy. Similarly, a psychophysiological assessment of dysfunctional respiratory activity, and of the resultant abnormalities in respiratory $CO_2$, can be helpful in treating panic disorder and other anxiety disorders. Exhaustive diagnosis includes an assessment of all dimensions of anxiety disorders shown in Figure 26.1.

## Medical Screening

Evaluation of anxiety disorders begins with a screening for medical conditions that trigger symptoms mimicking anxiety disorders (Gold, 1989). The initial exam should include a history, a physical, and lab work as indicated by symptoms and history. Family history should include special attention to cardiac disease, thyroid conditions, depression, and anxiety disorders in the past three generations. A family history of cardiac disorder, for example, can play a twofold role: (1) genetically by increasing the risk for cardiac illness that may have triggered current symptoms, and (2) psychologically by raising the fear of the patient for any heart irregularities, even those due to exertion or anxiety.

Table 26.2 lists medical illnesses that cause symptoms similar to anxiety. Careful screening for these conditions will accomplish three interrelated ends: to identify (and manage) any medical conditions contributing to anxiety symptoms, to medically reassure the patient in any unfounded fears of illness, and to reinforce the patient's acceptance of the anxiety diagnosis by emphasizing the physiological link between anxiety and the patient's current symptoms.

## Psychophysiological Assessment

The Psychophysiological Stress Profile (PSP) is a tool used to identify the profile of an individual's personal stress response (Wickramasekera, 1988) and to demonstrate convincingly for the patient the mind-body linkage. The PSP uses a variety of physiological sensors to monitor the body, first in a baseline condition, second in relaxation, third under stress conditions, and fourth on recovery. Table 26.3 shows a typical PSP format, using mental math to create the first stress trial and a visualization of a stressful situation to create the second stress trial. The third stress trial consists of hyperventilation or any another "challenge" activity that can

**Table 26.3**    Format for Psychophysiological Stress Profile

| Step | Duration (minutes) | Condition |
| --- | --- | --- |
| Baseline | 3 | Accommodation to room conditions |
| Relaxation | 3 | Relaxation without specific instructions |
| Mental math | 2 | Serial 7s, multiplication, division on demand |
| Recovery | 3 | Relaxation |
| Personal stressor | 2 | Visualization of stressful event |
| Recovery | 3 | Relaxation |
| Challenge trials | 1 | Therapist-guided activity to evoke anxiety symptoms |
| Recovery | 1 | Relaxation |
| Debriefing | | Discussion of patterns in psychophysiological stress profile |

trigger anxiety in the patient. For example, a patient with exertion-triggered panic might use a step-exercise machine for the challenge trial, or an individual who panics when light-headed might spin on a stool as a physiological challenge, in each case evoking the typical physiological accompaniments of an actual anxiety attack.

For anxiety, several physiological measures are relevant for the PSP. The electromyograph (EMG) measures muscle tension patterns accompanying fear and worry. The muscles of the upper torso, shoulders and neck, and the face are most likely to show the effects of anxiety. The skin conductance meter shows an immediate electrodermal increase when anxious thoughts occur. Temperature feedback units detect abnormally low skin temperatures, reflecting vasoconstriction as a measure of anxiety, fear, or hypervigilance. The pneumograph measures patterns in respiration, and provides a measure of the rate of breathing and a graphic picture showing how full or limited and how even or uneven each individual breath is. The pneumograph also shows whether the individual is relying on the muscles of the chest or the diaphragm for respiration. The electrocardiogram (EKG) and photoplethysmograph (PPG) measure heart rate and patterns in heart rhythms that frequently are affected by anxiety. When breathing is relaxed, slow, and full and the individual feels peaceful in both thoughts and feelings, then the respiratory and cardiovascular systems enter into a balance called the respiratory sinus arrhythmia (RSA), involving a parallel sinusoidal rise and fall in breathing and heart rate (Porges, 1986; Porges & Byrne, 1992).[1] This synchronous pattern also produces a coherent organization in the heart rhythms, evident in spectral analyses of the frequency distribution of heart rate changes. The patient can observe both the smooth RSA pattern and the heart rate variability patterns in the PSP if he or she can relax adequately either in the relaxation or recovery trials. (See Chapter 8 for a more detailed explanation of biofeedback modalities.)

After the patient has seen hand temperature drop, respiration and heart rates increase, and muscle tension rise each time she or he directs attention to job problems or marital strain, the involvement of psychosocial factors in physical symptoms becomes more plausible. Such a profile also indicates to the patient and the practitioner the physiologic systems most involved in symptom production and most relevant to symptom reduction. Later, relaxation and biofeedback training can focus on relaxing those physiological systems most activated on the PSP.

### Capnometric Assessment

The capnometric assessment is a useful tool, especially in panic disorder, to assess the presence of hyperventilation and the extent to which hypocapnia plays a role in the onset and maintenance of anxiety symptoms. The capnometer is an instrument that measures carbon dioxide in the exhaled breath. This measure is called end-tidal $CO_2$ ($etCO_2$) because it measures the level of carbon dioxide at the "end of the tide" of the respiration cycle. The carbon dioxide level is measured in millimeters of mercury, each unit known as a Torr. A nasal tube is inserted into the subject's nostril and taped into place. The capnometer provides a baseline value in Torrs for $etCO_2$. Normal breathing should maintain a fairly stable $etCO_2$ level at about 40 Torrs. Chronic hyperventilators, in contrast, show chronic unstable and low levels of $etCO_2$, often 33 Torrs or less. They are closer to the threshold of hypocapnia and recover less quickly to normal carbon dioxide levels.

A specialized PSP is conducted in a capnographic assessment, using a hyperventilation challenge as one trial. This assessment can be conducted conjointly with the PSP previously described. It is important to verify that the hyperventilation challenge actually involves hyperventilation. One criterion is to monitor the patient's respiration with both pneumograph and capnometer during the hyperventilation, ensuring that the subject breathes throughout the trial at a rate of at least 20 breaths per minute and that $etCO_2$ drops to a level of 33 Torrs or less.

Conway (1994) suggested the following criteria for hyperventilation syndrome, based on a PSP with capnometer:

1. Resting baseline of $CO_2$ of less than 30 mm Hg.

2. A fall in $CO_2$ of 20 percent or more from baseline level during hyperventilation challenge trials.

3. Failure of recovery to within 80 percent of baseline by three minutes after the cessation of hyperventilation.

### Neurometric Assessment

Neurometric assessment identifies electrocortical activation (brain-wave) patterns that contribute to anxiety and anxious thinking. Neurometric assessment examines the cortical EEG and assesses the amplitudes, relative powers, and frequency distribution of the EEG. Neurometric assessment can be based on EEG recording at a single site (such as the vertex, the site labeled Cz in the International 10-20 System) or at multiple sites. Topographical brain maps (quantitative EEGs, or QEEGs) are based on recordings of EEG at multiple sites (anywhere from 19 to 256 sites), enabling a sophisticated quantitative assessment of brain activation patterns, including the presence of asymmetries between left and right hemispheric activation and coherence and phase relationships among brain regions. (See Chapter 9 for further discussion of QEEG and neurometric assessment.)

### Cognitive Assessment

A number of behavior checklists are helpful in assessing the severity of anxiety symptoms, as well as in identifying specific fears and thoughts active in sustaining the patient's anxiety. The Hamilton Anxiety Scale, the Beck Anxiety Inventory, and the Spielberger State-Trait Anxiety Inventory provide a sampling of symptoms and numerical severity ratings. The Yale-Brown Obsessive-Compulsive Scale is useful in assessment and in sampling specific obsessions and compulsions. The Liebowitz Social Anxiety Scale not only provides a general severity index but also identifies specific social fear areas and related patterns of avoidance.

Careful identification of specific individual cognitive distortions is an important part of the assessment process. The patient is invited to voice specific fears accompanying the anxiety symptoms, to mentally relive that same fear in the interview room, and to report any physiological activation or recurrence of physiological tensions as the fear is experienced. The interviewer identifies typical cognitive schemas that frequently involve such fears. The interviewer need not aggressively confront the fears in the initial interview but should emphasize that similar thoughts and fears often keep individuals anxious and that treatment includes exploring such thoughts further and giving up or modifying many of them.

### Behavioral Assessment

Behavioral assessment focuses on identifying avoidance behaviors, safety (defensive) behaviors, and superstitious or symptomatic behaviors related to specific anxieties. The patient is invited to describe any behaviors or actions accompanying fears. Is the patient avoiding going anywhere that he or she used to go freely? Is the patient engaging in any superstitious behaviors or behaviors that don't make sense but that she or he cannot seem to stop?

In addition, behavioral assessment identifies patterns of stimulus generalization and environmental reinforcement of anxious behavior. The patient is asked whether his or her fears or anxious behaviors seem to be spreading to new situations and places. Does she or he feel any control over this spreading of symptoms? Does the patient think she or he can reverse the spread and resume entering situations recently avoided? What actions by other people might be enabling or encouraging the spread of avoidance behavior? Well-intentioned family members may be doing tasks for the patient, enabling her to become more helplessly trapped in self-isolation and inactivity.

### Conceptualizing the Patient's Anxiety Disorder

The multimodal assessment of anxiety culminates in a formulation that should integrate the several strands of the assessment and lead logically into a strategic treatment plan. For example, one might arrive at the following formulation:

A 31-year old woman presents with a recurrence of an obsessive-compulsive disorder (OCD). The patient's mother and two sisters have experienced similar OCD episodes, and she had a previous episode that focused on fear of germs and contamination. She is now afraid that she might see a sharp object and cut her young child. She becomes terrified of this possibility and begins to panic, with racing heart and hyperventilation. She has begun to avoid her child, avoids being home alone, and seeks family members to do child care. She has no desire to harm the child, only the intrusive obsessional thoughts that somehow she might do this. She has no history of violence, anger outbursts, or impulses toward abuse. Her assessment emphasizes the psychiatric diagnosis and family history of OCD, the cognitive schema that her impulses are out of control and she might do anything, behavior patterns of avoidance, and the physiological processes of hyperventilation and autonomic arousal. The treatment plan emphasizes medication (SSRI), reassurance that the obsessional ideas are symptoms of OCD, training in thought stopping and redirecting of her thoughts, and reassurance that she is a good mother and can resume care of the child. She is encouraged to practice her diaphragmatic breathing and relaxation exercises that she has previously mastered. The patient is also informed of neurofeedback protocols to modify cortical and subcortical patterns relevant to OCD, especially excessive activation in and over the anterior cingulate gyrus. She is a candidate for a QEEG assessment and neurofeedback training. She delays medication, resumes diaphragmatic breathing, and begins to redirect and talk back to her obsessional thoughts. With reassurance and encouragement, her intrusive ideas remit within less than a week after commencing treatment.

## TREATMENT PROTOCOLS

### *Pharmacotherapy*

Primary medical care for anxiety disorders begins most commonly with the selective serotonin reuptake inhibitor (SSRI) category of antidepressants. The SSRIs have a variety of FDA indications for anxiety. Paxil, for example, has indications for major depression, obsessive-compulsive disorder, social phobia, and posttraumatic stress disorder, yet the entire group of SSRIs is widely used for most anxiety disorders. The benzodiazepines are widely used for panic disorder but present difficulties with some medication dependency and complaints of sedation. The benzodiazepines should be used guardedly with anyone with a substance abuse history; fixed schedule regimens are helpful in reducing benzodiazepine abuse and dependency. Many primary care practitioners favor short-term (four- to six-week) use of a benzodiazepine to provide immediate relief from anxiety, in combination with long-term use of an SSRI. Buspirone (BuSpar) is an effective medication for many patients with generalized anxiety disorder, as is venlafaxine (Effexor). Obsessive-compulsive disorder is most responsive to the SSRIs and frequently requires significantly higher dosing.

Pharmacotherapy for posttraumatic stress disorders is often challenging. Patients with the disorder present a combination of anxiety and depressive symptoms, ongoing tension and vigilance, mood lability, and the characteristic reliving of traumatic experiences. Antidepressants and benzodiazepines can be helpful with the anxiety and depression, and mood stabilizers (e.g., lithium carbonate) and antiseizure medications can reduce mood lability and vigilance.

Patients not responsive to these medications may require a combination of benzodiazepines, two or more antidepressant medications, mood levelers, and neuroleptics. Psychiatric referral for evaluation and medication management should be considered whenever the patient is not responsive to first-line medications and wherever polypharmacy appears necessary.

### *Cognitive-Behavioral Therapies*

Today's treatment of anxiety disorders relies heavily on cognitive-behavioral interventions. Many patients benefit simply from a general orientation to the role of their thoughts and expectations in triggering anxiety. Aaron Beck (Beck & Emery, 1985) has identified a number of common cognitive distortions relevant to anxiety disorders. David Barlow (1994) has further identified critical cognitive and behavioral interventions useful in reducing anxiety. In addition, self-help books are widely available and can guide patients in mastering their own anxiety (Barlow & Craske, 1989; Burns, 1999; Craske, Barlow, & O'Leary, 1992; Ellis, 1998; Ellis & Harper, 1975; Weeks, 1978).

The therapist uses assessment to guide strategic, targeted cognitive-behavioral interventions with the following goals:

1. Modify cognitive schemas that elicit anxiety.

2. Modify specific thoughts and attributions that trigger anxiety.

3. Disrupt safety behaviors, including avoidance patterns, that preserve the cognitive distortions.

4. Teach adaptive coping skills.

5. Assist the individual to confront and master anxious situations.

Chapter 12 provides greater detail on the process and technique of cognitive-behavioral therapy.

## Relaxation Training and General Biofeedback

Relaxation training is useful in overcoming anxiety, tensions, and worry (Amar, 1995). Chapter 10 provides an introduction to progressive muscle relaxation, autogenic training, and clinically standardized meditation. Thermal biofeedback helps the patient learn general autonomic relaxation. EMG (muscle) biofeedback guides the individual to relax the expressive muscles of the face and upper torso. Anxiety, worry, and frustration typically produce tense muscles around the eyes and in the jaw, neck, shoulders, and arms. Skin conductance (electrodermal) biofeedback is useful in training the individual to decrease worrisome thinking and to quiet anxious thoughts.

## Respiratory and Heart Rate Variability Biofeedback

Breath retraining, respiratory biofeedback, and heart rate variability (HRV) biofeedback are useful tools in reducing anxiety disorders, especially panic disorder, and producing subjective calming (Berger & Gevirtz, 2001; Clark & Hirschman, 1990; von Scheele, 1998). Paced diaphragmatic breathing restores synchrony between the respiratory and cardiovascular systems (Gevirtz, 1999). Paced breathing produces RSA, in which low-frequency rhythms prevail in heart function at a frequency of about 0.1 Hz, or 6 cycles per minute. The heart rate gently increases with each in-breath and decreases with each out-breath at a rate of about 6 cycles of breathing and heart rate changes per minute. This RSA pattern produces greater homeostasis in the autonomic nervous system, reducing anxiety symptoms (Porges, 1995; Tiller, McCraty, & Atkinson, 1996). New software has been introduced to enable direct biofeedback training of heart rate variability, providing an additional tool to address the respiratory and cardiac

dysfunction accompanying anxiety states (McCraty & Singer, in press). Many patients report spontaneous reductions in their anxiety symptoms in everyday life once they have begun respiratory and HRV biofeedback. Others report that they are able to use their new breathing patterns when anxiety hits and quickly manage anxiety.

## Neurofeedback

A number of case studies and small research investigations have applied neurofeedback to generalized anxiety disorder, phobic disorders, obsessive-compulsive disorder, and posttraumatic stress disorder (Moore, 2000). The neurometric (QEEG) assessment identifies abnormal cortical activation patterns, and neurofeedback guides the patient to correct abnormal activation patterns. Typical cortical patterns in anxiety disorders include the following:

1. Excessive fast-wave activity that is high in the beta frequency range (24 to 32 Hz), often in combination with deficient amounts of slow-wave activation. This pattern calls for neurofeedback training to increase slow-wave (alpha) activity and suppress fast-wave activity.

2. Excessive slow-wave activity that is often in combination with deficient fast-wave activity. This pattern calls for a suppression of slow-wave activity and training to enhance fast-wave activity (Sattlberger & Thomas, 2000; Thomas & Sattlberger, 1997).

3. Excessive activity along the midline in central and frontal areas, reflecting probable subcortical overactivation in the anterior cingulate gyrus, driving obsessional thinking. This pattern calls for neurofeedback training to suppress the "hot spot" along the midline.

In each case, normalization of cortical activation patterns, as well as the implied normalization of subcortical processes,

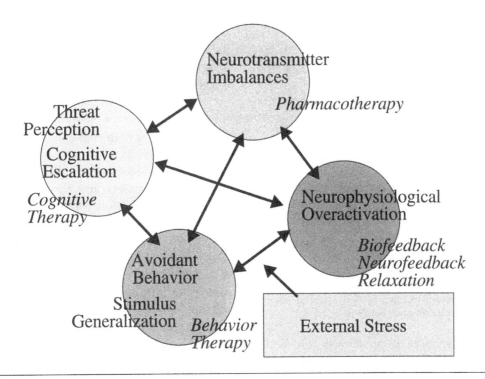

**Figure 26.2**   Comprehensive Treatment Model

serves to reduce anxiety, nervousness, and agitation and to enhance subjective feelings of relaxation and calming.

### Summary: Integrating Treatments

The various available medical and mind-body therapies for anxiety have been discussed separately, as though each were an entirely distinct path for treatment. However, both research and clinical experience show that therapies can have an interactive and synergistic effect (see Figure 26.2). For example, the combination of medication and cognitive-behavioral therapy produces faster recovery than therapy alone and lower relapse rates than medication alone (Gorman, 1997). Relaxation therapy, biofeedback, and neurofeedback can also facilitate the success of cognitive-behavioral therapy. For example, learning to reliably create a physiologically relaxed state makes it easier for patients to undertake exposure

therapy, which requires patients to enter anxiety-producing situations. On the other hand, research also shows that mind-body therapies can produce relatively positive results in isolation. For example, Berger and Gevirtz (2001) reported that breathing retraining alone produced as much improvement as cognitive-behavioral therapy alone.

### CONCLUSION: SELECTION OF CONVENTIONAL AND ALTERNATIVE TREATMENTS

The most critical task of the primary care provider is to *identify* anxiety disorders and distinguish them from their frequently somatic presentation. Next, the health care provider must *educate* the patient that anxiety disorders are troubling but common and manageable disorders. Patient education is critical in dispelling patient shame and denial, and in countering the common disposition to suspect organic medical illnesses, caused by the physiological symptoms of anxiety. Education serves to reassure the patient and, in milder cases of anxiety disorders, is frequently enough to elicit patient self-regulation and recovery. An example follows:

> You are showing today the typical symptoms of an anxiety disorder. Anxiety disorders are real medical disorders, with both biological and behavioral causes. Many people suffer similar anxiety; you are not alone. Help is available, and most patients with anxiety recover completely. I can teach you a few simple skills that will help you to cope with your anxiety. Medication can also help many patients. If skills and pills are not enough, I can arrange for an effective therapist to work with you and help you overcome your anxiety.

If reassurance is not enough, the health care provider can provide the patient with simple *anxiety management skills*, using printed brochures and audiotapes to teach relaxation skills, reassuring self-talk, and simple cognitive coping skills. At the same time, the patient should be encouraged to make changes in everyday life and to eliminate or reduce any stress load that is triggering or exacerbating anxiety symptoms. Stress management classes and individual sessions with nurse practitioners and health educators can assist stress management and provide self-regulation skills in a cost-efficient manner.

Medication can also reduce the frequency and intensity of anxiety symptoms. Patients should be reminded that appropriate medications work best in combination with increased use of self-regulation skills and lifestyle changes. Finally, when low-level interventions fail to reduce anxiety or when the patient's symptoms disrupt everyday life to a disabling degree, a referral to a specialist in cognitive behavioral and mind-body therapies is appropriate.

As depicted in Figures 26.1 and 26.2, both the anxiety disorders and their treatment form a complex structure with discrete neurobiological, neurophysiological, cognitive, behavioral, and environmental dimensions. The behavioral specialist should begin the treatment process with a thorough diagnostic assessment identifying *DSM-IV* diagnosis, relevant physiological activation patterns, the presence of dysfunctional breathing, abnormal neurocortical activation patterns, cognitive distortions serving to sustain anxiety, behavioral avoidance patterns, and any current environmental stressors. Assessment guides the selection of the mind-body therapies most likely to provide patient relief, with an initial focus on one or two sets of objectives. Patients with major stressors should be assisted in problem solving to eliminate or reduce the impact of the stressors. Patients with dysfunctional breathing patterns should undergo breath retraining. Patients with clear cognitive distortions will benefit from cognitive therapy. The availability of skilled effective behavioral or mind-body practitioners will also influence the choice of treatment interventions.

---

## NOTE

1. Physiologically, the paced diaphragmatic breathing induces a summated or composite frequency made up of both RSA and low-frequency baroreceptor activity, which some investigators are calling a resonant frequency (Gevirtz, 1999).

# REFERENCES

Abelson, J. L., Weg, J. G., Nesse, R. M., & Curtis, G. C. (2001). Persistent respiratory irregularity in patients with panic disorder. *Biological Psychiatry, 49*(7), 588–595.

Amar, P. B. (1995). Generalized anxiety disorder. In P. B. Amar & C. Schneider (Eds.), *Clinical applications of biofeedback and applied psychophysiology* (pp. 1–3). Wheat Ridge, CO: Association for Applied Psychophysiology and Biofeedback.

American Psychiatric Association. (1994). *The diagnostic and statistical manual of mental disorders,* (4th ed., *DSM-IV*). Washington, DC: Author.

Antai-Otong, D. (2000). The neurobiology of anxiety disorders: Implications for psychiatric nursing practice. *Issues in Mental Health Nursing, 21*(1), 71–89.

Barlow, D. H. (Ed.). (1994). *Clinical handbook of psychological disorders: A step-by-step treatment manual.* New York: Guilford.

Barlow, D. H., & Craske, M. G. (1989). *Mastery of your anxiety and panic.* Albany, NY: Graywind.

Beck, A. T., & Emery, G. (1985). *Anxiety disorders and phobias.* New York: Basic Books.

Berger, B. C., & Gevirtz, R. (2001). The treatment of panic disorder: A comparison between breathing retraining and cognitive behavioral therapy [Abstract]. *Applied Psychophysiology and Biofeedback, 26*(3), 227–228.

Bernstein, J. G. (1995). *Handbook of drug therapy in psychiatry.* St. Louis, MO: Mosby.

Bowen, R. C., Senthilselvan, A., & Barale, A. (2000). Physical illness as an outcome of chronic anxiety disorders. *Canadian Journal of Psychiatry, 45*(5), 459–464.

Burns, D. D. (1999). *The feeling good handbook.* New York: Plume.

Clark, D. M. (1986). A cognitive approach to panic. *Behaviour Research and Therapy, 24,* 461–470.

Clark, M. E., & Hirschman, R. (1990). Effects of paced respiration on anxiety reduction in a clinical population. *Biofeedback & Self-Regulation, 15*(3), 273–284.

Conway, A. (1994). Breathing and feeling: Capnography and the individually meaningful stressor. *Biofeedback & Self-Regulation, 19*(2), 135–139.

Craske, M. G., Barlow, D. H., & O'Leary, T. A. (1992). *Master of your anxiety and worry.* Albany, NY: Graywind.

Cummings, N. A., Cummings, J. L., & Johnson, J. N. (1997). *Behavioral health in primary care.* Madison, CT: Psychosocial Press.

Ellis, A. (1998). *How to control your anxiety before it controls you.* Secaucus, NJ: Carol Publishing Group.

Ellis, A., & Harper, R. A. (1975). *A new guide to rational living.* Englewood Cliffs, NJ: Prentice Hall.

Fried, R. (1990). *The breath connection.* New York: Plenum.

Fried, R. (1993). *The psychology and physiology of breathing in behavioral medicine, clinical psychology and psychiatry.* New York: Plenum.

Gevirtz, R. (1999). Resonant frequency training to restore autonomic homeostasis for treatment of psychophysiological disorders. *Biofeedback, 27*(4), 7–9.

Gold, M. S. (1989). *The good news about panic, anxiety, and phobias.* New York: Villard Books.

Gorman, J. M. (1997). The use of newer antidepressants for panic disorder. *Journal of Clinical Psychiatry, 58*(Suppl. 14), 54–58.

Gorman, J. M., Askanazi, J., Liebowitz, M. R., Fyer, A., Stein, J., Kinney, J., & Klein, D. F. (1984). Response to hyperventilation in a group of patients with panic disorder. *American Journal of Psychiatry, 14*(7), 857–861.

Jonas, B. S., Wagener, D. K., Lando, J. F., & Feldman, J. J. (1999). Symptoms of anxiety and depression as risk factors for development of asthma. *Journal of Applied Biobehavioral Research, 4*(2), 91–110.

Kessler, R. C., McGonagle, K. A., Zhao, S., Nelson, C. B., Hughes, M., Eshelman, S., et al. (1994). Lifetime and 12 month prevalence of DSM-III-R psychiatric disorders in the United States. *Archives of General Psychiatry, 51*(1), 8–19.

LeDoux, J. (1996). *The emotional brain: The mysterious underpinnings of emotional life*. New York: Simon & Schuster.

McCraty, R., & Singer, D. (in press). Heart rate variability: A measure of autonomic balance and physiological coherence. In A. Watkins & D. Childre (Eds.), *HeartMath: The science of emotional sovereignty*. Amsterdam: Harwood Academic Publishers.

Moore, N. C. (2000). A review of EEG biofeedback treatment of anxiety disorders. *Clinical Electroencephalography, 31*(1), 1–6.

Moss, D. (2001). Biofeedback. In S. Shannon (Ed.), *Handbook of complementary and alternative therapiesin mental health* (pp. 135–158). San Diego, CA: Academic Press.

Moss, D. (2002). Psychological perspectives: Anxiety disorders: Identification and intervention. In B. Horowitz (Ed.), *Communication apprehension: Origins and management* (pp. 74–113). San Diego, CA: Singular/Thomson Learning.

Nardi, A. E., Valenca, A. M., Nascimento, I., Mezzasalma, M. A., & Zin, W. A. (2001). Hyperventilation in panic disorder and social phobia. *Psychopathology, 34*(3), 123–127.

Narrow, W. E., Regier, D. A., Rae, D. S., Manderscheid, R., & Locke, B. Z. (1993). Use of services by persons with mental and addictive disorders: Findings from the National Institute of Mental Health Epidemiological Catchment Area Program. *Archives of General Psychiatry, 50*(2), 95–107.

Nixon, P. G. F. (1994). Effort syndrome: Hyperventilation and reduction of anaerobic threshold. *Biofeedback & Self-Regulation, 19*(2), 155–169.

Nutt, D. J., & Malizia, A. L. (2001). New insights into the role of the GABA-A-benzodiazepine receptor in psychiatric disorder. *British Journal of Psychiatry, 179*, 390–396.

Papp, L. A., Klein, D. F., & Gorman, J. M. (1993). Carbon dioxide hypersensitivity, hyperventilation, and panic disorder. *American Journal of Psychiatry, 150*(8), 1149–1157.

Porges, S. W. (1986). Respiratory sinus arrhythmia: Physiological basis, quantitative methods, and clinical implications. In P. Grossman, K. H. L. Janssen, & D. Vaitl (Eds.), *Cardiorespiratory and cardiosomatic psychophysiology* (pp. 101–115). New York: Plenum.

Porges, S. W. (1995). Orienting in a defensive world: Mammalian modifications of our evolutionary heritage. A polyvagal theory. *Psychophysiology, 32*(4), 301–318.

Porges, S. W., & Byrne, E. A. (1992). Research methods for measurement of heart rate and respiration. *Biological Psychology, 34*(2–3), 93–130.

Rachman, S. J. (1982). Fear and courage: Some military aspects. *Journal of the Royal Army Medical Corps, 128*(2), 100–104.

Rachman, S. J. (1996). Trends in cognitive and behavioural therapies. In P. M. Salkovskis (Ed.), *Trends in cognitive and behavioural therapies* (pp. 1–24). New York: Wiley.

Rachman, S. J. (1999, April). Fear and courage. A keynote address to the annual meeting of the Association for Applied Psychophysiology and Biofeedback, Vancouver, British Columbia.

Regier, D. A., Narrow, W. E., & Rae, D. S. (1990). The epidemiology of anxiety disorders. The epidemiological catchment area (ECA) experience. *Journal of Psychiatric Research, 24(2)*, 9–14.

Regier, D. A., Rae, D. S., Narrow, W. E., Kaelber, C. T., & Schatzberg, A. F. (1998). Prevalence of anxiety disorders and their comorbidity with mood and addictive disorders. *British Journal of Psychiatry, 173*(Suppl 34) 24–28.

Roth, W. T., Wilhelm, F. H., & Trabert, W. (1998). Voluntary breath holding in panic and generalized anxiety disorders. *Psychosomatic Medicine, 60(6)*, 1–9.

Salkovskis, P. M. (1996). *Trends in cognitive and behavioural therapies.* New York: Wiley.

Sattlberger, M.A., &. Thomas, J. E. (2000). Treatment of anxiety disorder with slow-wave suppression EEG feedback: A case study. *Biofeedback, 28(4)*, 17–19.

Schore, A. N. (1994). *Affect regulation and the origins of the self: The neurobiology of emotional development.* Hillsdale, NJ: Lawrence Erlbaum.

Thomas, J. E., & Sattlberger, E. (1997, Spring/Summer). Treatment of chronic anxiety disorders with neurotherapy. *Journal of Neurotherapy*, 14–19.

Tiller, W., McCraty, R., & Atkinson, M. (1996). Cardiac coherence: A new, non-invasive measure of autonomic nervous system order. *Alternative Therapies in Health and Medicine, 2(1)*, 52–65.

Timmons, B., & Ley, R. (1994). *Behavioral and psychological approaches to breathing disorders.* New York: Plenum.

Vila, G., Nollet-Clemencon, C., Vera, M., Robert, J. J., de Blic, J., Jouvent, R., et al. (1999). Prevalence of DSM-IV disorders in children and adolescents with asthma versus diabetes. *Canadian Journal of Psychiatry, 44(6)*, 562–569.

von Scheele, B. H. C. (1998). Respiratory sinus arrhythmia (RSA) and exhalation carbon dioxide (etCO$_2$) as pedagogical and biofeedback tools for treatment of anxiety disorders: Case reports. *Biofeedback & Self-Regulation, 23(2)*, 137.

von Scheele, B. H. C., & von Scheele, I. A. M. (1999). The measurement of respiratory and metabolic parameters of patients and controls before and after incremental exercise on bicycle: Supporting the effort syndrome hypothesis? *Applied Psychophysiology and Biofeedback, 24(3)*, 167–177.

Weeks, C. (1978). *Peace from nervous suffering.* New York: Bantam Books.

Wells, A. (1997). Cognitive therapy of anxiety disorders: A practice manual and conceptual guide. New York: Wiley.

Wickramasekera, I. (1988). *Clinical behavioral medicine: Some concepts and procedures.* New York: Plenum.

Wilhelm, F. H., Gerlach, A. L., & Roth, W. T (2001). Slow recovery from voluntary hyperventilation in panic disorder. *Psychosomatic Medicine, 63(4)*, 638–649.

Wilhelm, F. H., & Roth, W. T. (1998a). Taking the laboratory to the skies: Ambulatory assessment of self-report, autonomic and respiratory responses in flying phobia. *Psychophysiology, 35(5)*, 596–606.

Wilhelm, F. H., & Roth, W. T. (1998b). Using minute ventilation for ambulatory estimation of additional heart rate. *Biological Psychology, 49(1–2)*, 137–150.

Xiangcai, X. (2000). *Qigong for treating common ailments: The essential guide to self-healing.* Boston: YMAA Publication Center.

# CHAPTER 27

# Mood Disorders

Elsa Baehr and J. Peter Rosenfeld

**Abstract:** This chapter begins with a description of the types of mood disorders. The etiology of depression is presented in terms of psychosocial, genetic, and biological factors. A separate section reviews the neurobiology of depression, covering both neuroanatomical and neurophysiological factors. The epidemiology of the disorder is presented with a discussion of demographic factors. Diagnosis of depressive disorders, relying on clinical interview methods and standardized tests or inventories, is introduced. An overview of the standard treatments for depression covers pharmacotherapies as well as psychotherapies. Outcome study results are summarized for these treatments. Finally, the authors discuss recently studied, novel methods of treating depression, including biofeedback and light therapy.

## PROFILE OF THE DISORDER

### Depression Defined

In the past 20 years, there has been a shift in the way depressive disorders have been conceptualized, with less emphasis on specific etiologies and more on objective criteria. The first edition of the *Diagnostic and Statistical Manual of Mental Disorders (DSM-I)* published in 1952 was written as a manual for clinical use and contained descriptions of diagnostic categories. Many of the descriptions in that edition reflected a Freudian influence; for instance, depression was identified as a neurosis or depressive reaction to loss or internal conflict. Use of the term *reaction* in the descriptions of many mental disorders reflected the influence of Adolph Meyer, who viewed mental disorders as reactions to social, psychological, and biological conditions. This term was dropped in the second edition, *DSM-II.* Although the first and second editions contained short descriptions of each disorder, they did not present specific criteria for each type of depressive disorder. The need for more specific definitions was met in the 1974 publication of *DSM-III,* which included lists of symptoms defining each disorder. In a more recent edition of the manual, *DSM-IV* (American Psychiatric Association, 1994), and the subsequent revision, *DSM-IV-TR* (American Psychiatric Association, 2000), a dimensional model quantifies attributes assigned to each diagnostic category. In addition, specific syndromes define a boundary between normality and pathology. A multiaxial system was developed to take into account the degree of distress, the extent of disability, and the risk of experiencing loss of freedom, death, or pain. Other specifiers describe the course of recurrent mood disorders, such as seasonal affective disorders. The paradigm shift for depression occurred when criteria were defined more specifically in *DSM-III* and later refined in *DSM–IV.* The general category of mood disorders replaces depressive disorders, and the term *neurotic depression,* found in *DSM-III,* was replaced by *dysthymia* in *DSM-IV.* Roth and Montjoy (1997) argued for the continued inclusion of *neurotic depression* because the etiology and the treatment of this disorder differ from those of the chronic dysthymic disorders. Other clinicians have criticized the phenomenological approach for its emphasis on artificial distinctions and its failure to recognize the common elements in various depressive disorders (O'Connor, 1997). Nonetheless, the *DSM-IV* is currently the accepted diagnostic manual for clinicians and researchers.

## Etiology of Mood Disorders

There is no single factor underlying mood disorders. Most researchers agree that it is difficult to attribute mood disorders to any single cause and that a combination of biological, genetic, and/or psychosocial factors probably interact with each other and create pathological depressive states. The biological theories involve the thyroid and adrenal neuroendocrine axes, and the activities of noradrenergic and serotonergic biogenic amine systems. Hormonal disturbances have been observed in major depressive disorders, including low levels of melatonin (Levitt, Brown, Kennedy, & Stern, 1991; Rao, Mueller-Oberlinghausen, Mackert, & Strebel, 1992), elevated glucocorticoid secretions, and blunted growth hormone and thyroid stimulating hormone (American Psychiatric Association, 2000). Functional brain imaging studies have shown changes in cerebral blood flow and metabolism and changes in brain structure, including periventricular vascular change, when depression occurs later in life. These changes are not characteristic of or present in all major depressive disorders (American Psychiatric Association, 2000; Kaplan & Sadock, 1998).

There is agreement among researchers that mood disorders are associated with the dysregulation of biogenic amines, particularly norepinephrine and serotonin. Dysregulation of the dopamine, acetylcholine, and gamma-aminobutyric acid systems has also been found in mood disorders. Serotonin has been widely recognized to be involved in the pathophysiology of depression. Low levels of serotonin may precipitate depression and, in some cases, suicide. Many of the newer antidepressants are configured to help maintain the level of serotonin at the neuronal synaptic connection (Kaplan & Sadock, 1998).

Genetic studies have shown a strong relationship between the likelihood of unipolar and bipolar depression and a history of depression in the family (Roth & Montjoy, 1997). A first-degree relative of a patient diagnosed with bipolar disorder I or a major depressive disorder is 8 to 18 times more likely to have a mood disorder than is the general population. Monozygotic twins are 33 percent to 90 percent more likely to become depressed than the general population (Kaplan & Sadock, 1998). In a number of EEG studies, infants and young children were found to have asymmetric hemispheric brain activation patterns similar to those found in their depressed mothers, adding further support to genetic theories (Dawson, Klinger, Panagiotides, Hill, & Spieker, 1992; Field, Fox, Pickens, & Nawrocki, 1995; Jones, Field, Fox, Lundy, & Devalos, 1997).

Psychosocial factors include losses, family atmosphere, guilt, punitive cognitive styles, and interactions within a family when one family member is depressed (Arieti & Bemporad, 1978).

---

**Box 27.1** Some Major Subtypes of *DSM-IV* Mood Disorders

*Major depressive disorder*: Characterized by one or more major depressive episodes (at least two weeks of depressed mood or loss of pleasure or interest, plus four or more other symptoms of depression).

*Dysthymic disorder*: Characterized by depressed mood for a minimum of two years, plus at least four or more symptoms of depression.

*Bipolar disorder I*: Characterized by one or more manic or mixed episodes. A major depression usually accompanies bipolar disorder I.

*Bipolar disorder II*: Characterized by at least one hypomanic episode and one or more major depressive episodes.

*Cyclothymic disorder*: Characterized by at least one hypomanic episode and one or more major depressive episodes.

*Depressive disorder not otherwise specified*: Characterized by depressive features that do not meet the criteria for the preceding disorders, or an adjustment disorder with depression and/or depression and anxiety. Minor depressive disorder, recurrent brief disorder, and premenstrual dysphoric disorder are examples of depressive disorders included in this category.

*Mood disorder due to a general medical condition*: Characterized by a disturbance in mood caused by the effects of a general medical condition.

*Substance-induced mood disorder*: Characterized by mood disturbance caused by abuse of a drug, a medication, exposure to a toxin, or another somatic treatment for depression.

---

SOURCE: American Psychiatric Association (1994).

---

## DEPRESSION SCREENING AND DIAGNOSTIC EVALUATION

In the most recent edition of the best-known textbook designed for educating mental health practitioners, Kaplan and Sadock (1998) bring new concepts into focus when they describe mood as an affective expression that may be normal, depressed, or elevated. Normal people experience a wide range of moods; the difference between their affective states and those who suffer clinical depression and/or mania is the sense of ability to control affect. Using this model as the basis of screening for depression, Kaplan and Sadock explain that in mood disorders, the sense of control is lost, and the patient experiences a great deal of distress. Patients in a manic

(pathologically elevated) mood experience symptoms such as a flight of ideas, decreased need for sleep, heightened self-esteem, and grandiosity. Symptoms of a depressed mood include loss of energy, loss of appetite, poor self-esteem, feelings of guilt, sleep disturbances, inability to concentrate, and thoughts of death and/or suicide. Both types of mood disorders are characterized by impaired interpersonal, social, and occupational functioning. Mood disorders are considered forms of mental illness and are classified according to presenting symptoms in the *DSM-IV* (American Psychiatric Association, 1994). The three major categories are major depressive disorder, dysthymic disorder, and bipolar disorder. The major *DSM-IV* categories of mood disorders are shown in Box 27.1.

---

**Box 27.2**     Criteria for Major Depressive Disorder

Five or more of the following symptoms must be present during the same two-week period, and at least one is either depressed mood or loss of interest:

1. Depressed mood most of the day.
2. Diminished interest in daily activity.
3. Significant weight loss or change in eating habits.
4. Excessive sleepiness or insomnia.
5. Loss of energy or fatigue.
6. Daily feelings of worthlessness or inappropriate guilt.
7. Difficulty concentrating and thinking.
8. Psychomotor retardation/agitation.
9. Suicidal ideation.

SOURCE: American Psychiatric Association (1994).

---

**Box 27.3**     Criteria for Dysthymic Disorder

Depressed mood for most of the day, more days than not, for at least two years, and at least two of the following symptoms:

1. Change in eating pattern.
2. Insomnia.
3. Fatigue or lack of energy.
4. Low self-esteem.
5. Difficulty concentrating and in making decisions.
6. Feelings of hopelessness.

SOURCE: American Psychiatric Association (1994).

---

Patients who experience depression exclusively are identified as having a unipolar or major depressive disorder or a chronic dysthymic disorder, while those who experience manic and depressive episodes are identified as having a bipolar disorder I. Those who meet the criteria for major depressive disorder and also show hypomania are diagnosed as having a bipolar disorder II.

The *DSM-IV* criteria listed in Boxes 27.2, 27.3, and 27.4 may be used as the basis for identifying specific types of depression (American Psychiatric Association, 1994). The secondary symptoms of dysthymic disorder are similar to those of the major depressive disorder, except that psychomotor agitation/retardation and suicidal ideation are not listed, while low self-esteem is included. Dysthymic disorder is diagnosed when, during a two-year period (one year for children and adolescents), the individual has not been without the symptoms listed in

**Box 27.4**    Criteria for Bipolar Disorders

Bipolar disorders include episodes of major depressive disorders interspersed with periods of mania or hypomania

Manic Episode

A. A period of one week or more of abnormal elevated or irritated mood.

B. Three or more of the following symptoms in the same time frame:
   1. Decrease in need for sleep.
   2. More talkative than usual.
   3. Flight of ideas.
   4. Distractibility.
   5. Increased goal-directed activities or psychomotor activity.
   6. Excessive involvement in pleasurable activities, such as buying sprees.
   7. Increased sexual energy.
   8. Inflated self-esteem or grandiosity.

C. Mania may occur with or without psychotic symptoms.

Hypomanic Episode

A. Elevated or irritable mood for at least four days.

B. Three or more of the following symptoms must be present:
   1. Increased activity or restlessness.
   2. Increased talkativeness and overfamiliarity.
   3. Decreased ability to concentrate.
   4. Decreased need for sleep.
   5. Increased sexual energy.
   6. Reckless or irresponsible behavior, including mild overspending.

SOURCE: Adapted from Kaplan & Sadock (1998).

Box 27.3 for more than two months at a time. Patients are excluded from this category if they have had a major depressive episode during the first two years of the disorder or have been diagnosed as having one of the manic disorders. They are also excluded if the symptoms are the results of drugs, medication, or a general medication condition.

In addition to reviewing the factors just mentioned, the clinician who interviews a depressed person needs to obtain a complete developmental, family, social, and medical history. It is important to document when the mood disorder first occurred and to note the precipitating factors. The clinician doing the mental status examination should note factors such as hygiene and grooming, psychomotor retardation or agitation, the presence or absence of hallucinations and/or delusions, and the quality of speech and thought content. Attention should be paid to the rate of speech and whether the content of speech reflects feelings of hopelessness and guilt or suicidal and/or homicidal thoughts. The symptoms of depression, as listed in Box 27.5, can be divided into emotional, cognitive, and vegetative categories (Frohberg & Herting, 1997).

---

**Box 27.5**     Categories of Depressive Symptoms

1. Emotional: Dysphoria, irritability, withdrawal, lack of pleasure seeking.
2. Cognitive: Self-criticism, feelings of worthlessness or guilt, poor concentration, memory impairment, hallucinations or delusions.
3. Vegetative: Fatigue, decreased energy, sleep disorders, eating disorders, psychomotor retardation or agitation, impaired libido.

---

When the full criteria for a *DSM-IV* category are met, the clinician takes into account the number and intensity of the signs and symptoms and the impact on the social and occupational functioning. The level of impairment is then ranked as mild, moderate, severe, in partial remission, or in full remission (American Psychiatric Association, 1994).

Cassano and Savino (1997) introduced another perspective on depression. They describe mood disorders as being chronic and occurring on a continuum rather than as discrete episodes separated by periods of remission. This conceptualization encompasses the unipolar, bipolar, and subclinical disorders. Mood disorders are seen as enduring illnesses with an endogenous etiology. Chronicity, in this view, does not mean that symptoms are always present but that there is an underlying depressive temperament that could emerge as mild temperamental pathology or as a major depressive illness with manic episodes. This concept is consistent with the aforementioned fact that previously depressed individuals have the electroencephalograph (EEG) brainwave asymmetry trait for depression, whether they are currently depressed or not (Gotlib, Ranganath, & Rosenfeld, 1998; Henriques & Davidson, 1991).

Boxes 27.2 through 27.5 are helpful in screening and diagnosing patients for *DSM-IV* mood disorders. In addition to the clinical criteria previously mentioned, there are several objective rating scales commonly used as part of the assessment process. The Beck Depression Inventory (Beck, Ward, Mendelson, Mock, & Erbaugh, 1961) is a self-rating measure consisting of 21 items, with each item rated 0 to 3. Two measures are designed for therapists to administer during a clinical interview: The Hamilton Depression Scale (Hamilton, 1960) includes up to 24 items, each of which is rated 0 to 4; and the Inventory to Diagnose Depression (Zimmerman & Coryell, 1987) includes 22 questions based on *DSM-IV* criteria, with each item rated 0 to 4.

## EPIDEMIOLOGY

It has been estimated that between 2 percent and 25 percent of the population will have a lifetime predisposition for depression and that many more women than men will experience depression. From 10 percent to 15 percent of women and 5 percent to 12 percent of men will experience major depressive disorders. Women are more vulnerable to depression than are men and experience depressive episodes twice as frequently as their male counterparts (American Psychiatric Association, 2000).

Six percent of the population will experience the more chronic dysthymic disorders; less than 2 percent will experience either bipolar I or II disorder; and 5 percent to 15 percent of the population will experience a combination of bipolar I and II disorders with rapid cycling (Kaplan & Sadock, 1998).

The actual incidence of depression among children is not known; estimates range from a few tenths of a percent to between 15 percent and 20 percent of the adult rate of incidence. Approximately 10 percent of all children will experience some form of depression before age 12 (O'Connor, 1997).

## NEUROBIOLOGY OF DEPRESSION

Recently, excellent reviews of the neuroanatomy and physiology of depression were published by Davidson (2000) and Rolls (1999), the latter of which was recently rendered into a *precis* form that retains the superb "wiring diagram" of the original (Rolls, 2000). Some highlights abstracted from these reviews are presented here.

There is a great deal of data that implicates the prefrontal cortex (PFC) in the elaboration of emotion. In the primate, there are three important subdivisions of the PFC: the dorsolateral PFC, the ventromedial PFC, and orbitofrontal cortex. These cortical structures appear to be involved in a circuit of structures that interchange information as a basis for emotional experience. Other structures in the circuit include the amygdala, the hippocampus, the anterior cingulate, and insular cortices.

The differential involvement of right and left PFCs was first suggested by a series of studies of patients with damage to either the right or left PFC. It was noted that depressive symptoms tended to be associated with destruction of the left PFC rather than the right. Damage to the right PFC was associated with heightened affect. This suggested to Davidson (2000) that there was a positive or approach system in the left PFC (dampened by lesions) but an aversive/negative avoidance system in the right PFC. A series of experiments from Davidson's laboratory was consistent with this view: For example, depressed individuals showed greater activation in the right than in the left recorded anterior frontal EEG electrodes (overlying the PFC) in comparison with normal individuals.

Gotlib et al. (1998) extended this work by showing within one experiment that currently depressed and previously depressed individuals showed increased right-sided frontal activation relative to normal controls. (This result could suggest that EEG asymmetry marks a trait for vulnerability to depression, given the presence of life stressors, even though the person is not currently depressed. On the other hand, it could also suggest that once a depressive incident occurs, the brain is permanently changed to show the depressive asymmetry pattern.) The Davidson (2000) laboratory also evoked positive and negative moods with films; the positive-mood films increased left frontal activation, whereas the negative-mood films increased right-sided activation. These EEG studies were supported by positron emission tomography (PET) studies, which better localize regions of activation: When negative affect was induced, Davidson's group reported right-sided increases of metabolism in the orbitofrontal cortex and in the inferior frontal, middle frontal, and superior frontal gyri. The induction of positive affect, however, was associated with metabolic rate increases in the left pre- and postcentral gyri. Induced anxiety was also reported by the Davidson laboratory to induce right-sided EEG activation at anterior recording sites. There is little doubt regarding the involvement of the PFC in emotion. Further research is necessary, however, to associate specific subregions with particular affective functions.

A mass of evidence has been collected, mostly in rodents, that the amygdala is necessary for learning fear (Davidson, 2000; Fanselow & LeDoux, 1999; LeDoux, 1996). Humans with localized lesions of the amygdala show impairment in the recognition of facial expressions of fear (Adolphs, Damasio, Tranel, & Damasio, 1995, 1996). Bechara et al. (1995) reported impaired aversive conditioning in a human patient with amygdala damage, although the patient could accurately describe the contingencies of training. There are further suggestive findings that the amygdala may be necessary for the *expression* of previously learned fear. Recent studies with PET or functional magnetic resonance imaging show specific activation of the amygdala in humans with anxiety disorders in the presence of their specific anxiety-producing stimuli. Unpleasant pictures activate the amygdala, which is also activated during early aversive conditioning. Pleasant pictures do not have this same effect. A number of recent MRI studies have also reported decreases in hippocampal volume in association with disorders related to stress, including depression (see Davidson, 2000).

## TREATMENT PROTOCOLS FOR MOOD DISORDERS

The treatment of mood disorders is often a combination of medication and some form of psychotherapy. Hospitalization may be required for patients who are a danger to themselves or others, who lack support at home, or who have any complicating medical conditions. When these treatments are not effective, electroconvulsive shock therapy or transcranial magnetic stimulation (Kaplan & Sadock, 1998) may be tried. Artificial bright-light therapy (over 2,500 lux) may alleviate seasonal affective disorder (Kaplan & Sadock, 1998). In addition, a novel method in the treatment of depression, EEG neurofeedback (Baehr, Rosenfeld, & Baehr, 2001; Baehr, Rosenfeld, Baehr, & Earnest, 1999; Rosenfeld, 2000a, 2000b) is showing promise as a way of altering neuronal brainwave patterns associated with depression. These novel approaches are discussed later in the chapter.

## Conventional Therapies for Depression

Three main types of psychotherapy have been successfully used to treat depression: the psychodynamic approach, the cognitive approach, and the interpersonal approach. Karasu (1998) provides an excellent review of the three approaches. Discriminating features of the three are listed in Table 27.1.

The psychodynamic approach strives to heal by helping the patient to understand the past, to release feelings, and to use the transference aspects of the patient-therapist relationship. This point of view is based on concepts such as damaged self-esteem, loss, unresolved childhood conflicts, and anger turned inward. The goals of the cognitive approach are to change distorted thinking, which originated in learned negative views of the self and the world, and to promote self-control over thinking patterns. In most cases, cognitive therapy is combined with behavior therapy (cognitive-behavioral therapy) to induce change in both cognition and behavior. The interpersonal school views the dynamics of depression in relation to impaired interpersonal relationships. Interpersonal therapy aims to reduce stress in family life and at work and to improve communication skills.

Jones and Pulos (1993) compared the processes in psychodynamic and cognitive-behavioral therapy by analyzing verbatim transcripts and found few commonalities and significant differences between the two treatment strategies. Cognitive-behavioral therapy emphasizes intellectual, rational control over thoughts and feelings combined with enthusiastic support from therapists. Dynamic psychotherapy encourages the elicitation of emotions by bringing troublesome thoughts into awareness and relating previous life experiences to present issues. The relationship between the therapist and patient is thought to be a key agent of change in dynamic therapy.

**Table 27.1** Three Major Types of Psychotherapy for Depression: A Comparison of Features

| Approach | Major Theorists | Concept of Etiology | Major Goal |
| --- | --- | --- | --- |
| Psychodynamic | Freud, Abraham, and Kohut | Damaged self-esteem, unresolved conflicts due to disappointment and loss in childhood. | Use an understanding of the past to promote personality change. |
| Cognitive | Beck and Adler | Learned negative views about self, others, and the world result in distorted depressive thinking. | Provide symptom relief by promoting self-control over negative and self-destructive thinking patterns. |
| Interpersonal | Meyer, Sullivan, and Klerman | Impaired interpersonal relations and faulty social bonds. | Promote symptom relief by finding solutions for current interpersonal problems. Emphasis on stress reduction and improved communication skills. |

## Aerobic Exercise and Depression

During aerobic exercises such as running, biochemical changes occur in the body, including increased levels of endorphins and norepinephrine. Endorphins are the body's natural painkillers. Norepinephrine is an important neurotransmitter and is often deficient at the synaptic level in depressive states. A study of more than 100 college students compared those who jogged regularly with those who did not. The study showed that the depressed students who were joggers had more positive responses to an adjective checklist, than depressed students who did not participate in this type of exercise (Padus, 1986).

## Psychopharmacology

The most widely used antidepressant medications are selective serotonin reuptake inhibitors (SSRIs), which inhibit the central nervous system's neuronal uptake of serotonin (see Box 27.6). Atypical antidepressants include two drugs that combine SSRI effects with either norepinephrine reuptake blockade (Effexor) or serotonin receptor antagonism (Serzone). Another atypical antidepressant, Wellbutrin, has a mechanism of action involving inhibition of dopamine reuptake. Remeron is considered an effective alternative for SSRIs when anxiety is combined with depression. All atypical antidepressants are considered safer than the tricyclic and tetracyclic drugs. While there is support for using cyclic antidepressants for melancholic features, they may cause cardiotoxity and lethal overdose (Magellan Behavioral Health, 1999).

The monoamine oxidase inhibitors (MAOIs) are not widely prescribed because their use requires dietary restrictions and they may cause sedation as well as more adverse (including some life-threatening) effects compared with other antidepressants. Stimulants such as dextroamphetamine and methylphenidate may be used in combination with other antidepressants for rapid

---

**Box 27.6**     Antidepressant Medications

### Selective Serotonin Reuptake Inhibitors (SSRIs)

Citalopram (Celexa)
Fluoxetine (Prozac)
Fluvoxamine (Luvox)
Paroxetine (Paxil)
Sertraline (Zoloft)

### Cyclic Antidepressants

Amitriptyline (Elavil)
Clomipramine (Anafranil)
Doxepin (Sinequan)
Imipramine (Tofranil)
Trazodone (Desyrel)

### Atypical Antidepressants

Bupropion (Wellbutrin)
Mirtazapine (Remeron)
Nefazodone (Serzone)
Venlafaxine (Effexor)

### Monoamine Oxidase Inhibitors (MAOIs)

Isocarboxazid (Marplan)
Phenelzine (Nardil)
Tranylcypromine (Parnate)

---

SOURCE: Schatzberg (1997).

---

improvement of mood (Kaplan & Sadock, 1998). Lithium is used to augment MAOIs and cyclic antidepressants.

Alternative nonprescription medications, such as *Hypericum perforatum* (St. John's wort), have been compared to Prozac and have shown similar results with fewer side effects (Cass, 1998). The latest research, however, found some beneficial effects of this herbal medication on depression but casts doubt on its effectiveness for major depressive disorders (Shelton et al., 2001).

### Outcome Studies

Studies comparing the effectiveness of dynamically oriented therapy and cognitive therapy have shown that at the end of treatment, both groups were similar in the amount of improvement. Follow-up study one year posttherapy gave a slight advantage to the cognitive treatments as measured on the Beck Depression Inventory (Barkham, Shapiro, Hardy, & Rees, 1999; Shapiro, Barkham, et al., 1994; Shapiro, Rees, et al.,

1995). Factors such as pretreatment cognitive dysfunction and life stress have been taken into account when evaluating responsiveness to cognitive-behavioral therapy in depression. In a sample of 35 patients, these variables were found to have little effect on the predictability of outcome in therapy (Spangler, Simons, Monroe, & Thase, 1997). Cognitive-behavioral therapy may be successful without the facilitation of a therapist. A study comparing computer-administered cognitive-behavioral therapy for depression with therapist-administrated treatment and a waiting-room control group found that the two experimental groups showed improvement on tests for depression while the waiting-room group did not improve (Selmi, Klein, Greist, Sorrell, & Erdman, 1990). In another study (Burns, 1999), a self-help methodology called bibliotherapy was shown to be an effective way to practice cognitive-behavioral therapy. Scores on tests of depression improved for persons using a book with a specific cognitive approach, while scores of other depressed persons who read a placebo book, or no book at all, did not improve.

Treatment outcomes have been investigated in time-limited studies for both cognitive-behavioral and psychodynamic-interpersonal therapies. Patients were assigned to 8 or 16 weeks of one of the therapy types. There was little difference in the amount of improvement between groups at the end of therapy, except for slightly better scores by the cognitive-behavioral group on the Beck Depression Inventory (Shapiro, Barkham, et al., 1994). The results were different one year posttherapy: For both groups, mean scores on outcome measures were generally maintained, but only 29 percent of the clients were asymptomatic and needed no further therapy. For psychodynamic-interpersonal therapy, 8 sessions were not as effective as 16 sessions, whereas for cognitive-behavioral therapy, there was no measurable benefit of 16 sessions over 8 sessions, regardless of the severity of depression (Shapiro, Rees, et al., 1995).

## Choosing the Right Psychotherapy

Although research has shown that there are several effective ways to treat depression, few guidelines have been established for therapists regarding selecting the most effective treatment strategy for particular patients. As mentioned previously, outcome studies have shown little differences between psychodynamic-interpersonal and cognitive behavioral therapies. Keeping in mind that an alliance with the therapist is an important part of the healing process, the choice of therapist may be just as important as the type of treatment.

Efforts to evaluate factors associated with favorable outcome in psychotherapy have, for the most part, been inconclusive. Some researchers have addressed the issue of when and if medication should be used instead of cognitive-behavioral therapy. Research showed that the outcome was worse for tricyclic antidepressant medication than for either relaxation therapy or cognitive-behavioral therapy (Deckersback, Gershuny, & Otto, 2000; Murphy, Carney, Knesevitch, Wetzel, & Whitworth, 1995). Simons and Thase (1992) looked at biological markers, such as insomnia, and treatment outcome in endogenous depression in 53 patients. In a one-year follow-up study involving 53 patients receiving cognitive-behavioral therapy for depression, they found that they could not use the presence or absence of a sleep disorder to predict the outcome of short- or long-term therapy.

One factor was identified, however, that successfully predicted a favorable outcome for cognitive-behavioral therapy: 31 subjects in an experimental group were tested before receiving 16 weekly sessions of therapy. Researchers Bruder et al. (1997) found that persons who responded to cognitive-behavioral therapy had twice the right-ear (left-hemisphere) advantage for dichotic syllables than did those who did not respond to therapy. Both responders to cognitive-behavioral therapy and nonresponders scored the same on a nonverbal complex tone test. The findings suggest that persons with greater left-hemisphere advantage for verbal processing are more likely to have a favorable outcome of cognitive-behavioral therapy for depression than are persons who lack the left-hemisphere advantage.

## FUTURE DIRECTIONS FOR MIND-BODY TREATMENT OF DEPRESSION

The final section considers two novel treatments for depression—one behavioral and the other physiological.

### Neurofeedback and Asymmetry Training

The first approach is called EEG biofeedback, or neurofeedback. As mentioned earlier, there is a replicable EEG correlate of depression: Depressed individuals show an activation of the right frontal cortex, relative to the left, whereas normals tend to show the reverse asymmetry. Rosenfeld and colleagues (Baehr, Rosenfeld, Baehr, & Earnest, 1999; Rosenfeld, 2000a) developed an EEG training protocol intended to reverse this pathological asymmetry. *Inverse* activation, in the form of alpha (8- to 13-Hz) magnitude was the index used for training, inasmuch as Davidson's (1995) group used the same index in their seminal studies of EEG correlates of depression. Davidson used the inverse measure based on the traditional assumption that a great deal of alpha activity indicates an idling or relatively inactive cortex. Moreover, the use of beta (13- to 30-Hz) activity as a direct activation index would be

confounded by the possible presence of muscle activity (EMG) in this higher frequency range. Thus, relative *left* frontal activation (associated with positive affect) would be indexed by increased relative right frontal alpha magnitude. Depression would be indexed by increased relative left frontal alpha activity. The electrode sites defining left and right were F3 and F4, respectively (based on the International 10-20 System; see Chapter 9). The typical asymmetry score that depressed individuals were trained to increase was defined as $(F4 - F3)/(F4+F3)$, the difference between right and left alpha magnitude, relative to the sum of these scores (which corrects for undesirable, nonspecific, total alpha increases; see Rosenfeld, 2000a). The reference electrode used in these studies was Cz, because that was the reference used in the early Davidson studies (although it is problematic; see Rosenfeld 2000b).

To date, we have trained more than 50 patients presenting with depression to increase the alpha asymmetry score. For the first 5 of these patients, the training increased the asymmetry scores at least fivefold (Baehr, Rosenfeld, Baehr, & Earnest, 1999; Rosenfeld, 2000a). The Beck Depression Inventory scores were reduced by a comparable amount, as were the depression scale scores on the Minnesota Multiphasic Personality Index. The clinical pictures of these cases were all improved. We were able to do a follow-up study one to five years posttreatment on three of these cases (Baehr, Rosenfeld, & Baehr, 2001): EEG as well as clinical and behavioral indices indicated that the improvements were maintained. An independent replication was recently reported by Earnest (1999), in which an adolescent depressive was successfully treated. While these results with this novel, experimental treatment are encouraging, no formal controls have been run as yet, and until this is done, we cannot know whether or not the effects were specific to the neurofeedback protocol.

## *Light Therapy*

Another recently developed and still somewhat experimental therapy for a particular kind of depression is called light therapy. It involves using exposure to bright light to treat the subtype of depression known as seasonal affective disorder (SAD). This disorder is often seen in individuals who are deprived of light during shortened days in northern latitudes. Numerous studies have reported positive outcomes, and recently, Eastman, Young, Fogg, Liu, and Meaden (1998) reported positive effects in a placebo-controlled, double-blind trial of light therapy in 96 patients with SAD. (Other articles in the same journal volume also report effects of the therapy.) There were three groups: A group exposed to light in the morning, a group exposed to light in the evening, and a placebo group that received exposure to what appeared to be a light box but was, in fact, a sham negative-ion generator (externally indistinguishable from a light box). The percentage of patients with near complete remissions (i.e., achieving both a 50 percent decrease from baseline in the 24-item Structured Interview Guide for the Hamilton Depression Rating Scale, SAD version, and a score of 8 or lower on that instrument) were compared after three weeks of treatment.

The morning-light condition produced a higher rate of responders than did evening light, and evening light produced significantly more than did the placebo group. Light therapy produced a significantly higher rate of full remissions than did placebo.

There have been many studies of light therapy for SAD. (See the references in Eastman et al., 1998). One particularly interesting study was that of Allen, Iacono, Depue, and Arbisi (1993), who also reported a positive effect of light therapy (compared with placebo control) on SAD. The distinguishing feature of this study was the tracking of EEG correlates of the depression. The SAD patients showed the pathological activation asymmetry associated with depression as previously discussed. Moreover, consistent with studies previously cited, the pathological asymmetry persisted even as the Hamilton Rating Scale for Depression showed improvement. However, marking the state variable correlate of depression, right-hemisphere EEG coherence changed in SAD subjects, not in control subjects, following light therapy. Audiovisual entrainment, consisting of flashing lights and pulsing tones, was also found to be an effective treatment for seasonal affective disorder (Berg & Seiver, 2000). This is clearly a promising new therapy.

---

## REFERENCES

Adolphs, R., Damasio, H., Tranel, D., & Damasio, A. R. (1995). Fear and the human amygdala. *Journal of Neuroscience, 15,* 5879–5891.

Adolphs, R., Damasio, H., Tranel, D., & Damasio, A. R. (1996). Cortical systems for the recognition of emotion in facial expressions. *Journal of Neuroscience, 16,* 7678–7687.

Allen, J. J., Iacono, W. G., Depue, R., & Arbisi, P. (1993). EEG asymmetries in Seasonal Affective Disorder after exposure to bright light. *Biological Psychiatry, 33,* 642–646.

American Psychiatric Association. (1994). *Diagnostic and statistical manual of mental disorders* (4th ed., DSM-IV). Washington, DC: Author.

American Psychiatric Association. (2000). *Diagnostic and statistical manual of mental disorders* (4th ed., DSM-IV-TM). Washington, DC: Author.

Arieti, S., & Bemporad, J. (1978). *Severe and mild depression*. New York: Basic Books.

Baehr, E., Rosenfeld, J. P., & Baehr, R. (2001). Clinical use of an alpha asymmetry neurofeedback protocol in the treatment of mood disorders: Follow-up study one to five years post therapy. *Journal of Neurotherapy, 4*(4), 11–18.

Baehr, E., Rosenfeld, J. P., Baehr, R., & Earnest, C. (1999). Clinical use of an alpha asymmetry protocol in the treatment of mood disorders. In J. R. Evans & A. Abarbanel (Eds.), *Introduction to quantitative EEG and neurofeedback* (pp. 181–201). New York: Academic Press.

Barkham, M., Shapiro, D. A., Hardy, G. E., & Rees, A. (1999). Psychotherapy in two-plus-one sessions: Outcomes of a randomized controlled trial of cognitive-behavioral and psychodynamic-interpersonal therapy for subsyndromal depression. *Journal of Consulting and Clinical Psychology, 67*(2), 201–211.

Bechara, A., Tranel, D., Damasio, H., Adolphs, R. Rockland, C., & Damasio, A. R. (1995). Double dissociation of conditioning and declarative knowledge relative to the amygdala and hippocampus in humans. *Science, 269,* 1115–1118.

Beck, A., Ward, C., Mendelson, M., Mock, J., & Erbaugh, J. (1961). An inventory for measuring depression. *Archives in General Psychiatry, 4,* 561–571.

Berg, K., and Siever, D. (2000) Audio-visual entrainment as a treatment modality for seasonal affective disorder. In D. Siever, *The rediscovery of audio-visual entrainment technology* (pp. 15.5–16.5). Edmonton, Alberta, Canada: Comptronic Devices Ltd.

Bruder, G. E., Stewart, J. W., Mercier, M. A. S., Agosti, V., Leite, P., Donovan, S., et al. (1997). *Journal of Abnormal Psychology, 106*(1), 138–144

Burns, D. D. (1999). *The feeling good handbook*. New York: Penguin.

Cass, H. (1998). *St. John's wort*. Garden City, NY: Avery Publishing Group.

Cassano, G., & Savino, M. (1997). Chronic and residual major depressions. In H. S. Akiskal & G. Cassano (Eds.), *Dysthymia and the spectrum of chronic depression* (pp. 54–65. New York: Basic Books.

Davidson, R. J., (1995). Cerebral asymmetry, emotional and affective style. In R. J. Davidson & K. Hugdal (Eds.), *Brain asymmetry* (pp. 362–387). Cambridge, MA: MIT Press.

Davidson, R. J. (2000). Affective style, psychopathology, and resilience: Brain mechanisms and plasticity. *American Psychologist, 55,* 1196–1214.

Dawson, G., Klinger, H., Panagiotides, H., Hill, D., & Spieker, S. (1992). Frontal lobe activity and affective behavior of infants of mothers with depressive symptoms. *Child Development, 63,* 725–737.

Deckersback, T., Gershuny, B. S., & Otto, M. W. (2000). Cognitive-behavioral therapy for depression. Applications and outcome. *Psychiatric Clinics of North America, 34*(4), 795–809.

Earnest, C. (1999). Single case study of EEG asymmetry biofeedback for depression: An independent replication in an adolescent. *Journal of Neurotherapy, 3,* 28–35.

Eastman, C. I., Young, M. A., Fogg, L. F., Liu, L., & Meaden, P. M. (1998). Bright light treatment of winter depression: A placebo-controlled trial. *Archives in General Psychiatry, 55*(10), 883–889.

Fanselow, M. S., & LeDoux, J. E. (1999). Why we think plasticity underlying Pavlovian fear conditioning occurs in the basolateral amygdala. *Neuron, 23,* 229–232.

Field, T., Fox, N., Pickens, J., & Nawrocki, T. (1995). Relative right frontal EEG activation in 3- to 6-month-old infants of "depressed" mothers. *Developmental Psychology, 31,* 358–363.

Frohberg, N., & Herting, R. (1997). Psychiatry: Mood disorders. In M. A. Graber, P. P. Toth, & R. L. Herting (Eds.), *University of Iowa family practice handbook* (3rd ed., not paginated). St. Louis, MO: Mosby. Available online from http://www.vh.org/Providers/ClinRef/FPHandbook/FPContents.html

Gotlib, I. H., Ranganath, C., & Rosenfeld, J. P. (1998). Frontal EEG alpha asymmetry, depression, and cognitive functioning. *Cognition and Emotion, 12,* 449–478.

Henriques, J. B. & Davidson, R. J. (1991). Left frontal hypoactivation in depression. *Journal of Abnormal Psychology, 100, 534–545.*

Hamilton, M. (1960). Development of a rating scale for primary depressive illness. *British Journal of Social Clinical Psychology, 6, 178–196.*

Jones, E. E., & Pulos, S. M. (1993). Comparing the process in psychodynamic and cognitive-behavioral therapies. *Journal of Consulting Clinical Psychology, 61*(2), 306–316.

Jones, N., Field, T., Fox, N., Lundy, B., & Devalos, M. (1997). EEG activation in one month old infants of depressed mothers. *Development and Psychopathology, 9*(3), 491–505.

Kaplan, H. I., & Sadock, B. J. (Eds.). (1998). *Synopsis of psychiatry* (8th ed.). Baltimore: Williams & Wilkins.

Karasu, T. B. (1998). Scope of psychoanalytic practice. In H. I. Kaplan & B. J. Sadock (Eds.), *Synopsis of psychiatry* (8th ed., Table 34). Baltimore: Williams & Wilkins.

LeDoux, J. E. (1996). *The emotional brain: The mysterious underpinnings of emotional lift.* New York: Simon & Schuster.

Levitt, A., Brown, G., Kennedy, S., & Stern, K. (1991). Tryptophan treatment and melatonin response in a patient with seasonal affective disorder. *Journal of Clinical Psychopharmacology, 11*(1), 74–75.

Magellan Behavioral Health. (1999). *Clinical practice guideline for major depressive disorder in adults.* Chicago: Author.

Murphy, G. E., Carney, R. M., Knesevich, M. A., Wetzel, R. D., & Whitworth, P. (1995). Cognitive behavior therapy, relaxation training, and tricyclic antidepressant medication in the treatment of depression *Psychological Report, 77*(2), 403–20.

O'Connor, R. (1997). *Undoing depression.* Boston: Little, Brown.

Padus, E. (1986). *Your emotions and your health.* Emmaus, PA: Rodale Press.

Rao, M., Mueller-Oberlinghausen, B., Mackert, A., & Strebel, B. (1992). Blood serotonin, serum melatonin and light therapy in healthy subjects and in patients with nonseasonal depression. *Acta Psychiatrica Scandinavica, 86*(2), 127–132.

Rolls, E. T. (1999). *The brain and emotion.* New York: Oxford University Press.

Rolls, E. T. (2000). Precis of *The brain and emotion. Behavioral and Brain Sciences, 23,* 177–234.

Rosenfeld, J. P. (2000a). An EEG biofeedback protocol for affective disorders. *Clinical Electroencephalography, 31,* 7–12.

Rosenfeld, J. P. (2000b). Theoretical implications of EEG reference choice and related methodology issues. *Journal of Neurotherapy, 4,* 77–87.

Roth, M., & Montjoy, C. Q. (1997). A critical reappraisal of the concept of neurotic depression. In H. S. Akiskal & G. Cassano (Eds.), *Dysthymia and the spectrum of chronic depression* (pp. 96–129). New York: Basic Books.

Selmi, P. M., Klein, M. H., Greist, J. H., Sorrell, S. P., & Erdman, H. P. (1990). Computer-administered cognitive-behavioral therapy for depression. *American Journal of Psychiatry, 147*(1), 51–56.

Shapiro, D. A., Barkham, M., Rees, A., Hardy, G. E., Reynolds, S., & Startup, M. (1994). Effects of treatment duration and severity of depression on the effectiveness of cognitive-behavioral and psychodynamic-interpersonal psychotherapy. *Journal of Consulting and Clinical Psychology, 62*(3), 522–533.

Shapiro, D. A., Rees, A., Barkham, M., Hardy, G., Reynolds, S., & Startup, M. (1995). Effects of treatment duration and severity of depression on the maintenance of gains after cognitive-behavioral and psychodynamic-interpersonal psychotherapy. *Journal of Consulting and Clinical Psychology, 63*(3), 378–387.

Shelton, R. C., Keller, M. B., Gelenberg, A., Dunner, D. L., Hirschfeld, R., Thase, M. E., et al. (2001). Effectiveness of St. John's wort in major depression: A randomized controlled trial. *Journal of the American Medical Association, 285*(15), 1978–1986.

Simons, A. D, & Thase, M. E. (1992). Biological markers, treatment outcome, and 1-year follow-up in endogenous depression: electroencephalographic sleep studies and response to cognitive therapy. *Journal of Consulting Clinical Psychology, 60*(3), 392–401.

Spangler, D. L., Simons, A. D., Monroe, S. M., & Thase, M. E. (1997). Response to cognitive-behavioral therapy in depression: Effects of pretreatment cognitive dysfunction and life stress. *Journal of Consulting Clinical Psychology, 65*(4), 568–575.

Zimmerman, M., & Coryell, W. (1987). The inventory to diagnose depression, Lifetime version. *Acta Psychiatrica Scandinavia, 75,* 495–499.

# CHAPTER 28

# Sleep and Sleep Disorders

Suzanne Woodward

**Abstract:** Sleep disorders are widespread in the general population. This chapter reviews the neurophysiology of sleep, outlines the categories of sleep disorder established by the American Sleep Disorders Association, and summarizes the medical and behavioral treatment interventions effective for each. Women face a greater incidence of sleep disorders. Hormonal variations in the menstrual cycle, pregnancy, and menopause contribute to sleep problems in women; the greater incidence of mood disorders in women is also a factor. Hormone replacement therapy is critical in many sleep disorders of women. The author emphasizes the role of stimulus control therapy, sleep restriction therapy, behavioral sleep hygiene, relaxation skills training, and cognitive behavioral therapy in improving the quality of sleep for men and women.

## INTRODUCTION

The benefits of a good night's sleep are readily apparent. Approximately one third of our lives is spent sleeping. We organize our time for work and play to meet the demands of sleep. It is therefore not surprising that trouble sleeping for a few nights, weeks, months, or years can affect our health, our jobs, and almost every aspect of our lives. It has been estimated that more than 40 million people in the United States suffer from chronic complaints of sleep and wakefulness and that an additional 20 million to 30 million experience intermittent sleep-related problems (National Commission on Sleep Disorders Research, 1993, 1994). Considering these figures, it is amazing how few people actually consult their physicians about problems during sleep, leaving many of these problems undiagnosed and untreated.

## NEUROPHYSIOLOGY OF SLEEP

Sleep research has come a long way since 1935, when specific stages of sleep characterized by distinct electroencephalographic (EEG) patterns were first described (Loomis, Harvey, & Hobart, 1935). There are two distinct kinds of sleep: REM (rapid eye movement) and non-REM sleep. These phases of sleep are as different from each other as they are from waking, and can be measured by polysomnography.

Non-REM sleep has four stages, which together constitute close to 80 percent of a night's sleep.

• Stage 1 is the transition between wakefulness and sleep. A mixed-voltage pattern replaces the rhythmic alpha activity seen when eyes are closed, and people feel drowsy. Reaction to outside stimuli is decreased, and although mentation may occur, it is no longer based in reality. Short dreams may develop, but many people feel that they are still awake during stage 1 sleep.

• Stage 2 sleep is considered to be the first true stage of sleep and consists of a moderately low-voltage background EEG with sleep spindles and K complexes. Heart rate and respiration are slower and more regular than in stage 1, and thoughts are short and fragmented.

• Stages 3 and 4 consist of slow-wave sleep and are distinguished by the presence of slow delta waves. Heart and respiration rates are very slow and regular during these deeper stages of sleep.

About 70 to 100 minutes after sleep onset, the REM sleep period begins. The EEG pattern is similar to that of stage 1 sleep, except sawtooth waves are often seen. Rapid eye movements occur in REM sleep (as the term suggests), muscle activity is inhibited, and temperature regulation is for the most part suspended. Most people report vivid dreaming during REM sleep, and heart and respiration rates are increased and irregular.

REM sleep alternates with non-REM sleep at about 90- to 100-minute intervals in adults. A typical sleep cycle consists of a sequential merging of stages 1 through 4, which then reverses and is followed by the first REM period. A normal sleep pattern consists of three to five such cycles. As the night goes on, the frequency of stages 3 and 4 decreases, and the proportion of REM sleep tends to increase.

## THE IMPACT OF SLEEP DEPRIVATION

The amount of sleep needed to feel alert and refreshed varies from person to person, but research indicates that most people do not get enough sleep. Once a person reaches early adulthood, the sleep pattern stabilizes at about the eight hours considered normal. However, a survey by the National Sleep Foundation (1999) found that most Americans sleep less than seven hours during the week and that one in five American adults feel that to be successful in their careers, they must sacrifice sufficient sleep. The ability to maintain attention and react quickly is dependent on sufficient sleep. Driver drowsiness and fatigue are thought to be responsible for at least 100,000 automobile crashes every year (Institute for Traffic Safety Management and Research, 1996). Chronic sleep deprivation can also affect mood. Changes in mood are some of the noted indicators of sleep loss. It is possible to pay back this sleep debt, but this may take several nights of extended sleep. According to the *Wall Street Journal,* sleep disorder symptoms have actually worsened recently, and the pursuit of sleep through medical and alternative technologies has become a national priority, spawning a $14 billion a year business ("I Can't Sleep," 2002).

## SLEEP DISORDERS: ASSESSMENT, DIAGNOSIS, AND TREATMENTS

The American Sleep Disorders Association (1997) published a diagnostic classification of sleep and arousal disorders (see Box 28.1). Clinical polysomnography is used to confirm and diagnose these clinical sleep syndromes. This chapter includes a review of treatment interventions with the discussion of each type of sleep disorder.

Box 28.1    International Classification of Sleep Disorders, Classification Outline

1. Dyssomnias
   A. Intrinsic sleep disorders
   B. Extrinsic sleep disorders
   C. Circadian rhythm sleep disorders
2. Parasomnias
   A. Arousal disorders
   B. Sleep-wake transition disorders
   C. Parasomnias usually associated with REM sleep
   D. Other parasomnias
3. Sleep disorders associated with mental, neurological, or other medical disorders
4. Proposed sleep disorders

American Sleep Disorders Association (1997).

## Dyssomnias

Dyssomnias are the primary sleep disorders associated with disturbed sleep at night or impaired wakefulness. They are divided into three major groups: (1) intrinsic sleep disorders, (2) extrinsic sleep disorders, and (3) circadian rhythm sleep disorders.

### Intrinsic Sleep Disorders

Intrinsic sleep disorders originate or develop within the body and include psychophysiological insomnia, periodic limb movement disorder and restless legs syndrome, narcolepsy, and obstructive sleep apnea.

*Psychophysiological Insomnia.* Of the intrinsic sleep disorders, psychophysiological insomnia is the most common sleep-related complaint encountered in the general population. It is essentially a disorder of somatized tension and learned sleep-preventing associations. This interplay of factors results in the perception that sleep is inadequate or abnormal. During the night, these symptoms include difficulty initiating sleep, frequent awakenings during the night, a short sleep time, and nonrestorative sleep. Daytime symptoms of disturbed sleep (such as fatigue, daytime sleepiness, memory problems, anxiety, chronic pain, recent life stress, or even depression) also need to be considered to determine whether poor sleep is actually causing disturbed daytime functioning, or whether a psychological disorder such as depression is primary and the sleep disturbance is secondary.

A good initial step in evaluating someone with insomnia is considering the duration of the complaint. Both transient and short-term insomnia last less than three weeks and are usually situational; that is, they are related to an emotional problem, excitement, a schedule change such as jet lag, or a shift-work change. Chronic insomnia lasts for more than three weeks and begins with a clear precipitating event, but as the person deals with the resulting poor sleep, a maladaptive response to sleep disruption or inappropriate sleep habits develop and maintain the insomnia even after the precipitating factor has disappeared. When chronic psychophysiological insomnia develops as a result of perpetuating factors or somatized tension, it is best treated with behavioral techniques. When the insomnia is thought to be secondary to a medical or psychiatric disorder, treatment should be aimed at the underlying disorder, although behavioral techniques may prove helpful as an adjunctive treatment. The most commonly used behavioral therapies for the treatment of psychophysiological insomnia are stimulus control therapy, sleep restriction therapy, relaxation therapy and cognitive-behavioral therapy.

Stimulus control therapy was designed to promote the association of the bedroom with sleep rather than with frustration, anxiety, or wakefulness (Bootzin, 1979; Nicassio & Buchanan, 1981). Patients are told to go to bed only when sleepy, to reserve the bed only for sleeping and sex, to get up at the same time every morning regardless of how much sleep they got during the night, and not to nap during the day. If unable to sleep, patients should get out of bed and do something relaxing until they feel sleepy again, repeating this step as often as necessary throughout the night. Frequent contact with the therapist is necessary to encourage patients through the initial stages until proper associations are developed.

Sleep restriction therapy involves asking insomniacs to spend the same amount of time in bed as they report actually sleeping, but never less than four hours. The goal of this therapy is to increase sleep drive using partial sleep deprivation, thereby improving sleep quality (Spielman, Saskin, & Thorpy, 1987). The therapist computes each patient's moving average over five days from reports left on an answering machine of daily sleep time. When the average sleep efficiency (time in bed divided by actual time spent asleep) reaches at least 85 percent (80 percent for the elderly), time in bed is increased by 30-minute increments until the patient is sleeping through the night. Although this technique involves initial

sleep deprivation, the improvement in sleep quality can be significant.

Relaxation training techniques have also been shown to help with insomnia (Hauri & Linde, 1991). Regardless of the type of relaxation training, progressive muscle relaxation, meditation, deep breathing, self-hypnosis, or electromyograph (EMG) biofeedback, the technique must be overlearned, preferably in the daytime to avoid performance anxiety at bedtime. Hauri noted that although most insomniacs are muscularly tense, not all are. Relaxation training may actually worsen insomnia in patients who are already relaxed.

Cognitive-behavioral therapy (CBT), used for the treatment of psychological disorders such as anxiety and depression, has been adapted by sleep specialists for the treatment of insomnia (Stepanski & Perlis, 2000). This type of therapy is aimed at changing unrealistic beliefs and irrational fears regarding sleep or the loss of sleep and is typically combined with other behavioral therapies for insomnia. There is a strong emphasis on review of behavioral principles, compliance, and help with problems implementing these techniques (Morin, 1993). CBT has recently been shown to represent a viable intervention for primary sleep maintenance insomnia when compared to both behavioral treatment alone and a placebo therapy (Edinger, Wohlgenmuth, Radtke, Marsh, & Quillian, 2001).

*Periodic Limb Movement Disorder and Restless Legs Syndrome.* A complaint of poor sleep, particularly in the elderly, may be caused by periodic limb movement disorder. Patients are often unaware of this intrinsic disorder, which consists of repetitive muscle contractions, usually of the lower leg. These movements occur in rhythmic series throughout the sleep period and can result in arousals and complaints of disturbed or unrefreshing sleep. Restless legs is a disorder characterized by disagreeable leg sensations that occur while patients are awake and

---

**Box 28.2** Questions to Ask When Patients Complain of Excessive Daytime Sleepiness (Narcolepsy)

1. Have you ever had any unusual muscular experiences?
2. Do you snore?
3. Do your legs feel restless when you relax, or do they kick during sleep?
4. What medications have you used chronically in the past few months or years?
5. Do you sleep much longer on weekends than during the week?

---

Hauri (1992). Reprinted with permission.

---

relaxing. These sensations are present only at rest and may be ameliorated by moving the limbs vigorously (Hauri, 1992). The majority of patients with restless legs also have periodic limb movements, and the treatments for both are essentially the same. Dopaminergic agents as well as benzodiazepines or opioids are normally prescribed, and drug tolerance often develops.

*Narcolepsy.* The development of narcolepsy involves environmental factors acting on a specific genetic background, and the age of onset usually peaks in the 20s. Unlike insomnia, the primary symptom of narcolepsy is excessive daytime sleepiness. Auxiliary symptoms, including cataplexy, hypnogogic hallucinations, and sleep paralysis (Zarcone, 1973), are considered manifestations of REM sleep intruding into wakefulness and contribute to the diagnosis. Cataplexy is a sudden loss of muscle tone, usually triggered by an emotional event. A hypnogogic hallucination is a vivid dreamlike image occurring at sleep onset. Sleep paralysis is a total paralysis of voluntary muscles when falling asleep or waking up. Careful patient screening also aids in diagnosing narcolepsy (see Box 28.2). Since the etiology of narcolepsy is unclear, treatment is directed at the relief of symptoms. Short restorative naps taken during the day and stimulant medication can help relieve symptoms and allow a more normal lifestyle.

*Obstructive Sleep Apnea.* Another intrinsic sleep disorder with the main symptom of daytime sleepiness, obstructive sleep apnea can be life threatening. An obstruction of the airway occurs during sleep, often accompanied by a reduction in blood oxygen saturation and terminated by an arousal from sleep (Brassire & Guilleminault, 2000). Apneas and the accompanying arousals can occur numerous times during sleep, leading to the complaint of excessive daytime sleepiness. Obstructive sleep apnea is also associated with increased risk of automobile accidents and increased cardiovascular morbidity and mortality. The typical apnea sufferer is an obese, middle-aged male who snores. Apnea is much less common in women than in men until after the age of menopause. Naps are usually nonrestorative, and patients often complain of morning headaches, memory problems, and morning irritability. A clinical polysomnogram is helpful in assessing the frequency and severity of obstructive sleep apnea and in determining treatment protocols, which can range from weight loss to tracheostomy. However, nasally applied continuous positive airway pressure (CPAP) is

---

**Box 28.3**     Sleep Hygiene Suggestions

1. Try to get up at the same time every day, regardless of bedtime.
2. Avoid caffeine, alcohol, and nicotine close to bedtime.
3. Regular exercise in the late afternoon or early evening may be helpful, but try not to exercise strenuously right before bed.
4. A light snack of milk, crackers, or cereal may help promote sleep.
5. Keep the bedroom at a comfortable temperature, and reduce light and noise.
6. Keep naps relatively short, 30 to 40 minutes.
7. Find a time to worry before bedtime.
8. Keep clocks away from direct view to avoid "clock-watching."

---

now the established treatment for obstructive apnea syndrome.

### Extrinsic Sleep Disorders

Extrinsic sleep disorders originate from causes outside the body and include inadequate sleep hygiene, environmental sleep disorder, stimulant-dependent sleep disorder, alcohol-dependent sleep disorder, and altitude insomnia (American Sleep Disorders Association, 1997). Internal factors are important in the development and maintenance of all sleep disorders, including extrinsic sleep disorders. However, external factors are necessary for producing a sleep disorder (possibly in conjunction with internal factors), and their removal leads to the resolution of the sleep disorder.

*Inadequate Sleep Hygiene.* Activities or habits of daily living can promote sleep problems. Because an activity or habit that causes sleep disturbance in one person may not affect someone else, sleep logs are often used to help clarify inadequate sleep hygiene. Patients are asked to complete a daily log, noting when they went to bed, when they got up in the morning, napping behavior, alcohol or caffeine use, and stressful situations. The following week, one activity would be eliminated, such as daytime naps. The logs are then compared, and the patient can act as a co-investigator in determining the cause of the sleep disturbance. A list of sleep hygiene suggestions is included in Box 28.3. Attempting to follow every suggestion at once before a careful assessment of weekly sleep logs may only make the problem worse.

*Environmental Sleep Disorder.* Environmental factor can disturb sleep and results in the complaint of insomnia or daytime sleepiness. The elderly are often more sensitive to the impact of environmental factors on sleep such as excessive noise or light, hospitalization, a bed partner's sleep disorder, or death of a spouse. Asking on initial interview about any recent alterations in the sleep environment may be helpful when deciding what factors to include in weekly sleep logs.

*Stimulant-Dependent Sleep Disorder and Alcohol-Dependent Sleep Disorder.* Stimulant-dependent sleep disorder is characterized by a reduction of sleepiness or a suppression of sleep caused by the use of central stimulants. A diagnosis can be made when a stimulant medication has been identified in association with difficulty falling asleep or a cyclic pattern of sleep suppression and excessive sleepiness. A positive drug history or screening is also required for diagnosis. Alcohol-dependent sleep disorder is diagnosed when alcohol is used consistently as a hypnotic. Patients who use alcohol at bedtime to fall asleep usually have a sleep pattern of frequent awakenings that they may or may not be aware of.

*Altitude Insomnia.* Altitude insomnia is characterized by a complaint of insomnia when in high altitudes (usually greater than 4,000 meters). Other symptoms, including headaches, rapid heart rate, and fatigue, are thought to be the result of an instability of respiration during sleep and may become worse at higher altitudes. This sleep disorder usually abates at lower altitudes.

### Circadian Rhythm Sleep Disorders

The third type of dyssomnias are the circadian rhythm sleep disorders. Circadian rhythms are biological rhythms that repeat about every 24 hours, such as patterns of sleeping and waking, activity and rest, hunger and eating, and fluctuations in body temperature and hormone release (Ferber, 1985, 1990). Disorders of circadian rhythms share a common chronophysiological basis with the underlying problem usually one of misalignment between the patient's sleep pattern and the desired sleep pattern (American Sleep Disorders Association, 1997). The most common disorders of the circadian rhythm are advanced sleep phase syndrome, delayed sleep phase syndrome, and non-24-hour sleep-wake disorder.

Advanced sleep phase syndrome occurs more frequently in the elderly, who may find it difficult to stay awake after 7:00 or 8:00 in the evening and then find themselves wide awake at 3:00 or 4:00 in the morning. When this type of sleep-wake schedule fits into their lifestyles, complaints are rarely made to the physician, but when patients are required to maintain alertness for work or social reasons

chronic sleep deprivation and its associated symptoms may develop.

In delayed sleep phase syndrome, the sleep propensity shifts: The patient finds it difficult to fall asleep before 3:00 or 4:00 in the morning and has difficulty waking before 11:00 or noon. This slowing of the body clock is most common in teens and young adults. It may lead to difficulty getting to school or work on time and poor concentration and attention problems during the morning hours. Fortunately, as these patients age, their clocks speed up again and the disorder often dissipates.

Non-24-hour sleep-wake syndrome occurs when sleep onset and wake times are successively delayed each day. Patients exhibit periodically recurring problems with falling asleep, staying asleep, and rising, depending on the degree of synchrony between their internal clock and a normal 24-hour circadian rhythm (Turek & Zee, 1999). The majority of patients with this syndrome are totally blind, but a number of cases have been reported in sighted patients with various mental disorders (Klein et al., 1993).

A number of chronotherapies are currently in use for the treatment of circadian rhythm disorders; however, insurance companies often consider them experimental. The use of bright-light treatment in the early evening (7:00 to 9:00) is usually tried for elderly patients, resulting in a later sleep onset time and fewer awakenings (Campbell, Dawson, & Anderson, 1993). Treatment of delayed sleep phase syndrome involves the successive delay of sleep onset by three hours every day until the desired sleep time is achieved, followed by rigid adherence to a set sleep-wake schedule (Richardson & Malin, 1996). This type of chronotherapy has also proven successful in children, but patient compliance and a reduction in daylight exposure are necessary for success (Ferber, 1985, 1990). Studies looking at the use of bright-light exposure in the morning as well as the use of melatonin to shift the circadian clock are the most promising, but more clinical studies are needed (Lewy et al., 1992; Rosenthal et al., 1990). Melatonin appears to be the treatment of choice for non-24-hour sleep-wake syndrome in blind as well as sighted patients, given when the sleep phase period approaches the desired sleep onset time (Sack, Lewy, Blood, Stevenson, & Keith, 1991). In addition to chronotherapy, increasing research has been done on the field of chronomedicine for circadian rhythm disorders. Chronomedicine consists of diagnosis and treatment based on body time for specific disorders such as arthritis, asthma, diabetes, and depression (Smolensky & Lamberg, 2000).

## Parasomnias

The second major classification of sleep disorders comprises parasomnias, which are behaviors or movements that occur during sleep or are exacerbated by sleep. It is estimated that 5 percent of the general population suffers from some clinically significant parasomnia. This classification has been divided into arousal disorders, sleep-wake transition disorders, parasomnias usually associated with REM sleep, and other parasomnias.

Arousal disorders consist of impaired arousals that typically begin during slow-wave sleep (American Sleep Disorders Association, 1997). The most common arousal disorders are sleepwalking and night terrors. Sleepwalking is more common in children than in adults, and usually occurs in the first third of the night during slow-wave sleep. Episodes last 15 seconds to 30 minutes, and recall is sketchy the next day. Frequent sleepwalking in adults is more serious than in children because it is more often associated with dangerous activity. Night terrors, also called *pavor nocturnus,* are also characterized by an arousal from slow-wave sleep. Like sleepwalking, night terrors are more common

in children than adults. A night terror consists of an arousal along with agitation, sweating, and tachycardia. The patient looks terrified, often emits piercing screams, and is usually inconsolable. Night terrors can be differentiated from nightmares by the time of night and stage of sleep during which they occur and by the fact that night terrors are rarely associated with morning awareness of the event. In adults, night terrors are usually associated with psychopathology.

Sleep-wake transition disorders occur in otherwise healthy people during the transition from sleep to wakefulness. The most common of these disorders are rhythmic movement disorder, sleep starts, sleep talking, and nocturnal leg cramps. Rhythmic movement disorders such as head banging are more common in infants and children than in adults and consist of rhythmical forward-and-back head movements, sometimes accompanied by rocking body movements. This type of behavior is normal if it does not persist or begin in older children (Ferber, 1985, 1990). Sleep starts are brief muscle contractions that occur at sleep onset. Mild sleep starts are a normal feature of falling asleep and are seen in 60 percent to 70 percent of the population. Sleep talking is usually observed during non-REM sleep and, although it can be annoying to the bed partner, the patient has no subjective awareness of talking. Sleep talking is more common in males than females but is only listed as the sole diagnosis when it is the patient's primary complaint (Arkin, 1981). Nocturnal leg cramps are sustained painful contractions of the leg muscles and occur more often in the elderly and during pregnancy (Jacobsen et al., 1986). Massage, heat, or movement can help relieve cramps.

Parasomnias, usually associated with REM sleep, have a common underlying pathophysiological mechanism related to REM sleep (American Sleep Disorders Association, 1997). The most common of these are nightmares, sleep paralysis, and REM sleep behavior disorder. A nightmare is a frightening dream occurring during REM sleep that usually wakes the sleeper. Recall of a nightmare from REM sleep is often vivid and detailed. Although they are most common in children, nightmares can occur in adults under stress. Sleep paralysis occurs when there is a persistence of REM muscle atonia into wakefulness. Although eye movements and respiratory activity remain intact, somatic movements are not possible. Episodes of sleep paralysis may be accompanied by residual dream-related fear or with anxiety when a patient realizes that movement is not possible. Episodes may last one to several minutes and are often terminated by external touch (Schneck, 1970). REM sleep behavior disorder occurs during REM sleep when muscle atonia is absent. The symptoms are complex, often involving behaviors dangerous to themselves or bed partners and sometimes dream-like thoughts and images or vivid, unpleasant dreams. Patients who complain of these symptoms, should be evaluated by a sleep specialist. REM sleep behavior disorder usually occurs in the middle-aged or elderly, and a systematic evaluation needs to be conducted to eliminate seizure activity and verify REM sleep muscle activity. Sleep bruxism, sleep enuresis, primary snoring, and sudden infant death syndrome are all listed under the classification of other parasomnias.

### Sleep Disorders Associated with Mental, Neurological, and Other Medical Disorders

Sleep disorders associated with mental, neurological, and other medical disorders are the last major classification of sleep disorders (American Sleep Disorders Association, 1997). In general, the most common mental disorders associated with sleep problems are mood disorders, anxiety disorders, and panic disorder.

Most patients with major depression complain of insomnia, and episodes of recurrent depression may be preceded by several weeks of reported sleep disturbance (Benca, 1996, 2001). The American Sleep Disorders Association (1997) lists the inability to return to sleep after waking up too early as the cardinal insomnia complaint of patients with major depression. Excessive sleep or frequent napping is more common in milder bipolar depression and in some dysthymic patients. When mania symptoms are present, patients usually report sleeping less without feeling tired. Sleep complaints often covary with the severity of a mood disorder, and there is considerable polysomnographic evidence suggesting that sleep is biologically linked to mood disorders (Reynolds and Kupfer, 1987). When sleep tracings are conducted, at least 90 percent of patients with mood disorders exhibit sleep fragmentation, reduced stage 3 and stage 4 sleep, shortened REM latency, longer sleep latency (particularly in young patients), and increased REM activity. Once therapy for the mood disorder has been initiated, the subjective complaint of insomnia tends to improve more rapidly than does the mood disorder itself.

Sleep disturbance associated with anxiety disorders is characterized by difficulty falling asleep or inability to stay asleep due to excessive anxiety and apprehensive expectation about life circumstances (American Sleep Disorders Association, 1997). Patients often report that they cannot stop worrying, relax, or keep from thinking about problems at bedtime (Rosa, Bonnet, & Kramer, 1983). Treatment of the core symptoms of most anxiety disorders usually results in an improvement of the sleep disturbance. However, behavioral therapy for bad sleep habits that have developed may also be necessary. Since anxiety disorders tend to persist for months or years, the sleep problems may also become chronic, but if they continue after successful treatment of the anxiety, a sleep evaluation should be considered.

Nocturnal panic attacks are the most disturbing and disabling sleep problem experienced by 69 percent of individuals with panic disorder (Mellman & Uhde, 1989, 1990). Panic disorder patients with nocturnal panic report higher rates of insomnia, especially nonrestorative sleep and frequent awakenings, than do those without (Hauri & Linde, 1991). Panic attacks that occur during sleep have the typical symptoms of those that occur during the day but are associated with a sudden awakening and problems returning to sleep. Recommended treatment for patients with sleep panic includes an antipanic medication as well as normal sleep hygiene methods.

Neurological disorders associated with sleep disturbance include dementia, Parkinsonism, and fatal familial insomnia (American Sleep Disorders Association, 1997). Neurologically based sleep disturbances are often characterized by delirium, agitation, combativeness, wandering, and vocalization occurring during early evening or nighttime hours. Although patients with dementia present with frequent awakenings, difficulty falling asleep, and early morning awakening, by far the most troublesome symptom is sundown syndrome. *Sundowning* has been operationally defined as agitation that occurs only during evening or nighttime hours and is a major cause of institutionalization in the elderly patient with advanced dementia. Patients may wander outside, turn on kitchen appliances, or shout inappropriately (Pollak, Perlick, & Lisner, 1990). These types of sleep disturbances are very difficult to treat because they are secondary to the central nervous system changes, but reducing daytime napping, enhancing daylight exposure, and, if possible, restricting forced awakenings may be helpful.

Insomnia is the most common sleep-related symptom in patients with Parkinsonism. However, other sleep-related problems may also be present, such as the inability to get out of bed unaided, vivid dreams, daytime dozing, and pain (Aldrich, 2000). As happens with dementia, sleep disturbance worsens as the Parkinsonism progresses, and medications used to treat the disease may be a major factor in the sleep disturbance.

Fatal familial insomnia is a rare inherited, degenerative disorder that begins with trouble sleeping and progresses within months to a total lack of sleep and ultimately death (Dement, 1999).

A variety of medical disorders have features that occur during sleep or that cause sleep disturbance. They will not be detailed here but may include sleeping sickness, nocturnal cardiac ischemia, chronic obstructive pulmonary disease, sleep-related asthma, sleep-related gastroesophageal reflux, peptic ulcer disease, and fibromyalgia.

## SLEEP PROBLEMS IN WOMEN

Sleep complaints increase with age and are twice as prevalent among women of all ages as they are among men. Most of what we know about sleep is based on studies with male subjects. In fact, about 75 percent of all sleep research has been conducted with men. Recently, more researchers have been taking gender into consideration; these studies provide a better look at sleep and sleep disorders in women.

Hormones may set women up for special problems during sleep. Women of childbearing age report more difficulty with sleep during certain phases of the menstrual cycle. There is some evidence suggesting that the regular fluctuations of gonadal hormone levels during the menstrual cycle may be related to recurrent insomnia, particularly in women who experience mood and other physical symptoms characteristic of the premenstrual syndrome (Lee, Shaver, Giblin, & Woods, 1990). In addition, the elevated body temperature in the postovulary phase of the menstrual cycle may disrupt sleep stages and structure, as measured by REM sleep latency. However, a clear relationship between sleep disturbance and the menstrual cycle has not been established. It is possible that mood affects sleep as much as or more than the menstrual cycle does.

Mood disorders occur in both men and women, but the incidence is higher in women. Disturbances such as difficulty falling asleep, trouble maintaining sleep, and early-morning awakenings, are associated with major depressive disorder and in some cases may occur prior to an actual depressive episode. Research into the link between changes in sleep and depression indicates that treatment of sleep disturbances may help improve the course and management of depression.

Seasonal affective disorder occurs during the winter months and is a mood disorder diagnosed more frequently in women than in men. Bright-light treatment, either at night or in the morning, is believed to be helpful in reducing symptoms, but more studies are needed to determine the mechanism behind the antidepressant effect of bright-light treatment.

Reports of daytime fatigue and poor sleep during pregnancy are not new. What is new is that researchers are encouraging physicians to take sleep complaints during pregnancy more seriously. The high levels of progesterone during pregnancy may contribute to the feelings of tiredness that women may experience during pregnancy. Progesterone has also been shown to increase body temperature and to speed breathing, as well as to act on the smooth muscle of the urinary tract to cause frequent urination, which is potentially disruptive to sleep. Sleep disruption can begin as early as the third month of pregnancy and can persist at least eight months into the postpartum period. The need for attention to pregnancy-related sleep disruption is emphasized by the fact that the mood alterations often accompanying complaints of poor sleep both during and after pregnancy may constitute a risk factor for postpartum depression (Lee & DeJoseph, 1992).

Unfortunately, problems with sleep do not cease when menopause arrives. Complaints of disturbed sleep, daytime fatigue, and mood lability increase during the climacteric—the transition from the reproductive stage of life to the nonreproductive stage of life, which includes menopause. Hot flashes are the most common symptom of the climacteric and consist of intense feelings of heat, sweating, and (in some women) rapid heart rate and feelings of suffocation. They can occur frequently during both the day and night; those that occur during sleep almost always cause awakening. When nighttime hot flashes are particularly severe, they are called night sweats and may necessitate a change of nightclothes and bed linen. Even when hot flashes are relatively mild or do not occur at all, menopausal women still exhibit some signs of sleep disruption. On average, a menopausal woman's sleep is disrupted by brief arousals every 8 minutes if she is experiencing hot flashes and every 18 minutes if she is not. Interruption of the normal continuity of sleep by brief arousals has been shown to impair daytime functioning even when the length of sleep is not shortened. In addition to arousals from sleep, the thermoregulatory effects of hot flashes have the potential to alter sleep stage by increasing slow-wave sleep (Woodward & Freedman, 1994). Hot flashes and associated sleep disruption can continue for five years or more if untreated, so it is not surprising that complaints of insomnia are increased during the menopausal period.

The treatment most usually suggested for hot flashes and other menopausal symptoms is hormone replacement therapy (HRT)—either estrogen alone or a combination of estrogen and progesterone. However, HRT is often contraindicated, leaving some women with little relief of symptoms that may disturb sleep. Following the basic sleep hygiene, suggestions described earlier in this chapter may help prevent the insomnia that continues even when symptoms abate. Sleeping in a room with a thermoneutral temperature or even a slightly cool temperature may help. Cotton nightclothes and control of her side of the electric blanket may help as well.

As women age, their susceptibility to respiratory disturbance during sleep begins to increase. In fact, severe apnea, which (as noted earlier) consists of frequent brief episodes of breathing cessation during sleep, has been found to increase the mortality rate among women in nursing homes (Ford & Komerow, 1989). There is a strong prevalence of sleep-related respiratory disturbance in men throughout life. In women, the incidence of disordered breathing during sleep is very low before the age of 50 but increases dramatically following menopause. The prevalence of sleep-related breathing disturbance in middle-aged women is now estimated to be 9 percent, much higher than previously expected among women (Young et al., 1993). Suspicion of apnea or even heavy snoring should be evaluated.

## CONCLUSION

The fact that diagnosis of sleep disorders is often difficult reflects the numerous causes of poor sleep. However, research in the field of sleep medicine is expanding every day, and medical and behavioral interventions offer relief for the majority of sleep-disordered patients.

Approximately 50 percent more women than men report that daytime sleepiness interferes with their daily activities, and more women than men use sleep medications and report weekly insomnia (Chevalier et al., 1999; Hublin, Kaprio, Partinen, & Koskenvuo, 2001). Taking a woman's complaints of poor sleep seriously and providing appropriate treatment may result in not only improved sleep but also improved daytime functioning and mood.

## REFERENCES

Aldrich, M. S. (2000). Parkinsonism. In M. H. Kryger, T. Roth, & W. C. Dement (Eds.), *Principles and practices of sleep medicine* (pp. 1051–1057). Philadelphia: W. B. Saunders.

American Sleep Disorders Association. (1997). *International classification of sleep disorders, revised: Diagnostic and coding manual.* Rochester, MN: Author.

Arkin, A. M. (1981). *Sleep-talking: Psychology and psychophysiology.* Hillsdale, NJ: Lawrence Erlbaum.

Benca, R. M. (1996). Sleep in psychiatric disorders. *Neurological Clinics, 14*(4), 739–764.

Benca, R. M. (2001). Consequences of insomnia and its therapies. *Journal of Clinical Psychiatry, 62*(Suppl. 10), 33–38.

Bootzin, R. R. (1979). Effects of self-control procedures for insomnia. *American Journal of Clinical Biofeedback, 2*(2), 70–77.

Brassire, A., & Guilleminault, C. (2000). Clinical features and evaluation of obstructive sleep apnea-hypopnea syndrome. In M. H. Kryger, T. Roth, & W. C. Dement (Eds.), *Principles and practices of sleep medicine* (pp. 869–878). Philadelphia: W. B. Saunders.

Campbell, S. S., Dawson, P., & Anderson, G. W. (1993). Alleviation of sleep maintenance insomnia with timed exposure to bright light. *Journal of the American Geriatric Society, 41*, 829–836.

Chevalier, H., Los, F., Boichut, D., Bianchi, M., Nutt, D. J., Hajak, G., et al. (1999). Evaluation of severe insomnia in the general population: Results of a European multinational survey. *Journal of Psychopharmacology, 13*(4, Suppl. 1), S21–S24.

Dement, W.C. (1999). *The promise of sleep*. New York: Delacorte Press.

Edinger, J. D., Wohlgenmuth, W. K., Radtke, R. A., Marsh, G. R., & Quillian, R.E. (2001). Cognitive behavioral therapy for treatment of chronic primary insomnia. A randomized controlled trial. *Journal of the American Medical Association, 285*(14), 1856–1864.

Ferber, R. (1985). Sleep, sleeplessness, and sleep disruptions in infants and young children. *Annals of Clinical Research, 17*, 227–234.

Ferber, R. (1990). Sleep schedule-dependent causes of insomnia and sleepiness in middle childhood and adolescence. *Pediatrician, 17*(1), 13–20.

Ford, D. E., & Komerow, D. B. (1989). Epidemiologic study of sleep disturbances and psychiatric disorders: An opportunity for prevention? *Journal of the American Medical Association, 262*, 1479–1484.

Hauri, P. (1992). *Current concepts: The sleep disorders*. Kalamazoo, MI: Upjohn.

Hauri, P., & Linde, S. (1991). *No more sleepless nights*. New York: Wiley.

Hublin, C., Kaprio, J., Partinen, M., & Koskenvuo, M. (2001). Insufficient sleep: A population-based study in adults. *Sleep, 24*(4), 392–400.

I can't sleep. (2002, June 7). *Wall Street Journal*, p. W1.

Institute for Traffic Safety Management and Research. (1996, May). *New York State task force on drowsy driving status report*. Albany: New York State Governor's Traffic Safety Committee.

Jacobsen, J. H., Rosenberg, R. S., Hutenlocher, P. R., & Spire, J. P. (1986). Familial nocturnal cramping. *Sleep, 9*, 54–60.

Klein, T., Martens, H., Dijk, D. J., Kronauer, R. E., Seely, E. W., & Czeisler, C. A. (1993). Circadian sleep regulation in the absence of light reception: Chronic non-24-hour circadian rhythm sleep disorder in a blind man with a regular 24-hour sleep wake schedule. *Sleep, 16*, 333–343.

Lee, K. A., & DeJoseph, J. F. (1992). Sleep disturbances, vitality, and fatigue among a select group of employed childbearing women. *Birth, 19*, 208–213.

Lee, K. A., Shaver, J. R., Giblin, E. C., & Woods, N. F. (1990). Sleep patterns related to menstrual cycle phase and premenstrual affective disorders. *Sleep, 3*, 403–409.

Lewy, A. J., Ahmed, S., Jackson, J. M., & Sack, R. L. (1992). Melatonin shifts human circadian rhythms according to a phase-response curve. *Chronobiology International, 9*, 380–392.

Loomis, A. L., Harvey, E. N., & Hobart, G. (1935). Further observations on the potential rhythms of the cerebral cortex during sleep. *Science, 82*, 198–200.

Mellman, T. A., & Uhde, T. W. (1989). Sleep panic attacks: New clinical findings and theoretical implications. *American Journal of Psychiatry, 146*(9), 1204–1207.

Mellman, T. A., & Uhde, T. W. (1990). Patients with frequent sleep panic: Clinical findings and response to medication treatment. *Journal of Clinical Psychiatry, 51*(12), 513–516.

Morin, C. (1993). *Insomnia: Psychological assessment and management.* New York: Guilford.

National Commission on Sleep Disorders Research. (1993). *Executive summary and executive report. Wake up, America: A national sleep alert* (Vol. 1). Washington, DC: Author.

National Commission on Sleep Disorders Research. (1994). *Wake up, America: A national sleep alert* (Vol. 2). Washington, DC: Author.

National Sleep Foundation. (1999). *Omnibus sleep in America poll.* Washington, DC: Author.

Nicassio, P. M., & Buchanan, D. C. (1981). Clinical application of behavior therapy for insomnia. *Comprehensive Psychiatry, 22,* 512–521.

Pollak, C. P., Perlick, D., & Lisner, J. P. (1990). Sleep problems in the community elderly as predictors of death and nursing home placement. *Journal of Community Health, 15,* 123–135.

Reynolds, C. F., III, & Kupfer, D. J. (1987). Sleep research in affective illness: State of the art circa 1987. *Sleep, 10*(3), 199–215.

Richardson, G. S., & Malin, H. V. (1996). Circadian rhythm sleep disorders: Pathophysiology and treatment. *Journal of Clinical Neurophysiology, 13*(1), 17–31.

Rosa, R. R., Bonnet, M. H., & Kramer, M. (1983). The relationship of sleep and anxiety in anxious subjects. *Biological Psychology, 16*(1–2), 119–126.

Rosenthal, N. E., Joseph-Vanderpool, J. R., Levendosky, A. A., Johnston, S. H., Allen, R., Kelly, K. A., et al. (1990). Phase-shifting effects of bright morning light as treatment for delayed sleep phase syndrome. *Sleep, 13,* 354–361.

Sack, R. L., Lewy, A. J., Blood, M. L., Stevenson, J., & Keith, L. D. (1991). Melatonin administration to blind people: Phase advances and entrainment. *Journal of Biological Rhythms, 6,* 249–261.

Schneck, J. M. (1970). Sleep paralysis and spontaneous hypnotic paralysis. *Perceptual and Motor Skills, 31,* 16.

Smolensky, M., & Lamberg, L. (2000). *The body clock guide to better health.* New York: Henry Holt.

Spielman, A. J., Saskin, P., & Thorpy, M. J. (1987). Treatment of chronic insomnia by restriction of time in bed. *Sleep, 10,* 45–46.

Stepanski, E. J., & Perlis, M. L. (2000). Behavioral sleep medicine: An emerging subspecialty in health psychology and sleep medicine. *Journal of Psychosomatic Research, 49*(5), 343–347.

Turek, F. W., & Zee, P. C. (Eds.). (1999). Regulation of sleep and circadian rhythms. New York: M. Dekker.

Woodward, S., & Freedman, R. R. (1994). The thermoregulatory effects of menopausal hot flashes on sleep. *Sleep, 17,* 497–450.

Young, T., Palta, M., Dempsey, J., Skatrud, J., Weber, S., & Badr, S. (1993). The occurrence of sleep-disordered breathing among middle-aged adults. *New England Journal of Medicine, 328,* 1230–1235.

Zarcone, V. (1973). Narcolepsy. *New England Journal of Medicine, 288,* 1156–1166.

# CHAPTER 29

# Rheumatoid Arthritis

## Cheryl Bourguignon and Diana Taibi

**Abstract:** The authors overview the pathophysiology of rheumatoid arthritis, review assessment and diagnostic procedures, and identify cognitive and psychological processes that influence the severity of the symptoms of the disorder. A program including education for disease management, relaxation training, and cognitive-behavioral therapy can assist the patient in reducing the severity of the symptoms, reducing medical utilization, and improving functional capacity.

## PROFILE OF THE DISORDER

Rheumatoid arthritis (RA) is a chronic, inflammatory autoimmune disease that affects approximately 1 percent of the adult population worldwide but is approximately three times more prevalent in women than in men (Da Silva & Hall, 1992). RA is characterized by joint stiffness in the morning, symmetrical joint swelling, and generalized fatigue. The disease occurs most commonly between the ages of 30 and 60. Patients with rheumatoid arthritis may have periods of remission, but because the disease is inflammatory and not curable, individuals must manage flares of symptoms and disease throughout their lives.

### Pathophysiology

Although the full pathophysiology of RA remains unclear, several processes have been suggested in its pathogenesis. A key factor in the development of the disorder is the loss of immune self-tolerance. The etiology of the loss of self-tolerance is unknown, but there are several possible contributing factors. One theory proposes that environmental exposure to certain infectious agents might precipitate the autoimmune process. Research findings have indicated that Epstein-Barr virus and parvovirus may contribute to the development of RA, but no evidence definitively links these agents to the pathogenesis of the disease (Harris, 1986). There is also strong evidence supporting the involvement of genetic factors in RA. The high concordance rate of RA in monozygotic twins indicates that certain genotypes may have a greater risk of developing the disorder (Silman, 1994). In addition, studies have found that many HLA class II alleles, which affect antigen presentation and the subsequent

AUTHOR'S NOTE: The development of this chapter was supported by the grant award T32AT00052 funded by the National Center for Complementary and Alternative Medicine, National Institutes of Health.

immune response, are involved in RA susceptibility and severity (Zanelli, Breedveld, &
de Vries, 2000). Since no single environmental
or genetic cause has been identified, it is
postulated that RA is a syndrome resulting
from a complex combination of environmental and genetic factors.

The known pathogenesis of RA is highly
complex, involving many different cell lines
and various cellular communication pathways. Within the synovium, T lymphocytes,
macrophages, and fibroblast-like synovio-
cytes (FLSs) produce cytokines, particularly
interleukin-1β (IL-1β) and tumor necrosis
factor-α (TNF-α), and growth factors that
promote the pathological processes in RA
(Fox, 2001). Formation of blood vessels in
the normally avascular synovium allows
infiltration of inflammatory cells and promotes destructive proliferation of the synovial membrane (Harris, 1986). Abnormally
proliferating FLSs at the cartilage-bone junc-
tion, called pannus, invade the articular capsule, causing deformity. T lymphocytes also
enhance the activity of B lymphocytes, which
produce autoantibodies and rheumatoid
factor (Weyand, 2000). Eventually, these
processes result in structural damage, joint
deformity, functional disability, and pain.

Several factors outside the synovium are
involved in RA, including gonadal hormones, which contribute to the fluctuations
in disease activity. First, more women are
diagnosed with RA disease than are men.
The overall female-to-male prevalence is
approximately 3.5:1 (Da Silva & Hall,
1992); however, the ratio is exaggerated during reproductive years at about 5:1 and then
moves closer to 2:1 in postmenopausal years
(Masi, Feigenbaum, & Chatterton, 1995).
Second, at times of the largest shifts in estrogen and progesterone, during pregnancy and
postpartum, symptoms and disease activity
change. At least 75 percent of women with
RA have decreased symptoms and disease

activity or full remission during pregnancy,
with 62 percent of them experiencing a
return of their prepregnancy symptoms
during the postpartum period (Ostensen,
Aune, & Husby, 1983). Smaller fluctuations
in estrogen and progesterone during the course
of the menstrual cycle may also contribute to
symptom severity (Goldstein, Duff, & Karsh,
1987; Latman, 1983). Third, the proinflam-
matory cytokines that are increased in RA,
TNF-α, IL-1β, and IL-6, may vary depending
on levels of estrogen and progesterone
(Cutolo, 1999).

Also involved in the disease process, the
hypothalamic-pituitary-adrenal (HPA) axis
and autonomic nervous system (ANS), which
are essential in the process of adapting to stressors, respond abnormally in RA. The HPA
axis normally produces cortisol, a steroid hormone that suppresses inflammation. HPA production of cortisol is blunted in RA, which
allows joint inflammation to continue unop-
posed (Cutolo, 1999). This unchecked inflammation increases pain, sleepiness, and fatigue
(Payne & Krueger, 1992). An imbalance often
exists in the ANS between the sympathetic nervous system (SNS) and parasympathetic nervous system (Baerwald, Panayi, & Lanchbury,
1997). Some individuals with RA have heightened SNS activity with increased catecholamines (norepinephrine and epinephrine)
(Baerwald et al., 1997), and abnormalities of
the parasympathetic nervous system
(Bekkelund, Jorde, Husby, & Mellgren, 1996).
Abnormal parasympathetic activity, demonstrated by decreases in heart rate variability,
has been found in those with RA. In other
chronic conditions, decreased heart rate variability was found to increase risk of sudden
cardiac arrest and mortality (Burr et al., 1994).
This is significant for patients with RA because
cardiovascular complications are significant
contributors to mortality in the disorder
(Myllykangas-Luosujarvi, Aho, Kautiainen, &
Isomaki, 1995).

## Diagnosing Rheumatoid Arthritis

### Symptoms

Pain, fatigue, sleep disturbances, and depression are the most prevalent symptoms described by people who have rheumatoid arthritis, and these symptoms are closely related. Most people with RA experience joint pain and stiffness with a usual remitting-recurring pattern. When disease flares occur, joint pain and stiffness are significantly increased. Approximately 40 percent of men and women with RA experience fatigue, and women experience greater levels of fatigue than do men (Wolfe, Hawley, & Wilson, 1996). Fatigue is associated with sleep disturbances, greater pain, and depression, as well as lower functional abilities in RA patients. Sleep disturbances, which include prolonged sleep latency (time to sleep onset), increased number of awakenings, and lowered sleep efficiency (ratio of total sleep time to total time in bed) are prevalent. In people with RA, sleep latency estimates range from 23 to 76 minutes, and sleep efficiency ranges from 76 percent to 81 percent; below 90 percent is considered poor sleep efficiency (Hirsch et al., 1994; Moldofsky, Lue, & Smythe, 1983). Pain often increases sleep disturbances (Drewes, 1999). The prevalence of depression in people with RA has been estimated to be from 15 percent to 40 percent (Pincus, Griffith, Pearce, & Isenberg, 1996), and individuals with more depression have higher levels of joint pain, greater fatigue, and more sleep disturbance (Affleck, Tennen, Urrows, & Higgins, 1992).

### Pattern of Joint Involvement

The pattern of joint involvement is distinctive in rheumatoid arthritis. Symmetrical involvement commonly presents in several of the following joint areas: the metacarpophalangeal and proximal (but not the distal) interphalanges (joints) of the hands, wrists, knees, hips, feet, ankles, shoulders, elbows, neck, and jaw. If the disease has progressed and joint destruction is present, hand deformities, such as ulnar drift and swan neck, may be apparent. Ulnar drift is evident when the fingers "drift" or slant toward the ulnar side of the hand. Swan neck is observed when flexion of the distal interphalanges and metacarpophalanges is present, along with hyperextension of the proximal interphalanges.

### Laboratory Tests

Laboratory tests that are usually performed include erythrocyte sedimentation rate (ESR), C-reactive protein (CRP), rheumatoid factor, and antinuclear antibodies. ESR and CRP are general measures of inflammation. Rheumatoid factor, an antibody specific to rheumatoid arthritis, is not always positive but if present usually indicates more severe disease. Antinuclear antibodies, which indicate an autoimmune process, are present in only 20 percent of cases.

### X Rays

X rays are taken on all affected joints when first diagnosed to establish a baseline and then periodically repeated to determine progression of joint involvement and destruction. Typically, the X rays of people with RA depict soft tissue swelling, marginal erosions, narrowing of joint spaces, hand and wrist deformities, and articular osteoporosis.

Although no definitive laboratory analysis or X-ray finding alone can diagnose RA, the American College of Rheumatology has published criteria that can be used to establish the diagnosis of RA (Arnett et al., 1988) as well as functional classifications of the disease (see Tables 29.1 and 29.2).

**Table 29.1** 1987 Criteria for the Classification of Rheumatoid Arthritis

| *Criteria* | *Definition* |
| --- | --- |
| 1. Morning stiffness | Stiffness in and around joints that starts on arising in the morning and lasts an hour or more |
| 2. Arthritis of three or more joints | At least three joint areas simultaneously have had soft-tissue swelling or fluid (not bony overgrowth alone) observed by physician. Joint areas include right or left proximal interphalangeal, metacarpophalangeal, wrist, elbow, knee, ankle, and metatarsophalangeal joints |
| 3. Arthritis of hand joints | At least one area swollen in a wrist, metacarpophalangeal, or proximal interphalangeal joint. |
| 4. Symmetric arthritis | Simultaneous involvement of the same joint areas on both sides of the body. |
| 5. Rheumatoid nodules | Subcutaneous nodules, over bony prominences, or extensor surfaces, or in juxta-articular regions, observed by physician. |
| 6. Serum rheumatoid factor | Abnormal amounts of serum rheumatoid factor. |
| 7. Radiographic changes | Radiographic changes typical of rheumatoid arthritis on posteroanterior hand and wrist radiographs, which must include erosions or unequivocal bony decalcification localized in or most marked adjacent to the involved joints (osteoarthritis changes alone do not qualify). |

SOURCE: The American Rheumatism Association 1987 revised criteria for the classification of rheumatoid arthritis. Arnett, F. C., Edworthy, S. M., Bloch, D. A., McShane, D. J., Fries, J. F., Cooper, N. S., Healey, L. A., Kaplan, S. R., Liang, M. H., & Luthra, H. S. In *Arthritis and Rheumatism*, Copyright © 1988 American College of Rheumatology. Reprinted by permission of Wiley-Liss, Inc., a subsidiary of John Wiley & Sons, Inc.
NOTE: To be diagnosed with rheumatoid arthritis, a patient must satisfy at least four of the seven criteria, and criteria 1 through 4 must have been present for at least six weeks.

**Table 29.2** Classification of the Functional Status in Rheumatoid Arthritis

| *Class* | *Definition* |
| --- | --- |
| Class I | Able to perform usual activities of daily living (self-care, vocational, avocational) |
| Class II | Able to perform usual self-care and vocational activities but limited in avocational activities |
| Class III | Able to perform usual self-care activities, but limited in vocational and avocational activities |
| Class IV | Limited in ability to perform self-care, vocational, and avocational activities |

SOURCE: The American College of Rheumatology 1991 revised criteria for the classification of global functional status in rheumatoid arthritis. Hochberg, M. C., Chang, R. W., Dwosh, I., Lindsey, S., Pincus, T., & Wolfe, F. In *Arthritis & Rheumatism*, Copyright © 1992 American College of Rheumatology. Reprinted by permission of Wiley-Liss, Inc., a subsidiary of John Wiley & Sons, Inc.
NOTES: Self-care activities = feeding, bathing, dressing, grooming, and toileting; vocational activities = work, school, or homemaking; avocational activities = recreational and/or leisure events.

## COGNITIVE BELIEFS AND PSYCHOLOGICAL PROCESSES

An increasing number of studies indicate that arthritis pain cannot be solely explained by physiological causes (Keefe & Bonk, 1999; Keefe & Caldwell, 1997). Internal psychological phenomena related to individual characteristics and coping patterns have been found to act in a cyclical manner with the experience of musculoskeletal pain. An individual's experience of pain influences cognitive patterns, which in turn modify the pain experience. Psychological processes can modify pain by creating muscle tension, activating the sympathetic nervous system, influencing mood states, impacting pain beliefs, and altering the perception of painful sensations (Keefe & Gil, 1986). Given the importance of psychological factors in the experience of RA pain and the failure of traditional medical approaches to consistently control pain, cognitive-behavioral approaches are highly appropriate and useful in RA (Bradley & Alberts, 1999).

Cognitive beliefs, such as catastrophizing, helplessness, and self-efficacy, may influence the symptoms of RA. A maladaptive coping strategy, catastrophizing is a cognitive distortion characterized by negative self-talk and negative ideas about one's future. Catastrophizing involves perceiving small problems as major disasters and is associated with low self-efficacy and high levels of pain, functional disability, and depression (Keefe, Kashikar-Zuck, et al., 1997).

Helplessness is the belief that one's efforts will not be successful in achieving a goal (Keefe & Bonk, 1999). In people with RA, helplessness is associated with high levels of pain, depression, functional disability, and the use of passive coping strategies (Bradley & Alberts, 1999; Keefe & Bonk, 1999). Helplessness at baseline was found to be a significant predictor of RA disease flares at three months in one study (Nicassio et al., 1993) and of mortality at five years in another study (Callahan, Cordray, Wells, & Pincus, 1996).

Self-efficacy is at the opposite end of the beliefs continuum from helplessness. Self-efficacy is the belief that one's efforts will be successful in accomplishing a particular goal (Bandura, 1997). Interest in this concept has grown with the recognition that self-efficacy is consistently associated with improvements in pain, mood, and coping (Lefebvre et al., 1999). Testing an intervention to enhance self-efficacy, Smarr et al. (1997) found that as participants increased their self-efficacy for dealing with RA, subsequent pain, depression, and helplessness decreased and disease activity improved. After controlling for demographic variables and disease duration, arthritis self-efficacy remained a significant predictor, explaining 28 percent (out of a total of 49 percent) of the variance in daily joint pain (Lefebvre et al., 1999). Riemsma et al. (1998) found that pain and self-efficacy explained 37 percent of the variance in fatigue; patients with higher self-efficacy scores had less fatigue. Thus, self-efficacy is an important factor affecting symptom management in RA.

## PSYCHOEDUCATIONAL AND COGNITIVE-BEHAVIORAL THERAPY PROGRAMS

Understanding the contribution of catastrophizing, helplessness, and self-efficacy to the experience of pain and other symptoms in RA has contributed greatly to the development of effective cognitive-behavioral interventions. The purpose of cognitive-behavioral therapy (CBT) is to help individuals understand the relationships between cognitive, affective, and physiological processes with the goal of teaching them skills to manage their symptoms through reconceptualization of their experiences and through an application of active coping strategies (Keefe, Dunsmore, & Burnett, 1992). CBT is designed to teach people to use effective self-management and coping skills, positive cognitive strategies, and stress reduction techniques to decrease SNS activation.

The decrease in SNS responsiveness should in turn decrease inflammation, promote pain control, and improve sleep. Thus, cognitive-behavioral therapy is highly appropriate for RA because it targets the pathophysiology of the disease as well as coping with symptoms of the disease. The general protocol of cognitive-behavioral therapy for RA includes (1) teaching individuals the effects of cognitions, feelings, and behaviors on the experience of pain and other symptoms; (2) helping individuals understand their role in controlling their pain and other symptoms through cognitive-behavioral approaches; and (3) teaching individuals the skills for managing their symptoms (Keefe & Caldwell, 1997).

A CBT program often includes relaxation and imagery training, self-management and coping skills for dealing with rheumatoid arthritis, assertiveness and interpersonal training, problem-solving, and cognitive restructuring. Cognitive restructuring focuses on correcting erroneous and distorted perceptions of oneself and one's disease to reduce catastrophizing. Patients can be taught to self-monitor for negative thoughts and recognize situations that prompt automatic thoughts. Cognitive restructuring can be an effective intervention for pain and mood disturbance as well, since these factors have been found to be associated with catastrophizing (Keefe, Kashikar-Zuck, et al., 1997).

Initially, efforts to improve management of arthritis symptoms focused on two types of interventions: psychoeducational programs and cognitive-behavioral therapy (Broderick, 2000). Research has shown that education alone improved knowledge but did not produce strong results in symptom and disease outcomes, and that education in conjunction with CBT produced positive results in patients' abilities to manage their symptoms (Keefe & Van Horn, 1993). Therefore, many of the successful interventions have included both CBT and educational components. It is not entirely known if CBT alone is effective, because most CBT studies include a certain amount of self-management education.

The Arthritis Self-Management Program (ASMP), designed by Lorig (1986) at the Stanford Arthritis Center, combines education and some of the cognitive-behavioral strategies previously discussed. This program is intended to be widely disseminated and taught by lay people. The most significant later revision of the program added interventions for improving self-efficacy, because addressing self-efficacy had been found to be associated with reduced pain and increased behavior change compared to education alone (Lorig & Holman, 1993). Rather than focusing solely on providing information, the ASMP aims to provide individuals with CBT skills for managing their arthritis.

The ASMP is a six-week course taught in weekly two-hour sessions (Lorig & Holman, 1993). The topics covered by the course include information about arthritis, appropriate use of medications, physical exercise, relaxation training, joint protection techniques, nutrition, successful interaction with physicians, and evaluation of nontraditional treatments. Teaching methods used include group discussion, practice, self-contracting, and diaries. Studies investigating the outcomes of the ASMP have found that the program produces improved knowledge, decreased pain, greater use of relaxation and exercise, and increased self-efficacy (Lorig, Konkol, & Gonzalez, 1987). In addition, the changes in coping have been found to persist at follow-up four years after the beginning of the intervention, and periodic reinforcement is unnecessary for the maintenance of these changes (Lorig & Holman, 1993). Other researchers have investigated interventions similar to the ASMP and found comparable results. Taal et al. (1993) implemented a program designed using the ASMP as a model and found improvement in knowledge, self-efficacy, and the use of physical and relaxation exercises. Lindroth, Bauman, Brooks, and Priestley (1995) implemented a program similar to the ASMP in Australia and reevaluated participants at 12 months and five years. Improvement of knowledge, reduction of pain, and development of an internal locus of control persisted at the five-year follow-up.

The most prominent cognitive-behavioral aspect of these programs is relaxation training, but this particular intervention appears to be well accepted and may contribute to the positive outcomes of the interventions. Given the effectiveness and persistent effects of CBT programs for arthritis self-management, these programs, especially the thoroughly studied ASMP, are effective first-line interventions to help individuals with RA develop effective cognitive and behavioral coping skills.

## OUTCOME STUDIES

### Treatment Outcomes

CBT alone or with education has been demonstrated to decrease pain and helplessness while increasing self-efficacy. The outcomes of ASMP were presented in the previous section, thus this section focuses on other CBT programs. Overall, the evidence strongly supports the effectiveness of CBT for controlling the pain of rheumatoid arthritis, improving sleep, decreasing depressive symptoms, reducing disease activity and functional disability, increasing self-efficacy, and improving coping (Bradley et al., 1988; National Institutes of Health, 1996; O'Leary, Shoor, Lorig, & Holman, 1988). Some studies have demonstrated that treatment gains last for at least a year (Bradley et al., 1988; Goeppinger, Arthur, Baglioni, Brunk, & Brunner, 1989); however, O'Leary et al. found that treatment gains were not sustained at four months. Parker et al. (1995) found that treatment gains (decreased pain and helplessness as well as increased self-efficacy and coping) could be maintained by giving CBT treatment boosters every three months.

### Economic Outcomes

Attention to the economic outcomes of CBT for rheumatoid arthritis is needed to provide support for common use of these therapies. The economic impact of the disorder is significant, despite the limited prevalence of the disease. In the United States, direct medical costs for an individual with RA are estimated at $4,798 annually (Singh, Ramey, & Terry, 1997). Among individuals who are working when diagnosed, 60 percent to 70 percent experience work-related disability after five years, which results in loss of income and disability financial support (Callahan, 1998; Yelin, Meenan, Nevitt, & Epstein, 1980). Furthermore, individuals with RA have been found to earn only 50 percent of what their projected income would be without the disease (Meenan, Yelin, Nevitt, & Epstein, 1981).

Few studies have examined the socioeconomic impact of CBT, but the findings of these studies have been favorable. A study by Lorig and Holman (1993) examined outcomes four years after patients participated in the ASMP and found that outpatient clinic visits were reduced by 43 percent. This study also found that, while their program cost $54 per participant, it saved approximately $647 per participant by reducing physician visits. Similarly, Young, Bradley, and Turner (1995) found that a CBT program reduced outpatient clinic visits, inpatient hospital days, and the costs of outpatient and inpatient treatments. After the intervention, total RA-related expenses exclusive of medications were reduced by 54 percent in the CBT group, whereas expenses declined only 5 percent in the group that received social support and remained almost unchanged in the control group.

A meta-analysis conducted by Superio-Cabuslay, Ward, and Lorig (1996) compared educational and CBT intervention studies for RA to placebo-controlled trials of non-steroidal anti-inflammatory medications (NSAIDs). Comparing the effectiveness of education and NSAIDs, this analysis found that educational interventions were 25 percent as efficacious as NSAIDs for pain, 30 percent to 40 percent as efficacious for functional disability, and 60 percent to 80 percent as efficacious for tender-joint count. In a separate analysis, the researcher found that interventions that used CBT produced even larger effects on pain, functional disability, and tender-joint counts than did education alone. Although more evidence is needed, these studies provide strong support for the cost-effectiveness of cognitive-behavioral interventions for rheumatoid arthritis.

## CONCLUSION

Rheumatoid arthritis is a chronic, inflammatory, autoimmune disease found in 1 percent of the adult population worldwide, causing joint stiffness, joint swelling, and generalized fatigue. There is no available cure, and patients are faced with learning to manage the condition and painful periodic flares of symptoms. Standard medical treatment consists primarily of the use of nonsteroidal anti-inflammatory drugs. Self-regulation-oriented approaches can further reduce symptoms, improve functional capacity, and reduce negative cognitive patterns. The combination of education for disease management and cognitive-behavioral therapy has been shown to substantially reduce pain, improve sleep, and improve everyday functioning. The cognitive-behavioral therapy programs typically include relaxation training designed to reduce sympathetic nervous system activation, along with other cognitive interventions.

## REFERENCES

Affleck, G., Tennen, H., Urrows, S., & Higgins, P. (1992). Neuroticism and the pain-mood relation in rheumatoid arthritis: Insights from a prospective daily study. *Journal of Consulting and Clinical Psychology, 60*(1), 119–126.

Arnett, F. C., Edworthy, S. M., Bloch, D. A., McShane, D. J., Fries, J. F., Cooper, N. S., et al. (1988). The American Rheumatism Association 1987 revised criteria for the classification of rheumatoid arthritis. *Arthritis and Rheumatism, 31*(3), 315–324.

Baerwald, C. G., Panayi, G. S., & Lanchbury, J. S. (1997). Corticotropin releasing hormone promoter region polymorphisms in rheumatoid arthritis. *Journal of Rheumatology, 24*(1), 215–216.

Bandura, A. (1997). *Self-efficacy: The exercise of control.* New York: W. H. Freeman.

Bekkelund, S. I., Jorde, R., Husby, G., & Mellgren, S. I. (1996). Autonomic nervous system function in rheumatoid arthritis. A controlled study. *Journal of Rheumatology, 23*(10), 1710–1714.

Bradley, L. A., & Alberts, K. R. (1999). Psychological and behavioral approaches to pain management for patients with rheumatic disease. *Rheumatic Diseases Clinics of North America, 25*(1), 215–232, viii.

Bradley, L. A., Young, L. D., Anderson, K. O., Turner, R. A., Agudelo, C. A., McDaniel, L. K., et al. (1988). Effects of cognitive-behavioral therapy on rheumatoid arthritis pain behavior: One-year follow-up. In R. Dubner, G. F. Gebhart, & M. R. Bond (Eds.), *Proceedings of the Vth World Congress on Pain* (pp. 310–314). New York: Elsevier Science.

Broderick, J. E. (2000). Mind-body medicine in rheumatologic disease. *Rheumatic Diseases Clinics of North America, 26*(1), 161–176, xi.

Burr, R., Hamilton, P., Cowan, M., Buzaitis, A., Strasser, M. R., Sulkhanova, A., et al. (1994). Nycthemeral profile of nonspectral heart rate variability measures in women and men. Description of a normal sample and two sudden cardiac arrest subsamples. *Journal of Electrocardiology, 27*(Suppl.), 54–62.

Callahan, L. F. (1998). The burden of rheumatoid arthritis: Facts and figures. *Journal of Rheumatology, 25*(Suppl. 53), 8–12.

Callahan, L. F., Cordray, D. S., Wells, G., & Pincus, T. (1996). Formal education and five-year mortality in rheumatoid arthritis: Mediation by helplessness scale scores. *Arthritis and Rheumatism, 9*(6), 463–472.

Cutolo, M. (1999). Macrophages as effectors of the immunoendocrinologic interactions in autoimmune rheumatic diseases. *Annals of the New York Academy of Sciences, 876*, 32–41; discussion 41–32.

Da Silva, J. A. P., & Hall, G. M. (1992). The effects of gender and sex hormones on outcome in rheumatoid arthritis. *Bailliere's Clinical Rheumatology, 6*(1), 193–219.

Drewes, A. M. (1999). Pain and sleep disturbances with special reference to fibromyalgia and rheumatoid arthritis. *Rheumatology (Oxford), 38*(11), 1035–1038.

Fox, D. A. (2001). The role of T lymphocytes in rheumatoid arthritis. In G. S. Firestein, G. S. Panayi, & F. A. Wollheim (Eds.), *Rheumatoid arthritis* (pp. 89–100). London: Oxford University Press.

Goeppinger, J., Arthur, M. W., Baglioni, A. J., Jr., Brunk, S. E., & Brunner, C. M. (1989). A reexamination of the effectiveness of self-care education for persons with arthritis. *Arthritis and Rheumatism, 32*(6), 706–716.

Goldstein, R., Duff, S., & Karsh, J. (1987). Functional assessment and symptoms of rheumatoid arthritis in relation to menstrual cycle phase. *Journal of Rheumatology, 14*(2), 395–397.

Harris, E. D., Jr. (1986). Pathogenesis of rheumatoid arthritis. *American Journal of Medicine, 80*(4B), 4–10.

Hirsch, M., Carlander, B., Verge, M., Tafti, M., Anaya, J.-M., Billiard, M., et al. (1994). Objective and subjective sleep disturbances in patients with rheumatoid arthritis: A reappraisal. *Arthritis and Rheumatism, 37*(1), 41–49.

Hochberg, M. C., Chang, R. W., Dwosh, I., Lindsey, S., Pincus, T., & Wolfe, F. (1992). The American College of Rheumatology 1991 revised criteria for the classification of global functional status in rheumatoid arthritis. *Arthritis & Rheumatism, 35*(5), 498–502.

Keefe, F. J., & Bonk, V. (1999). Psychosocial assessment of pain in patients having rheumatic diseases. *Rheumatic Diseases Clinics of North America, 25*(1), 81–103.

Keefe, F. J., & Caldwell, D. S. (1997). Cognitive behavioral control of arthritis pain. *Medical Clinics of North America, 81*(1), 277–290.

Keefe, F. J., Dunsmore, J., & Burnett, R. (1992). Behavioral and cognitive-behavioral approaches to chronic pain: Recent advances and future directions. *Journal of Consulting and Clinical Psychology, 60*(4), 528–536.

Keefe, F. J., & Gil, K. M. (1986). Behavioral concepts in the analysis of chronic pain syndromes. *Journal of Consulting and Clinical Psychology, 54*(6), 776–783.

Keefe, F. J., Kashikar-Zuck, S., Robinson, E., Salley, A., Beaupre, P., Caldwell, D., et al. (1997). Pain coping strategies that predict patients' and spouses' ratings of patients' self-efficacy. *Pain, 73*(2), 191–199.

Keefe, F. J., & Van Horn, Y. (1993). Cognitive-behavioral treatment of rheumatoid arthritis pain: Maintaining treatment gains. *Arthritis Care and Research, 6*(4), 213–222.

Latman, N. S. (1983). Relation of menstrual cycle phase to symptoms of rheumatoid arthritis. *American Journal of Medicine, 74*, 957–960.

Lefebvre, J. C., Keefe, F. J., Affleck, G., Raezer, L. B., Starr, K., Caldwell, D. S., et al. (1999). The relationship of arthritis self-efficacy to daily pain, daily mood, and daily pain coping in rheumatoid arthritis patients. *Pain, 80*(1, 2), 425–435.

Lindroth, Y., Bauman, A., Brooks, P. M., & Priestley, D. (1995). A 5-year follow-up of a controlled trial of an arthritis education programme. *British Journal of Rheumatology, 34,* 647–652.

Lorig, K. (1986). Development and dissemination of an arthritis patient education course. *Family and Community Health, 9*(1), 23–32.

Lorig, K., & Holman, H. (1993). Arthritis self-management studies: A twelve-year review. *Health Education Quarterly, 20*(1), 17–28.

Lorig, K., Konkol, L., & Gonzalez, V. (1987). Arthritis patient education: A review of the literature. *Patient Education and Counseling, 10*(3), 207–252.

Masi, A. T., Feigenbaum, S. L., & Chatterton, R. T. (1995). Hormonal and pregnancy relationships to rheumatoid arthritis: Convergent effects with immunologic and microvascular systems [Review]. *Seminars in Arthritis & Rheumatism, 25*(1), 1–27.

Meenan, R. F., Yelin, E. H., Nevitt, M., & Epstein, W. V. (1981). The impact of chronic disease: A sociomedical profile of rheumatoid arthritis. *Arthritis and Rheumatism, 24*(3), 544–549.

Moldofsky, H., Lue, F. A., & Smythe, H. A. (1983). Alpha EEG sleep and morning symptoms in rheumatoid arthritis. *Journal of Rheumatology, 10*(3), 373–379.

Myllykangas-Luosujarvi, I., Aho, K., Kautiainen, H., & Isomaki, H. (1995). Cardiovascular mortality in women with rheumatoid arthritis. *Journal of Rheumatology, 22,* 1065–1067.

National Institutes of Health. (1996). Integration of behavioral and relaxation approaches into the treatment of chronic pain and insomnia. NIH technology assessment panel on integration of behavioral and relaxation approaches into the treatment of chronic pain and insomnia. *Journal of the American Medical Association, 276*(4), 313–318.

Nicassio, P. M., Radojevic, V., Weisman, M. H., Culbertson, A. L., Lewis, C., & Clemmey, P. (1993). The role of helplessness in the response to disease modifying drugs in rheumatoid arthritis. *Journal of Rheumatology, 20*(7), 1114–1120.

O'Leary, A., Shoor, S., Lorig, K., & Holman, H. R. (1988). A cognitive-behavioral treatment for rheumatoid arthritis. *Health Psychology, 7*(6), 527–544.

Ostensen, M., Aune, B., & Husby, G. (1983). Effect of pregnancy and hormonal changes on the activity of rheumatoid arthritis. *Scandinavian Journal of Rheumatology, 12,* 69–72.

Parker, J. C., Smarr, K. L., Buckelew, S. P., Stucky-Ropp, R. C., Hewett, J. E., Johnson, J. C., et al. (1995). Effects of stress management on clinical outcomes in rheumatoid arthritis. *Arthritis and Rheumatism, 38*(12), 1807–1818.

Payne, L. C., & Krueger, J. M. (1992). Interactions of cytokines with the hypothalamus-pituitary axis. *Journal of Immunotherapy, 12*(3), 171–173.

Pincus, T., Griffith, J., Pearce, S., & Isenberg, D. (1996). Prevalence of self-reported depression in patients with rheumatoid arthritis. *British Journal of Rheumatology, 35,* 879–883.

Riemsma, R. P., Rasker, J. J., Taal, E., Griep, E. N., Wouters, J. M., & Wiegman, O. (1998). Fatigue in rheumatoid arthritis: The role of self-efficacy and problematic social support. *British Journal of Rheumatology, 37*(10), 1042–1046.

Silman, A. J. (1994). Epidemiology of rheumatoid arthritis. *Apmis, 102*(10), 721–728.

Singh, G., Ramey, D., & Terry, R. (1997). Direct costs of medical care in rheumatoid arthritis: Patterns and role of rheumatology care. *Arthritis and Rheumatism, 40*(9, Suppl.), S170.

Smarr, K. L., Parker, J. C., Wright, G. E., Stucky-Ropp, R. C., Buckelew, S. P., Hoffman, R. W., et al. (1997). The importance of enhancing self-efficacy in rheumatoid arthritis. *Arthritis Care and Research, 10*(1), 18–26.

Superio-Cabuslay, E., Ward, M. M., & Lorig, K. R. (1996). Patient education interventions in osteoarthritis and rheumatoid arthritis: A meta-analytic comparison with antiinflammatory drug treatment. *Arthritis Care and Research, 9*(4), 292–301.

Taal, E., Riemsma, R. P., Brus, H. L., Seydel, E. R., Rasker, J. J., & Wiegman, O. (1993). Group education for patients with rheumatoid arthritis. *Patient Education and Counseling, 20*, 177–187.

Weyand, C. M. (2000). New insights into the pathogenesis of rheumatoid arthritis. *Rheumatology (Oxford), 39*(Suppl. 1), 3–8.

Wolfe, F., Hawley, D. J., & Wilson, K. (1996). The prevalence and meaning of fatigue in rheumatic disease. *Journal of Rheumatology, 23*(8), 1407–1417.

Yelin, E., Meenan, R., Nevitt, M., & Epstein, W. (1980). Work disability in rheumatoid arthritis: Effects of disease, social, and work factors. *Annals of Internal Medicine, 93*(4), 551–556.

Young, L. D., Bradley, L. A., & Turner, R. A. (1995). Decreases in health care resource utilization in patients with rheumatoid arthritis following a cognitive behavioral intervention. *Biofeedback & Self-Regulation, 20*(3), 259–268.

Zanelli, E., Breedveld, F. C., & de Vries, R. R. (2000). HLA association with autoimmune disease: A failure to protect? *Rheumatology (Oxford), 39*(10), 1060–1066.

# CHAPTER 30

# Premenstrual Syndrome and Premenstrual Dysphoric Disorder

## ANNABAKER GARBER

**Abstract:** Premenstrual syndrome and premenstrual dysphoric disorder affect up to 80 percent of women by causing physical, psychological, and social disturbances. This chapter reviews the symptomatology of these disorders and introduces effective mind-body treatments, including dietary changes, nutritional supplements, and a comprehensive program of cognitive and stress management training.

## PROFILE OF THE DISORDERS

Premenstrual syndrome (PMS) refers to the mild to moderate symptoms that occur in the luteal phase of the menstrual cycle (Korzekwa & Steiner, 1997; Pearlstein & Stone, 1998). The time between ovulation and menstruation is called the luteal phase. The time between the end of menstruation and ovulation is the follicular phase. Usually, the follicular phase is defined as day 7 to day 11 *after* flow begins. (The first day of the period is day 1.) The late luteal phase is usually defined as day 6 to day 2 *before* menstrual flow begins (Korzekwa & Steiner, 1997). Common symptoms include irritability, mood swings, increased appetite with food cravings, fatigue, breast tenderness, bloating, difficulty concentrating, avoidance of social activities, changes in sleep, or headaches (Kessel, 2000; Pearlstein & Stone,

1998). In one study, women with PMS identified irritability, backaches or muscle pain, and bloating as the symptoms experienced most often as severe or extreme (Deuster, Adera, & South-Paul, 1999).

Premenstrual dysphoric disorder (PMDD) is a severe form of PMS characterized by significant functional impairment and a significant mood component (Korzekwa & Steiner, 1997; Ling, 2000; Pearlstein & Stone, 1998). Between 3 percent and 8 percent of women experience the severe symptoms of PMDD (Korzekwa & Steiner, 1997; Pearlstein & Stone, 1998).

Patterns of symptom activity may vary (Ling, 2000). Symptoms begin some time after ovulation and during the luteal phase. For some women, symptoms end early in the menstrual flow. For others, symptoms last through the duration of the flow. Some women also experience a brief period of symptoms during ovulation. However, in all cases, there is a symptom-free period during the follicular phase.

PMS and PMDD are likely to be influenced by a host of physiological, psychological, cultural, and social factors (Kessel, 2000). In a population-based study, Deuster et al. (1999) found that PMS was more prevalent in blacks, in women younger than 34 years old, and in women whose menses lasted longer than six days. Women whose menarche was before 10 years old had a much higher incidence of PMS than women who started menstruation after 13 years. Women with a body mass index greater than 27 kg/m$^2$ were almost twice as likely to suffer from PMS. In addition, Deuster's study found that perception of stress is one of the primary factors associated with PMS. Woods, Lentz, Mitchell, Heitkemper, et al. (1998) also found that women with PMS had a higher correlation between perception of stress and symptom activity.

## SCREENING QUESTIONS AND DIAGNOSTIC ASSESSMENT

PMDD is a diagnostic classification in the *Diagnostic and Statistical Manual of Mental Disorders (DSM-IV;* American Psychiatric Association, 1994), replacing the late luteal phase dysphoric disorder in the *DSM-III-R.* As shown in Box 30.1, the *DSM-IV* specifies that the chief complaints must include irritability, tension, dysphoria, or lability of mood and 5 of 11 possible symptoms, and that symptoms are missing before or during ovulation and in the follicular phase (see also Korzekwa & Steiner, 1997; Pearlstein & Stone, 1998; Steiner, 2000). To meet the diagnostic criteria, the symptoms must be documented in a daily log over two menstrual periods. As shown in Box 30.2, for diagnosis of PMS, the *International Statistical Classification of Diseases and Related*

*Health Problems (ICD-10;* World Health Organization, 1996) requires a history of only one symptom occurring in a cyclic fashion (see also Kessel, 2000; Ling, 2000).

Because of the difficulty in recalling a symptom pattern, the patient must keep a rating scale, diary, or log to identify the symptom pattern (Kessel, 2000; Pearlstein & Stone, 1998; Steiner, 2000). Commonly used scales include the Menstrual Distress Questionnaire (Moos, 1969, 1991), Premenstrual Tension Scales (Steiner, Haskett, & Carroll, 1980), the Calendar of Premenstrual Experiences (COPE; Mortola, Girton, Beck, & Yen, 1990), and the Prospective Record of the Impact and Severity of Menstruation (PRISM; see Box 30.3). Each scale asks the patient to rate the severity of a number of symptoms over the course of the menstrual period. The total number of symptoms and the total severity can be scored. It has been suggested that there should be at least a 30 percent change in symptoms between the follicular and luteal phases to diagnose PMDD, regardless of the instrument (Kessel, 2000; Steiner, 2000).

Instead of a formalized scale, a patient can keep a log, rating her most prominent symptoms over her cycle (Ling, 2000). It is important to use a severity scale that the patient understands and then rate each symptom daily. A visual analog scale can also be used to track the symptom(s) of interest (Korzekwa & Steiner, 1997). In this way, a severity score can be obtained and changes over time will be documented. Any daily recording should also include a description of medications and concurrent life events, which can have a major influence on symptom activity (Korzekwa & Steiner, 1997).

It is important to assess symptoms during the entire menstrual cycle, especially to document the absence of symptoms during the follicular phase. Symptoms present during the follicular phase may be indicative of a chronic disorder, such as anemia, thyroid disease,

---

**Box 30.1**    Diagnosis of Premenstrual Dysphoric Disorder (PMDD)

A. In most menstrual cycles during the past year, five (or more) of the following symptoms were present for most of the time during the last week of the luteal phase, began to remit within a few days after the onset of the follicular phase, and were absent in the week postmenses, with at least one of the symptoms being either 1, 2, 3, or 4:

1. Markedly depressed mood, feelings of hopelessness, or self-deprecating thoughts.
2. Marked anxiety, tension, feelings of being "keyed up" or "on edge."
3. Marked affective lability (e.g., feeling suddenly sad or tearful or increased sensitivity to rejection).
4. Persistent and marked anger or irritability or increased interpersonal conflicts.
5. Decreased interest in usual activities (e.g., work, school, friends, hobbies).
6. Subjective sense of difficulty in concentrating.
7. Lethargy, easy fatigability, or marked lack of energy.
8. Marked change in appetite, overeating, or specific food cravings.
9. Hypersomnia or insomnia.
10. A subjective sense of being overwhelmed or out of control.
11. Other physical symptoms, such as breast tenderness or swelling, headaches, joint or muscle pain, a sensation of "bloating," weight gain.

B. The disturbance markedly interferes with work or school or with usual social activities and relationships with others (e.g., avoidance of social activities, decreased productivity and efficiency at work or school).

C. The disturbance is not merely an exacerbation of the symptoms of another disorder, such as major depressive disorder, panic disorder, dysthymic disorder, or a personality disorder (although it may be superimposed on any of these disorders).

D. Criteria A, B, and C must be confirmed by prospective daily ratings during at least two consecutive symptomatic cycles. (The diagnosis may be made provisionally prior to this confirmation.)

---

SOURCE: American Psychiatric Association (1994).

---

hypoglycemia, or autoimmune disorders (Korzekwa & Steiner, 1997; Pearlstein & Stone, 1998; Steiner, 2000). Gynecological factors such as perimenopausal symptoms, postpartum status, irregular cycles, polycystic disease, and endometriosis can also have overlapping symptoms with PMS or PMDD (Korzekwa & Steiner, 1997). The menstrual cycle can exacerbate migraines, asthma, rheumatoid arthritis, irritable bowel syndrome, diabetes, psychiatric disorders, seizures, systemic lupus erythematosus, anemia, and endometriosis (Case & Reid, 1998; Ling, 2000; Sigmon et al., 2000).

A psychosocial or psychiatric interview should include a history of depression,

---

**Box 30.2     Diagnosis of Premenstrual Syndrome (PMS)**

A. Does not meet DSM-IV criteria for PMDD but does meet ICD-10 criteria for PMS.

B. Symptoms occur only in the luteal phase, peak shortly before menses, and cease with menstrual flow or soon after.

C. Presence of one or more of the following symptoms:
1. Mild psychological discomfort.
2. Bloating or weight gain.
3. Breast tenderness.
4. Swelling of hands or feet.
5. Aches and pains.
6. Poor concentration.
7. Sleep disturbance.
8. Change in appetite.

SOURCE: World Health Organization (1996). Adapted from Ling (2000).

---

**Box 30.3     Symptoms Listed in the PRISM Assessment Tool**

| | |
|---|---|
| Irritability | Bowels, constipated or loose |
| Fatigue | Appetite, up or down |
| Inward anger | Drive, up or down |
| Labile mood (crying) | Chills/sweats |
| Depressed | Headaches |
| Restless | Craving, sweet or salt |
| Anxious | Feel unattractive |
| Insomnia | Guilty |
| Lack of control | Unreasonable behavior |
| Edema or tight rings | Low self-image |
| Breast tenderness | Nausea |
| Abdominal bloating | Menstrual cramps |

SOURCE: Reid (1985). Adapted from Ling (2000).

---

hypomania or mania, anxiety, panic, eating and personality disorders, and alcohol and drug abuse (Korzekwa & Steiner, 1997). Approximately 45 percent to 70 percent of women with PMDD also have had an episode of major depression (Altshuler, Hendrick, & Parry, 1995; Pearlstein et al., 1990). Women with anxiety disorders, including panic attack (Sigmon et al., 2000), agorophobia, and social phobia may experience increases in their symptoms premenstrually (Pearlstein & Stone, 1998).

PMDD and depression are thought to be different entities, although they may be found concurrently. Differences in PMDD and depression include distinct circadian rhythms of cortisol and pharmacological responses. PMDD responds to selective serotonin reuptake inhibitors (SSRIs) but not tricyclic antidepressants. Depression responds to both types of drugs (Kessel, 2000; Korzekwa & Steiner, 1997).

## ANATOMY AND PHYSIOLOGY

Studies have failed to show differences between levels of estradiol and progesterone in patients with PMS and controls (Kessel, 2000; Korzekwa & Steiner, 1997). However, Woods and colleagues found a complex interrelationship among symptoms, ovarian hormones, cortisol, and catecholamines in women with PMS (Woods, Lentz, Mitchell, Heitkemper, et al., 1998; Woods, Lentz, Mitchell, Shaver, & Heitkemper, 1998). It appears that normal ovarian function sets off a complex chain of events that can trigger an abnormal psychoneuroendocrine response (Korzekwa & Steiner, 1997). Two hypotheses are that the central nervous system metabolism of sex steroids may be different in patients with PMS or that the sensitivity of central nervous system neurotransmitters to sex steroids may be different in patients with PMDD (Kessel, 2000).

The research efforts of Kessel (2000) and Korzekwa and Steiner (1997) have identified the neurohormonal basis of PMS and PMDD, focusing on the serotonin system. Both researchers found much evidence for the interrelationship between serotonin, estradiol, and progesterone. Women with PMDD were found to respond differently to various pharmacological challenges to the serotonin system. Further, although depression, anxiety, and PMDD are different

disorders, the researchers found that all three disorders share many features that have been linked to serotonin disregulation, and SSRIs were shown to be a useful, therapeutic tool for PMDD. All these observations point to a central role for serotonin.

Rapkin et al. (1997) suggest that women with PMS or PMDD may have a difference in the metabolism of progesterone. Progesterone is metabolized into allopregnanolone and pregnenolone. Both these metabolites interact with the gamma-aminobutyric acid A (GABA-A). Allopregnanolone enhances GABA-A and tends to reduce anxiety. A deficiency of allopregnanolone may produce a predisposition toward anxiety. Pregnenolone, on the other hand, appears to antagonize GABA-A and promote anxiety. Rapkin hypothesizes that women with PMS may process progesterone differently to produce either a deficiency of the metabolite that reduces anxiety or too much metabolite that increases anxiety.

## PHARMACOLOGICAL TREATMENTS

Pharmacological treatment for PMS and PMDD deserves mention. For severe symptoms of PMS and PMDD, selective serotonin reuptake inhibitors have been shown to be effective. SSRIs interact with allopregnanolone, independently from their effect on serotonin receptors (Steiner & Pearlstein, 2000). This may explain why SSRIs are effective for PMDD and tricyclic antidepressants are not. In a meta-analysis of 15 randomized controlled studies, Dimmock, Wyatt, Jones, and O'Brien (2000) concluded that SSRIs were effective in treating physical and behavioral symptoms. There was no significant difference between continuous and intermittent dosing. However, discontinuation of medication due to side effects is a significant problem.

---

**Box 30.4    Alternative Therapies for PMDD**

In Chapter 27, the authors introduced a specialized neurofeedback training protocol for depression. Research reveals that many depressed patients show a pattern of relatively greater activation of the right frontal cortex and lower activation of the left frontal cortex. The asymmetry protocol calls for training the depressed individual to "reverse this pathological asymmetry." One of the authors of Chapter 27, Elsa Baehr, has applied this asymmetry protocol to 75 women with PMDD and reported improvements in mood (Baehr, 2001). Baehr applied asymmetry training in combination with several other therapies to treat PMDD. She used electromagnetic stimulation and audiovisual stimulation, experimental neurotherapy procedures aimed at "entraining" the cortex to a different dominant frequency. She also included cognitive therapy, light therapy, and nutritional supplements such as tryptophan, calcium, vitamins B6 and B12, omega 3, and gamma-aminobutyric acid (GABA). This is an interesting experimental approach integrating several alternative therapies. Further research is necessary to document the efficacy of the overall approach and to measure the relative contribution of the various components in the protocol to the overall therapeutic effect. [Editor's note]

---

SOURCE: Baehr (2001).

---

## LIFESTYLE AND BEHAVIORAL TREATMENT PROTOCOLS AND OUTCOME STUDIES

Once serious gynecological, endocrine, or psychiatric conditions have been ruled out, lifestyle and behavioral programs can begin (Korzekwa & Steiner, 1997; Steiner & Born, 2000). Behavioral treatments or programs that have been shown to be effective include daily charting of symptoms, dietary changes, exercise, and self-management training, including cognitive therapy and stress management. Box 30.4 describes an alternative-therapies approach for PMDD.

As in the behavioral treatment of any other disorder, daily charting is useful to both the clinician and the patient. It provides a record that is not dependent on long-term recall, which can serve as a basis for charting changes over time. A daily record of self-observation is a crucial way to get the patient involved in her treatment. It provides a sense of self-awareness and self-efficacy.

Dietary recommendations include reducing salt, caffeine, and alcohol, especially in the luteal phase (Korzekwa & Steiner, 1997; Steiner, 2000). Salt reduction may affect the tendency to retain water, which contributes to edema. Caffeine and alcohol worsen irritability and sleep disturbances. Small, frequent, carbohydrate-rich meals may also be helpful (Sayegh et al., 1995). In women with PMS, 1,000 to 1,200 mg per day of calcium carbonate (e.g., Tums EX) significantly reduced total symptoms within three months compared with placebo in a randomized, controlled, double-blind study. Symptoms of negative affect, water retention, food cravings, and pain were reduced significantly (Thys-Jacobs, Starkey, Bernstein, & Tian, 1998). Other supplements that may be useful include vitamin E, vitamin B6, magnesium, and tryptophan (Korzekwa & Steiner, 1997; Pearlstein & Steiner, 2000; Steiner & Born, 2000). In a meta-analysis of nine studies, Wyatt, Dimmock, Jones, and Shaughn O'Brien (1999) found an overall odds ratio in favor of a benefit from vitamin B6, although no dose response curve could be identified. The dosage in the studies was 50 to 100 mg per day.

Exercise as a treatment has not been tested in a well-controlled study. However, it is often recommended in the popular literature. Women who exercise regularly report fewer physical and psychological symptoms across the whole menstrual cycle (Aganoff & Boyle, 1994). It also appears that regular exercise is related to a decrease in PMS symptoms (Steege & Blumenthal, 1993). Certainly, regular exercise has been associated with a host of salutary benefits, and these may include an improved mood.

Cognitive therapy, either alone or as part of a comprehensive self-management program, has been shown to improve severe PMS symptoms significantly (Blake, Salkovskis, Gath, Day, & Garrod, 1998; C. A. Morse, Dennerstein, Farrell, & Varnavides, 1991; G. Morse, 1999; Taylor, 1999). In a study with a treatment group (*n* = 40) and a waiting-list control (*n* = 51), Taylor offered a comprehensive treatment program to a group of women with severe PMS symptoms. The treatment consisted of self-monitoring, behavioral and cognitive stress reduction techniques, time and role management techniques, interpersonal competency training, diet, exercise, and vitamin supplementation. Individualized plans were developed for each subject, depending on professional guidance and personal choice. Treatment was conducted by a nurse-facilitator and delivered in a group setting, 10 to 15 women in each group, meeting for three hours weekly over four consecutive weeks. The subjects were expected to practice exercises, maintain a symptom record, and do weekly homework assignments. Measures of PMS symptom type and severity using the Menstrual Symptom Severity List, personal demands using the Symptom Checklist–90, and personal resources using eight different questionnaires were taken at two baseline points and 3, 6, 12, and 18 months postbaseline. The scores of

depression and well-being for the participants at baseline were well above the cutoff for depression, reflecting the distress of the subjects. Using repeated measures on the treatment subjects, this program reduced PMS severity by 75 percent, reduced depression and general distress by 30 percent to 54 percent, and increased well-being by 22 percent and self-esteem by 14 percent over the 18 months of follow-up. Most changes occurred within the 3-month follow-up period, and these changes were maintained at 18 months. The waiting-list controls showed no change in symptom activity or general distress while in the waiting period. This comprehensive program's outcomes compare favorably with drug treatment studies.

Blake et al. (1998) reported another waiting-list-controlled study looking at the effects of cognitive therapy only. The subjects (*n* = 11 in treatment; *n* = 12 on the waiting list) monitored symptoms using the Menstrual Distress Questionnaire (Moos, 1969, 1991) for two cycles. In addition, the subjects were assessed for anxiety, depression, personality, social adjustment, and marital status. Follow-up measures were obtained at two and four months after completing treatment. Treatment included 12 one-hour sessions conducted by a psychiatrist, focusing on identifying problems, precipitating and perpetuating factors, and attitudes. The subjects were asked to try new behaviors between sessions as homework and focus on specific problems or incidents. Attention was drawn to specific links between thoughts, feelings, behaviors, and physical symptoms and how changing thoughts or behaviors can lead to more helpful behavior. Subjects kept a log of "thought records" in relation to specific incidents and a diary of PMS symptoms. Treatment subjects showed significant improvement at two- and four-month follow-ups compared with waiting-list controls in depression, anxiety, global interference of symptoms, interference of symptoms in home life, and interference in general relationship with partners. Compared

---

**Box 30.5**    Components of Effective Nonpharmacological Treatment for PMS

A. Charting
   1. Daily log of symptom activity
B. Diet
   1. Reduction of salt, caffeine, alcohol
   2. Addition of calcium carbonate, vitamin B6
   3. Small, frequent meals of complex carbohydrates
C. Cognitive training
   1. Problem-solving
   2. Reframing
   3. Stress management
   4. Interpersonal competency
   5. Education about PMS
D. Exercise
   1. Moderate, regular aerobic exercise

---

SOURCE: Adapted from Steiner (2000).

---

with waiting-list subjects, there was a significant decrease in physical symptoms premenstrually. Treatment was associated with a progressive decrease of psychological symptoms premenstrually.

G. Morse (1999) conducted a waiting-list-controlled study using positive reframing, a type of cognitive therapy. Treatment included four two-hour sessions of education on PMS, diet, exercise, and stress reduction. Each session included the positive reframing component to change the subject's perceptions of the menstrual cycle experience. There were 17 subjects in treatment and 11 in the waiting-list group. There was a significant improvement in premenstrual symptoms in the control group over time, whereas the waiting-list group showed no improvement. There were no differences over time in anxiety or depression.

C. A. Morse et al. (1991) compared cognitive treatment with hormone treatment. Coping-skills training was provided over ten 90-minute sessions to a group of four subjects at a time (total $n = 16$). Training included understanding the link between thinking, feeling, and emotions, along with cognitive restructuring techniques, problem solving, and responsible assertiveness. As a control group, other subjects ($n = 12$) were taught relaxation training using Benson's method on audiotape. The hormone therapy group ($n = 14$) was given dydrogesterone, a synthetic progestin. At two months of treatment, the cognitive treatment group and the hormone therapy group showed significant improvement on both physical and psychological symptoms, whereas the relaxation group showed a worsening of symptoms. Two-thirds of the relaxation group dropped out of treatment and were dropped from analysis. Both the hormone therapy and cognitive treatment significantly improved physical symptoms. Cognitive treatment also improved psychological and anxiety symptoms. Gains were maintained at three-month follow-up.

Comprehensive programs, such as those recommended by Taylor (1999) or Steiner (2000), appear to be effective for women with mild to severe PMS. The components of these programs are summarized in Box 30.5.

## CONCLUSION

Premenstrual syndrome and premenstrual dysphoric disorder are common disorders that affect large numbers of women on a cyclic basis, disrupting their lives to varying degrees. The disorders are influenced by hormonal, physiological, psychological, cultural, and environmental factors. Medication treatment, primarily using SSRIs, can be helpful. Self-monitoring, diet, cognitive training, and exercise can assist many women in recovering some self-regulatory control over these conditions.

## REFERENCES

Aganoff, J. A., & Boyle, G. J. (1994). Aerobic exercise, mood states and menstrual cycle symptoms. *Journal of Psychosomatic Research, 38*(3), 183–192.

Altshuler, L. L., Hendrick, V., & Parry, B. (1995). Pharmacological management of premenstrual disorder. *Harvard Review of Psychiatry, 2*(5), 233–245.

American Psychiatric Association. (1994). *Diagnostic and statistical manual of mental disorders* (4th ed., *DSM-IV*). Washington, DC: Author.

Baehr, E. (2001, October 27–30) Premenstrual dysphoric disorder and changes in prefrontal alpha asymmetry. Conference abstracts (pp. 3–4). Monterey, CA: Society for Neuronal Regulation.

Blake, F., Salkovskis, P., Gath, D., Day, A., & Garrod, A. (1998). Cognitive therapy for premenstrual syndrome: a controlled trial. *Journal of Psychosomatic Research, 45*(4), 307–318.

Case, A. M., & Reid, R. L. (1998). Effects of the menstrual cycle on medical disorders. *Archives of Internal Medicine, 158*(13), 1405–1412.

Deuster, P. A., Adera, T., & South-Paul, J. (1999). Biological, social, and behavioral factors associated with premenstrual syndrome. *Archives of Family Medicine, 8*(2), 122–128.

Dimmock, P. W., Wyatt, K. M., Jones, P. W., & O'Brien, P. M. (2000). Efficacy of selective serotonin-reuptake inhibitors in premenstrual syndrome: A systematic review. *Lancet, 356*(9236), 1131–1136.

Kessel, B. (2000). Premenstrual syndrome. Advances in diagnosis and treatment. *Obstetric and Gynecologic Clinics of North America, 27*(3), 625–639.

Korzekwa, M. I., & Steiner, M. (1997). Premenstrual syndromes. *Clinical Obstetrics and Gynecology, 40*(3), 564–576.

Ling, F. W. (2000). Recognizing and treating premenstrual dysphoric disorder in the obstetric, gynecologic, and primary care practices. *Journal of Clinical Psychiatry, 61*(Suppl. 12), 9–16.

Moos, R. (1969). The development of a menstrual distress questionnaire. *Psychosomatic Medicine, 30*, 853–867.

Moos, R. (1991). *Menstrual distress questionnaire manual.* Los Angeles: Western Psychological Services.

Morse, C. A., Dennerstein, L., Farrell, E., & Varnavides, K. (1991). A comparison of hormone therapy, coping skills training, and relaxation for the relief of premenstrual syndrome. *Journal of Behavioral Medicine, 14*(5), 469–489.

Morse, G. (1999). Positively reframing perceptions of the menstrual cycle among women with premenstrual syndrome. *Journal of Obstetrical, Gynecological, and Neonatal Nursing, 28*(2), 165–174.

Mortola, J. F., Girton, L., Beck, L., & Yen, S. S. (1990). Diagnosis of premenstrual syndrome by a simple, prospective, and reliable instrument: The calendar of premenstrual experiences. *Obstetrics and Gynecology, 76*(2), 302–307.

Pearlstein, T., Frank, E., Rivera-Tovar, A., Thoft, J. S., Jacobs, E., & Mieczkowski, T. A. (1990). Prevalence of axis I and axis II disorders in women with late luteal phase dysphoric disorder. *Journal of Affective Disorders, 20*(2), 129–134.

Pearlstein, T., & Steiner, M. (2000). Non-antidepressant treatment of premenstrual syndrome. *Journal of Clinical Psychiatry, 61*(Suppl. 12), 22–27.

Pearlstein, T., & Stone, A. B. (1998). Premenstrual syndrome. *Psychiatric Clinics of North America, 21*(3), 577–590.

Rapkin, A. J., Morgan, M., Goldman, L., Brann, D. W., Simone, D., & Mahesh, V. B. (1997). Progesterone metabolite allopregnanolone in women with premenstrual syndrome. *Obstetrics and Gynecology, 90*(5), 709–714.

Reid, R. (1985). Premenstrual syndrome. *Current Problems in Obstetrics and Gynecology, 8,* 1–57.

Sayegh, R., Schiff, I., Wurtman, J., Spiers, P., McDermott, J., & Wurtman, R. (1995). The effect of a carbohydrate-rich beverage on mood, appetite, and cognitive function in women with premenstrual syndrome. *Obstetrics and Gynecology, 86*(4, Pt. 1), 520–528.

Sigmon, S. T., Dorhofer, D. M., Rohan, K. J., Hotovy, L. A., Boulard, N. E., & Fink, C. M. (2000). Psychophysiological, somatic, and affective changes across the menstrual cycle in women with panic disorder. *Journal of Consulting and Clinical Psychology, 68*(3), 425–431.

Steege, J. F., & Blumenthal, J. A. (1993). The effects of aerobic exercise on premenstrual symptoms in middle-aged women: a preliminary study. *Journal of Psychosomatic Research, 37*(2), 127–133.

Steiner, M. (2000). Premenstrual syndrome and premenstrual dysphoric disorder: guidelines for management. *Journal of Psychiatry and Neuroscience, 25*(5), 459–468.

Steiner, M., & Born, L. (2000). Diagnosis and treatment of premenstrual dysphoric disorder: an update. *International Clinical Psychopharmacology, 15*(Suppl. 3), S5–S17.

Steiner, M., Haskett, R. F., & Carroll, B. J. (1980). Premenstrual tension syndrome: The development of research diagnostic criteria and new rating scales. *Acta Psychiatrica Scandavica, 62*(2), 177–190.

Steiner, M., & Pearlstein, T. (2000). Premenstrual dysphoria and the serotonin system: Pathophysiology and treatment. *Journal of Clinical Psychiatry, 61*(Suppl. 12), 17–21.

Taylor, D. (1999). Effectiveness of professional-peer group treatment: symptom management for women with PMS. *Research in Nursing and Health, 22*(6), 496–511.

Thys-Jacobs, S., Starkey, P., Bernstein, D., & Tian, J. (1998). Calcium carbonate and the premenstrual syndrome: Effects on premenstrual and menstrual symptoms. Premenstrual syndrome study group. *American Journal of Obstetrics and Gynecology, 179*(2), 444–452.

Woods, N. F., Lentz, M. J., Mitchell, E. S., Heitkemper, M., Shaver, J., & Henker, R. (1998). Perceived stress, physiologic stress arousal, and premenstrual symptoms: Group differences and intra-individual patterns. *Research in Nursing and Health, 21*(6), 511–523.

Woods, N. F., Lentz, M. J., Mitchell, E. S., Shaver, J., & Heitkemper, M. (1998). Luteal phase ovarian steroids, stress arousal, premenses perceived stress, and premenstrual symptoms. *Research in Nursing and Health, 21*(2), 129–142.

World Health Organization. (1996). Mental, behavioral and developmental disorders. *International statistical classification of diseases and related health problems (ICD-10).* Geneva, Switzerland: Author.

Wyatt, K. M., Dimmock, P. W., Jones, P. W., & Shaughn O'Brien, P. M. (1999). Efficacy of vitamin B-6 in the treatment of premenstrual syndrome: Systematic review. *British Medical Journal, 318*(7195), 1375–1381.

# CHAPTER 31

# Caring for the Person
# With a Chronic Condition

SHARON WILLIAMS UTZ

**Abstract:** Chronic conditions represent the most prevalent health problems for all age groups in developed nations around the globe. In the United States, more than 90 million Americans are living with one or more chronic conditions. Several trends are likely to increase the prevalence of chronic illness in the future: longer life span, the aging of the population, survival of young and old with previously untreatable conditions, and technological medical advancements that prolong life. Because of these trends, large numbers of individuals will require health care providers who can give comprehensive care across the life span and across health care settings. Primary care clinicians are called on to provide optimal medical management considering the illness or disability while enhancing quality of life. A holistic approach is needed that (1) reflects understanding of the illness experience, (2) establishes a therapeutic partnership, (3) recognizes the tasks required of the chronically ill, (4) uses evidence-based practice guidelines while tailoring the treatment plan to the individual, (5) incorporates appropriate complementary therapies, (6) enhances self-care, and (7) monitors outcomes while continually refining therapeutic approaches. Each of these elements of quality care for the chronically ill is examined in this chapter.

## INTRODUCTION

Everyone who is born holds dual citizenship, in the kingdom of the well and in the kingdom of the sick. Although we all prefer to use only the good passport, sooner or later each of us is obliged, at least for a spell, to identify ourselves as citizens of that other place. (Sontag, 1978, p. 3)

As the quotation by writer Susan Sontag indicates, every human being experiences sickness sometime in life. For those with a chronic, noncurable illness, the "kingdom of the sick" becomes the place where they must dwell for an indefinite time. The care of those with chronic conditions is complex and challenging but ultimately satisfying to those primary care clinicians who do it well. The purpose of this chapter is to provide primary care clinicians with the insights and knowledge necessary to succeed in the challenging task of enhancing the lives of those with incurable conditions.

## PROFILE OF THE DISORDER

For purposes of this chapter, *chronic illness* is defined as a condition that

> is neither curable nor reversible; is of a long-term duration; requires ongoing contact, supervision and care over a long period of time; imposes new self-care requirements (e.g., monitoring condition, taking medications, performing treatments); potentially can affect the physical, emotional, socioeconomic, and spiritual well-being of the client and the client's family. (Eliopoulos, 1999, p. 17)

Chronic illnesses are the most prevalent health problems around the world (Institute for Health and Aging, 1996; Lubkin & Larson, 1998). In the United States, it is estimated that over 45 percent of noninstitutionalized Americans have one or more chronic conditions and that their direct health care costs account for three fourths of U.S. health care expenditures (Hoffman, Rice, & Sung, 1996). Although children with chronic conditions constitute a larger number than at any previous time in history, rates of chronic illness tend to rise with age; thus the vast majority of the chronically ill are older adults (Donnelly, 1993). Studies indicate people aged 60 years and older have on average 2.2 chronic conditions (Lorig, Sobel, et al., 1999). The most prevalent chronic conditions are arthritis, hypertension, heart disease, and pulmonary disease. Some chronic diseases such as diabetes, chronic obstructive pulmonary disease, and arthritis have increased during the last decade by 100 percent (Lorig, Stewart, et al., 1996). A number of trends make it likely that chronic illnesses and disability will continue to increase in the future: a longer life span, the aging of the population, survival of young and old with previously untreatable conditions, the sedentary lifestyle associated with economic development, and medical and technological treatments that prolong life (Eliopoulos, 1999; Lubkin & Larson, 1998).

Although chronic conditions are the most common health problems treated by health care providers, more often than not, the incentives within the health care system continue to support an acute care approach, focusing on an immediate solution to an acute problem (Etzwiler, 1997). The current chaotic health care nonsystem has not provided incentives for consistent management across settings or prevention of complications, nor has it created accessible, integrated care across settings—all elements required by those with chronic conditions (Thorne, 1993). Most often, individuals with complex chronic conditions receive "quick-fix solutions [that] usually fall far short of the fundamental changes needed to enhance long-term care" (Etzwiler, 1997, p. 569).

There are indications that the health care system is continuing to change because of rising costs and consumer demand. For example, costs continue to rise for the complex, technical care now being provided, while at the same time, consumer demand is increasing for health care that provides appropriate use of technology, effective medical management, and a caring presence (Eliopoulos, 1999). Consumers are increasingly knowledgeable about their health problems due to easy access to information from bookstores, libraries, and the Internet. Consumers are also "voting with their feet" by seeking health care from those who offer the caring approach missing in highly technical, medically focused care. Studies have shown that the use of complementary modalities in the United States (such as acupuncture, massage, or herbal remedies) as alternatives to Western medical therapies increased from 34 percent to 42 percent between 1990 and 1997 (Eisenberg et al., 1998; Westley, 2000). These findings reflect the fact that many individuals with chronic conditions wish to be involved in treatment decisions and seek care that is holistic—that is, care that respects their crucial role and establishes a partnership to find acceptable therapies. Another important finding of Eisenberg's study was that less than 40 percent of patients interviewed told their primary care clinicians about the alternative therapies they were using. Studies have shown that many patients with long-term chronic conditions become skilled in knowing what works for them and are resentful of health care providers who ignore and dismiss the knowledge they have gleaned from experience dealing with their own bodies (Thorne, Nyhlin, & Paterson, 2000). They seek care that considers the illness in the overall context of their life goals rather than making the illness the center of their lives (Eliopoulos, 1999).

## ASSESSMENT OF THE CHRONICALLY ILL

To deliver more effective and comprehensive care, primary care clinicians need to focus on goals appropriate to those with noncurable conditions, such as managing the disease, promoting the patient's own healing capacities, preventing complications, and achieving optimal quality of life and ultimately a peaceful and dignified death (Eliopoulos, 1999). In addition to these broad goals, Lorig, Sobel, et al. (1999) and Miller (2000) each proposed a set of common tasks that people with chronic conditions must master, such as diabetics learning to inject insulin (see Table 31.1).

While recognizing that there are unique tasks to particular diseases, primary care clinicians find these general lists of tasks useful as a broad framework for assessment or as a beginning checklist to identify overall needs of the person with a chronic condition. During the initial evaluation and subsequent follow-up visits, either list can provide a way of identifying the needs of each person as

well as help in identifying problem areas for more detailed assessment and intervention.

One of the key elements for successful assessment and management of a chronic illness is the establishment of a trusting relationship or therapeutic partnership between the clinician and patient (Brown, 2000). An extensive review of studies on patient participation in decision making concluded that the majority of patients want to be informed of treatment alternatives and participate in decisions about treatment (Guadagnoli & Ward, 1998). Primary care clinicians need to recognize that the person with the illness is truly in charge of her or his fate and that most chronic care is self-care (Lubkin & Larson, 1998). Given this reality, clinicians are only successful to the extent that they work *with* the person who has the illness to enhance self-care and therapeutic goals. The alternative is "mutual alienation in chronic illness care relationships if professionals are unable to value patient expertise" (Thorne, Nyhlin, & Paterson, 2000). As previously noted, studies of people with long-term conditions have shown that over the years of living with a chronic condition, patients often develop expertise in knowing their bodies and what works for them (Thorne, Nyhlin, & Paterson, 2000). Primary care clinicians also hold essential information from professional knowledge and training about the disease and options for care. To meet the challenges of a chronic illness, both professional and patient expertise are needed to arrive at the best solutions—solutions that are effective medically and are acceptable to the person with the illness. Box 31.1 summarizes the elements of a positive working relationship in the care of individuals with chronic illness.

The initial assessment lays the foundation for the therapeutic partnership essential to successful care of the person with a chronic illness. As noted, the initial evaluation should focus not only on the medical aspects of the

**Table 31.1**    Two Lists of Common Tasks for People with Chronic Conditions

| List 1[a] | List 2[b] |
|---|---|
| <ul><li>Recognizing and acting on symptoms</li><li>Using medication correctly</li><li>Managing emergencies</li><li>Maintaining nutrition and diet</li><li>Maintaining adequate exercise</li><li>Giving up smoking</li><li>Using stress reduction techniques</li><li>Interacting effectively with health care providers</li><li>Using community resources</li><li>Adapting to work</li><li>Managing relations with significant others</li><li>Managing psychological responses to illness</li></ul> | <ul><li>Maintaining a sense of normalcy</li><li>Modifying daily routine and/or adjusting lifestyle</li><li>Obtaining knowledge and skill for continuing self-care: maintaining a positive concept of self</li><li>Adjusting to altered social relationships</li><li>Grieving over losses concomitant with chronic illness</li><li>Dealing with role change</li><li>Handling physical discomfort</li><li>Complying with prescribed regimen</li><li>Confronting the inevitability of one's own death</li><li>Dealing with social stigma of illness or disability</li><li>Maintaining a feeling of being in control</li><li>Maintaining hope despite an uncertain or downward course of health</li></ul> |

SOURCES: a. Lorig, Sobel, et al. (1999, p. 6); b. Miller (2000, p. 29).

disease but also on the context of the person's life and how the illness impacts the person and the family (Kuyper & Wester, 1998). Several studies have shown the importance of eliciting the individual's cultural and personal perspectives about the illness, including the person's belief about what caused the illness, what it means to have this illness, and what treatments would be most effective (Kleinman, Eisenberg, & Good, 1978; Strain, 1996; Turner, 1996). Identifying the patient's beliefs from the outset can prevent miscommunications and problems that arise due to different beliefs by the health professional and the patient. The problem often termed "noncompliance" by clinicians reflects a tendency to blame the patient for problems such as not taking medications or not exercising. If the patient does not value the medication or believes that rest is needed rather than exercise, this problem of inadequate medical management and self-care cannot be solved.

In acknowledging the importance of cultural and individual perspectives to the success of chronic illness management, one

should note that the "partnership" approach is not appropriate in all cultures, with all individuals, or in all environments (Thorne & Paterson, 1998). Several studies have shown that individuals vary in their desire and/or ability to be involved in decisions about their health care and that this preference may vary at different times or settings (Guadagnoli & Ward, 1998). For example, Utz et al. (2001) found that many subjects undergoing invasive cardiovascular procedures did not wish to make decisions but preferred to put themselves in the hands of clinicians. To be effective, primary care clinicians need to be skillful in eliciting the preferences for each person's involvement in decisions. Clinicians can provide opportunities and education to promote self-care, while at the same time realizing that some individuals may find this burdensome either generally or during acute illness (Thorne & Paterson, 1998). In summary, "there is an onus on the part of nurses [caregivers] to understand the chronic illness from the patient's perspective. Only in doing so are

**Box 31.1**    Features of the New Paradigm of Health and Medical Care

The Client

- Is viewed as an autonomous individual who has an active role in health promotion and illness-related care
- Assumes responsibility for self-care, health promotion, and illness management
- Utilizes inner and external resources to promote wellness, manage illness, and heal
- Is seen as a dynamic member of other systems (e.g., family, community) that influence and are influenced by the client's health status

The Health Care Professional

- Promotes a relationship with the client in which they are partners in the achievement of health-related goals
- Appreciates the client's mind, body, and spirit as interrelated variables affecting health and illness and considers these variables in assessing, planning, delivering, and evaluating services to clients
- Values subjective data as a highly important adjunct to objective data in assessment and evaluation
- Utilizes natural, noninvasive techniques before employing aggressive, high-tech, or high-risk interventions
- Respects the client's self-healing capabilities, and strengthens and assists the client in healing
- Recognizes that the health care professional's self and energy play a part in the therapeutic relationship and uses these factors to facilitate the client's healing

SOURCE: Eliopoulos (1999, p. 3).

they likely to be trusted as carers [sic] and in turn to influence behaviour in constructive ways" (Price, 1996, p. 276).

## MEDICAL, BEHAVIORAL, AND PSYCHOSOCIAL INTERVENTIONS

Once a therapeutic relationship is established, primary care clinicians can begin to address the elements of the medical regimen that significantly affect the goals of managing the disease and enhancing healthy behaviors and self-care. Achieving these goals requires different kinds of clinical knowledge, yet they are both integral factors of attaining good health outcomes.

### *Principles of Medical Management for the Chronically Ill*

Specific approaches to medical management are unique to each disease and may involve medications, dietary prescriptions, use of splints, and so forth. Clinicians find the law of averages useful in understanding and predicting general patterns within specific disease entities, but they must balance scientifically based "norms" with the principles of human variation and diversity (Thorne, 1999). The principle of stepped care is emerging in the current literature as relevant to decisions by primary care clinicians caring for the chronically ill. The approach called individualized stepped care follows the principle that "simpler interventions

**Table 31.2**   Indicators of Disparities in Health Behavior Among Adults in the United States

| U.S. Population | Total | White | Black |
|---|---|---|---|
| Percentage who are obese | 16.6 | 15.6 | 26.4 |
| Percentage told they have high blood pressure | 23.0 | 23.0 | 30.9 |
| Percentage told they have diabetes | 4.8 | 4.4 | 7.6 |
| Percentage report no leisure-time physical activity | 28.0 | 25.1 | 38.2 |
| Percentage who report binge drinking | 14.4 | 14.3 | 8.7 |
| Percentage who smoke | 23.3 | 23.6 | 22.8 |
| Percentage who have no health care coverage | 12.0 | 10.8 | 16.4 |

SOURCE: Bolen, Rhodes, Powell-Griner, Bland, and Holtzman (2000).

are tried first, with more intensive interventions reserved for when a good outcome is not achieved" (Von Korff & Tiemens, 2000, p. 134). The "simpler" intervention is the one that is the least invasive in the patient's everyday life and the least costly and complex to administer. Stepped care recognizes that individuals require different levels of care, finding the right level depends on monitoring the results, and moving systematically from a lower-level to a higher-level intervention (while monitoring outcomes) enhances quality of life and is cost-effective (Von Korff & Tiemens, 2000). Successful stepped care requires continuity of the care provider's relationship and accurate records to document results of treatment approaches and self-care measures.

## Enhancing Healthy Behaviors and Self-Care

Much of the current literature on chronic illness emphasizes that daily health behaviors play a major role in both the causes and treatments of prevalent chronic conditions (Department of Health and Human Services, 2000; Lubkin & Larson, 1998). There is also increasing awareness that health behaviors contribute significantly to disparities in health status among various socioeconomic, racial and ethnic groups in the United States (Appel & Harrell, 2001; Department of Health and Human Services, 2000). Table 31.2 provides an example of indicators

of disparities in health behavior that relate directly to the development of chronic illness.

Primary care clinicians need to become skillful in helping individuals find ways to be successful at health behavior change. Daily health behaviors have profound effects on the development and management of chronic illnesses, yet behavior patterns such as smoking, a high-fat diet, and a sedentary lifestyle are very difficult to change. It is abundantly clear to clinicians that knowledge is necessary but not sufficient to bring about behavior change. Patient education can provide the foundational knowledge needed to make changes, and some individuals have the abilities and resources to move quickly to change behavior. Others require more time, more energy, more support, and/or more resources for successful change.

One of the most useful approaches to help clinicians enhance health behavior change is using the "stages of change" framework (Prochaska, DiClemente, & Norcross, 1992). Based on this approach, the clinician recognizes that individuals typically experience differing stages of readiness to change at various points in time. For example, when an individual is first diagnosed with asthma, he or she may initially be unable to take actions to quit smoking or use an inhaler but at another time be willing to do so. The stages that individuals typically experience are acknowledged to be nonlinear and cyclical but generally reflect the five stages in Box 31.2.

---

**Box 31.2**    Stages of Change

- Precontemplation
- Contemplation
- Preparation
- Action
- Maintenance

---

SOURCE: Prochaska, DiClemente, and Norcross (1992).

---

**Table 31.3**    Stages of Change in Which Particular Processes of Change Are Emphasized

| *Precontemplation* | *Contemplation* | *Preparation* | *Action* | *Maintenance* |
|---|---|---|---|---|
| Consciousness raising | | | | |
| Dramatic relief | | | | |
| Environmental reevaluation | | | | |
| | Self-reevaluation | | | |
| | | Self-liberation | | |
| | | | Reinforcement management | |
| | | | Helping relationships | |
| | | | Counterconditioning | |
| | | | Stimulus control | |

SOURCE: Prochaska, DiClemente, and Norcross (1992).

Given that an individual may be at a particular stage of willingness to change, the challenge to the clinician is to identify the level of readiness for change and approach the person in a way that enhances readiness. Tailoring interventions is important to capture the person's ability to move forward. Table 31.3 shows the various stages of change with examples of the kinds of interventions that clinicians might use to encourage behaviors to manage illness, promote health within illness, and improve self-care.

For example, if the person is in the precontemplation stage and insists that he is not ready to quit smoking, the goal of the clinician is to encourage the person to begin thinking about change and to keep the door open to future readiness. Techniques that may be successful include those shown in Table 31.3—consciousness raising, dramatic

relief, and environmental reevaluation (Cassidy, 1999; Prochaska, DiClemente, & Norcross, 1992). Clinicians could ask patients, "What would have to happen for you to know this is a problem?" or "Have you tried to change in the past?" (Zimmerman, Olsen, & Bosworth, 2000). Another technique is a visual aid called the "Readiness to Change Ruler," in which the clinician asks the patient to indicate where she or he is on a line that stretches between two poles of "not prepared to change" and "already changing" (see Figure 31.1). This visual experience can increase awareness and start the person down the road of thinking about change.

If the person is at the stage of contemplating change, the goal is to help him or her examine benefits and barriers to change and to begin exploring solutions for barriers. The

Changing Behavior for Your Health

On the line below, mark where you are now on this line that measures change in behavior. Are you not prepared to change, already changing, or someplace in the middle?

Not prepared to change                                        Already Changing

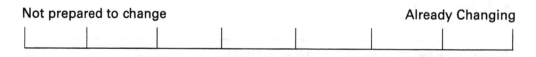

**Figure 31.1**    Readiness-to-Change Ruler

SOURCE: Zimmerman et al. (2000, p. 1413).

intervention of self-reevaluation is appropriate and could be encouraged by clinicians by asking, "What do you want to change at this time?" or "What might keep you from changing at this time?" (Zimmerman et al., 2000, p. 1413). As with all stages, preparation for change overlaps with contemplation, so approaches by the clinician may be similar in both and can emphasize the strategies previously described as well as self-liberation (Prochaska, DiClemente, & Norcross, 1992). The goal in this stage is to help the patient discover elements necessary for decisive action by encouraging these efforts, exploring strategies, and setting a date for change (Zimmerman et al., 2000).

The stages of action and maintenance require interventions that involve promoting skills in behavioral self-management. The goals during these stages are to help the patient take decisive action and to incorporate change into one's daily lifestyle (Zimmerman et al., 2000). Specific strategies, as shown in Table 31.3, include reinforcement management, helping relationships, counterconditioning, and stimulus control (Prochaska, DiClemente, & Norcross, 1992). As previously noted, a trusting therapeutic relationship is the foundation of all aspects of caring for those with chronic conditions. Once established, the ability to

empower the person to act on his or her own behalf is greatly enhanced. Given that a sense of powerlessness and feelings of uncertainty are frequently experienced by the chronically ill (Germino, Mishel, & Belyea, 2001; Miller, 2000), promoting empowerment is far from simple. Success at empowering individuals to act requires helping them experience success by skillful encouragement, goal setting, and self-reinforcement (Funnell et al., 1991). Individuals can learn to manage their own behavior by planning self-rewards—for example, deciding to keep a log of blood sugar levels for one week and then treating themselves to a movie. With counterconditioning, the person structures her or his experiences to encourage and support the desired behavior—for example, listening to music when taking a vigorous 30-minute walk. The strategy of stimulus control involves teaching the individual to structure the environment in ways that will enhance or stimulate the targeted healthy behavior, such as having tasty low-fat vegetables and fruits cut up and ready to eat as snacks instead of high-fat chips or candy. Another important intervention in the action and maintenance stages is promoting the use of social support. Studies have shown that individuals benefit enormously from support by others and often need help soliciting the right kind of support from significant others or organized groups (Beckerman & Northrop, 1996; Burks, 1999). From support groups, individuals can learn new problem-solving strategies as well as the hope of a better quality of life. An ongoing challenge that individuals face during this time is often referred to as relapse prevention. It is important that individuals understand that occasional relapses are "normal," are to be expected, and should not be interpreted as total failure. Individuals should be urged to consider this as a temporary slip and to resolve to return to healthy ways rather than to feel hopeless. Encouraging patients to use their support systems is one of the best strategies for overcoming relapse (Cassidy, 1999).

In summary, successful intervention by primary care clinicians requires attention to both the skillful management of the disease and the development of the person's abilities to engage in healthy self-care. By careful tailoring of interventions using a stepped-care approach to medical management and by using the stages of change model to address health behaviors, the goals of quality care and optimal quality of life can both be achieved.

## USE OF COMPLEMENTARY AND ALTERNATIVE THERAPIES

As previously mentioned, nearly half the population of the United States use alternative therapies without informing their primary care clinicians because they think it's unimportant or fear being criticized (Eisenberg et al., 1998). Individuals with chronic conditions are especially likely to use alternative therapies while searching for effective symptom management and/or cure. In recent years, the National Institutes of Health recognized the importance of such therapies by establishing a National Center for Complementary and Alternative Medicine (NCCAM) to

study them. The NCCAM has described complementary and alternative medicine (CAM) as "a broad range of healing philosophies (schools of thought), approaches, and therapies that mainstream Western (conventional) medicine does not commonly use, accept, study, understand, and make available" (National Center for Complementary and Alternative Medicine, 2000). Examples of alternative approaches include homeopathy, bioelectromagnetism, aromatherapy, reflexology, massage therapy, and acupuncture, to name a few.

### Encouraging Disclosure and Evaluation of Complementary Therapies

The principle that a trusting relationship forms the foundation of caring for individuals with chronic conditions is highly relevant if primary care clinicians are to determine and prescribe adequate therapies for those selecting CAM approaches. Clinicians should incorporate specific questions into the health history that will solicit information about CAM therapies without implying criticism or judgment. One approach is a self-completed form that includes space for writing all treatments that are used, herbs or supplements taken, and what does and does not help (Westley, 2000). During the oral interview, clinicians can invite information by asking, "What do you do to maintain or improve your health?" (Westley, 2000, p. 224). Such matter-of-fact approaches can help create an atmosphere of acceptance, opening up the conversation about therapies while considering the conventional treatment being prescribed.

### OUTCOMES IN CHRONIC ILLNESS

Numerous studies on chronic illness have shown that there are common goals and tasks that challenge those with chronic, noncurable conditions (see Table 31.1). These goals and tasks can serve as a framework for clinicians to follow when evaluating the progress of individual patients, as well as for an entire population of patients. Clinicians can work with patients to prioritize the tasks and refer to the list of tasks at each office visit as a "checklist" for overall care. Such a framework is holistic, providing a comprehensive approach rather than merely evaluating one piece of the treatment plan (for example, "Did the medication work to decrease blood sugar?"). The stepped-care approaches and tailoring interventions require establishing individual outcomes or goals for successful therapy, while at the same time using the template of national standards and evidence-based clinical protocols. Nationally established evidence-based guidelines are available from the Web sites for the National Guideline Clearinghouse (http://www.guidelines.gov) and the Agency for Healthcare Research and Quality (http://www.ahrq.gov). In selecting interventions for individual patients, clinicians should keep in mind the evidence that patients who are most vulnerable—that is, members of lower socioeconomic groups and minority groups, and those in the highest and lowest age groups—benefit most from tailored interventions that are comprehensive in scope for multiproblem situations and address their individual needs (Mishel, 2001; Kingston & Smith, 1997).

## SUMMARY

Caring for persons with chronic conditions requires clinicians to develop a working relationship that honors the experience of the person while at the same time offering the best that conventional and complementary therapies can offer. This holistic approach helps the person meet the daily challenges, select effective therapies to manage the disease, and enhance healthy behaviors to meet life goals. Clinicians can use nationally established clinical protocols and guidelines readily available on the Internet and tailor recommended therapies using the principles of stepped care and outcome evaluation. Effective care of the chronically ill can best be achieved through a working relationship that empowers the person to be successful in the daily behaviors required for effective self-care. This empowering approach by clinicians recognizes the person's right to make choices while providing information, skill building, and support to promote behaviors that enhance health and quality of life and provide hope for the future.

## REFERENCES

Appel, S. J., & Harrell, J. S. (2001, February). *Racial and socio-economic differences in risk factors for cardiovascular disease among southern rural women.* Proceedings of the 15th Anniversary Conference of the Southern Nursing Research Society, Baltimore, MD.

Beckerman, A., & Northrop, C. (1996). Hope, chronic illness and the elderly. *Journal of Gerontological Nursing, 22*(5), 19–25.

Bolen, J. C., Rhodes, L., Powell-Griner, E. E., Bland, S. D., & Holtzman, D.(2000, March 24). State-specific prevalence of selected health behaviors, by race and ethnicity—Behavioral risk factor surveillance system, 1997. *Morbidity and Mortality Weekly Report, 49*(SS02), 1–60. Retrieved April 19, 2000, from http://www.cdc.gov/mmwr/preview/mmwrhtml/ss4902a1.htm

Brown, S. J. (2000). Direct clinical practice. In A. Hamric, J. Spross, & C. Hanson (Eds.), *Advanced nursing practice* (2nd ed. pp. 137–182). Philadelphia: Saunders.

Burks, K. J. (1999). A nursing practice model for chronic illness. *Rehabilitation Nursing, 24*(5), 197–200.

Cassidy, C. A. (1999). Using the transtheoretical model to facilitate behavior change in patients with chronic illness. *Journal of the American Academy of Nurse Practitioners, 7*(11), 281–287.

Department of Health and Human Services. (2000). *Healthy people 2010* (Conference edition in two volumes). Washington, DC: Author.

Donnelly, G. F., (1993). Chronicity: Concept and reality. *Holistic Nursing Practice, 8*(1), 1–7.

Eisenberg, D. M., Davis, R. B., Ettner, S. L., Appel, S., Wilkey, S., Van Rompay, M., et al. (1998). Trends in alternative medicine use in the United States, 1990–1997: Results of a follow-up national survey. *Journal of the American Medical Association, 280*(18), 1569–1575.

Eliopoulos, C., (1999). *Integrating conventional alternative therapies: Holistic care for chronic conditions.* St. Louis, MO: Mosby.

Etzwiler, D. D. (1997). Chronic care: A need in search of a system. *The Diabetes Educator, 23*(5), 569–573.

Funnell, M. M., Anderson, R. M., Arnold, M. S., Barr, P. A., Donnelly, M., Johnson, P. D., et al. (1991). Empowerment: An idea whose time has come in diabetes education. *The Diabetes Educator, 17*(1), 37–41.

Germino, B. B., Mishel, M. H., & Belyea, M. (2001, February). *Moderators of an uncertainty management intervention for family care providers of men with early stage prostate cancer.* Proceedings of the 15th Anniversary Conference of the Southern Nursing Research Society, Baltimore, MD.

Guadagnoli, E., & Ward, P. (1998). Patient participation in decision-making. *Social Science Medicine, 47*(3), 329–339.

Hoffman, C., Rice, D., & Sung, H. (1996). Persons with chronic conditions: Their prevalence and costs. *Journal of the American Medical Association, 276*(18), 1473–1479.

Institute for Health and Aging. (1996). *Chronic care in America: A 21st century challenge.* Princeton, NJ: The Robert Wood Johnson Foundation.

Kingston, R. S., & Smith, J. P. (1997). Socioeconomic status and racial and ethnic differences in functional status associated with chronic diseases. *American Journal of Public Health, 87*(5), 805–810.

Kleinman, A., Eisenberg, L., & Good, B. (1978). Culture, illness, and care: Clinical lessons from anthropologic and cross-cultural research. *Annals of Internal Medicine, 88,* 251–258.

Kuyper, M. B., & Wester, F. (1998). In the shadow: The impact of chronic illness on the patient's partner. *Qualitative Health Research, 8*(2), 237–253.

Lorig, K. R., Sobel, D. S., Stewart, A. L., Brown, B. W., Bandura, A., Ritter, P., et al. (1999). Evidence suggesting that a chronic disease self-management program can improve health status while reducing hospitalization: A randomized trial. *Medical Care, 37*(1), 5–14.

Lorig, K. R., Stewart, A. L., Ritter, P., Gonzalez, V., Laurent, D., & Lynch, J. (1996). *Outcome measures for health education and other health care interventions.* Thousand Oaks, CA: Sage.

Lubkin, I. M., & Larson, P. D. (1998). *Chronic illness: Impact and interventions* (4th ed.). Sudbury, MA: Jones & Bartlett.

Miller, J. F. (2000). *Coping with chronic illness: Overcoming powerlessness* (3rd ed.). Philadelphia: Davis.

Mishel, M. H. (2001, February). *How to improve who benefits from an intervention: The use of moderator effects.* Proceedings of the 15th Anniversary Conference of the Southern Nursing Research Society, Baltimore, MD.

National Center for Complementary and Alternative Medicine. (2000, June). *General information about CAM and the NCCAM* (Publication No. 3008). Retrieved August 2000 from http://nccam.nih.gov/an/general

Price, B. (1996). Illness careers: the chronic illness experience. *Journal of Advanced Nursing, 24*(2), 275–279.

Prochaska, J. O., DiClemente, C. C., & Norcross, J. C. (1992). In search of how people change. *American Psychologist, 47,* 1102–1114.

Sontag, S. (1978). *Illness as a metaphor.* New York: Vintage Books.

Strain, L. A. (1996). Lay explanations of chronic illness in later life. *Journal of Aging and Health, 8*(1), 3–26.

Thorne, S. E. (1993). *Negotiating health care: The social context of chronic illness.* Newbury Park, CA: Sage.

Thorne, S. E. (1999). The science of meaning in chronic illness. *International Journal of Nursing Studies, 36,* 397–404.

Thorne, S. E., Nyhlin, K. T., & Paterson, B. L. (2000). Attitudes toward patient expertise in chronic illness. *International Journal of Nursing Studies, 37,* 303–311.

Thorne, S., & Paterson, B. (1998). Shifting images of chronic illness. *Image—The Journal of Nursing Scholarship, 30*(2), 173–178.

Turner, D. C. (1996). The role of culture in chronic illness. *American Behavioral Scientist, 39*(6), 717–728.

Utz, S. W., Padgett, L., Blank, M., Guarini, J., Morton, S., Wilson, J., et al. (2001). Comparisons of specific illness beliefs of rural and urban blacks and whites. *Southern On-Line Journal of Nursing Research, 2* (7), www.snrs.org.

Von Korff, M., & Tiemens, B. (2000). Individualized stepped care of chronic illness. *West Journal of Medicine, 172,* 133–137.

Westley, C. J. (2000). What to say when your patients ask you about complementary and alternative medicine. *Lippincott's Case Management, 5*(6), 221–225.

Zimmerman, G. L., Olsen, C. G., Bosworth, M. F. (2000). A "stages of change" approach to helping patients change behavior. *American Family Physician, 61*(5), 1409–1416.

# Part IV

# EDUCATION FOR
# MIND-BODY MEDICINE

# CHAPTER 32

# Medical Education for Mind-Body Medicine

## MARGARET DAVIES AND OLAFUR S. PALSSON

**Abstract:** An increasing number of medical educators are recognizing that medical schools do not adequately prepare physicians to manage the complex disorders of multifactorial origin that constitute the majority of problems seen in modern health care. Although education about psychosocial problems has been increased within the medical school curriculum, this does not translate into adoption of a biopsychosocial model of care in everyday medical practice. The authors identify key elements necessary for effective training in mind-body medicine and provide an example of how improvements in this important teaching area were accomplished at their institution.

## THE MIND-BODY GAP IN MEDICAL EDUCATION

After more than a century of resounding technological and pharmacological victories over infection and trauma, the remaining major challenge facing modern medicine in the Western world is the treatment and prevention of chronic disease of multifactorial origin and psychosomatic conditions. Three quarters of the U.S. health care budget currently goes toward care for chronic conditions such as heart disease, cancer, and diabetes (Hoffman, Rice, & Sung, 1996). Behavioral, social, and psychophysiological factors are recognized as contributing substantially to the etiology and prognosis of these and other chronic disorders.

Medical educators have in recent years become increasingly concerned that current medical education does not prepare future physicians to handle such complex and chronic varieties of illness. This was brought to the attention of the medical profession and medical schools in 1977 by Engels in his classic paper on the need to teach and adopt a comprehensive biopsychosocial approach rather than a purely biomedical one.

Despite the fact that this paper was widely read and promoted within the medical establishment, medical schools continue to graduate a majority of physicians who have been prepared to practice within a biomedical frame of reference, with little consideration for the mind-body connection. This is a matter for concern because it reduces the effectiveness of medical management for the majority of patients in the health care system. It is also a problem for the physicians themselves: Without adequate training in psychosocial and mind-body aspects of medicine, physicians are prone to frustration and feelings of impotence when attempting to manage the many chronic and psychosomatic patients that inevitably seek their care. Moreover, if they fail to address patients' problems, physicians must subsequently deal with dissatisfied patients and families.

Undoubtedly, reasons other than shortcomings in medical education contribute to the failure of physicians to address in practice the important behavioral and mental factors contributing to physical health problems. These other obstacles include (1) the structure of the U.S. health care system, which has made access to psychophysiological treatment difficult for many patients and has traditionally separated mental health care from biomedicine; and (2) the ever increasing pressures of physicians to do more in less time, especially in primary care (Palsson & Davies, 1999).

Many physicians have voiced the opinion, however, that medical schools still contribute to the perpetuation of the narrow biomedical focus of medical practice and have argued that this problem can only be resolved through changes in medical education. If physicians are to embrace psychosocial and mind-body methods of care, medical schools must lead the way by training physicians differently. In response to these concerns, the education of medical students has been strengthened nationwide in psychosocial areas. Medical schools now incorporate didactic material about psychotherapy and various mind-body therapies into their curriculum and educate their students about psychosocial problems that affect health. However, evidence is accumulating that these efforts have had limited impact on the ability of physicians to use this learning in their treatment of complex psychosocial problems (Mann et al., 1996; Merrill, Laux, & Thornby, 1990; Reid and Glasser, 1997; Staropoli, Moulton, & Cyr, 1997).

Based on our experience and observations as medical educators, we believe that the reasons for the discrepancy between medical education and practice are twofold. First, psychosocial issues are generally not taught in a way that makes them relevant to the rest of the medical curriculum, and second, the education of physicians typically does not include the learning of skills or pragmatic knowledge relating to mind-body interventions.

## ESTABLISHING THE PHYSICAL AND MEDICAL RELEVANCE OF THE MIND

Although the relationship between mind and body receives repeated mention in the education of most physicians, its physiological reality is rarely discussed or explained. In our teaching experience, we have found that senior medical students, residents, and sometimes even medical school faculty are often surprised by the revelation that the influences of the mind on the body have clearly delineated anatomical and physiological pathways (from the brain's cortex through the limbic system and out to the body via the hypothalamus) that are no more mysterious than those governing respiration or renal functioning. An outdated Cartesian dualism continues to be promoted unknowingly in medical schools by the omission of psychophysiology in the teaching of psychosocial influences on health. Students have difficulty seeing the mind as relevant to physical health because no conceptual link is provided between the two.

The isolation of the mind from the physical reality of health and illness is promoted further by the context within which mind-body medicine is presented within the medical school curriculum. Traditionally, education about mind-body therapies such as biofeedback, relaxation training, or hypnosis has primarily been in the domain of psychiatric lectures and courses. This gives many students the unfortunate impression that mind-body therapies are mostly relevant to psychopathology rather than to the average medical patient.

More recently, complementary and alternative medicine (CAM) has become a popular topic in society in general, and CAM is finding its way into medical school curricula. Mind-body medicine and mind-body interventions are classified by the National Center for Complementary and Alternative Medicine (2002), part of the National Institutes of Health, as one category of alternative medicine. Accordingly, mind-body treatments are now increasingly placed within alternative or complementary medicine curriculum components, along with methods such as acupuncture, herbal medicine, and homeopathy. Although broadening the scope of medical education by incorporating alternative medicine is a positive development, mind-body medicine is probably ill served by being placed in the teaching category of alternatives to regular medical care. It obscures the fact that the mind is no less a part of the patient than the arms or legs and is contrary to the aim of making the consideration of a patient's mental and psychophysiological health a standard in mainstream medical practice rather than an alternative (which in medical practice generally means "use if conventional approaches fail").

To close the mind-body gap in medical education, mind-body teaching must be incorporated into the courses and topics that concern regular medical practice. In addition to didactic teaching, demonstrations and first-hand experiences of mind-body connection are also important to make its relevance to medicine apparent to students. Psychophysiological demonstrations with biofeedback equipment can be a potent educational tool to build solid mind-body bridges in the minds of medical students, demonstrating that cognitions and emotions reliably and measurably affect physical activity (Davies & Palsson, 1999). Once that conceptual bridge is built, students can understand—without having to abandon the skepticism and scientific reasoning of medicine—how emotions, such as those surrounding loss of a loved one, family conflict, domestic violence, and sexual abuse, can cause stress (sympathetic autonomic arousal), which in turn can produce or exacerbate illness through neural, endocrine, and immunological pathways.

## TEACHING PRACTICAL MIND-BODY SKILLS

Medical schools have typically failed to provide practical clinical knowledge of how physicians can help patients by using mind-body treatment methods and how to identify patients suited for referrals for specialized psychological and psychophysiological interventions. Generally, students have not had the opportunity to observe and try these treatment methods in hands-on experience, which is a critical part of learning any practical medical skill. It is unlikely, for example, that surgery would be practiced much in modern medicine if future physicians only heard about it in lectures, as is generally the case for mind-body therapies. Medical schools must impart practical treatment skills to future physicians beyond the use of pills and scalpels and teach the student reliable ways to influence the mediation of healthful and harmful effects of the mind on the body.

We believe that education on mind-body medicine in medical schools must include the following four elements to ensure that students graduate with the skills necessary for translating mind-body knowledge into medical practice:

1. Teach students that an ill patient seen for any reason is affected by her or his attitude toward the illness, which in turn is derived from her or his family background coupled with events before or surrounding the current illness.

2. Train students to detect and assess presenting problems in which psychosocial issues are likely to play a prominent role

3. Provide students with empirically based knowledge documenting which mind-body treatments are suitable, and teach them how to successfully refer patients for such treatment.

4. Train students in the basic skills of specific mind-body approaches that can be incorporated into physicians' everyday work, such as relaxation training and hypnosis.

## CLOSING THE MIND-BODY GAP IN MEDICAL EDUCATION: THE EXAMPLE OF EASTERN VIRGINIA MEDICAL SCHOOL

In 1992, a small team of faculty at Eastern Virginia Medical School set out to improve the psychosocial education of students at the school, under the direction of Dr. Margaret Davies. That year the team implemented a 20-hour course called "The Doctor—The Patient" designed to encourage and support first-year medical students in their personal and professional growth and increase their self-understanding of psychological issues. The course included a two-hour workshop on biofeedback and self-relaxation techniques (Davies & Wickramasekera, 1996).

In 1993, in the third-year family medicine clerkship, five standardized patient practice cases were added to enhance clinical interpersonal and psychosocial skills. Each student had to complete five structured encounters with highly trained actors who simulated specific medical problems. These interviews were videotaped, and students

received feedback and suggestions about their interviewing performance.

Analysis of the collective results of the videotaped encounters showed that in the two practice cases in which patients had purely biomedical presentations with no psychosocial problems, the students performed very well, not missing an accurate diagnosis and giving adequate management and treatment. In the other three cases, in which the simulated patients had significant underlying psychosocial problems, the students often ignored the contributing psychosocial factors and performed at a significantly lower level of effectiveness. We interpreted this discrepancy as students' inability to make practical use of their knowledge of the psychosocial aspects of medical problems. Therefore, we further increased the teaching time devoted to detection of psychosocial problems, with special attention to practical training and clarifying further the close relationship between mind and body.

In 1996, we added a lecture on somatization to the second-year pathophysiology course—a course traditionally limited to only a biomedical approach. This lecture, now taught annually, included a brief description of the more common presentations of somatization, followed by clinical examples emphasizing the importance of detecting and managing the psychological problem of somatization instead of taking a strictly pathophysiological approach.

In 1997, students were sent for half-day visits in groups of two or three to the Eastern Virginia Medical School Behavioral Medicine Clinic during their third-year clerkship. In the course of each academic year, all third-year students at the school completed this experience (approximately 100 students a year). In the course of their half-day visit, the following topics were covered:

1. The technology and methods used to apply biofeedback, and the clinical problems responsive to such treatment.

2. A group demonstration of biofeedback that typically included biological monitoring of skin temperature, skin conductance, heart rate, muscle tension, and brain-wave activity.

3. The nature of physiological stress and its effects on health and diseases.

4. Success rates and the nature of various behavioral medicine treatments

5. Completion of individual physiological stress profiles on each student, followed by individual interpretation of their psychophysiological reactivity.

In 1997, we offered a month-long fourth-year elective in behavioral medicine, in response to increasing student demand for more hands-on experience with mind-body medicine methods due to our previously instituted teaching components in this area. In this elective, students, working together with a clinical psychologist, assessed patients, helped make decisions about treatment, and had opportunities to conduct such therapies as biofeedback, relaxation training, hypnosis, and breathing exercises.

In 1998, in the third-year clerkship in family medicine, we created and implemented 15 interactive computer training modules focusing on some of the most common psychosocial problems of medical patients. These modules gave targeted training in five problem areas: depression, anxiety, domestic violence, somatization, and sexual abuse. We concluded that students had previously not been adequately trained in the effective diagnosis and management of these five problems. We also added specific lecture content to the curriculum in the first three academic years addressing these problems. The interactive training modules are on a Web site and easily accessible to the students, who can work on them from home with a borrowed laptop computer.

Each computer training module provides the case of a patient presenting a complaint.

Students are free to explore the case in as much detail as they want, through questions and corresponding answers from the patient's case history, the history of the present illness, past medical history, family history, psychosocial problems, relationships, health risk factors, review of systems, current medications, and the results of the physical examination. Then students must extract from this case material a working diagnosis, choose appropriate tests, and devise a management and treatment plan. The aim is for them to develop the ability to balance appropriately their psychosocial and biomedical perspective in assessment, treatment, and patient management. Students receive automated feedback on the first 10 modules so that they can learn and improve with each case. On the remaining 5 modules, they receive no feedback but are assigned a score that counts as 15 percent of their final grade.

In summary, we have introduced a substantial emphasis on mind-body medicine education at the Eastern Virginia Medical School over the past eight years. These changes have been made in several incremental steps, and we have come to recognize that this gradual pace is necessary for long-term success. Medical schools have highly structured and very condensed curricula and generally do not accommodate sudden major revisions or additions to the educational content or methods. We have been fortunate to obtain federal grant support to aid our efforts, without which our progress would certainly have been slower. However, we feel that our work has demonstrated that mind-body education can be enhanced substantially with persistence and dedication over time and the collaboration of a few medical school faculty.

Finally, we have also come to see, through trial and error along the way, that behavioral scientists and academic physicians must work hand in hand to accomplish effective mind-body teaching in medical schools. The behavioral educators have valuable psychological knowledge and mind-body techniques to teach the students, but the academic physicians have the crucial responsibility of being the ultimate role models for medical students to learn how to adopt a biopsychosocial model of patient care and incorporate it into their everyday work.

## REFERENCES

Davies, S. M., & Palsson, O. S. (1999). Building mind-body bridges in medical school: A model. *Biofeedback*, 27(1), 21–23.

Davies, S. M., & Wickramasekera, I. E. (1996). Enhancing the credibility of the applied psychophysiologic approach via a stress reduction program for medical students. *Biofeedback*, 24(1), 12–25.

Engels, G. L. (1977). The need for a new medical model: A challenge for biomedicine. *Science, 196*, 129–136.

Hoffman, C., Rice, D., & Sung, H-Y. (1996). Persons with chronic conditions: Their prevalence and costs. *Journal of the American Medical Association, 276*, 1473–1479.

Mann, B. D., Sachdeva, A. K., Nieman, L. Z., Nielan, B. A., Rovito, M. A., & Damsker, J. I. (1996). Teaching medical students by role-playing: A model for integrating psychosocial issues with disease management. *Journal of Cancer Education, 11*(2), 65–72.

Merrill, J. M., Laux, L. F., & Thornby, J. I. (1990). Why doctors have difficulty with sex histories. *Southern Medical Journal, 83*, 613–617.

National Center for Complementary and Alternative Medicine. (2002). *What is complementary and alternative medicine?* (NCCAM Publication No. D156). Retrieved May 31, 2002, from http://nccam.nih.gov/health/whatiscam/

Palsson, O. S., & Davies, T. C. (1999). Behavioral health providers and primary care: Innovative models for intervention and service delivery. *Biofeedback*, 27(1), 14–20.

Reid, S. A., & Glasser, M. (1997). Primary care physicians' recognition of an attitude toward physical violence. *Academic Medicine*, 72(1), 51–53.

Staropoli, C. A., Moulton, A. W., & Cyr, M. G. (1997). Primary care internal medicine training and women's health. *Journal of General Internal Medicine*, 12(2), 129–131.

# CHAPTER 33

# Nursing Education for Mind-Body Nursing

## DEBRA E. LYON AND ANN GILL TAYLOR

**Abstract:** Nursing science has historically advocated a holistic mind-body view of the patient and of the nurse-patient relationship. Although nursing education has, in the recent past, limited curricula to more conventional and mainstream patient care interventions, there is currently a rapid evolution in nursing education toward incorporating mind-body views into curricula in both undergraduate and graduate programs. The chapter examines current moves to broaden nursing practice and nursing education, specifically including mind-body medicine and evidence-based complementary and alternative therapies. Approaches appropriate for future nursing practice, including therapeutic touch, guided imagery, cognitive behavioral therapy, hypnotherapy, aromatherapy, and massage therapy are discussed.

## INTRODUCTION: HISTORICAL ASPECTS OF MIND-BODY APPROACHES IN NURSING

Nursing science has long promoted the principles of mind-body interaction. Beginning with Florence Nightingale (1820–1910), the first nurse to have a scientific background, a foundation was laid for the caring-healing consciousness of the nurse as a potentiator for mind-body-spirit unity (Watson, 1995). However, 20th-century nurses and physicians eschewed the concept of holistic health care for fear that it would impede the scientific process (Achterberg, 1985). The Cartesian approach became dominant, except within

the religious communities that educated women as nurses. In the late 20th century, however, mind-body integration reemerged as a significant paradigm in nursing discourse. Martha E. Rogers (1990), one of many nurses who theorized about the essence of nursing during the 1960s and 1970s, reemphasized the mind-body unity proposed by Nightingale. Rogers wrote that every person's body is considered an energy field that interacts with other energy fields and the global energy field. She refuted the Cartesian dualism that mind and body are separate and proposed a Science of Unitary Human Beings. Another prominent nursing theorist, Jean Watson (1994), proposed that nursing care

AUTHOR'S NOTE: This chapter was written with partial support from grants T32-AT-00052-01 and K-30-AT00060-01 from the National Center be based on a metaphysical and spiritual orientation that draws on Eastern philosophy.

Currently, many nurse researchers embrace the psychoneuroimmunological (PNI) paradigm to explain mind-body interactions. PNI proposes that relationships exist among stress, immunological impairment, and health outcomes. PNI studies have attempted to ascertain and define the extensive links among susceptibility to disease, stress, and the progression of disease (Lovejoy & Sisson, 1989). Intervention modalities in the PNI paradigm focus on decreasing stress by altering cognitive perception and/or modulating neuroendocrine and sympathetic reactivity (Robinson, Mathews, & Witek-Janusek, 2000).

## MIND-BODY PRINCIPLES IN NURSING EDUCATION

Although mind-body principles are a dominant theme of academic discourse, incorporating mind-body principles in traditional undergraduate and graduate education has been slowed by professional role restrictions and educational programs focused on meeting accreditation standards. In addition, state regulations often prohibit nurses from practicing selected complementary therapies without additional training and certification. However, as evidence-based data accumulate to support selected complementary modalities, changes in practice standards will likely include these modalities within diverse nursing practice specialties.

There have been several recent events that make it more likely that selected complementary and alternative therapies will become more integrated into nursing curricula and practice. In response to the societal trend toward acceptance and adoption of complementary and alternative medicine, the National League for Nursing recently listed ten trends to watch in nursing education (Heller, Oros, & Durney-Crowley, 2000). Alternative therapies and genetics were listed

as the fourth trend. In addition, the American Association of Colleges of Nursing adopted a standard explicitly requiring students of nursing to be aware of complementary modalities and the usefulness of evidence-based practices and products in promoting health, and the Joint Commission on Hospital Accreditation added standards specific to complementary and alternative modalities in the practice setting. The actions by these organizations help remove major barriers to successful education and practice of mind-body interventions.

At the advanced-practice level, there is growing emphasis in the practice-oriented nursing organizations for the integration of evidence-based mind-body interventions. In fact, in a survey of 266 schools of nursing— the Collaborative Curriculum Survey sponsored by the American Association of Colleges of Nursing (AACN) and the National Organization of Nurse Practitioner Faculty (NONPF)—more than 99 percent of surveyed schools reported that they either had a separate course on CAM (7.7 percent) or integrated CAM modalities in other nurse-practitioner courses (91.5 percent; Berlin, Harper, Werner, & Stennett, 2002). Consequently, the NONPF prepared guidelines for the curricular implications of integrating complementary and alternative modalities in nurse practitioner programs (Quinn, 2002). These changes are likely to further spur curricular development in mind-body modalities.

## REQUIRED KNOWLEDGE AND SKILLS

Preparation for mind-body modalities requires an independent attitude and a desire to expand the boundaries of one's nursing practice skills. Because much of the training in complementary and alternative therapy is available by continuing education courses and conferences, nurses at both the registered nurse (RN) level and at the advanced-practice level can obtain these skills outside traditional nursing education arenas. While the practice of nurses working in inpatient or outpatient settings may be limited by traditional boundaries, with continued education and certification, nurses can augment their traditional nursing practice skills to enhance clinical nursing care.

Therapies such as aromatherapy; guided imagery and other forms of visualization; massage; acupressure; music listening combined with vibrotactile, cutaneous stimulation; meditation; and other relaxation techniques have been within the domain of nursing practice and research since Nightingale's times. At the low-tech end of the spectrum, there is great demand by consumers for complementary practices and products to enhance health and healing, which has begun to influence mainstream health care delivery. Across the country, major health systems are seeking ways to provide the best of conventional Western medicine while offering evidence-based complementary therapies to their patients. Consequently, nursing education and practice is expanding to include the implications of the emerging evidence-based information from both the emerging field of complementary health care practices and products and genetic research while managing ethical conflicts and questions that might arise (Heller et al., 2000).

## CURRICULA AND PROGRAMS INCORPORATING MIND-BODY PRINCIPLES

The American Holistic Nurses' Association has published AHNA Standards of Holistic Nursing Practice, which form the basis for curricula in holistic nursing adopted by several universities (Dossey, Quinn, Frisch, & Guzzetta, 2000). The AHNA has also published a position statement on the role of nurses in the practice of complementary therapies (American Holistic Nurses' Association, 2001) and currently offers a four-phase certificate program, which typically takes 18 months to complete and includes a self-designed practicum. The certificate program is based on a foundation of holistic philosophy and nursing theory, and course work covers a range of topics, including nutrition and its effect on the immune system and beliefs about health and illness and the influences of these on the healing process. Approximately 4,000 nurses have completed one or more phases of the AHNA holistic nursing certificate program (Trossman, 1998).

The New York College of Health Professions is chartered by the Board of Regents of the University of the State of New York, and all its programs are registered with the New York State Education Department. Graduates of the holistic nursing program are eligible to sit for the national certification exam in oriental bodywork therapy established by the National Certification Commission for Acupuncture and Oriental Medicine. The master's program in nursing at Tennessee State University (2001), fully accredited by the National League for Nursing, offers a major concentration in holistic nursing as a specialty. Recently, the University of California at San Francisco (2001) was awarded a grant by the Department of Health and Human Resources to offer a program leading to certification as an adult health nurse practitioner with an integrated complementary healing focus. This novel curriculum will focus on the contribution of nursing to complementary healing in a primary care setting and includes studies in imagery, energy healing, relaxation therapies, and the use of herbs and other supplements.

Faculty at the University of Texas Medical Branch in Galveston, with grant support from the National Center for Complementary and Alternative Medicine (part of the National Institutes of Health), are designing for future dissemination a core curriculum in integrative health care in which nursing faculty are participating. The faculty will adapt components of the curriculum for nursing and allied health students, which will include mind-body modalities as cost-effective and safe therapies that must be taught in the nursing curriculum. Teaching about such evidenced-based therapies as relaxation response, meditation, hypnosis, biofeedback, and massage will lessen the conventionally perceived duality between mind and body modalities.

Several national centers offer training in mind-body modalities. For example, the Center for the Study of Complementary and Alternative Therapies at the University of Virginia (2001) offers an interdisciplinary research training program in which selected mind-body modalities are studied by both pre- and postdoctoral trainees interested in research in the emerging field of integrative health care. Trainees, including nurses, can focus on research related to mind-body modalities and complete a course in evidence-based complementary therapies that contains a component on mind-body modalities.

## EXAMPLES OF MIND-BODY INTERVENTIONS FOR INCLUSION IN NURSING EDUCATION AND TRAINING

### Imagery

Imagery, a cognitive intervention used to alleviate responses to noxious stimuli, can be defined as using one's imagination to create healing mental images that involve all the senses. The Iowa Nursing Interventions Classification defines imagery as the purposeful use of imagination to achieve relaxation and/or direct attention away from

undesirable sensations (McCloskey & Bulechek, 1996). Use of imagery has been recommended as an independent nursing intervention that uses psychoneuroimmunology principles. However, research examining the effects of imagery has yielded mixed results. One possible explanation for inconsistencies is that the ability to imagine may determine one's capacity to use imagery successfully. Two measurable factors have been suggested as possible correlates of imaging ability: the ability to generate mental images and absorption, a personality factor associated with the capacity for focused attention and mind-body awareness (Owens, Taylor, & DeGood, 1999).

Imagery as an intervention has many potential uses to reduce anxiety for nurses themselves. At the University of Hawaii, imagery is taught to nursing students to help them reduce anxiety, manage stress, and transfer psychomotor skill performance from the learning laboratory to the clinical setting (Contrades, 1991).

The literature reflects a number of terms, including *visualization* and *imagination*, to convey the concept of imagery. Authors use a number of modifiers to convey techniques and strategies used to apply imagery in practice, including *guided, interactive guided,* and *mental*. Widely used imagery techniques include Carl Simonton's imagery for wellness (Simonton, Mathews-Simonton, & Creighton, 1978), Jeanne Achterberg's (1985) healing imagery, Deirdre Brigham's Getting Well Program (Brigham, Davis, & Cameron-Sampey, 1994), and the Interactive Guided Imagery approach. For example, Interactive Guided Imagery is designed to help individuals connect with their deeper resources at the cognitive, affective, and somatic levels. (Chapter 10 describes autogenic training, which also draws heavily on visualization.) The Academy for Guided Imagery (AGI) educates practicing clinicians in their uses of imagery and imagery-related approaches to therapy and healing. AGI is an accredited postgraduate training provider for health professionals, including nurses, and has received approval from the California Board of Registered Nursing for its total program on continuing education for nurses.

## Cognitive-Behavioral Therapy

Nurses have used cognitive-behavioral techniques to decrease negative thinking in patients and to reduce anxiety in clinical situations. However, as a psychotherapeutic modality, cognitive-behavioral therapy requires extensive training and clinical supervision (Freeman & Reinecke, 1995). The National Association of Cognitive-Behavioral Therapists, which provides opportunities for national certification, requires a master's or doctoral degree in psychology, counseling, social work, or a related field (such as nursing) and three years of postgraduate supervision with course work in cognitive-behavioral ther-apy. In addition, prospective applicants for certification as cognitive-behavioral therapists must pass written and oral exams (National Association of Cognitive-Behavioral Therapists).

## Hypnosis

Registered nurses prepared at the basic level and those prepared for advanced practice may become certified in hypnosis or clinical hypnotherapy through 120 hours or more of formal education in hypnosis. To become a clinical hypnotherapist, 220 hours or more of formal education in hypnosis and clinical hypnotherapy are required. National certification is available through the American Council of Hypnotist Examiners, a national organization that has certified more than 9,000 hypnotherapists, including numerous health professionals. (Chapter 11 describes additional certification programs in hypnosis.)

## Aromatherapy

Aromatherapy is the use of essential oils for the improvement of physical/mental health and well-being. In the United States, aromatherapy is not a curricular offering in most schools of nursing, although training and education in aromatherapy are offered through continuing education programs. For instance, the Institute of Integrative Aromatherapy in Colorado and the Colorado Center for Healing Touch offer continuing education workshops that include holistic practitioner norms and techniques for integrating aromatherapy in a variety of health care settings. Also, the Australasian College of Herbal Studies in Lake Oswego, Oregon, offers comprehensive distance education and residential programs on aromatherapy approved by the California Board of Registered Nursing for continuing education units. In the United Kingdom, the prominent Oxford Brookes University offers a bachelor's degree in clinical aromatherapy for health care professionals.

## Massage Therapy

Nurses have used massage extensively in clinical settings in a variety of specialties to promote relaxation and to decrease stress. Massage has been shown to have calming effects on premature infants (Field, 1995; Wheeden et al., 1993), infants and children (Watson, 1999), women in labor and childbirth (Simkin, 1995), and medical patients in inpatient settings (Gauthier, 1999). Although the benefits of massage are among the most well supported by empirical data of any complementary modality, nursing education programs typically have not focused on the specifics of massage over the past three decades. Today, few nursing schools teach massage other than as a clinical skill to augment bathing and positioning patients in the inpatient setting. Nurses with a special interest in massage pursue additional training and certification through the National Certification Examination for Therapeutic Massage and Bodywork (2000). Certification as a massage therapist generally requires at least 500 in-class hours of formal training at an established school of massage. Although certification is necessary in some states to practice as a massage therapist, the clinical use of massage has been a traditional nursing care technique in many clinical settings.

## Therapeutic Touch and Healing Touch

Therapeutic touch and healing touch are forms of energy therapy. Therapeutic touch is mutual interaction that is thought to involve a transfer of energy from nurse to patient, with resultant changes in energy fields (Krieger, 1975). Therapeutic touch was developed by Dolores Krieger, Ph.D., RN, a professor at New York University, and Dora Kunz, a spiritual healer said to possess unusual abilities for perceiving what occurred energetically during the healing process (Leadbeater, 1967). Practitioners of therapeutic touch believe that keeping the body's energy in a balanced state is germane to maintaining health. The practitioner seeks to help the individual rebalance energy in the body by stimulating, unblocking, or dispersing it (Alternative Medicine Foundation, 2000).

## CONCLUSION

Nursing education has long-promoted the principles of mind-body interaction. Until recently, mind-body therapeutic modalities have been somewhat limited in conventional, highly technical inpatient hospital settings. However, as health care professionals and the general public alike renew their focus on therapies that complement conventional health care, more formal nursing education programs have begun to incorporate evidence-based mind-body modalities into the curriculum to ensure nurse preparation in these therapies. Thus it is likely that mind-body principles will receive greater emphasis in nursing education, and the least controversial among the complementary practices and products will be integrated into advanced practice nursing in a variety of settings. The American Association of Colleges of Nursing has made several recommendations to the White House Commission on Complementary and Alternative Medicine Policy (2001), including expanding the databases on mind-body interventions and on the emerging evidence of the efficacy of these interventions. These recommendations will do much to foster the integration of the mind-body therapies.

## REFERENCES

Achterberg, J. (1985). *Imagery in healing*. Boston: New Science Library.

American Holistic Nurses' Association. (2001). *AHNA position statement on the role of nurses in the practice of complementary and alternative therapies*. Flagstaff, AZ: Author.

Alternative Medicine Foundation. (2000). *Energy work. An alternative and complementary medicine resource guide*. Bethesda, MD: Author.

Berlin, L. E., Harper, D., Werner, K. E., & Stennett, J. (2002). *Master's level nurse practitioner educational programs: Findings from 2000-2001 collaborative curriculum survey*. Washington, DC: National Organization of Nurse Practitioner Faculty.

Brigham, D. D., Davis, A., & Cameron-Sampey, D. C. (1994). *Imagery for getting well: Clinical applications of behavioral medicine.* New York: Norton.

Contrades S. (1991). Guided imagery use in nursing education. *Journal of Holistic Nursing, 9*(2), 626–628.

Dossey, B. M., Quinn, J. A., Frisch, N. C., & Guzzetta, C. E. (2000). *AHNA standards of holistic nursing: Guidelines for caring and healing.* New York: Aspen.

Field, T. (1995). Massage therapy for infants and children. *Journal of Developmental Behavioral Pediatrics, 16*(2), 105.

Freeman, A., & Reinecke, M. (1995). Cognitive therapy. In A. Gurman & S. Messer (Eds.), *Essential psychotherapies* (pp. 182–225). New York: Guilford.

Gauthier, D. M. (1999). The healing potential of back massage. *Online Journal of Knowledge Synthesis for Nursing, 6*(5).

Heller, B. R., Oros, M. T., & Durney-Crowley, J. (2000). The future of nursing education. Ten trends to watch. *Nursing & Health Care Perspectives. 21*(1), 9–13.

Krieger, D. (1975). Therapeutic touch: The imprimatur of nursing. *American Journal of Nursing, 75*(5), 784–787.

Leadbeater, C. W. (1967). *The inner life* (4th ed., Vol. 2). Wheaton, IL: Theosophical Publishing House.

Lovejoy, N. C., & Sisson, R. (1989). Psychoneuroimmunology and AIDS. *Holist Nurse Practice, 3*(4), 1–15.

McCloskey, J., & Bulechek, G. (1996). Iowa nursing interventions classification [Classification term]. *Nursing interventions classification: Iowa intervention project* (2nd ed.). St. Louis, MO: Mosby-Year Book.

National Association of Cognitive-Behavioral Therapists. (n.d.). NACBT's applications and forms central. Retrieved June 14, 2002, from http://www.nacbt.org/applications.htm

National Certification Board for Therapeutic Massage and Bodywork. (2000). *Candidate handbook.* McLean, VA:Author.

New York College of Health Professions. (n.d.). Division of Holistic Health, Education, and Research. Retrieved June 14, 2002, from http://www.nycollege.edu/index.html

Owens, J. E., Taylor, A. G., & DeGood, D. (1999). Complementary and alternative therapies (CAT) and psychological factors: Toward an individual differences model of CAT uses and outcomes. *Journal of Alternative and Complementary Medicine, 5*(6), 529–541.

Quinn, A. A. (2002, April). Complementary/alternative modalities: Curriculum implications for nurse practitioners. In National Organization of Nurse Practitioner Faculty (Eds.), *Advanced nursing practice: Building curriculum for quality nurse practitioner education* (pp. 87–96). Washington, DC: Author.

Robinson, F. P., Mathews, H. L., & Witek-Janusek, L. (2000). Stress reduction and HIV disease: A review of intervention studies using a psychoneuroimmunology framework. *Journal of the Association of Nurses in AIDS Care, 11*(2), 87–96.

Rogers, M. E. (1990). Nursing: Science of unitary, irreducible, human beings: Update 1990. In E.A.M. Barrett (Ed.), *Visions of Rogers' science-based nursing* (pp. 5-11). New York: National League for Nursing.

Simkin, P. (1995). Reducing pain and enhancing progress in labor: A guide to non-pharmacologic methods for maternity caregivers. *Birth, 22*(3), 161–171.

Simonton, O. C., Mathews-Simonton, S., & Creighton, J. (1978). *Getting well again.* Los Angeles: Tarcher.

Tennessee State University. (2001, July 5). Master's program in nursing. Retrieved June 14, 2002, from http://www.tnstate.edu/nurs/MSN2.htm

Trossman, S. (1998). Holistic nursing: The goal is the whole person. *The American Nurse, 30*(5), 11.

University of California at San Francisco. (2001, June). Adult nurse practitioner: Integrated complementary healing. Retrieved June 14, 2002, from http://nurseweb.ucsf.edu/www/anpich.htm

University of Virginia Health System. (2001, February). Center for the study of complementary and alternative therapies. Retrieved June 14, 2002, from http://www.med.virginia.edu/cscat

Watson, J. (Ed.). (1994). *Applying the art and science of human caring*. New York: National League for Nursing.

Watson, J. (1995). Nursing's caring-healing paradigm as exemplar for alternative medicine? *Alternative Therapies in Health and Medicine, 1*(3), 64–69.

Watson, S. (1999). Using massage in the care of children. *Pediatric Nursing, 10*(10), 27–29.

Wheeden, A., Scafidi, F. A., Field, T., Ironson, G., Valdeon, C., & Bandstra, E. (1993). Massage effects on cocaine-exposed pre-term neonates. *Developmental Psychobiology, 14*(5), 318.

White House Commission on Complementary and Alternative Medicine Policy. (2001, February 23). Meeting on training, education, credentialing and licensing of CAM practice, Part 1. Retrieved June 14, 2002, from http://www.whc-camp.hhs.gov/meetings/transcript_022300.html

# The Professional Role and Education of Physician Assistants in Mind-Body Medicine

Robert W. Jarski

**Abstract:** Physician assistants are educated in the traditional medical mode but emphasizing primary care, and interviewing and communication skills. Approximately half of all physician assistants recommend and use mind-body approaches as complementary therapies, but these modalities are not systematically included in program curricula. With additional education in mind-body approaches to diagnosis and treatment, physician assistants appear especially suited to integrate mind-body modalities with conventional medical and surgical treatment options. The chapter introduces some practical tools for a new practice paradigm: (1) an educational model based on psychoneuroimmunology, relaxation training, patient empowerment, and the role of belief and placebo effects; and (2) specific mind-body educational components.

## APPROPRIATE EDUCATION AND TRAINING

Physician assistants (PAs) are health care professionals licensed to practice medicine with physician supervision. PAs are educated in a broad-based approach to primary care medicine that prepares them to practice in a variety of health care settings. They are employed in hospitals, HMOs, physicians' offices, nursing homes, military installations, correctional facilities, public health agencies, community clinics, VA medical centers, educational institutions, research centers, and the White House as well as inner-city, rural

health, and industrial clinics. PAs take medical histories, perform physical exams, order laboratory and imaging studies, counsel and advise patients, and diagnose and treat illnesses, including suturing minor wounds, setting fractures, and first-assisting in surgery. PAs have prescriptive authority in 47 states and the District of Columbia (Association of Physician Assistant Programs, 1999). As in the medical education model, most PA programs do not have formal, standardized curricula for teaching mind-body medicine and its various behavioral, physical, and herbal disciplines (Wetzel, Eisenberg, & Kaptchuk, 1998).

Since its inception, the American Academy of Physician Assistants (the formal PA professional organization) and PA educators have worked very closely with medical educators and medical professional organizations. In 1971, four years after the first PA class graduated from Duke University, a system for PA program accreditation was established through a joint effort of the American Medical Association, the American Academy of Family Physicians, the American Academy of Pediatrics, the American College of Physicians, and the American Society of Internal Medicine (Association of Physician Assistant Programs, 1999). Currently, all PA programs must be accredited by the Accreditation Review Commission on Education for the Physician Assistant (ARC-PA). The mission of ARC-PA is to set quality standards and accredit PA programs based on their classroom, laboratory, and library facilities; clinical affiliations; faculty qualifications; admissions procedures and policies; record keeping; and administration (Association of Physician Assistant Programs, 1999).

There are 129 accredited entry-level PA programs, 62 of which are master's degree programs that take two to three years to complete following preprofessional studies (for a list of and links to current programs, see American Academy of Physician Assistants, n.d.). Approximately 22 postgraduate PA programs offer degrees in specialties such as surgery, emergency medicine, and psychiatry and take between one and two years to complete. Currently, there are no nationwide standards for teaching mind-body medicine in the entry-level or graduate programs.

The general philosophy of PA education involves intensive preparation in primary care medicine in a biopsychosocial context that emphasizes clinical sciences rather than the basic sciences. On average, approximately 75 percent of the curriculum is devoted to the medical sciences and 124 contact hours to behavioral and social sciences that include bioethics, cross-cultural medicine, and death and dying (Hooker & Cawley, 1997).

Hallmarks of PA education include program curricula that are competency based, socially responsive, practical, and multidisciplinary. Although some of these factors are difficult to measure, most indicators have shown that PAs are cost-effective, less expensive to hire than physicians, spend more time with patients, and have a humanistic orientation to medical practice (Hooker & Cawley, 1997). For these reasons, PAs with proper preparation in mind-body medicine appear especially well prepared for integrating unconventional modalities into conventional medical/surgical care, and they tend to spend the time necessary to counsel patients regarding the risks and benefits of integrative treatment options.

## REQUIRED KNOWLEDGE AND SKILLS

As a requirement for certification, all graduates must complete the primary care essentials of the didactic and clinical curricula. In addition, all 50 states require for practice a satisfactory performance on the rigorous national certification exam administered by the National Commission on Certification of Physician Assistants (NCCPA). PAs must complete a cycle of recertification consisting of 100 hours of continuing medical education every two years and reexamination every six years. Whether PAs practice in primary or specialty care, primary care competency must be certified for licensure. There are certification and recertification exams in general surgery, but these exams are *in addition to* primary care certification and recertification. Presently there are no certifying examinations in mind-body or complementary medicine.

How does PA education differ from that of a physician? Medical or osteopathic education typically involves four years. The basic and clinical sciences are usually emphasized during the first two years and clinical rotations the second two years. PA education typically involves two to three years, with clinical sciences emphasized over the first half of the curriculum and clinical rotations the second half.

Do PA services differ from those of primary care physicians? A review of eight published studies have shown that 60 percent to 100 percent of the services provided by primary care physicians can be performed at the same level by PAs without consultation (Hooker & Cawley, 1997). It may be assumed that the competencies PAs require for integrating mind-body techniques into traditional practice do not differ to a large degree from those required by primary care physicians (see Chapter 32). However, because PAs usually spend more time with patients and are educated to provide increased patient education and counseling, PAs may have more opportunities to include mind-body options in developing therapeutic plans with patients.

Like medical education, PA curricula should include the systematic study of nontraditional therapies; this need is being met somewhat by approximately 64 percent of U.S. medical schools (Wetzel et al., 1998). A survey has provided evidence that nearly half of PAs use complementary medicine themselves and recommend some form of it to patients. However, 80 percent reported that their knowledge of and preparation for complementary medicine is "poor" or only "fair" (Houston, Bork, Price, Jordan, & Dake, 2001).

Increasing complementary medicine curricular content seems appropriate. However, some faculty may argue that the PA curriculum is already overcrowded and omitting the study of topics that have been deemed essential to the practice of primary care, such as diabetes, would be unacceptable. Although

patients with diabetes present very frequently to primary care PAs, approximately 42 percent of all patients may be expected to use complementary medicine (Eisenberg et al., 1998). Thus it would be unacceptable for PA knowledge and preparation about either diabetes or complementary medicine to be "poor" or only "fair," and room must be made in PA curricula for teaching complementary mind-body medicine.

Most PAs agree that complementary medicine is not merely a placebo. However, whether a modality is unconventional or conventional, it could serve patients well if it elicits a beneficial placebo effect and is safe (Brody, 2000). Potential problems regarding safety include (1) negative side effects, (2) patients withholding information about their use of mind-body interventions, and (3) misuse (e.g., overdosage and chronic use; Jarski, 2001). Primary care PAs should consult evidence-based references for treatment interactions and possible side effects, and as a means to facilitate patients' informed decisions.

Side effects can be systematically reported only when a clinician is familiar with the modality and aware that a patient is using it. Eisenberg et al. (1998) found that 72 percent of patients who use complementary medicine do not inform their conventional health care providers. In addition, more than 83 percent of individuals who use complementary medicine also use conventional therapies. For example, a patient may take St. John's wort (*Hypericum perforatum*) for mild depression in addition to prescribed digoxin for heart disease. This combination may decrease digoxin blood levels and produce digoxin toxicity on withdrawing the herb (Medical Economics Company, 2000). PAs familiar with both conventional and unconventional modalities should be alerted to possible problems when taking a medical history and reviewing patients' charts.

## OPTIMAL EDUCATIONAL MODELS

Because PAs are educated in traditional medical and surgical therapies with an additional emphasis on patient education, communication, and interviewing skills, those with the appropriate background and interest in mind-body approaches appear especially suited as integrative medical practitioners. This role involves adding mind-body approaches to conventional medical and surgical interventions with the goal of providing patients with viable treatment options. This empowers patients to intelligently select modalities that are compatible with their belief systems by offering the best evidence-based conventional and unconventional approaches. The safest, most efficacious, least toxic, and least costly modalities should be discussed and made available to patients.

The PA should serve as an information resource facilitating informed patient decisions. To do this, PAs must be educated in mind-body complementary approaches that include the breadth of behavioral, physical, and herbal modalities. Because new information about mind-body approaches is constantly evolving, effective education should include (1) a conceptual framework that serves as an enduring foundation and encompasses presently known facts; (2) evidence-based content that is likely to enhance current practice; and (3) skills in reading, interpreting, and evaluating new information so safe and effective modalities can be recommended and harmful ones avoided.

## PROBLEMS WITH PRESENT MIND-BODY EDUCATIONAL METHODS

More than half of all PA programs and U.S. medical schools include some instruction on topics related to mind-body therapies. However, within medical curricula that have been studied, mind-body topics were found to be nonstandardized and far from uniform in their content, duration, and placement in the curriculum (e.g., within psychiatry, family medicine, or internal medicine; Wetzel et al., 1998). Although not extensively studied, PA curricula appear to similarly lack standardized complementary medicine content.

Although the increased interest and curricular emphasis is gratifying, most programs include only a small sample of the numerous unconventional disciplines. This approach often lacks a unifying theme or conceptual framework and has several additional inherent problems: (1) It cannot possibly represent the range of mind-body approaches; (2) it does not equip practitioners as lifelong learners with the tools necessary for evaluating new information over a professional lifetime; (3) no practical model is taught for integrating mind-body modalities into conventional practice; and (4) the theoretical underpinnings and rationale that help students internalize mind-body approaches to diagnosis and treatment are routinely lacking. Students are generally not prepared to build bridges between Eastern and Western traditions or to justify the practical uses of mind-body approaches vis-à-vis modern science. Rather than being prepared to integrate complementary modalities, mind-body concepts may appear to lack relevance to medical practice in today's technological world.

The following section describes a conceptual model to help students integrate the range of mind-body content into practice. The section also describes specific curricular components that apply across medical specialties to patients with their unique family, social, occupational, and lifestyle interactions and their relationship to their disease or state of health.

## A CONCEPTUAL MODEL FOR MIND-BODY EDUCATION

The Oakland University Complementary Medicine and Wellness Program has developed a model of mind-body medicine that helps clinically oriented students structure a coherent and useful foundation from information that is evidence-based, interdisciplinary, and from conventional and unconventional orientations derived from Eastern and Western traditions. This model may be conceptualized as a table with four legs: (1) the principles of psychoneuroimmunology, (2) the health benefits of the relaxation response, (3) patient empowerment, and (4) placebo effects (Oakland University, 2001).

Psychoneuroimmunology (PNI) is the study of the body's integrated organ systems involved with health and disease behavior. It is often considered the science of the mind-body connection. The hormonal and nervous system effects of the relaxation response (Benson, Beary, & Carol, 1974) are the physiological opposite of those of the fight-or-flight response. The relaxation response controls excessive sympathetic nervous arousal and is the basis of many clinically useful stress management methods (see Chapter 10). Counseling and education regarding health care options empower patients by helping them incorporate PNI mechanisms, stress management, and other health-promoting strategies into their lifestyles. Patients become informed consumers able to make their own health care choices, while providers become information resources and partners in health maintenance. Using techniques and behaviors that are consistent with a patient's belief system helps maximize placebo effects that are frequently synergistic with other treatment modalities.

Those who enroll in the Oakland University Complementary Medicine and Wellness Program develop a new paradigm of health and disease by becoming knowledgeable about the scientific basis of mind-body phenomena and the potential benefits of the psychoimmune system. When health is conceptualized as merely the absence of disease, the practice model is the interventional "patch and fix" approach. The new paradigm conceives health as a dynamic movement toward realizing one's full physical, psychological, social, environmental, and spiritual potential. A clinician's mode of practice changes when the patient is seen as a developing "mind-body entity" that is not static but always striving to improve following disease or exposure to noxious physical and psychological conditions. For example, a record of normal physical and laboratory findings despite occasional headaches and an unfulfilling employment situation is not necessarily "healthy." But the cancer patient who experiences his or her full potential as an interactive family member while eating wholesome foods and exercising regularly can be a model for life's meaning.

Some PAs exposed to this educational model have expressed that they will "never see their patients the same way again." Others have indicated they will empower patients to choose more of their treatment options and provide them with more opportunities to "heal themselves" through behavioral and lifestyle methods when it is safe and efficacious to do so. To apply this new practice model, PAs should develop specific skills in (1) relaxation training, (2) counseling patients about mind-body or complementary medicine, and (3) facilitating health-promoting behavior and lifestyle modification.

## SPECIFIC COMPETENCIES FOR PRACTICING MIND-BODY MEDICINE

PAs practicing a mind-body approach to health and disease should be skilled in the specific competencies described in the following paragraphs. These competencies are subsumed under the four-legged-table conceptual model previously described and have been derived from articles published in the *Journal of the American Academy of Physician Assistants* (Jarski, 2001) and *Family Medicine* (Kligler, Gordon, Stuart, & Sierpina, 1999). The former reference provides some succinct and useful practice guidelines. Because it comprehensively lists knowledge, skills, and attitudes appropriate for family physicians as well as PAs, the latter reference should be consulted by PA program faculty as they develop future curricula and by practicing PAs for guidance in selecting continuing education materials and programs.

*1. Respecting and learning about the cultural, religious, and ethnic beliefs of patients.* It is also necessary to examine one's own core beliefs and values and how these may influence treatment recommendations. Biases should be recognized and thoughtfully evaluated using available evidence-based information regarding therapeutic safety and efficacy.

*2. Eliciting an accurate medical history that includes a patient's use or desire to use mind-body approaches.* Most patients do not inform their conventional health care providers about their use or interest in unconventional therapies (Eisenberg et al., 1998). Knowing this information will help the PA develop a constructive discussion about therapeutic options and promote a patient-centered approach to treatment. A nonjudgmental and nonthreatening query should be routinely included in the medical history; for example, "In addition to the health concerns we have discussed, are there any other treatments or approaches you would like to know about, are using, or would like to use?" This manner of inquiry shows the clinician's interest and astuteness

about mind-body treatment options and opens the door to further discussion.

*3. Becoming familiar with the most common known conventional and unconventional treatment interactions, both synergistic and potentially harmful.* The text by Jonas and Levin (1999) devotes an entire section to patient safety and the *PDR for Herbal Medicines* (Medical Economics Company, 2000) and contains an entire section on herb-drug interactions. These references are highly recommended for PAs.

*4. Critically evaluating information sources and reading on a regular basis the most current refereed articles pertaining to mind-body medicine and complementary therapies.* As research increases, primarily due to the National Institutes of Health's National Center for Complementary and Alternative Medicine (NCCAM), evidence-based assessments should be consulted. Alerts and advisories may be accessed free of charge from NCCAM's Web site, http://altmed.od.nih.gov/. In addition, http://www.cochranelibrary.com/ provides among the most rigorous evidence-based evaluations of both unconventional and conventional therapeutics, and PubMed, http://www.ncbi.nlm.nih.gov/entrez/query.fcgi, provides access to refereed medical literature catalogued by the National Library of Medicine.

Most popular media, including books, magazines, and the Internet, are notoriously unreliable. They are often major sources of misinformation about both conventional and unconventional modalities. Popular media are seldom useful for PAs except for assessing the magnitude of misinformation to which our patients are exposed (Jarski, 2001).

*5. Becoming skilled in evaluating clinical studies.* This involves, at a minimum, familiarity with using the principles of evidence-based medicine and recognizing the power and limitations of various study designs and biostatistics. Within the past few years, PA educators have recognized this, and research education is a program accreditation requirement. Two highly recommended succinct references are Blessing (2001) and Ballweg, Stolberg, and Sullivan (2002).

Selecting information published in refereed information sources and placing some degree of confidence in reviews by reputable authorities can guide clinicians attempting to evaluate new mind-body medical information. However, this approach is not sufficient and does not apply to most popular (mis)information that patients bring to their health care providers. Because of the errors that are inherent in the best review systems (Jarski, 1999) and the fact that most scientific information is statistically derived, only the research-savvy provider can properly educate patients and intelligently determine how group statistical information may be appropriate for the individual patient who has unique life circumstances, values, and interactions with a disease.

*6. Experiencing several forms of mind-body therapies that are potentially useful in one's own practice.* Examples include biofeedback, guided imagery, hypnosis, massage, and acupuncture. For both students and practicing PAs, there is no substitute for the knowledge gained by first-hand experience of the techniques they will discuss with or recommend to patients.

*7. Seeking out reliable alternative practitioners to whom patients can be referred for specialized therapies.* Scheduling an experiential session with several providers in the community will help the PA evaluate the quality of care provided and begin collaborative relationships that help ensure patients' access to quality care.

*8. Becoming familiar with legal issues, documentation, and reimbursement schedules regarding alternative therapies.*

*9. Electing continuing education courses in mind-body modalities that complement conventional care and provide opportunities for building on existing clinical skills.* Providers skilled in one or two areas of complementary medicine can better educate patients about some of the benefits, precautions, and contraindications of using unconventional therapeutic options as adjuncts to conventional practice (Kligler et al., 1999).

*10. Assisting patients to integrate mind-body techniques with conventional practices for maximal benefit.* Some mind-body interventions are clearly beneficial and supported by quality evidence-based data. Others have documented side effects that should be avoided. According to the first rule of practice, "do no harm," safety should be documented for any treatment, conventional or unconventional. If unconventional approaches are used to replace conventional ones, they should be tested through phases I, II, and III for safety and efficacy as required by the FDA. Many believe that patients have the right to use therapies that have not been proved effective but are not harmful. But at a minimum, safety should be documented through the equivalent of phase I FDA testing (Jarski, 2001).

## PROFESSIONAL ROLES

Many patients ask for advice regarding modalities that, to them, may hold promise but have no documented efficacy to validate their use. How can PAs help patients balance a sense of hope with reliable scientific information?

Hope is the feeling that a desired outcome is possible. Is there such a thing as "false hope," or holding out as possible desired outcomes that are unlikely? Ideally, medical information is based on information obtained from randomized, controlled clinical trials using large samples of subjects that represent the population to which a conclusion is to be generalized. Conclusions are made using inferential statistics and statistical tests that help decipher between-group differences. By design, study results do not necessarily apply to all subjects in a population where only a representative sample was tested. Yet clinicians are forced to make important decisions on individual patients based on group studies.

The exceptional patient may be the one out of one thousand about whom a clinician is attempting to make a decision based on what appears to be a good scientific study with a statistical $p$ value of .001, where the error rate is 1 in 1,000. Good practice is based on the art of healing and good scientific studies that have built-in (and disclosed) error rates (probabilities, or $p$ values). All study results, diagnoses, and prognoses are necessarily probability statements. Therefore, we can never predict with certainty the outcome for any given individual patient, and we must not (and in fact *cannot*) eliminate the possibility of an unexpected outcome. Hope is hope; statistically there is no such thing as "false hope" in the clinical setting. PAs should reinforce patients' efforts to achieve health and at the same time guide their enthusiasm toward interventions that have a high probability of efficacy.

PA education already prepares professionals with primary care knowledge and skills in conventional medicine and surgery. Patients will be best served when treatment options from the best of both worlds—conventional and unconventional—are made available to them. Future curricula should include additional education in evidence-based mind-body modalities. The array of treatment modes should be validated and reinforced through a conceptual model that has as its foundation the science of mind-body interactions, stress management training, and the principles of belief and placebo effects that are likely to augment practice and significantly benefit patients—and providers.

## REFERENCES

American Academy of Physician Assistants. (n.d.). Physician assistant programs. Retrieved June 14, 2002, from http://www.aapa.org/pgmlist.php3

Association of Physician Assistant Programs. (1999). *1999 Physician assistant programs directory* (17th ed.). Alexandria, VA: Author.

Ballweg, R., Stolberg, S., & Sullivan, E. M. (Eds.). (1999). Physician's assistant: A guide to clinical practice. Philadelphia: W. B. Saunders.

Benson, H. B., Beary, J. F., & Carol, M. P. (1974). The relaxation response. *Psychiatry, 37,* 37.

Blessing, J. D. (2001). *Physician assistant's guide to research and medical literature.* Philadelphia: F.A. Davis.

Brody, H. (2000). *The placebo response.* New York: Cliff Street Books.

Eisenberg, D. M., Davis, R. B., Ettner, S., Appel, S., Wilkey, S., Van Rompay, M., et al. (1998). Trends in alternative medicine use in the United States 1990–1998. *Journal of the American Medical Association, 280,* 1569–1575.

Hooker, R. S., & Cawley, J. F. (1997). *Physician assistants in American medicine.* New York: Churchill Livingstone.

Houston, E. A., Bork, C. E., Price, J. H., Jordan, T. R., & Dake, J. A. (2001). Physician assistants' perceptions and use of complementary and alternative medicine. *Journal of the American Academy of Physician Assistants, 14,* 29–34.

Jarski, R. W. (1999). Using the medical literature: Life-long learning skills. In R. Ballweg, E. M. Sullivan, & S. Stolberg (Eds.), *Physician assistant: A guide to clinical practice.* Philadelphia: W. B. Saunders.

Jarski, R. W. (2001). PAs are recommending and using CAM. *Journal of the American Academy of Physician Assistants, 14,* 29–34.

Jonas, W. B., & Levin, J. S. (1999). *Essentials of complementary and alternative medicine.* Philadelphia: Lippincott, Williams & Wilkins.

Kligler, B., Gordon, A., Stuart, M., & Sierpina, V. (1999). Suggested curriculum guidelines on complementary and alternative medicine: recommendations of the Society of Teachers of Family Medicine Group on Alternative Medicine. *Family Medicine, 32* (1), 30–33.

Medical Economics Company. (2000). *PDR for herbal medicines.* Montvale, NJ: Author.

Oakland University. (2001). *Oakland University Graduate Catalog 2001-2003.* Rochester, MI: Author.

Wetzel, M. S., Eisenberg, D. M., & Kaptchuk, T. J. (1998). Courses involving complementary and alternative medicine at U.S. medical schools. *Journal of the American Medical Association, 280,* 784–787.

# CHAPTER 35

# The Behavioral Health Provider in Mind-Body Medicine

RICHARD GEVIRTZ

**Abstract:** This chapter provides information on training models for behavioral health practitioners in mind-body medicine. The author focuses on the acquisition of skills in applied psychophysiology and biofeedback, which are especially relevant for primary care patients with mind-body problems. The chapter reviews training and educational options, necessary skill sets and knowledge, emerging professional roles, innovative practice models, and currently available certification and credentialing pathways.

## THE NEED FOR BEHAVIORAL HEALTH PROVIDERS IN PRIMARY CARE

It has long been recognized that more than 40 percent of patient visits to primary care physicians are related to mind-body disorders. There is a growing awareness of the need for practitioners who are trained to effectively manage this subpopulation of the general medical practice. These patients are known to overuse the heath care system, and new opportunities are emerging for behavioral health providers.

Training models for practitioners in behavioral health have been varied and interdisciplinary until now. The chapter focuses on the acquisition of skills and knowledge in applied psychophysiology and biofeedback (AP/B), because this is a particularly relevant approach for behavioral intervention with the primary care patient.[1] Applied psychophysiology involves using interventions based on a scientific understanding of the mind-body link and drawing on the research fields of behavioral psychology, psychophysiology, cognitive psychology, and biofeedback. Biofeedback is the use of electronic instruments to monitor biological processes as a way to increase the individual's awareness and control over body and mind. There is a growing body of literature showing effective outcomes for applied psychophysiology and biofeedback with the disorders of primary care (Moss, 1999; Schwartz & Associates, 1995).

Biofeedback has often been described in the past as a tool only to be used in the hands of an independently licensed practitioner. While this makes sense at many levels, it may no longer be in tune with the realities of the emerging managed health care environment. For AP/B to have a truly meaningful impact in primary care medicine, professionals with specific skills will be needed, including practitioners at various levels of education and training.

## APPROPRIATE EDUCATION AND TRAINING

Practitioners can be trained at three different levels: unlicensed, master's level, and doctoral level. Some practitioners begin their practice with an undergraduate degree and some external training. Others complete training in a master's level program with some connection to AP/B, while many practitioners are fully licensed in another discipline such as psychology or medicine.

### Practitioners Without Independent Licensure

For many years AP/B services have been delivered by individuals who are not independently licensed and do not belong to any commonly known professional group. They call themselves biofeedback therapists, stress management specialists, or other similar titles and come from a variety of backgrounds, although most have a bachelor's degree in one of the behavioral or health sciences. Within the AP/B community, unlicensed practitioners have been a source of controversy. One view holds that there neither is nor should be a profession of AP/B but that AP/B tools should only be used by individuals licensed within their own profession (physicians, doctoral level clinical psychologists, nurse practitioners, licensed social workers, physical therapists, etc.). Although this view has much to support it, it is not practical. Since mind-body medicine is itself a largely unregulated field, few strictures have been enforced that would prevent an unlicensed practitioner from being involved in treatment.

Furthermore, the field of AP/B has historically been greatly influenced by unlicensed practitioners. Thus both the Association for Applied Psychophysiology and Biofeedback (AAPB), the largest professional association in this practice area, and the Biofeedback Certification Institute of America (BCIA), the most widely recognized AP/B credentialing body, have accepted these practitioners as valid members of the AP/B community. Of the approximately 2,000 members listed in the AAPB directory in 2000, 29 percent listed themselves as unlicensed. Furthermore, licensure bills for independent biofeedback practitioners have been discussed in several states; as of this writing, one such licensure bill is in the New York legislature.

Training at the unlicensed level can take many forms. Some practitioners have only informal training, but most have attended freestanding workshops or training programs, a university course, or an offering from the AAPB or a state association. The workshops are typically offered in an intense 8- to 10-day format, cost between $1,500 and $3,000, and follow the BCIA blueprint for required knowledge and skills. Instructors are usually experienced professionals, and much hands-on work is expected. To some degree, the marketplace has ensured that the better programs have survived. AAPB's published certification exam results are available for consumer observation. AAPB also offers a biofeedback home study program, following the BCIA blueprint and providing the necessary 50 hours of didactic credit for certification. The most current BCIA blueprint and additional authorized training programs preparing an individual for BCIA certification are available on the BCIA Web site at http://www.bcia.org.

## Master's-Level Training

A second training model consists of formal university training programs culminating in a master's degree or a specialized undergraduate degree. These programs vary widely but usually have a core curriculum similar to that described in this section.

Students can be trained to deliver AP/B in a yearlong, full-time training program that incorporates a practicum in a clinical setting. Typically, the goal of the program is to train professionals who can deliver protocol-driven services within health care settings under supervision from physicians, physicians' assistants, or psychologists.

This training approach usually emphasizes the development of a psychophysiological mediation path model for most disorders. Students are asked to formulate a path model for each patient using interview data and stress profiles, allowing students to conceptualize how the patient's symptoms are affected by sympathetic and parasympathetic nervous system factors and by respiratory patterns (Gevirtz, 2000). In turn, cognitive and emotional factors are explored for their effects on physiology, and developmental histories are assessed for their impact on cognitive factors.

To socialize the students into the medical culture, students take a sequence in clinical medicine. Often taught by physicians, these courses emphasize medical anatomy, physiology, pathophysiology, and especially medical terminology.

The master's programs offer direct training in applied psychophysiology through courses with an accompanying practicum in real-life settings. These courses follow the BCIA blueprint, as discussed later. The first semester usually emphasizes electronics, autonomic and respiratory physiology, and basic common treatment modalities such as cultivated low arousal, Jacobson's progressive muscle relaxation, and autogenic training.

Students work on biofeedback systems until they have mastered all the common modalities, including surface electromyography (SEMG), temperature, heart rate, respiration (rate and pattern), electrodermal response (EDP), electrencephalography (EEG), and sometimes capnometry (measuring end-tidal respiratory carbon dioxide, or $etCO_2$), and heart rate spectral modalities (see Chapter 8 for more information on basic biofeedback modalities).

Later semesters shift the focus to clinical syndromes. The medical background is reviewed and protocols are presented. Disorders covered typically include headache (tension and migraine), hypertension, temporomandibular disorders, Raynaud's disease, anxiety disorders, chronic pain, irritable bowel syndrome, tinnitus, functional cardiac syndrome, and others. Since the students in these programs are not usually licensed professionals, the disorders are presented in the form of a structured protocol. Ability to diagnose is not assumed. Students continue to practice these protocols in their practicum settings.

Pelvic floor rehabilitation for disorders of urinary and fecal incontinence, and neurofeedback for attention deficit hyperactivity disorder are also often covered in separate courses, using well-established protocols to present the fundamentals of these complex areas. It is assumed that further training will be necessary for most of the students planning to work in these areas. However, it is hoped that each student receives a solid foundation.

In addition to the specialized curriculum in AP/B, students usually take a full load of behavioral science courses, including behavioral medicine, behavioral/social learning theory, introduction to psychotherapy, and social psychology. These courses are designed to supplement the AP/B training and allow students to progress to advanced degrees if they desire.

The curriculum is usually designed to allow the student to progress through a series of competencies. In theory, no one progresses to the next level without first achieving competency at the lower level. This is done using traditional assessments such as exams and papers as well as through oral presentations, practical exams, and clinical materials (such as client tapes). Integration is, of course, critical and should occur within the practicum over the course of the year.

### Doctoral-Level Training

A third training model is the professional model for candidates intending to become independently licensed in their respective disciplines. These programs are not common but exist in a few graduate and medical schools. Presently, it is not clear whether this specialty training will grow to be more popular or remain in only a few institutions. The existing programs are found in doctoral programs in clinical health psychology, behavioral medicine, and counseling, and at least one family medicine residency has some AP/B training. Candidates are trained primarily in the traditional disciplines but are allowed enough time for the specialty courses previously discussed. Modern concepts in psychology or psychiatry such as cognitive therapy, family systems, and interpersonal psychology are often included.

Many traditionally trained clinical psychologists and psychiatrists think they can expand to treat these psychophysiological or functional disorders, but this attitude ignores the inherently interdisciplinary nature of the disorders. In fact, too much emphasis on the psychological or even cognitive aspects of the disorders seems to diminish the treatment efficacy of psychophysiological intervention.

The doctoral training models that do exist with specialty AP/B training provide the core clinical psychology curriculum, so that licensure in psychology is possible, and add course work and practical training in medical settings. The course work follows traditional American Psychological Association (APA) guidelines with basic behavioral science courses and statistics/design courses in the first two years, followed by clinical psychology courses (psychopathology, assessment, therapies, etc.). However, from the first semester on, students are trained to function in medical settings with patients with or without psychiatric diagnoses.

The second-year practicum placements (16 hours per week) are typically in a medical setting. Pain clinics, cancer treatment centers, AIDS response clinics, behavioral medicine hospital services, and the school's own AP/B clinic are typical of the settings. Students quickly become socialized into these settings and often work alongside physicians, nurses, physical therapists, physician assistants, and others.

The remaining internship can be in traditional mental health settings or APA-approved internship settings. As in clinical psychology or other health psychology programs, there are many settings around the country available with at least a health rotation.

The dissertation requirement ensures students' research competency. Most students complete research in applied areas that are relevant to their future professional activities. Thus the dissertation becomes an integral part of the training, not a "hoop" to jump through to get through the program.

## REQUIRED KNOWLEDGE AND SKILLS

The national and state organizations in AP/B have struggled to create an accepted and universal set of knowledge and skills for the field. In accordance with the trend toward increasing specialization, AP/B has subspecialties—including neurofeedback, general rehabilitation, and pelvic floor rehabilitation—that define competencies very differently. For the general practitioner, however, the BCIA blueprint represents a good consensus of the domains of knowledge and skill. Eleven domains of skills and knowledge are identified:

1. *Introduction to biofeedback*: general definitions, concepts, and history of the field.

2. *Preparation for clinical intervention*: assessment skills, periodic evaluation, integrating background, psychophysiological and psychological data.

3. *General neuromuscular interventions*: central nervous system, somatic/motor system, and neuromuscular disorders.

4. *Specific neuromuscular interventions*: anatomy, physiology, and treatment protocols for neck and low-back pain, rehabilitation protocols, tension headache, temporomandibular disorders, and torticollis and pelvic floor rehabilitation.

5. *General central nervous system interventions*: brain anatomy and neurofeedback applications for attention deficit hyperactivity disorder and epilepsy.

6. *General autonomic nervous system (ANS)*: ANS anatomy and physiology, endocrine physiology, electrodermal, temperature, and heart rate measures and feedback modalities.

7. *Specific ANS interventions*: migraine, Raynaud's disease, hypertension, and respiratory interventions.

8. *Biofeedback and distress*: general adaptation syndrome, and stress and distress models.

9. *Instrumentation*: basic electronics as applied to biofeedback.

10. *Adjunctive techniques*: relaxation, autogenic, cognitive, and other therapeutic interventions as integrated with biofeedback.

11. *Professional conduct and ethics*.

## Documented Competencies

At the end of the training period, students are expected to be able to articulate and explain several areas of acquired knowledge, demonstrate the mastery of skills and procedures, and conduct assessment and treatment following standardized protocols. Examples of expected knowledge and skills include the following:

1. The student will conduct and analyze a physiological stress profile assessing four physiological domains:
   a. Sympathetic nervous activity (monitoring sympathetic nervous activity via the electrodermal response, peripheral temperature, very low frequency heart rate spectral activity, and heart rate).
   b. Parasympathetic nervous activity (using high-frequency heart rate spectral activity).
   c. Respiratory parameters (using abdominal/thoracic respiratory patterning, $etCO_2$ levels and patterns, respiration rate, and variability).
   d. Voluntary striate muscle activity (SEMG, both static and dynamic).

2. The student will present case intake material using the psychophysiological mediation path model.
   a. For each disorder, the student will present a basic mediation model, identifying physiological, cognitive, and behavioral mechanisms that mediate the disorder and allowing for intervention at several levels.
   b. The student will be able to implement each of the treatment protocols derived from the mediation model.

3. The student will present an explanation at the patient's level of understanding that will assist the patient to shift his or her causal attribution for the disorder. In other words, the student will convincingly reframe the patient's disorder so that the patient can modify his or her personal understanding of what factors influence the disorder and what personal strategies might relieve the disorder.

4. The student will pass the BCIA written and practical tests.

5. The student will interpret a continuous performance test for attention problems while using EEG to monitor and assess the significance of beta–theta range brain activity at a specific scalp site (Cz).

6. The student will analyze a urodynamic assessment provided by a urologist and implement pelvic floor retraining using a vaginal or anal probe. This implementation includes conducting an assessment, analyzing the information gathered, and designing home training exercises.

7. The student will know enough about psychopathology, counseling, or psychotherapy to make an appropriate referral.

8. The student will define general electronics terminology and give a rudimentary explanation of the elements involved in a basic thermal or EMG device.

Beyond these areas of curriculum content, there are many other adjunctive fields in mind-body studies. For example, many professionals are convinced that psychological constructs such as hypnotic susceptibility are critical to the understanding of functional disorders. Others focus on specific therapy techniques from behavioral to psychoanalytic. And of course developments in the neurosciences, pharmacology, and medical science constantly add to the understanding of the brain and body and their interactions.

## PROFESSIONAL ROLES

Practitioners of applied psychophysiology in mind-body medicine function in a wide variety of professional roles, reflecting the three levels of professional training previously discussed:

1. Unlicensed professionals work in settings ranging from independent practice to salaried employment in a medical environment. Despite the difficulties with third-party payments, many practitioners have been successful in fee-for-service practices, with fees ranging from $40 to $120 per hour session. Referrals are obtained from physicians, psychologists, and the general public; thus the therapist must manage a diverse client base. Practitioners should be aware of the limitations of their training and consult with appropriately licensed professionals. Based on a sample of the listings in the directory of the AAPB (2000), problem areas most often seen include anxiety disorders, stress management, stress-related disorders, pain control, and EEG applications.

2. Master's-level practitioners work in similar settings and roles as unlicensed practitioners but can be independently licensed. Social workers, marriage and family therapists, counselors, and master's-level psychologists are representative of this category. Nurses, occupational therapists, and physical therapists might also be included in this broad category. Some of these practitioners are independently based, some work in medical or mental health settings, and some become specialists in areas such as urinary incontinence or rehabilitation.

3. Licensed professionals (doctoral level) constitute the largest share of AP/B practitioners. This group includes psychologists (Ph.D. or Psy.D.), physicians, chiropractors, and dentists. Within medicine, the most common specialties are family medicine, psychiatry, rehabilitation or physical medicine, neurology, and internal medicine. Practitioners in this category deliver services directly to patients; supervise unlicensed or master's-level practitioners; and provide various combinations of service, consulting, and supervision.

## INNOVATIVE USES OF APPLIED PSYCHOPHYSIOLOGY AND BIOFEEDBACK

As mentioned earlier, more than 40 percent of patient visits to primary care physicians are related to mind-body disorders. With the growth of managed care, the economic impact of this fact has become central to potential cost savings. A variety of disorders have been mentioned and are probably worth some attention, but five groups of disorders seem especially ripe for AP/B interventions: irritable bowel syndrome, functional cardiac disorder, fibromyalgia, chronic fatigue syndrome, myofascial pain disorders, and anxiety disorders with somatic features. In addition, migraine headache may be a candidate since its prevalence is growing rapidly and pharmacological management is expensive and often disappointing. Each of these disorders has associated screening and diagnostic tests, poor outcomes using traditional medical interventions, and high medical utilization rates. The presence and cost of functional disorders in primary medicine has led to many innovative models using AP/B and other behavioral techniques.

## Applied Psychophysiology in Primary Care

Given these costs, the opportunities for behavioral health providers trained in applied psychophysiology are emerging. Training models for practitioners in AP/B have been varied and interdisciplinary until now. Biofeedback has often been described as a tool only to be used in the hands of an independently licensed practitioner. Many primary care patients, however, could benefit greatly from an in-clinic biofeedback practitioner at the bachelor's or master's level, using standardized treatment protocols for common disorders. The more challenging cases can still be referred to the doctoral level specialist.

## The Trojan Horse

By labeling the service "biofeedback," the clinic removes the stigma for the patient of being referred to a behavioral health professional. The patient accepts the biofeedback practitioner, dressed in a lab coat, as one more health practitioner, using biomedical devices to assess and retrain physiologic processes (Wickramasekera, 1988). Yet once the patient accepts the practitioner, biofeedback treatment can include many other treatment components, including traditional psychotherapy, hypnosis, stress management, and relaxation training. Within this milieu, AP/B practitioners can be successful in improving outcomes and cost-benefit ratios. In their research, Ryan and Gevirtz (2001) found that patients receiving biofeedback-based treatment saved an average of $72 per patient per month compared with a control group.

## Chronic Pain Care

Multidisciplinary pain centers commonly use AP/B practitioners. For the more functional disorders like headache, temporomandibular disorders, irritable bowel syndrome, and myofascial pain, the interventions are usually successful. For more intractable problems such as neuropathy, radiculopathy, or complex regional pain syndrome, these behavioral interventions are less effective (see Association for Applied Psychophysiology and Biofeedback, 1995).

## Incontinence Care

The disorders of urinary incontinence and vulvodynia represent areas where AP/B has been used innovatively. Recently, the Health Care Finance Administration has recognized biofeedback as an efficacious treatment for these disorders.

## Cardiac Rehabilitation

Another area of emerging interest is cardiac rehabilitation. *Cardiac psychology* is a term used to refer to the important role that psychological or emotional processes play in the recovery process and the etiology of heart disease (Clay, 2001). AP/B will probably play an important role in this area.

### Electronic Innovation

The recent emerging areas of multimedia therapy, virtual reality in mental health, and telemedicine are ripe for AP/B applications (Wiederhold & Wiederhold, 1998).

### Pediatrics

Finally, pediatric settings have always been compatible with AP/B protocols. Humphreys and Gevirtz (2000) showed that even simple biofeedback procedures are effective in the treatment of recurrent abdominal pain in children.

## CERTIFICATION AND CREDENTIALING

Schwartz and Associates (1995) provide a comprehensive history of the credentialing process for AP/B. In 1981, the AAPB (then known as the Biofeedback Society of America) authorized funding for an independent credentialing organization, the Biofeedback Certification Institute of America (BCIA). This organization has survived as the leading AP/B credentialing authority in the world. Through the use of educational requirements, exams, and continuing education, individuals are credentialed as possessing "minimal competency" in AP/B. The credential is used as a requirement for many institutions hiring AP/B practitioners. Beyond this, most AP/B practitioners are independently licensed in their disciplines (e.g., medicine, psychology, etc.). Some also have specialty board certification or additional certification in adjunctive techniques such as hypnosis and pain management.

## CONCLUSION

Based on current evidence and the continued need to ration health care, it appears inevitable that mind-body medicine will take its rightful place in the health sciences. Too many patients have primary complaints that would be better served by behavioral health practitioners with solid mind-body approaches. The shape of this new profession depends on those of us who have recognized the folly of mind-body dualism and can coherently put forth a scientifically based model that recognizes the nature of the problems that increasingly plague modern cultures.

Such a model requires that gold standard research accompany the training of clinical practitioners. Each of the curriculum elements and competencies in behavioral health training programs should derive from ongoing research on mechanisms causing functional disorders and from the most current evidence-based research on effective treatment protocols. There is certainly no lack of public fascination for the mind-body connection, but much remains to be done before mind-body medicine achieves a respectable position in the hallowed halls of academics and in the National Institutes of Health.

## NOTE

1.   The graduate programs described in the chapter are based on those created at Alliant University, formerly the California School of Professional Psychology, in San Diego by the author and his colleague, Perry Nicassio, Ph.D.

## REFERENCES

Association for Applied Psychophysiology and Biofeedback. (1995). *Clinical applications of biofeedback and applied psychophysiology: White papers.* Wheat Ridge, CO: Author.

Association for Applied Psychophysiology and Biofeedback. (2000). *2000 membership directory.* Wheat Ridge, CO: Author.

Clay, R. (2001). Research to the heart of the matter. *Monitor on Psychology,* 32(1), 42–49.

Gevirtz, R. (2000). Physiology of stress. In D. Kenney, J. Carlson, J. Sheppard, & F. J. McGuigan (Eds.), *Stress and health: Research and clinical applications* (pp. 53–72). Sydney, Australia: Harwood Academic Publishers.

Humphreys, P. A., & Gevirtz, R. N. (2000). Treatment of recurrent abdominal pain: Components analysis of four treatment protocols. *Journal of Pediatric Gastroenterology and Nutrition, 31*(1), 47–51.

Moss, D. (1999). Biofeedback, mind-body medicine, and primary care. *Biofeedback, 27*(1), 4–11.

Ryan, M., & Gevirtz, R. N. (2001, March). The effects of biofeedback on cost effectiveness in primary care settings. Poster presented at the 32nd annual meeting of the Association for Applied Psychophysiology and Biofeedback, Raleigh/Durham, NC.

Schwartz, M., & Associates. (1995). *Biofeedback: A practitioner's guide* (2nd ed.). New York: Guilford.

Wickramasekera, I. (1988). *Clinical behavioral medicine: Some concepts and procedures.* New York: Plenum.

Wiederhold, B., & Wiederhold, M. (1998). A review of virtual reality as a therapeutic tool. *CyberPsychology and Behavior, 1*(2), 45–52.

# CHAPTER 36

# Existential and Spiritual Dimensions of Primary Care: Healing the Wounded Soul

## Donald Moss

**Abstract:** Human beings are both physical and metaphysical beings. In every breath, they are anchored in accidents of anatomy and physiological process yet actively yearn to reach the farthest limits of the imagination. Illness transforms the world and the everyday experience of the sick. Driven by the human need to discover meaning in every event, injured, ill, and disabled individuals display a special need to make sense of their suffering and to discover a deeper purpose beneath illness. Participation in inward spiritual activities and outward religious activities may enhance wellness and buffer individuals against illness. Spiritual texts, liturgies, and wisdom offer additional tools for the health practitioner in reducing suffering, guiding the troubled, and bringing depth to the lives of the well. Empirical research today is clarifying the health-enhancing and health-debilitating effects of religious and spiritual involvement.[1]

## INTRODUCTION

> The great malady of the twentieth century, implicated in all our troubles and affecting us individually and socially, is "loss of soul." (Moore, 1992, p. xi)

Most chapters in this book have emphasized a self-regulation and self-efficacy approach—that is, the acquisition of knowledge and skills to increase self-mastery over illness. The present chapter is a reminder to the health care provider that illness nevertheless involves a suffering component, a loss of mastery and control over one's body and life, that compels the sufferer to search for meaning and for acceptance. The psychology of illness is also a psychology of loss, with consequent mood and identity problems. Compassion and understanding increase the health care provider's ability to be with the patient in that search for meaning amidst pain and loss. This chapter examines the following perspectives, each of which argues for attention to existential and spiritual perspectives in mind-body practice and in general health care:

- Illness, especially when chronic, disabling, or life threatening, brings human beings into the "kingdom of the sick," a transformed world of narrowing horizons and personal loss.
- Health care practice brings clinicians into the midst of sick, suffering, and dying individuals who are led by their illness and disability to raise existential and spiritual questions and to seek spiritual meaning.
- Many mind-body interventions, such as meditation, relaxation exercises, and biofeedback, cultivate a mental attitude of "letting go" and teach a physiological and emotional self-quieting to create meditative conditions conducive to spiritual experiences.
- By training patients to modify brain states, mind-body approaches like neurofeedback and meditation induce states of consciousness conducive to spiritual awakening and personal transformation.
- Spiritual concepts, texts, liturgies, symbols, and music are powerful tools for transformation and increase the effectiveness of conventional relaxation training and self-regulation-oriented therapies.
- Spiritual traditions, Eastern and Western, offer guidance for living, wisdom for coping, and values that orient troubled, ill, and dying individuals.
- Current empirical research suggests that prayer and involvement in religious activities may positively enhance health and wellness.
- Spiritual experiences are mind-body phenomena and invite one to apply the scientific tools of psychophysiology.

## THE KINGDOM OF THE SICK: THE PHENOMENOLOGY OF ILLNESS

*Illness, especially when chronic, disabling, or life threatening, brings human beings into the "kingdom of the sick," a transformed world of narrowing horizons and personal loss.*

In Chapter 31, Sharon Utz speaks of the chronically ill individual as entering the kingdom of the sick. Becoming ill or disabled dramatically changes the patient's experience of the world. The longer an illness or disability lingers, the more radically the patient's world is transformed. If a health professional wishes to understand the patient's perspective, it is crucial to come to understand the flavor and texture of the world of illness.

Initially, patients often experience illness or injury as a "violation." Illness breaks into the individual's life uninvited. The entrance may be abrupt, in a violent injury or heart attack, or it may be more gradual. One day, the individual feels too ill to go to the office or to play tennis as expected. Unless the onset of illness is violent, most patients cling to the expectation of acute illness. The patient may take a few vitamins, get some extra sleep, or take a medication left over from a previous illness. There is a momentary retreat from life in order to recover, but the expectation remains that, in a few hours or days, one will resume a normal life and get back to normal priorities.

When illness worsens or lingers, patients turn to health professionals, usually family-practice physicians. Patients in mainstream cultures in the United States are typically thoroughly acculturated in the acute medicine model. They visit the physician, looking for a specific diagnostic process leading to medication and recovery. The typical primary care visit will not produce a conclusive diagnosis, but the patient remains oriented to a process of brief treatment of symptoms and a return to life as usual in short order.

As illness lingers or progresses, patients often become more emotionally invested in the process of diagnosis and a search for a cure. If the diagnostic process is prolonged, uncertainty grows, and all too often, primitive fears arise that one is not cared about. The common assumption that one is entitled to treatment and a quick cure slowly breaks down. Emergence of chronicity challenges much favored beliefs about self and life.

## The Medical World

For the severely or chronically ill, physicians and other health care providers become a secondary social circle. Medical appointments structure one's schedule, medications punctuate one's day, and laboratory tests become markers for personal hopes and disappointments. Over time, the patient role becomes for many a kind of substitute social role and even identity. Today many patients with chronic illnesses, especially those with few effective medical treatments, turn to self-help groups, Internet chat rooms, and self-help books in search of both emotional support and alternative treatment options.

## Perception of Threat in Chronic Illness and Disability

There are a multitude of threats, stressors, and losses that burden the chronically ill and disabled individual. The individual faces threats to life, comfort, and physical well-being, along with threats to the integrity of the body. For example, those with chronic diabetes may face potential loss of limb(s). Patients often face stressful or painful diagnostic procedures and treatments and medications with uncomfortable side effects. Many face threats to independence, privacy, autonomy, and control over their bodies and lives. Longer-term illness brings threats to identity, social roles, career, and income. Illness often feels like a falling out of time and out of life. Life goes on around the ill or disabled without his or her participation. The patient can no longer visualize a life progressing toward goals. Time itself can feel congealed and broken to the extent that the patient declares, "I have no future."

## Changes in the Patient's World Mirror Changes in the Body

Many illnesses and chronic conditions produce weariness, lethargy, and weakness in the body. The patient begins to perceive the surrounding world as full of obstacles, distances, and challenges. Stores begin to seem too far from the car, stairs appear too steep and dangerous, and so on. Continued illness brings a reluctance to go out, to initiate activities, or to tackle new tasks. The ill individual feels no momentum, no progress, only exertion and fatigue. Prosthetic devices and aids, such as motorized wheelchairs and canes, can enable renewed participation in everyday life; yet they also stand out as visible symbols of illness and disability.

## Chronic Illness Through the Life Cycle

Age and stage of life also shape the meaning of the illness for the individual. Illness and disability can interfere with developmentally critical activities. Cancer in adolescence, for example, disrupts normal dating and emancipation. For the elderly, personal identity may be less dependent on work, yet physical disability still hastens dependence on family and professional caregivers.

## ILLNESS AND THE SPIRIT

*Health care practice brings clinicians into the midst of sick, suffering, and dying individuals who are led by their illness and disability to raise existential and spiritual questions and to seek spiritual meaning.*

Health care work unfolds amidst pain and suffering. Human beings who face illness, pain, and death seek the meaning of their being. They ask themselves and their health care providers metaphysical questions such as the following:

"Why me, God?"

"Did I commit some terrible sin to bring this illness on myself?"

"Is my illness part of a larger design?"

"Has the purpose of my living ended?"

"Can I discover a worth in simply being, when I can no longer achieve?"

These are universal and ultimate human questions. Karl Jaspers (1932), the German existential psychiatrist and philosopher, called critical situations in life, such as illness, suffering, crises, and death, "limit situations." In such moments, human beings wake up from the usual absorption with schedules, tasks, and the trivia of life, to once again view their lives as a whole and to ask questions about purpose. In such moments, many formulate their struggles and their solutions in spiritual language.

The English poet Milton (1608–1674), when he had lost his vision, wrote a poem expressing his struggle to find meaning in a life without his sight.

> When I consider how my light is spent,
> E're half my days, in this dark world and
> wide,
> And that one talent which is death to hide,
> Lodged with me useless
> (Sonnet XIX, in Quiller-Couch, 1939,
> p. 352)

His timeless answer expresses the kind of "cognitive reframing" that we seek to teach our disabled patients today.

> God doth not need
> Either man's work or his own gifts, who
> best
> Bear his mild yoke, they serve Him
> best . . .
> Thousands at his bidding speed
> And post o'er Land and Ocean without
> rest:
> They also serve who only stand and waite.
> (Sonnet XIX, in Quiller-Couch, 1939,
> p. 353)

Rabbi Harold Kushner (1981) drew on Hebrew and Christian scriptures, especially the story of Job and his suffering, to address the meaning of suffering. His text reminds the reader that in all historical eras, human beings have struggled to understand why "bad things happen to good people." Kushner's guiding principle seems to be that sick, injured, and impaired individuals will benefit from hearing the classic spiritual formulations in biblical texts, while searching for their own answers and personal formulations of meaning.

## MIND-BODY THERAPIES, STILLNESS, AND THE SOUL

*Many mind-body interventions, such as meditation, relaxation exercises, and biofeedback, cultivate a mental attitude of "letting go" and teach a physiological and emotional self-quieting to create meditative conditions conducive to spiritual experiences.*

Mind-body medicine rests on a holistic approach dedicated to a unitary understanding of mind, body, and spirit. Mind-body therapists regularly use therapies, such as meditation, visualization, and imagery therapies, that are conducive to spiritual awareness.

The Hebrew psalmist counseled individuals to find their God in silence: "Be still and know that I am God" (Psalm 46:10). Biofeedback, relaxation, and meditation teach the skills necessary to bring about inner physiological, mental, and emotional quieting. In the stillness many individuals find emotional release and the presence of spirit.

Biofeedback and relaxation therapies teach a physiological and emotional letting go and letting be. Both Wolfgang Luthe (1969) and Herbert Benson (1975) advocated a passive volition or passive attitude of mind. This same process of relinquishing personal control and detaching from effortful striving is a part of most meditative traditions, from Buddhism to Christianity. The Christian mystics, such as the German Rhineland mystics Meister Eckhart and Johannes Tauler, saw this letting go as the first step toward an inner encounter with God (Moss, 1980). Biblical texts in the Judaic-Christian tradition support a pursuit of inwardness and stillness: "Thou dost keep him in perfect peace, whose mind is stayed on thee, because he trusts in thee" (Isaiah 26:3-4).

Biofeedback and relaxation training overlap with non-Western traditional spiritual practices, cultivating a deep and full diaphragmatic breathing. Traditional Chinese philosophy teaches that "mind and breathing are interdependent, and regular respiration produces a serene mind" (Yue Yanggui, cited by Xiangcai, 2000, p. 7). Yue, living during China's Qing Dynasty, further taught that "the tranquility of the mind regulates the breathing naturally and, in turn, regulated breathing brings on concentration of the mind naturally" (p. 7).

## BRAIN STATES AND ALTERED STATES OF CONSCIOUSNESS

*By training patients to modify brain states, mind-body approaches like neurofeedback and meditation induce states of consciousness conducive to spiritual awakening and personal transformation.*

In 1969, Joe Kamiya published his classic text, "Operant Control of the Alpha EEG Rhythm," as a chapter in Charles Tart's book, *Altered States of Consciousness.* Kamiya's research showed that with feedback a human subject could modify his or her cortical state at will and thereby modify the state of consciousness. Alpha rhythms in the cortex are accompanied by a creative, open awareness and a meditative, receptive attitude of mind. Kamiya's work coincided with the 1960s countercultural interest in pursuing higher states of consciousness through drugs. EEG appeared to offer a drug-free pathway toward higher states of

mind, and a new industry quickly emerged, offering inexpensive and often shoddy alpha home-training machines.

A recent hot topic in the popular media is the concept of "neurotheology," an approach that emphasizes that certain cortical or subcortical brain centers are the basis for spiritual experiences. A recent book, *Why God Won't Go Away,* points to the "orientation association" area in the parietal lobe (Newberg, D'Aquili, & Rause, 2001). SPECT brain-imaging studies show that this area becomes less active during meditation, when the meditator feels one with the universe. Hypothetically, when this cortical area is inhibited, it facilitates mystical, oceanic feelings of harmony and unity with being.

> We saw evidence of a neurological process that has evolved to allow us humans to transcend material existence and acknowledge and connect with a deeper, more spiritual part of ourselves perceived by us as an absolute, universal reality that connects us to all that is. (Newberg et al., 2001, p. 9)

Many years ago Carl Jung observed that there was little hope for psychological treatment for alcoholism. He then added that most of the recovered alcoholics he had encountered had experienced some kind of a spiritual transformation process. Today neurofeedback guides patients to enter altered states of consciousness and to experience a deep process of existential and spiritual transformation. The widely adapted Peniston protocol combines temperature biofeedback-assisted relaxation training, alpha-theta brain-wave training, breathing training, and the use of imagery to assist addicts and alcoholics to visualize and experience themselves as powerfully changed (Peniston & Kukolsky, 1989). This protocol is also the basis for therapies for individuals with posttraumatic stress disorder, dissociative disorders, and a variety of other disorders.

## SPIRITUAL WORDS AS TOOLS FOR TRANSFORMATION

*Spiritual concepts, texts, liturgies, symbols, and music are powerful tools for transformation and increase the effectiveness of conventional relaxation training and self-regulation therapies in health care.*

On a wintry Tuesday morning early last year, I conducted a chronic pain class on the use of imagery and visualization for pain management. I was not enthusiastic about conducting this session, because one member of the pain group was a blustery and angry policeman with a spinal injury and severe head and back pain. He had expended enormous amounts of energy informing me, the other therapists in the program, and the patient group how useless he found each of the self-regulation strategies that we had taught him. He had already rejected progressive muscle relaxation, autogenic training, and diaphragmatic breathing. In his mind, the cognitive reframing we taught the class was "snake oil," and he didn't know why he was wasting his time in the pain management program.

After an introduction to the role of imagery in pain reduction and pain management, I guided the group through an imagery exercise as follows:

> You are in a beautiful, lush, green garden. The sun is shining on you and around you. You can feel its warmth on your face and all over your body. You feel the serenity of this place, its peacefulness and comfort. Now picture yourself becoming tinier and tinier. Imagine yourself scooped up very gently and carefully. You are resting in the hands of the Lord. His hands are so large and strong, and you are cradled securely and gently in his palms. He is gazing down upon you with love and acceptance. You feel a healing light from His face wash over your body. You feel relieved of all burdens. Your pain is lighter now, soothed by His presence. Allow yourself to remain quiet for several minutes now, and feel the comfort of His caring for you.

As I looked around the group after the imagery exercise, I was surprised to find my skeptical patient in tears and smiling warmly at the group. He asked us why we hadn't done this wonderful exercise right away and told us it was the only worthwhile lesson in three weeks. He reported feeling less pain and a new sense of lightness in his body. He began to talk about how he had been feeling abandoned by God and had been asking himself what he had done to bring such suffering on himself. The exercise relieved that sense of being spiritually cut off and comforted him. This was also a turning point in his cooperation with other strategies, as he felt a new confidence that the pain management curriculum had something to offer him.

Many religiously oriented individuals use hymns, prayer, and Bible reading to cope with their illness, pain, and suffering. A contemporary Christian "praise song" includes the following lines: "I'm trading my sickness, I'm trading my pain, I'm laying them down for the joy of the Lord" (Evans, 1998, track 1).[2] The melody and rhythm are rousing and support the sentiment expressed. The individual who is able to sing such hymns with feeling, especially in a church crowded with like-minded persons, participates in a communal and shared celebration of hope over despair.

## SPIRITUALITY AND LIFE WISDOM

*Spiritual traditions, Eastern and Western, offer guidance for living, wisdom for coping, and values that orient troubled, ill, and dying individuals.*

Patients turn to their health care professionals not only for physiological evaluation and technical interventions but also for guidance for life. Yet psychophysiological science offers no great wisdom or life direction. Many mind-body practitioners have taken the concepts of self-regulation, relaxation, and holism and extended them metaphorically to create a philosophy of living.

That philosophy emphasizes self-direction, responsibility for one's own health, and harmony with one's body, nature, and fellow humans. It also encourages respect for the integral physical, emotional, and spiritual needs of human beings. But there are many moments in clinical practice when a patient is seeking "true north"—ultimate directions and priorities in dealing with their personal challenges. Ultimate directions include the challenge to make peace with suffering and to accept changes in one's body that one cannot reverse.

Each religious tradition accumulates a set of sacred texts, prayers, hymns, and spiritual disciplines that convey pathways and priorities for living. Traditional pastoral counseling in health settings provides an abundance of consolation and direction in health care settings. Pastoral care has been grappling with the problem of human suffering since the time of Job. Chaplains are ideal individuals to teach self-regulation and wellness practices to patients because of their credibility and holistic orientation. Many churches and synagogues now employ "parish nurses" to reach out to ailing members and to optimize the wellness of healthy persons. Parish nurses are also ideally suited to integrate body, mind, and spirit as well as spirituality and medical lessons into one holistic outreach (Clark & Olson, 2000; Solari-Twadell & McDermott, 1999).

The spiritual wisdom that informs chaplaincy work can also provide guidance to the health care professional dealing with a troubled medical patient. A number of spiritual authors have advocated a revival of spiritual disciplines as tools for coping with contemporary life problems and stress. Richard Foster (1978), a Quaker, richly described traditional Christian disciplines as sources for contemporary wellness. He lists the following "spiritual disciplines" and explores their present-day relevance:

| | | |
|---|---|---|
| Meditation | Simplicity | Confession |
| Prayer | Solitude | Worship |
| Fasting | Submission | Guidance |
| Study | Service | Celebration |

Numerous authors have explored Western and Eastern religious traditions for life wisdom. For example, Henri Nouwen (1981) and Thomas Merton (1961) both explored the wisdom of the "desert fathers," Christian hermits who lived lives of prayer in the Egyptian desert. These fifth- and sixth-century hermits contribute surprisingly contemporary perspectives to the modern search for a meaningful life.

Similarly Jon Kabat-Zinn (1990) describes a way of life based on Buddhist mindfulness meditation, and Ken McLeod (2001) describes the "Buddhist path of attention" as an orientation for contemporary life.

## SOUL, SPIRIT, AND HEALTH CARE

*Current empirical research suggests that prayer and involvement in religious activities may positively enhance the health and wellness.*

Larson and Larson (1994) assembled a compendium summarizing current empirical research on the impact of religious involvement and practices on health care.

If you heard that research had demonstrated a factor which could lower your blood pressure, help you recover from surgery, provide a greater sense of well-being, add years to your life and help protect your children from drug abuse, alcohol abuse or suicide, would you be interested in discovering what it might be? (pp. 1, 63–84)

Their point is that a growing body of research shows correlations between active church attendance (or involvement in church-related activities) and positive health.

Both inward spiritual experiences and outward religious practices appear to have health value.

Levin and Vanderpool (1987) cited more than two dozen studies showing that regular attendance at church or synagogue has documented health-promoting effects. Koenig, Hays, et al. (1999) reported that individuals with high "intrinsic religiousness" show more rapid remission of depression and that religious involvement predicts successful coping with physical illness. Religious people are generally healthier, lead healthier lifestyles, possess better social support networks, exhibit more positive worldviews, and require fewer health services (Koenig, 1999, 2000; Koenig, McCullough, & Larson, 2001). Helm, Hays, Flint, Koenig, and Blazer (2000) reported that private religious activity (prayer, meditation, or Bible study) prolonged the survival of intact older adults. Koenig, Larson, et al. (1998) showed that religious involvement can prolong life in spite of illness, and Koenig, Hays, et al. (1999) reported that the magnitude of the impact of religious involvement on physical health is almost as great as that of abstaining from cigarette smoking. Hummer, Rogers, Nam, and Ellison (1999) reported that religious involvement can add 7 to 14 years to life.

Larry Dossey (1993, 1999) summarized the growing body of research on the role of prayer in healing and wellness. The present chapter can only allude to the enormous literature that is accumulating. Braud (1990) showed that healing visualizations minimized negative effects on red blood cells when the blood was exposed to salt solution. Research at the Spindrift Institute in Oregon documented positive effects of prayer on the germination and growth of seeds (Dossey, 1993, p. 135). Randolph Byrd (1988) documented the practical effect of prayer by assigning 393 coronary care patients randomly to prayed-for and not-prayed-for conditions. The patients in the prayed-for condition were five times less likely to receive antibiotics, three times less likely to have pulmonary edema, and overall were less likely to die than were their counterparts in the non-prayer condition. Dossey emphasized that Christian, Jewish and Buddhist prayer similarly facilitates improved healing. The distance between the individual praying and the individual being prayed for has little effect, and positive effects can be measured even when the individual prayed for has no awareness of the prayer. This latter fact rules out a simple placebo explanation for the empirical effects of prayer.

Although some have criticized the methodology in the investigations on the empirical effects of prayer (Sloan & Bagiella, 2002), others raise the "best practices" question: If evidence continues to accumulate showing that prayer enhances health and optimizes survival, will future physicians be liable if they fail to pray for a patient?

Nevertheless, all prayer and all religious exercises are not exactly the same, and do not have the same effects. Elkins, Anchor, and Sandler (1979) compared the effects of relaxation and prayer. Subjects practicing relaxation reduced their EMG readings (muscle tension levels), while those practicing prayer did not affect either the EMG levels or their scores on the State-Trait Anxiety Inventory. Shaffer, Malone, Callahan, and Lipps (2001) studied the physiological effects of silent Bible reading and silent self-composed prayer. The silent self-composed prayer lowered accessory EMG significantly but did not lower other physiological measures. Silent Bible reading had no significant physiological effect. Research like this is critical, as believers should not mistakenly assume that prayer replaces all other relaxation and meditation strategies.

There can also be a dark side to religion and religious preoccupations that is not conducive to health. Pargament, Koenig,

Tarakeshwar, and Hahn (2001) studied elderly individuals with "religious struggles" and found that those who endorsed the following questionnaire items had an increased risk for death: "Wondered whether God had abandoned me," "Questioned God's love for me," and "Decided the devil made this happen." So the manner of involvement with religion can turn a potentially positive health factor into a health risk factor.

# THE PSYCHOPHYSIOLOGY OF THE SOUL

*Spiritual experiences are mind-body phenomena and invite one to apply the scientific tools of psychophysiology.*

Philosophers today no longer think about soul as some insubstantial entity that, added to a physical body, makes up a complete human being. Such Cartesian dualistic notions have fallen by the wayside. Our everyday language use of *soul* often refers to something deep and essential about the person. When I say that a person in my life "touched me in my soul," I mean that this person reached or affected me in some very special and lasting way, having to do with who I am.

Our sense of soul is rooted in the individual and collective histories of the person. Soul is neither abstract nor ethereal; rather, soul reverberates in memory with the resonance of childhood and personal roots. Soul has a sensory richness that is first auditory, with sounds and voices; second visual, with snapshot memories and images of primordial places of one's life; and third olfactory, with the rich fragrance of childhood. My spiritual roots resonate with the childhood echoes of Gregorian chants, glimpses of colorful priestly vestments, and the fragrance of incense. Another's roots are called up with the sensory richness of the seder celebration at Passover, the taste of bitter herbs, the

vision of family around the table, and the memory of the oldest son opening the door for the wandering prophet Elijah.

Some physiological functions, especially respiration, appear to be closer to the human experience of spirit. The word *spirit* derives from the Latin *spiritus*, with a root meaning of breath. The Greek *pneuma*, or breath, is also the soul. In Genesis, Yahweh breathed life into the man and "thus man became a living being" (Genesis 2:7). For the Hindu, the individual soul is *atman*, from the Sanskrit for breath. Previous research has found low serum lipid rates and low rates of cardiovascular disease in Buddhist monastic communities (Kita et al., 1988; Lehrer, Sasaki, & Saito, 1999; Ogata, Ikeda, & Kuratsune, 1984). Zen monks spend hours a day in meditation with very slow breathing, and Rinzai monks place special emphasis on *tanden* breathing— breathing slowly, focusing each breath, and meditating on an area below navel. In one illustrative psychophysiological investigation, Lehrer et al. reported on research on Zen monks and nuns in Japan. They found that during meditation, the monks' respiration rates slowed to a range associated with "low frequency" heart rate variability (0.05–0.15 Hz), and higher-frequency (0.15–0.4 Hz) heart rate variability decreased. One Rinzai master, who breathed at the slow rate of one breath per minute, showed an increase in very low frequency (less than 0.05 Hz) cardiac waves. Lehrer et al. interpreted this study as supporting the theory that slow breathing "resonates" with cardiac function and produces low-frequency cardiac oscillation with benefits for cardiac health.

# CLOSING: A CAUTION FOR PRACTICE

The take-home message from this article is not simply that health professionals should order their patients to "go to church and ask for God to heal them." Many of my patients have experienced a lifetime's worth of that kind of abusive advice, with the implication that perhaps their problems are due to their lack of faith or spiritual failures.

Optimal spirituality in health care does not consist of an evangelical Christian surgeon telling a Buddhist patient to follow Jesus Christ for a better outcome. No health care provider has a right to push a personal religious preference on a patient. Post, Puchalski, and Larson (2000) discuss appropriate and ethical professional approaches to patients' spirituality and suggest four questions to open discussion:

"Is faith (religion, spirituality) important to you in this illness?"

"Has faith been important at other times in your life?"

"Do you have someone to talk to about religious matters?"

"Would you like to explore religious matters with someone?"

Koenig (2000) offered a position on prayer with patients, suggesting that requests for prayer should come from the patient, and when the patient is comfortable, prayer can be deeply meaningful.

Our calling as physicians is to cure sometimes, relieve often, *comfort always*. If a distressed and scared patient asks for a prayer and the physician sees that such a prayer could bring comfort, then it is difficult to justify a refusal to do so. The comfort conveyed when a physician supports the core that gives the patient's life meaning and hope is what many patients miss in their encounters with caregivers. (p. 1708)

## NOTES

1. This chapter is expanded and modified from an earlier article, with permission of *Biofeedback* (Moss, 2001).
2. Reprinted with permission of Integrity Music. Copyright held by Integrity's Hosanna! Music/ASCAP, c/o Integrity Music, Inc., 1000 Cody Road, Mobile, AL 36695.

## REFERENCES

Benson, H. B. (1975). *The relaxation response.* New York: Morrow.
Braud, W. G. (1990). Distant mental influence on rate of hemolysis of human red blood cells. *Journal of the American Society for Psychical Research, 84*(1), 1–24.
Byrd, R. C. (1988). Positive therapeutic effects of intercessory prayer in a coronary care unit population. *Southern Medical Journal, 81*(7), 826–829.
Clark, M. B., & Olson, J. K. (2000). *Nursing within a faith community: Promoting health in times of transition.* Thousand Oaks, CA: Sage.
Dossey, L. (1993). *Healing words: The power of prayer and the practice of medicine.* San Francisco: HarperSanFrancisco.
Dossey, L. ( 1999). *Reinventing medicine: Beyond mind-body to a new era of healing.* San Francisco: HarperSanFrancisco.

Elkins, D., Anchor, K. N, & Sandler, H. M. (1979). Relaxation training and prayer behavior as tension reduction techniques. *Behavioral Engineering, 5*(3), 81–87.

Evans, D. (1998). Trading my sorrows. On *Freedom* [CD]. Mobile, AL: Integrity Music.

Foster, R. J. (1978). *The celebration of discipline.* NY: Harper & Row.

Helm, H. M., Hays, J. C., Flint, E. P., Koenig, H. G., & Blazer, D. G. (2000). Does private religious activity prolong survival? A six-year follow-up study of 3,851 older adults. *Journals of Gerontology. Series A, Biological Sciences and Medical Sciences, 55*(7), M400–M405.

Hummer, R., Rogers, R., Nam, C., & Ellison, C. (1999). Religious involvement and U.S. adult mortality. *Demography, 36,* 273–285.

Jaspers, K. (1932). *Philosophie* (4 volumes). Berlin: Springer-Verlag.

Kabat-Zinn, J. (1990). *Full catastrophe living.* New York: Bantam.

Kamiya, J. (1969). Operant control of the alpha EEG rhythm. In C. Tart (Ed.), *Altered states of consciousness* (pp. 507–515). New York: Wiley.

Kita, T., Yokode, M., Ishii, K., Nagano, Y., Mikami, A., Kita, M., et al. (1988). The concentration of serum lipids in Zen monks and control males in Japan. *Japanese Circulation Journal, 52,* 99–104.

Koenig, H. G. (1999). *The healing power of faith: Science explores medicine's last great frontier.* New York: Simon & Schuster.

Koenig, H. G. (2000). Religion, spirituality, and medicine: Application to clinical practice. *Journal of the American Medical Association, 284*(13), 1708.

Koenig, H. G., Hays, J., Larson, D., George, L. K., Cohen, H. J., McCullough, M. E., et al. (1999). Does religious attendance prolong survival? A six-year follow-up study of 3,968 older adults. *Journals of Gerontology. Series A, Biological Sciences and Medical Sciences, 54*(7), M370–M377.

Koenig, H. G., Larson, D. B., Hays, J. C., McCullough, M. E., George, L. K., Branch, P. S., et al. (1998). Religion and survival of 1010 male veterans hospitalized with medical illness. *Journal of Religion and Health, 37,* 15–29.

Koenig, H. G., McCullough, M. E., & Larson, D. B. (2001). *Handbook of religion and health.* New York: Oxford University Press.

Kushner, H. S. (1981). *When bad things happen to good people.* New York: Schocken Books.

Larson, D. B., & Larson, S. L. (1994). *The forgotten factor in physical and mental health: What does the research show? An independent study seminar.* Rockville, MD: National Institute for Healthcare Research.

Lehrer, P. M., Sasaki, Y., & Saito, Y. (1999). Zazen and cardiac variability. *Psychosomatic Medicine, 61,* 812–821.

Levin, J. S., & Vanderpool, H. Y. (1987). Is frequent religious attendance really conducive to better health? Toward an epidemiology of religion. *Social Science and Medicine, 24*(7), 589–600.

Luthe, W. (1969). *Autogenic therapy* (6 volumes). New York: Grune & Stratton.

McLeod, K. (2001). *Wake up to your life : Discovering the Buddhist path of attention.* San Francisco: HarperSanFrancisco.

Merton, T. (Ed. & Trans.). (1961). *The wisdom of the desert: Sayings from the Desert Fathers of the fourth century.* New York: New Directions.

Moore, T. (1992). *Care of the soul: A guide for cultivating depth and sacredness in everyday life.* New York: HarperCollins.

Moss, D. (1980). Transformation of self and world in Johannes Tauler's mysticism. *Revision: A Journal of Knowledge and Consciousness, 3*(2), 18–26. Revised version in R. Valle, and R. Von Eckartsberg (Eds.), *The metaphors of consciousness* (pp. 337–357). New York: Plenum.

Moss, D. (2001). Soul and spirit in health care. *Biofeedback, 29* (3), 4–7, 27.

Newberg, A., D'Aquili, E. G., & Rause, V. (2001). *Why God won't go away: Brain science and the biology of belief.* New York: Ballantine.

Nouwen, H. J. M. (1981). *The way of the heart: Desert spirituality and contemporary ministry.* New York: Seabury Press.

Ogata, M., Ikeda, M., & Kuratsune, M. (1984). Mortality among Japanese Zen priests. *Journal of Epidemiology and Community Health, 38,* 161-166

Pargament, K. I., Koenig, H. G., Tarakeshwar, N., & Hahn, J. (2001). Religious struggle as a predictor of mortality among medically ill elderly patients: A 2-year longitudinal study. *Archives of Internal Medicine, 161,* 1881–1885.

Peniston, E. G., & Kukolski, P. J. (1989). Alpha-theta brainwave training and beta-endorphin levels in alcoholics. *Alcoholism: Clinical and Experimental Research, 13,* 271–279.

Post, S. G., Puchalski, C., & Larson, D. (2000). Physicians and patient spirituality: Professional boundaries, competence, and ethics. *Annals of Internal Medicine, 132,* 578–583.

Quiller-Couch, A. (Ed.). (1939). *The Oxford book of English verse, 1250–1918.* New York: Oxford University Press.

Shaffer, F., Malone, E., Callahan, C., & Lipps, A. (2001). Is prayer relaxing? [Abstract]. *Applied Psychophysiology and Biofeedback, 26*(3), 246.

Sloan, R. P., & Bagiella, E. (2002). Claims about religious involvement and health outcomes. *Annals of Behavioral Medicine, 24* (1), 14-21.

Solari-Twadell, P. A., & McDermott, M. A. (Eds.). (1999). *Parish nursing: Promoting whole person health within faith communities.* Thousand Oaks, CA: Sage.

Xiangcai, X. (2000). *Qigong for treating common ailments: The essential guide to self-healing.* Boston, MA: YMAA Publication Center.

# Author Index

Aaron, L. A., 339, 340
Abbey, S. E., 335, 336
Abelson, J. L., 362
Abrahamsson, J., 342
Abrams, P., 315
Abreu, J., 241
Achterberg, J., 196, 449, 452
Adam, K., 252
Addis, M. E., 171
Ader, R., 9, 46, 70, 72, 76, 77, 114
Adera, T., 419, 420
Ad Hoc Committee on Classification
    of Headache, 207
Adolphs, R., 383, 384
Affleck, G., 409, 411
Agachan, F., 304
Aganoff, J. A., 425
Agosti, V., 387
Agudelo, C. A., 413
Ahern, D. K., 265
Ahlbom, A., 254
Ahles, T., 324
Ahmed, S., 400
Ahn, D. K., 280
Ahn, H., 123, 127
Alberts, K. R., 411
Alboukrek, D., 324
Aldag, J., 324
Alexander, C. N., 289
Alexander, F. M., 138
Alexander, R. W., 339, 340
Ali, A., 305, 307
Alkalay, D., 323
Allen, J. J., 389
Allen, R., 400
Allenback, G., 118
Allison, D. B., 291
Alper, K. R., 127
Alpert, J. J., 20
Altenmüller, E. O., 126
Alternative Medicine Foundation, 454
Altrocchi, J., 6
Alvarez, A., 127

Amar, P. B., 115, 370
Amen, D. G., 348
American Academy of Family Physicians
    (AAFP), 85, 458
American Academy of Physician Assistants, 458
American Association of Orofacial Pain, 228
American Diabetes Association, 276, 277,
    278, 279, 284
American Gastroenterological Association, 301
American Holistic Nurses' Association, 451
American Psychiatric Association, 194, 197, 347,
    364, 377, 378, 379, 380, 382, 420, 421
American Psychological Association (APA), 12,
    96, 97, 128, 194, 470
American Sleep Disorders Association, 393, 394,
    395, 398, 399, 400, 401
Amoroso-Camarata, J., 288, 289
Anaya, J.-M., 409
Anchor, K. N., 484
Anda, R., 254
Andersen, J. T., 315
Andersen, M. S., 155
Anderson, B. J., 283, 287
Anderson, G., 261
Anderson, G. W., 399
Anderson, J., 323, 324
Anderson, K. O., 413
Anderson, R. M., 283, 436
Andersson, L., 342
Anderton, C. H., 153, 155, 156
Andrasik, F., 4, 51, 74, 113, 116, 212, 216, 327
Andreski, P., 6
Andreychuk, T., 153
Andruzzi, E., 299
Angst, J., 211
Antai-Otong, D., 361
Antonuccio, D., 6
Apfel, R. J., 153, 155
Apfel-Savitz, R., 25
Appel, L. J., 289
Appel, S., 13, 14, 58, 60, 87, 430, 431,
    434, 437, 459, 462
Appelbaum, K. A., 4, 208

Appell, R. A., 317, 318, 319
Appels, A., 254
Applegate, W. B., 289
Arbanel, A., 65
Arbisi, P., 389
Arena, J. G., 74
Arendt-Nielsen, L., 151, 154
Arieti, S., 378
Arkin, A. M., 400
Arnett, F. C., 409, 410
Arnold, L. M., 6
Arnold, M. S., 283, 436
Aronne, L. J., 275
Arthur, M. W., 413
Asai, M., 282
Ashina, M., 114
Askanazi, J., 361
Asser, S. M., 197
Association for Applied Psychophysiology and
     Biofeedback, 66, 128, 468, 472, 473, 474
Association of Physician Assistant
     Programs, 457, 458
Astin, J., 60
Atkinson, G., 29, 75, 154
Atkinson, M., 254, 370
Atkinson, R., 21, 22, 153
Aune, B., 408
Austin, B. J., xviii
Avants, S. K., 184
Ax, S., 339

Babyak, M., 289
Bacchetti, P., 59
Badr, S., 404
Baehr, E., 384, 388, 424
Baehr, R., 384, 388
Baer, L., 155
Baerwald, C. G., 408
Bagby, J., 342
Bagiella, E., 484
Baglioni, A. J., Jr., 413
Baharloo, L., 229
Bailey, B. K., 289
Bakal, D. A., 209, 217
Baker, D., 254
Baker, J., 317
Baker, S., 243
Bakheit, A. M., 339, 340
Bakow, H., 304
Balint, E., 5
Balint, M., 5
Ballweg, R., 463
Bandstra, E., 453
Bandura, A., 411, 412, 430, 431, 432
Bangdiwala, S. I., 300
Banhamou, S., 184
Baptista, M. A., 73, 76
Barabasz, A. F., 153, 154, 155, 157
Barabasz, M., 153, 154, 155, 157

Barale, A., 364
Barber, J., 154
Barber, T. X., 72, 73, 76, 151
Bargh, J. A., 28
Barkham, M., 386, 387
Barkley, G., 206
Barkley, R. A., 347, 350, 351
Barlow, D. F., 369
Barlow, D. H., 8, 176, 218, 369
Barlow, W., 226
Barnes, V. A., 51, 289
Barnhart, H. X., 14
Barr, P. A., 436
Barrett-Connor, E., 276, 278
Barron, F. X., 196
Barsky, A., 85
Barsky, A. J., 45, 51
Barton, K. A., 208
Bartsokis, T., 253
Basham, R. B., 30
Baskin, S., 206, 209, 212
Baskin, S. M., 116
Basmajian, J., 328
Basmajian, J. V., 110, 118, 265
Bass, C., 44, 300
Bass, E. B., 20
Bassett, M. T., 280
Bassman, L., 59, 65
Basta, R., 6
Bates, D. W., 336
Batitucci, E., 228
Battafarano, D., 323, 324
Battie, M. C., 259
Beary, J. F., 461
Beaupre, P., 411, 412
Bechara, A., 383
Beck, A. T., 138, 168, 171, 176, 218, 363, 369, 382
Beck, J. S., 168, 169, 172, 174, 176
Beck, L., 420
Beck, W. S., 342
Becker, D. J., 281
Beckerman, A., 437
Beckles-Wilson, N. R., 214
Beckman, R. J., 291
Beecher, H. K., 70, 76
Behan, P. O., 339, 340
Bekkelund, S. I., 408
Belicki, D., 22, 153, 155
Belicki, K., 22, 153, 155
Bell, D. S., 335
Bell, R. A., 281
Belles, D. R., 231
Belyea, M., 436
Bemporad, J., 378
Benca, R. M., 401
Bendtsen, L., 114
Benness, C., 317
Bennett, H. L., 151
Bennett, P. H., 276

Bennett, R. M., 323, 329
Bennett, R., 324, 330, 335
Bennett, R. T., 50
Benoit, J., 335, 339
Benotsch, E. G., 151, 156
Benson, H., 50, 113, 137, 138, 146, 147
Benson, H. B., 461, 480
Benson, K., 355
Bentin, S., 28
Berbaum, K. S., 151, 156
Berbaum, M. L., 151, 156
Berch, H., 333, 334, 335, 336
Berg, J. E., 184
Berg, K., 389
Berger, B. C., 370, 371
Berger, H., 123
Bergin, A., 70
Bergin, A. E., 98, 195
Berglund, G., 282
Bergman, A., 316, 317
Berkelmans, I., 300
Berkson, D. M., 276
Berlin, L. E., 450
Bernal, G. A. A., 291
Bernier, C., 300
Bernstein, D., 424
Bernstein, D. I., 4, 244
Bernstein, I. L., 4, 244
Bernstein, J. G., 359
Bernstein, L., 244
Bernstein, R., 114
Berntson, G. G., 45
Beyer, H., 265
Beyerstein, B. L., 13
Bhat, K., 253
Bhat, N., 253, 255
Bhatia, N. N., 316
Bhatnagar, S. O. D., 243, 289
Bianchi, A., 26
Bianchi, M., 404
Biederman, H. J., 265
Bigos, S. J., 259
Billiard, M., 409
Billiot, K., 327
Birbaumer, N., 114, 126, 128, 129, 325
Bishop, G. D., 196
Bishop, K. R., 317
Bittencourt, M., 228
Bjerring, P., 151, 154
Bjork, R. A., 145
Black, R., 300
Black, S., 154, 155
Blackburn, J., 124
Blackwood, S. K., 341
Blair, T., 131
Blaivas, J. G., 315, 317, 318, 319
Blake, F., 425
Blanchard, E. B., 4, 5, 9, 74, 116, 131, 168,
    208, 211, 214, 290, 291, 305, 306, 307

Bland, S. D., 434
Blank, M., 432
Blankenhorn, V., 128
Blazer, D. G., 484
Bleijenberg, G., 307
Blessing, J. D., 463
Bliss, E. L., 22, 153
Bloch, D. A., 409, 410
Blonshine, S., 4
Blood, M. L., 400
Bloom, J. R., 156, 157, 197
Blount, A., 5
Blum, G. S., 154
Blum, K., 348
Blumenfeld, A., 338
Blumenthal, J. A., 250, 253, 254, 289, 425
Bo, S., 283
Bocher, P., 127
Boersma, J., 324
Bogart, R. K., 230
Bogduk, N., 325
Boichut, D., 404
Bolen, J. C., 434
Bolocofsky, D. N., 155
Boltwood, E., 253
Bombardiare, C., 323, 329
Bond, A., 44
Bond, E. F., 300
Bond, J. A., 28
Bonk, V., 410, 411
Bonnet, M. H., 401
Boone, J. L., 49
Bootzin, R. R., 396
Borcherding, S., 207, 212
Bork, C. E., 459
Borkovec, T. D., 145
Born, L., 424
Bornstein, R. F., 70
Borus, J. F., 45, 51, 85
Borysenko, J., 50
Bosworth, M. F., 435, 436
Bouchard, C., 275
Bouchard, T. J., Jr., 24, 155
Bou-Houlaigah, L., 335, 339
Boulard, N. E., 421, 422
Bourey, R. E., 276
Bourguignon, E., 197
Boushey, H. A., 235
Bouter, L. M., 281, 282
Boutros, N. N., 207, 212
Bowden, C. A., 338
Bowen, M., xiii
Bowen, R. C., 364
Bower, P., 88
Bowers, K. S., 151, 154
Bowers, P. E., 24
Bown, R., 300
Boyle, G. J., 425
Braddom, R. L., 261

Bradley, L. A., 339, 340, 411, 413
Brakel, L. A., 28
Branch, P. S.. 484
Brann, D. W., 423
Brassire, A., 397
Braud, W. G., 484
Brauer, D., 265
Braun, C., 114, 325
Braun, G. G., 153
Braunwald, E., 251
Braunwald, W., 252
Bray, G. A., 275
Bray, J. H., 12
Breasure, J., 198
Breedveld, F. C., 407
Brenner, G. F., 44
Breslau, N., 6, 211
Bridges, K. W., xv
Brigham, D. D., 452
Brim, S., 124
Broderick, J. E., 412
Brodie, H., xv
Brody, D., xv, 43
Brody, H., 459
Brook, R. D., 282
Brooke, R., 22, 153, 155
Brooks, P. M., 412
Brown, B., 110
Brown, B. W., 430, 431, 432
Brown, D., 123, 127
Brown, D. P., 153
Brown, D. T., 229
Brown, G., 378
Brown, J. S., 313
Brown, J. W., 20
Brown, M., 154
Brown, S. J., 431
Brownell, K. D., 156
Bruce, B. K., 300
Bruce, R. A., 70, 76
Bruder, G. E., 387
Brunet, A., 24
Brunk, S. E., 413
Brunner, C. M., 413
Bruno, O., 211
Brus, H. L., 412
Brutsaert, D. L., 49
Buceta, J. M., 241, 242
Buchanan, D. C., 396
Buchwald, D., 333, 334, 335, 336
Buckelew, S. P., 343, 411, 413
Buckley, J., 167
Budd, M., 50
Budzynski, T., 327
Budzynski, T. H., 65
Buick, D. L., 167
Buijs, R. J. C., 265
Buki, V. M., 45, 287
Bulechek, G., 452

Bull, J., 77
Bullock, M. L., 184
Burckhardt, C., 324, 330
Burg, M., 253
Burgio, K. L., 318
Burkhart, K. S., 315
Burks, K. J., 437
Burleson, M. H., 45
Burnet, R. B., 342
Burnett, C. K., 307
Burnett, R., 411
Burns, D. D., 170, 172, 369, 387
Burns, P. A., 318
Burr, R., 408
Burt, V. L., 277
Burton, E., 229
Burton, J. R., 318
Busch, S., 129
Bush, C., 74
Buskila, D., 323
Bustros, J., 317, 318
Butler, P. M., 283
Button, J., 154
Buzaitis, A., 408
Byers, A. P., 270
Byrd, R. C., 484
Byrne, E. A., 26, 366

Cacioppo, J. T., 45, 46
Cadusch, P. J., 126
Cailliet, R., v
Cain, K. C., 300
Calabrese, L. H., 335
Caldwell, D. S., 410, 411, 412
Calfas, K. J., 51
Calkins, D. R., 58, 60
Calkins, H., 335, 339
Callahan, C., 484
Callahan, J. C., 94, 95, 99
Callahan, L. F., 411, 413
Callanan, P., 94, 95, 97, 98, 99
Callegari, S., 244
Calne, D. B., 70
Cameron-Sampey, D. C., 452
Camilleri, M., 300
Camp, B. W., 130
Campbell, M. J., 342
Campbell, S., 324
Campbell, S. S., 399
Cancro, R., 127
Canelones, P., 241
Canter, A., 27
Cardena, E., 194
Cardozo, L., 317
Carlan, S. J., 319
Carlander, B, 409
Carlson, B., 154
Carlson, V., 241, 242
Carlsson, A., 276

Carlsson, G. E., 225
Carlsson, S. G., 226
Carmichael, B. D., 348
Carnes, M., 319
Carney, R. M., 387
Carol, M. P., 461
Carpenter, M. E., 26
Carr, R. E., 242, 243, 244
Carrington, P., 138, 146, 147
Carroll, B. J., 420
Case, A. M., 421
Cash, J. M., 335
Cass, H., 386
Cassano, G., 382
Cassell, E. J., 4, 89
Cassidy, C. A., 435, 437
Cassisi, J. E., 231, 265
Castés, M., 241
Castillo, J., 205
Cavagnini, F., 282
Cavallo-Perin, P., 283
Cawley, J. F., 458, 459
Cedercreutz, C., 155
Celentano, D. D., 205
Centers for Disease Control and Prevention,
    237, 276, 278, 279, 334, 335, 336, 339
Ceresoli, A., 317, 318
Cha, G., 131
Chabot, R. J., 127, 353
Chabriat, H., 210
Chaffin, D., 261
Chalder, T., 340
Challis, G. B., 24, 73, 155
Chamberlin, J., 43
Chambers, L. A., 291
Chambless, D. L., 128
Chang, P., 184
Chang, R. W., 410
Charest, J., 75
Chatterton, B. E., 342
Chatterton, R. T., 408
Chaturvedi, N., 280
Chavira, J. A., 193
Chenard, J. R., 75
Cheney, P. R., 333, 334, 335, 336, 341
Chernigovskaya, N. V., 243
Cheskin, L. J., 291
Chesney, M., 253
Chester, T. D., 24, 153
Chestnut, W. N., 184
Chevalier, H., 404
Chila, A. G., 74
Chilcoat, H., 6
Child, C., 59
Chiotakakou-Faliakou, E., 307
Chiverton, S. G., 184
Christensen, J. F., 49
Christie-Seely, J., xiii
Chrousos, G. P., 46, 333, 335, 339

Chung, D. G., 335, 336
Cigada, M., 26
Clapp, A. J., 341, 343
Clapp, L. L., 341, 343
Clare, A., 305
Clark, D. A., 168
Clark, D. M., 363
Clark, L. A., 30
Clark, M. B., 483
Clark, M. E., 370
Clark, M. L., 300
Clark, M. M., 44
Clark, R., 330
Clark, S., 324
Clark, S. C., 335
Clarke, L., 214
Claros, A. G., 229
Clavel-Chapelon, F., 184
Clay, R., 473
Clayborne, B. M., 289
Clemence, C., 184
Clemmey, P., 411
Cliver, S. P., 319
Clouse, R. E., 282, 288, 292
Cluff, L. E., 27
Cobb, I. A., 70, 76
Cobbe, S. M., 286, 287
Coderre, T., 325
Coffey, P., 50
Cohen, H. D., 71, 74
Cohen, H. J., 484
Cohen, M., 59, 60, 63, 64
Cohen, M. J., 349
Cohen, N., 9, 46, 72, 114
Cohen, S., 46, 48, 51
Cohn, N., 250
Colditz, G. A., 283
Coleman, G., 72, 76
Colgan, S. M., 151, 156, 300, 304, 305, 307
Collette, P., 276
Collings, G. H., 146, 147
Collins, J. F., 169
Collins, J. K., 154
Collins, R. W., 301, 308
Collison, D. A., 155
Colson, R., 300
Compas, B. E., 168
Con, A. H., 290
Concato, J., 355
Conners, C. K., 350
Conroy, A. M., 24, 153
Consensus Trial Study Group, 250
Constantini, S., 26
Contrades, S., 452
Conway, A., 367
Conway, R., 343
Coogler, C., 14
Cook, M. R., 71, 74
Cooper, N. S., 409, 410

Cooper, P., 305, 307
Cooper, R., 276
Coran, A., 304
Corao, A., 241
Corazziari, E., 299, 300, 301, 303
Corcoran, C., 47
Cordingley, G., 205, 211
Cordingley, G. E., 207, 209, 212, 215
Cordingley, G. F., 215
Cordray, D. S., 411
Corey, G., 94, 95, 97, 98, 99
Corey, M. S., 94, 95, 97, 98, 99
Corney, R. H., 305
Corning, W. C., 123, 127
Cornwell, N., 214
Corry, D. B., 235
Coryell, W., 382
Cosire, F., 22, 153, 155
Costa, P. T., Jr., 75
Coulter, A., 284
Coulter, I., 187
Coulthard-Morris, L., 155
Council, J. R., 154, 265
Couper, J., 168, 340, 341
Cowan, M., 408
Cox, I. M., 342
Coyne, J., 6
Cram, J. R., 212
Craske, M. G., 145, 176, 369
Crawford, G., 127, 353
Crawford, H. J., 154
Crawford, S., 59
Creed, F., 305
Creer, T. L., 242, 244
Creighton, J., 452
Crider, A. B., 230
Cripps, H. A., 304
Criqui, M. H., 276, 278
Critelli, J. W., 140
Crits-Christoph, P., 168
Croci, M., 282
Crockett, J. E., 70, 76
Crouch, M., xiii
Crowne, D. P., 21
Crowson, J. J., 24, 153
Cruikshanks, P., 305, 307
Csikszentmihalyi, M., 24
Culbertson, A. L., 411
Culligan, P. J., 315, 316
Culliton, P. D., 184
Culter, J. A., 277
Cummings, J., 11
Cummings, J. L., 364
Cummings, N., 11
Cummings, N. A., 364
Curtis, G. C., 362
Cutcomb, S., 154
Cutner, A., 317
Cutolo, M., 408

Cyr, M. G., 444
Cyr-Provost, M., 207, 212
Czeisler, C. A., 399

Dafter, R. E., 29
Dahlström, L., 226
Dahme, B., 242, 243, 244
Dailey, J., 324
Dake, J. A., 459
Dale, J. K., 335, 339, 340
Dalessio, D. J., 116, 206
Damasio, A. R., 28, 29, 83, 84, 152, 383, 384
Damasio, H., 383, 384
Dams, P.-C., 8
Damsker, J. I., 444
Danchot, J., 210
D'Andrea, G., 206
Danning, C., 323, 324
Danton, W. G., 6
Dantzer, R., 45
D'Aquili, E. G., 481
Das, J. P., 23, 27, 72, 73, 76
Da Silva, J. A. P., 407, 408
Davenport, T. L., 127
Davert, E. C., 155
David, S. V., 128
Davidson, M., xii, 341
Davidson, R. J., 138, 382, 383, 384, 388
Davies, M., 10, 21, 25, 28, 30, 33
Davies, S. M., 445, 446
Davies, T., 10, 21, 25, 30, 33, 212
Davies, T. C., 84, 90, 444
Davies, W. H., 288, 289
Davis, A., 452
Davis, G. C., 211
Davis, H., 51, 289
Davis, K., 88
Davis, M. K., 218
Davis, R. B., 13, 14, 58, 60, 87, 430, 431, 437, 459, 462
Dawson, A. A., 156
Dawson, D., 305
Dawson, G., 378
Dawson, P., 399
Day, A., 425
D'Costa, A., 241
Deale, A., 340
DeBecker, P., 341
DeBenedittis, G., 26, 153, 210, 211
de Blic, J., 364
De Chant, H., 20, 49
Deckersback, T., 387
Deckro, J. P., 291
de Courten, M. P., 275
DeGood, D., 452
DeGruy, F. V., III, xv, 6, 20, 21, 43, 88
DeJoseph, J. F., 403
de Kloet, R., 324
DeLaCruz, M., 51

de la Fuente-Fernandez, R., 70
Delbanco, T. L., 58, 60
DeLeeuw, I., 341, 342
De Lorgeril, M., 283
De Luca, C., 328
DeLuca, C. J., 265
DeLuca, J., 341
DeMarco, G., 51
Dembroski, T., 253
DeMeirleir, K., 341
Demitrack, M. A., 335, 339, 340
Dempsey, J., 404
Denis, P., 300
Dennerstein, L., 425, 426
Dennett, D., 29
Dennis, C., 253
Denollet, J., 49
Dentinger, M. P., 116, 208, 211
Department of Health and Human
     Services, 434
DePascalis, V., 153
DePasqua, V., 207, 212, 212
Depue, R., 389
Deriu, F., 139
de Rivera, J. L. G., 241
Derman, S., 323, 324
Derogatis, L., 330
Derogatis, L. R., 20
DeRubeis, R. J., 168, 169, 171, 172
Descartes, R., 59
Deshields, T. L., 225
Desotelle, P., 318
Deuser, W. E., 343
Deuster, P. A., 419, 420
Devalos, M., 378
Devaul, R. A., 27
Devine, D. A., 153
Devlin, M. J., 44, 281, 291
De Vries, H., 281, 282
de Vries, R. R., 407
Devroede, G., 300
Deyo, R. A., 8, 70, 71
Diabetes Research Working Group, 278
Diamant, N. E., 300, 304
Diamond, S., 214
Diclemente, C. C., 50, 434, 435, 436
Diener, H. C., 209, 210
Dietrich, A. J., 47
Diez-Rouz, A. V., 280
DiGasbarro, I., 305, 307
Dijk, D. J., 399
Dill, L., 20, 49
Dillard, D. H., 70, 76
Dimmock, P. W., 423, 424
Dimond, E. G., 70, 76, 182
Dimsdale, J. E., 46, 281
Dinan, T. G., 339, 340
Ditto, B., 74
Dixon, D. C., 230

Dixon, M., 24
D'Lugoff, B. C., 290
Dmochowski, R. R., 317, 318, 319
Dobbins, J. G., 336, 337
Dobson, K. S., 168, 171
Dolce, J. J., 265
Donaldson, C. C. S., 323, 324, 325, 326,
     327, 328, 329, 330
Donaldson, M., 326, 328
Donaldson, M. S., xi, xv
Donchin, Y., 26
Dondershine, H., 22, 153
Donnelly, G. F., 430
Donnelly, M., 436
Donovan, S., 387
Doolittle, T., 336
Dorhofer, D. M., 421, 422
Dossey, B. M., 451
Dossey, L., 61, 87, 254, 484
Dougherty, M., 317
Downing, B., 28
Dowson, D., 342
Doyle, W. J., 46
Dozois, D. J. A., 168
Drane, J. R., 101
Dreher, H., 11
Dresselhaus, T. R., 90
Drewes, A. M., 409
Drossman, D. A., 299, 300, 301, 303, 304
Dryden, W., 168
Dryehag, L. E., 342
Dubos, R., xii
Duckro, P. N., 225
Duff, S., 408
Duffy, F. H., 128
DuHamel, K., 22, 26, 35, 153
Duke, D. L., 187
Duncan, R., 184
Dundee, J. W., 184
Dunner, D. L., 386
Dunni, W. J., 230
Dunsmore, J., 411
Durney-Crowley, J., 450, 451
Duvall, K., 243
Dworkin, S. F., 224, 225, 226, 227, 228, 229
Dworkind, M., 44
Dworschak, M., 210
Dwosh, I., 410
Dyer, A., 276
Dykes, S., 300
D'Zurilla, T. J., 168

Eaker, E., 254
Earnest, C., 388
Eastman, C. I., 389
Easton, P., 65, 123, 127, 353
Eaton, K. K., 343
Eccleston, C., 168
Edelberg, R., 242

Edinger, J. D., 396
Edkins, G., 5
Edmeads, J., 205
Edworthy, S. M., 409, 410
Ee, J. S., 140
Egolf, G., 254
Ehde, D. M., 151, 156
Eisenberg, D. M., 13, 14, 58, 60, 87, 430,
    431, 437, 457, 459, 460, 462
Eisenberg, L., 432
Eisman, E., 315, 318
Ekelund, P., 317, 319
Elbert, T., 114, 325
El-Galley, R. E., 319
Elger, C. E., 124
Elia, G., 317
Eliopoulos, C., 430, 431, 433
Eliot, R., 253, 254
Elkin, I., 169, 171
Elkins, D., 484
Elkins, D. N., 191
Ellenberg, S. S., 129
Ellis, A., 168, 170, 196, 369
Ellison, C., 484
Ellsworth, N., 291
Elswick, R. K., 318
Emery, G., 176, 363, 369
Emley, M., 265
Emmott, S. D., 176
Emmott, S., 305, 307
Enck, P., 300, 304, 305, 306
Endre, T., 282
Engel, B. T., 290, 318
Engel, G. L., xii, 11, 86, 87, 443
England, R., 324
Engstrom, D. R., 75, 157
Epping-Jordan, J. E., 90
Epstein, H., 127
Epstein, W. V., 413
Erbaugh, J., 382
Erdman, H. P., 387
Eriksen, B. C., 317
Ernest, C., 384, 388
Ernst, E., 8, 12
Eshelman, S., 359
Esparza, J., 276
Espeland, M. A., 289
Ettinger, W. H., 289
Ettner, S., 13, 14, 58, 60, 87, 459, 462
Ettner, S. L., 430, 431, 437
Etzwiler, D. D., 430
Evans, D., 482
Evans, D. D., 4, 50
Evans, F. J., 22, 70, 71, 72, 76, 153, 154
Evans, J. R., 65
Evans, M. D., 169
Ewer, T. C., 151, 155
Expert Committee, 276
Expert Panel, 277, 278

Fabrizi, P., 211
Fahrion, S., 144
Fahy, J. V., 235
Faillace, L. A., 27
Fairclough, P., 305
Faith, M. S., 291
Fall, M., 317, 319
Fanselow, M. S., 383
Fantl, J. A., 316, 318
Faragher, E. B., 151, 156, 307
Farrar, D. J., 339, 340
Farrell, E., 425, 426
Feeley, M., 172
Feigenbaum, S. L., 408
Feinglos, M. N., 288
Feinman, C., 75
Feinstein, A. R., 89
Feixas, G., 172
Feld, J. M., 26
Feldenkrais, M., 138
Feldman, J. J., 364
Feldman, J. M., 345
Felt, B., 304
Felten, D., 46
Fenger, T. N., 349
Fennis, J. F., 307
Ferber, R., 399, 400
Ferrara, A., 306
Feste, C. C., 283
Feuerstein, M., 74
Fick, L. J., 151, 156
Field, T., 378, 453
Findlay, H., 205
Fine, T. H., 290
Fink, C. M., 421, 422
Fisch, B. J., 124
Fish, L., 244
Fisher, E. B., 283, 287
Fisher, J. G., 74
Fisher, S., 22, 26, 35, 69, 70, 153
Fitzgerald, J. T., 283
Flaws, B., 64, 65
Fleshner, M., 46
Fletcher, E., 324
Fletcher, E. M., 338
Flint, E. P., 484
Flor, H., 114, 126, 128, 212, 325
Florin, I., 241
Flotzinger, D., 128
Fogg, L. F., 389
Folen, R. A., 340
Folkman, S., 45
Follick, M. J., 265
Fonseca, V., 283
Fontaine, K. R., 291
Forbes, M., 229
Ford, D. E., 404
Ford, I., 286, 287
Fordyce, W. E., 70, 71

Forrest, K. Y. Z., 281
Forsblom, C., 276
Fortney, J., 6
Foster, C., 58, 60
Foster, R. J., 483
Fotopoulos, S. S., 71, 74
Fouad-Tarazi, F. M., 335
Fox, D. A., 408
Fox, N., 378
Fox, S., 127
Foxhall, K., 12
France, C. R., 114, 207, 209, 212
France, J. L., 114
Frank, E., 422
Frank, J. B., 193
Frank, J. D., 76, 193
Frank, R. G., 12
Frankel, F. H., 25, 153, 155
Franks, P., 281, 282
Fraser, R. J., 276
Frederick, J., 124
Freedland, K. E., 288, 292
Freedman, R. R., 116, 144, 403
Freeman, A., 453
Freeman, D. J., 287
Freeman, L. J., 250, 251, 252
Freeman, L. W., 13
Freeman, R., 335
French, M., 51
Freud, S., 28
Fricton, J. R., 225
Fridman, J., 65
Fried, R., 361
Friedberg, F., 340
Friedman, J., 353
Friedman, M., 252
Friedman, R., 291
Fries, J. F., 409, 410
Frisch, N. C., 451
Fritsche, G., 210
Frohberg, N., 381
Frolich, M., 287
Fromm, E., 157
Frymoyer, J., 261
Fujita, T., 290
Fukuda, K., 336, 337
Fulkerson, W. J., 235
Fuller, J. H., 280
Funnell, M. M., 283, 436
Furst, M., 114, 325
Fuster, J. M., 347
Fyer, A., 361

Gaarder, K. R., 290
Gaeddert, A., 59
Gaffney, R. D., 342
Gaist, D., 210
Galeta, G., 318
Galli, C., 211

Galli, F., 211
Gallitano, A., 47
Galloway, N. T., 319
Galuska, D. A., 291
Galvin-Nadeau, M., 339
Gantz, N. M., 336
Garada, B. M., 335, 336
Garcia, F. O., 197
Garfield, S., 70
Garfinkel, P. E., 22, 28
Garrod, A., 425
Garvey, M. J., 169
Gasser, T., 127
Gath, D., 425
Gaudet, E. L., 229
Gauthier, D. M., 453
Gavard, J. A., 282
Geiger, A., 333, 334, 335, 336
Geisler, F. H., 127
Gekoski, W. L., 154
Gelenberg, A., 386
Gellhorn, E., 139, 242
Generelli, P., 242
Gentile, L., 283
George, L., xv
George, L. K., 484
Georgiades, A., 289
Gerard, P., 207, 212, 212
Gerardi, M. A., 290, 291
Gerardi, R. J., 290, 291
Gerdes, J. L., 90
Gerin, W., 254
Gerlach, A. L., 362
Germgard, T., 342
Germino, B. B., 436
Gershuny, B. S., 387
Gerson, I., 127
Gevirtz, R., 366, 370, 371, 372, 469
Gevirtz, R. N., 473, 474
Geyman, J. P., 8
Ghaly, R. G., 184
Ghanayim, N., 128
Giardino, N. D., 245
Gibbs, F. A., 123, 127
Giblin, E. C., 403
Gick, M., 153
Gil, K. M., 411
Gill, D., 44
Giller, E. L., Jr., 46
Gilmore, S. L., 289
Gimotty, P., 317
Girton, L., 420
Glaros, A. G., 129, 225, 226, 227, 228, 229, 230
Glaser, R., 11
Glasgow, M. S., 290
Glasgow, R. E., 283, 287
Glasman, A., 254
Glass, E. G., 225, 226, 227, 228, 229, 230

Glass, G. V., 151, 155, 156
Glasser, M., 444
Glaun, D. E., 244
Glaus, K. D., 242
Glavind, K., 318
Gleit, M., 335, 336
Goadsby, P. J., 206
Gobel, H., 210
Godfrey, C., 13
Goebel, M., 117, 290
Goeppinger, J., 413
Gold, D. M., 304
Gold, M. S., 365
Gold, P. W., 46, 333, 335, 339
Goldberg, D., 88
Goldberg, D. P., xv
Goldberg, M. L., 151, 156
Goldberg, R. J., 90
Goldenberg, D. L., 323, 329, 339
Goldensohn, E. S., 126
Goldfine, I. D., 281
Goldman, L., 423
Goldstein, A., 154
Goldstein, M. G., 51
Goldstein, R., 408
Gollan, J. K., 171
Gonsalkorale, W. M., 305, 307
Gonzalez, J. J., 349
Gonzalez, V., 412, 430
Gonzalez-Martin, I. J., 241
Good, B., 432
Good, M. P., 289
Goodall, T. A., 282
Goodman, B. M., 319
Goodman, M., 253
Goodnick, P. J., 45, 287, 340
Goodwin, F. K., 86
Goodwin, G. M., 341
Gordon, A., 462, 463
Gorlib, I. H., 131
Gorman, J. M., 8, 361, 371
Gortner, E., 171
Gotlib, I. H., 382, 383
Gottehil, E., 156, 157, 197
Goupil, G., 300
Grady, D., 313
Grady, E., 323, 324
Graffin, N. F., 153
Graham, C., 71, 74
Graham, G., 289
Gram, L., 210
Gramling, S. E., 230
Grammith, F. C., 341
Granella, F., 211
Grassi, C., 139
Gray, B., 335, 336
Gray, C. E., 339, 340
Grayson, R., 230
Greeley, A. M., 197

Green, A. M., 10, 109, 110
Green, E., 10, 109, 110
Green, G., 127, 349
Green, J., 117, 154
Greenberg, M. D., 70
Greenberg, R. P., 69, 70
Greenberger, D., 174, 175, 176
Greene, B., 305, 307
Greene, C. S., 225
Greenleaf, M., 22, 26, 35, 153
Greenwald, A. G., 28
Gregg, V. H., 339
Greineder, D. K., 244
Greist, J. H., 387
Griep, E., 324
Griep, E. N., 411
Griffith, J., 409
Griffith, L. S., 282, 288, 292
Grillmayr, H., 292
Grof, C., 193
Grof, S., 60, 193
Grollman, A. P., 8
Groop, L., 278, 280
Grootenhuis, P. A., 281, 282
Gross, J. J., 50
Gross, M., 348
Grossman, P., 254
Groth-Marnat, G., 5
Group, L. C., 276
Grove, J. R., 24
Grove, W. M., 169
Grubb, B. P., 46
Gruzalier, J., 131
Guadagnoli, E., 431, 432
Guarini, J., 432
Guarneri, A., 317, 318
Guerra, S., 228
Guidetti, V., 211
Guilleminault, C., 397
Guitera, V., 205
Gulledge, A. D., 300
Gullette, E. C., 289
Gunary, R. M., 151, 156
Guthrie, E., 305
Guzzetta, C. E., 451
Gwaltney, J. M., Jr., 46

Haaga, D. A. F., 168
Haanen, H. C. M., 156
Haas, L. J., 102
Habib, K. E., 333, 335, 339
Habib, T., 352
Hackman, A., 340
Hadley, E. C., 318
Hadley, H. R., 317, 318, 319
Haffner, S. M., 276
Hagel, I., 241
Haggerty, C., 230
Hahn, E. G., 241

Hahn, I., 317, 319
Hahn, J., 485
Hahn, S. R., xv, 43
Hains, A. A., 288, 289
Hajak, G., 404
H'ajek, P., 153, 155
Haken, J., 317
Haley, W. E., 12
Halford, W. K., 282
Hall, G. M., 407, 408
Hall, J. R., 74
Hall, M. J., 243
Hall, R. C. W., 27
Hallas, J., 210
Hallowell, E. M., 351
Halstead, W. C., 348
Hamer, R., 242
Hamilton, D., 151
Hamilton, L., 156
Hamilton, M., 382
Hamilton, P., 408
Hand, G. A., 139
Haney, T. L., 253
Hanington, E., 214
Hannerz, J., 214
Hanninen, O., 265
Harden, H., 243
Hardy, G. E., 386, 387
Harkins, S. W., 318
Harmon, R. L., 50
Harper, D., 450
Harper, R. A., 369
Harrell, J. S., 434
Harris, E. D., Jr., 407, 408
Harris, M. J., 127, 353
Harris, R. M., 26
Harrison, G. L., 313
Hart, J. T., 75, 157
Harth, M., 323, 324, 326
Hartz, A. J., 355
Harver, A., 242
Harvey, E. N., 393
Harvey, R. F., 151, 156
Harvey, W., 75
Harwood, M. K., 318
Hashish, L., 75
Haskell, W. L., 291
Haskett, R. F., 420
Hasselmark, L., 214
Hatch, J. P., 74, 207, 212, 226
Haupt, J., xv
Hauri, P., 396, 397
Hawley, D. J., 409
Hawton, K., 340
Hayden, W. J., 226, 227
Haynes, R. B., 7
Hays, J. C., 484
He, D., 184
He, Y., 127

Headache Classification Committee, 205, 206, 207, 208
Health Care Finance Administration, 9, 317, 319, 473
Heath, G. W., 291
Heather, N., 51
Heaton, K., 300, 303, 304
Hebert, L., 323, 324
Heetderks, W. J., 128
Heger, M., 66
Heide, F., 145
Heine, R. J., 281, 282
Heinze, A., 210
Heit, M., 315, 316
Heitkemper, M., 300, 420, 422, 423
Hekster, G. B., 156
Heldring, M., 12
Heller, B. R., 450, 451
Hellman, C. J. C., 50
Helm, H. M., 484
Helms, J. M., 182, 185
Helstad, C. P., 51
Hemond, M., 300
Hendrick, V., 422
Henk, H. J., 51
Henker, B., 347
Henker, R., 420, 423
Henning, K., 50
Henriksson, L., 317, 318, 319
Henriques, J. B., 382
Henry, J. H., 45, 287
Henry, M., 241
Henry, P., 210
Herbs, D., 291
Herkenham, M., 196
Herman, J., 171
Herman, J. L., 6
Hernstein, R. J., 72
Hertel, R. K., 28
Herting, R., 381
Herzog, A. R., 313
Hewett, J. E., 413
Heymen, S., 300
Hickie, I., 336, 337
Hida, W., 237
Higgins, J. T., 291
Higgins, J. T., Jr., 117, 290, 291
Higgins, M., 277
Higgins, P., 409
Hilgard, E. R., 23, 73, 76, 152, 154, 155
Hilgard, J. R., 23, 154, 155
Hill, C., 75
Hill, D., 378
Hill, K., 205, 211
Hinderstein, B., 225
Hinterberger, T., 128
Hinton, R. A., 151, 156
Hirsch, M., 409
Hirschfeld, R., 386

Hirschman, R., 370
Hobart, G., 393
Hochberg, M. C., 410
Hochron, S., 155, 241, 242
Hoenderdos, T. W., 156
Hoffman, C., 430, 443
Hoffman, R. W., 411
Hoizey, D., 187
Hoizey, M. J., 187
Hollaender, J., 241
Hollander, B., 153
Holley, R. L., 319
Hollingshead, W. H., 259
Hollon, S. D., 128, 169
Holloszy, J. O., 276
Holm, J. E., 74, 116, 210, 215
Holman, E. A., 44, 50
Holman, H., 412, 413
Holmes, G. P., 336
Holmes, R. H., 30
Holroyd, K. A., 74, 114, 116, 205, 207, 208, 209,
      211, 212, 213, 215, 217
Holtzman, D., 434
Holzapfel, S., 128
Holzman, A. D., 168
Home, L., 22
Homma, M., 237
Honkoop, P., 211
Hooker, R. S., 458, 459
Hop, W. C. J., 156
Horan, M. J., 277
Horie, H., 124
Horne, L., 153, 154
Horne, R., 167
Horne, R. L., 22, 153, 154
Horner, J., 289, 291
Horowitz, M., 276
Horowitz, R., 355
Hostmark, A. T., 184
Hotovy, L. A., 421, 422
Hou, Y., 127
Houghton, L. A., 153
Houlsby, W. T., 214
House, J. S., 30
Houston, E. A., 459
Hovell, M., 71, 76
Howd, A., 195, 199
Howorka, K., 292
Hoyt, I. P., 29, 154
Hoyt, W. T., 50
Hrybyk, M., 126
Hu, F. B., 283
Hu, S., 341
Hu, T. W., 313
Hu, Y. J., 300
Hublin, C., 404
Hudspeth, W., 125, 127
Hughes, M., 359
Hulihan, D., 153

Hulthén, U. L., 282
Hummer, R., 484
Humphreys, P. A., 474
Hunt, R. H., 184
Hunt, T., 22, 153
Hunter, C., 230
Hurewitz, A., 241
Hursey, K. G., 74, 116, 215
Hurwitz, E. L., 187
Husby, G., 408
Hutenlocher, P. R., 400
Hynd, G. W., 349

Iaccarino, G., 282
Iacono, W. G., 389
Ianni, P., 116
Ichise, M., 335, 336
Ikeda, M., 485
Imber, S. D., 169
Imboden, J. B., 27
Inglis, J., 265
Ingram, D. D., 281, 282
Institute for Health and Aging, 430
Institute for Traffic Safety Management
      and Research, 394
Institute of Medicine, xi, xv 152
Intermediate Visual and Auditory (IVA)
      Continuous Performance Test, 350
Invitti, C., 282
Ironson, G., 253, 453
Irvine, E. J., 300, 303, 304
Isenberg, D., 409
Isenberg, S., 241, 242
Ishii, K., 485
Isles, C. G., 286
Isomaa, B., 276
Isomaki, H., 408
Iversen, I., 128

Jabon, S. L., 289
Jaccard, J., 208
Jackson, A., 242
Jackson, D., 215
Jackson, J. L., 43
Jackson, J. M., 400
Jacobs, E., 422
Jacobs, J. J., 59
Jacobsen, J. H., 400
Jacobson, E., 110, 137, 138, 139, 140, 148
Jacobson, N. S., 171
Jain, D., 253
Jain, S. C., 243, 289
Jakoubek, B., 153, 155
James, J. Y., 305
James, L. C., 339
James, T., 252
Jamner, L. D., 27
Jarrett, J., 280
Jarrett, M., 300

Jarski, R. W., 459, 462, 463
Jarvis, G. J., 318
Jason, L. A., 335, 340
Jaspers, K., 480
Javors, M. A., 338
Jaynes, J., 84
Jeejeebhoy, K. N., 22, 28
Jennen-Steinmetz, C., 127
Jensen, J. P., 98
Jensen, M. R., 27
Jensen, R., 207, 212
Jerome, A., 215
Jha, U. K., 243
Jobe, P., 324
Johansson, C., 25
John, E. R., 65, 123, 127, 353
John, R., 153
Johnson, D. A., 307
Johnson, J. C., 413
Johnson, J. N., 364
Johnson, P., 317, 318, 319
Johnson, P. B., 86
Johnson, P. D., 436
Johnson, S. B., 12, 283, 287
Johnson, S. K., 341
Johnston, J. C., 70
Johnston, S. H., 400
Joint National Committee, 276, 277, 283, 284
Joire, J., 210
Jolesz, F. A., 335, 336
Jonas, B. S., 281, 282, 364
Jonas, G., 114
Jonas, W. B., 7, 8, 12, 13, 14, 462
Jones, A., 339
Jones, D., 254, 339
Jones, E. E., 384
Jones, L., 284
Jones, N., 378
Jones, P. W., 423, 424
Jordan, A. E., 93
Jordan, K. M., 335, 340
Jordan, T. R., 459
Jorde, R., 408
Jorge, C. M., 340
Jorge, J. M., 301
Jorgensen, K., 265
Joseph-Vanderpool, J. R., 400
Jouvent, R., 364
Joyce, J., 151
Julius, S., 277, 280, 281, 282
Jung, C. G., 28, 481
Jupp, J. J., 154
Juptner, M., 207
Jurek, I. E., 290
Jurish, S. E., 4

Kabat-Zinn, J., 146, 483
Kaelber, C. T., 359
Kaiser, J., 128

Kamiya, J., 110, 481
Kamm, M. A., 307
Kan, J., 335, 339
Kandel, J., 351
Kantrowitz, F. G., 339, 340
Kaplan, G., 187
Kaplan, H. I., 378, 379, 381, 382, 384, 386
Kaplan, J., 250, 254
Kaplan, J. E., 336
Kaplan, K. H., 339
Kaplan, R. M., 89
Kaprio, J., 404
Kaptchuk, T. J., 187, 457, 459, 460
Karasek, R., 254
Karasu, T. B., 195, 384
Karkowski, L. M., 49
Karlin, R., 155
Karmel, B. Z., 123, 127
Karpel, C., 194
Karram, M. M., 316
Karsh, J., 408
Kashikar-Zuck, S., 411, 412
Kashkarova, O. E., 243
Katon, W. J., 46, 49
Katsarava, Z., 210
Katz, J., 325
Katzelnick, D. J., 51
Kaube, H., 207
Kautiainen, H., 408
Kawachi, L., 254
Kaye, H., 127
Kazdin, A. E., 70
Kee, W. G., 118
Keefe, F. J., 168, 410, 411, 412
Kegel, A. H., 317
Keith, L. D., 400
Keith-Spiegel, P., 95, 102
Kelleher, W. J., 230
Keller, M. B., 386
Keller, M. L., 167
Kelley, R. L., 154
Kelley, S. F., 153, 155
Kelly, K. A., 400
Kelly, S. F., 153
Kelvin, W. T., 89
Kemeny, M. E., 46
Kendler, K. S., 49
Kenkel, M. B. , v, 30, 74
Kennedy, S., 378
Kentsmith, D. K., 102
Kermit, K., 153
Kern, D. E., 20, 49
Kerns, R. D., 168
Kesavalu, L. N., 243
Kessel, B., 419, 420, 423
Kessler, B. H., 304
Kessler, R. C., 58, 60, 359
Kewman, D. G., 71, 76
Khoury, J. M., 313, 315

Kiecolt-Glaser, J. K., 11, 45
Kihlstrom, J. F., 24, 28, 29, 154
Kikuchi, Y., 237
Kim, J. A., 73, 76
Kim, N., 230
King, A. C., 348
King, D. R., 23, 72, 76, 154
King, D. S., 276
King, J., 251
King, T. K., 44
Kingham, J. G., 300
Kingston, R. S., 438
Kinney, J., 361
Kinsman, R. A., 237
Kipchik, G. L., 218
Kirk, J., 13
Kirmayer, L. J., 44
Kirsch, I., 72, 151, 152, 154, 156
Kirsh, J. C., 335, 336
Kirshnite, C., 253
Kirwan, J. P., 276
Kita, M., 485
Kita, T., 485
Kitamura, S., 282
Kitchener, K. S., 93, 95, 96, 97, 98, 99, 100, 101, 102
Kith, P., 336
Kittle, C. F., 70, 76
Klapow, J. C., 90
Klausner, J., 227
Kleber, H. D., 7
Kleijnen, J., 184
Klein, D. F., 361
Klein, K. B., 153
Klein, M. H., 387
Klein, T., 399
Kleinman, A., 197, 432
Kligler, B., 462, 463
Klimes, I., 340
Kline, S. S., 284, 291
Klinger, H., 378
Klinger, M. R., 44
Kloner, R. A., 252
Knesevich, M. A., 387
Knipschild, P., 184
Knott, J. R., 123, 127
Knowles, W., 276
Knox, V. J., 154
Kochhar, P., 304
Koenig, H., 13
Koenig, H. G., 50, 192, 195, 196, 197, 484, 486
Koerner, K., 171
Kogan, L. G., 22, 153, 154
Kohen, D. P., 243
Kohrt, W. M., 276
Kojima, T., 127
Kolm, P., 23, 24, 25, 26, 28, 153
Kolodner, K., 20, 49
Komaroff, A. L., 335, 336, 337
Komaroff, L. A., 336

Komerow, D. B., 404
Kondwani, K., 289
Konefal, J., 184
Konen, J. C., 281
Konkol, L., 412
Konstantinov, M. A., 243
Koocher, C. P., 95, 102
Koocher, G. P., 95, 96, 97, 98
Korbee, L., 4, 244
Korszun, A., 225
Korzekwa, M. I., 419, 420, 421, 422, 423, 424
Kosa, J., 20
Kosinski, D. J., 46
Koskenvuo, M., 404
Kosten, T. R., 184
Kostis, J. B., 289
Koszer, S., 126
Kotchen, T. A., 282
Kotchoubey, B., 128, 129
Kotses, H., 4, 242, 244
Kouba, R. B., 75
Kovacs, M., 171
Koyama, E., 22, 28
Kraemer, H. C., 156, 157, 197, 280
Kramer, M., 401
Krasner, L., 154
Kraus, H. M., 287
Krause, P. J., 126
Krauss, H. H., 13
Krieger, D., 454
Krippner, S., 191, 192, 194, 196
Krishanan, R., 254
Kriss, M. R., 169
Kroenke, K., xv, 5, 6, 43, 47, 51, 85
Kronauer, R. E., 399
Kroner-Herwig, B., 116
Krueger, J. M., 408
Kruesi, M. J., 335, 339, 340
Kruger, D. F., 282, 283
Kubiszyn, T., 88
Kubler, A., 128
Kuboki, T., 124, 290
Kudrow, L., 211
Kuhajda, M. C., 44
Kukolski, P. J., 481
Kulkosky, P. J., 353
Kuller, L. H., 281
Kumano, H., 124
Kunzel, M., 116
Kupfer, D. J., 401
Kuratsune, M., 485
Kuriyama, S., 59
Kurtz, R. M., 154
Kushner, H. S., 480
Kussin, P. S., 235
Kutner, M., 265
Kutner, N. G., 14
Kuyper, M. B., 432
Kvaal, S. A., 114, 207, 209, 212

Laakso, M., 276
Labarthe, D., 277
Laferrere, B., 275
LaGreca, A., 283, 287
Lagro-Janssen, T., 319
Lake, J., 64, 65
LaManca, J. J., 341
Lamberg, L., 400
Lanchbury, J. S., 408
Landis, K. R., 30
Lando, J. F., 281, 364
Lane, J. D., 288
Lang, A. J., 145
Lang, E. V., 151, 156
Lange, G., 341
Lao, L., 187
Lapidos, S., 51
Lapp, C. W., 335, 341, 342
Larach, S. W., 306
Larkins-Pettigrew, M., 317
Larsen, S., 154
Larson, D. B., 50, 192, 195, 196, 197, 483, 484, 486
Larson, P. D., 430, 431, 434
Larson, S. L., 483
Laser-Wolston, N., 265
Lasker, J., 254
Laskin, D. M., 225
Lasoski, A. M., 241, 242
Latini, D., 244
Latman, N. S., 408
Laue, L., 335, 339, 340
Laurence, J. R., 24
Laurencelle, L., 75
Laurent, D., 430
Lausten, L., 230
Laux, L. F., 444
La Vaque, T. J., 117, 124, 128, 129, 130, 352
Lavignolle, G., 75
Lawlis, G. F., 9, 13
Lawrie, S. M., 341
Layman, M., 325, 327, 330
Lazarus, R. S., 45
Leach, G. E., 317, 318, 319
Leadbeater, C. W., 454
Lechnyr, R., 7
Ledermann, H. M., 276
LeDoux, J., 362
LeDoux, J. E., 383
Lee, C. K., 127
Lee, J., 336
Lee, K. A., 403
Lee, K. K., 151
Lee, M. H. M., 187
Lefebvre, J. C., 411
Legatte, A. D., 126
Lehrer, P. M., 137, 138, 140, 146, 147, 155, 241, 242, 243, 245, 244, 485
Lehto, M., 276
Leigh, H., 27

Leite, P., 387
Leitenber, H., 168
Leitenberg, H., 50
Leitman, D., 47
Lembo, G., 282
Lentz, M. J., 420, 422, 423
Lenz, J. W., 290
Leplow, B., 243
LeResche, L., 224, 225, 226, 227, 228, 229
Leroi, A. M., 300
Leserman, J., 291
Levendosky, A. A., 400
Leventhal, E. A., 167
Leventhal, H., 167
Levin, B., 77
Levin, J. S., 12, 13, 14, 462, 484
Levine, H. M., 30
Levine, J., 304
Levine, M. D., 304
Levine, M. S., 304
Levi-Strauss, C., 193
Levitt, A., 378
Levitt, E. E., 153, 155, 156
Levitt, S. R., 229
Levy, J. R., 306
Levy, R., 254
Lewicki, P., 28
Lewinsohn, P. M., 173, 174
Lewis, C., 411
Lewis, D. C., 7
Lewis, M. A. E., 24
Lewis, P., 44
Lewis-Fernandez, R., 197
Lewy, A. J., 400
Ley, R., 361
Li, H., 276
Li, J., 75, 139
Li, Y., 184
Li, Z., 299
Liao, S. J., 187
Liebowitz, M. R., 361
Limmroth, V., 207, 210
Linde, K., 7, 8
Linde, S., 396
Linden, M., 127, 349, 352
Linden, W., 51, 138, 290, 291
Lindroth, Y., 412
Lindsey, S., 410
Ling, F. W., 419, 420, 421
Linzer, M., xv, 43
Lipchik, G. L., 114, 205, 207, 209, 211, 212
Lipkin, M., 86
Lipowski, Z., 252
Lipowski, Z. J., 21
Lipps, A., 484
Lipton, R. B., 205, 206, 208, 209, 211
Listwak, S., 335, 339, 340
Litchman, H., 265
Littman, B., 324

Liu, L., 389
Loane, K. C., 244
Locke, B. Z., 86, 364
Locke, S. E., 339, 340
Loenig-Baucke, V., 305, 306
Loes, L. M., 244
Loeser, J. D., 70, 71
Loew, T. H., 241
Lohr, N., xi, xv
Lokken, C., 210
London, P., 75, 157
Long, D. W., 75
Longstreth, G., 300, 303, 304
Lookingbill, D. P., 22, 153, 155
Loomis, A. L., 393
Lorenzetti, A., 210, 211
Lorig, K. R., 412, 413, 430, 431, 432
Lorimer, A. R., 286
Los, F., 404
Lovejoy, N. C., 450
Low, P. A., 335
Lowery, S. P., 304, 305, 307
Lu, F., 192
Lu, G. D., 187
Lubar, J. F., 117, 124, 127, 128, 347, 349, 352, 354
Lubar, J. O., 347, 352
Luber, K. M., 317, 318, 319
Lubkin, I. M., 44, 430, 431, 434
Lue, F. A., 409
Lukoff, D., 192, 194
Lundy, B., 378
Lundy, R., 153
Luparello, T., 237
Lusebrink, V. B., 139
Lustman, P. J., 282, 288, 292
Lutgendorf, S., 151, 156
Luthe, W., 110, 137, 139, 144, 145, 148, 480
Lutzenberger, W., 114, 325
Lykken, D. T., 24, 155
Lynas, A. G., 184
Lynch, D., 43, 44, 153
Lynch, D. J., 155
Lynch, J., 430
Lynch, N. R., 241
Lynch, P. M., v
Lynn, D. J., 338
Lynn, S., 154
Lynn, S. J., 194

MacCallum, R. C., 11
Macdonald, H., 154
MacDougall, J. M., 253
Macera, C., 254
Macfarlane, P. W., 286
MacHale, S. M., 341
MacInnis, A. L., 327
MacKay, I. R., 276
Mackert, A., 383
Mackey, S., 291

MacLennan, A. H., 313, 314
MacMillan, M., 265
Madrid, A., 156
Magellan Behavioral Health, 385
Mahesh, V. B., 423
Mahler, H., 192
Mahtani, M. M., 276
Maier, S. F., 46
Maigne, R., 259
Majani, G., 244
Malarkey, W. B., 45
Malaspina, D., 47
Malin, H. V., 399
Malinoski, P., 217
Malizia, A. L., 359
Mallee, C., 156
Malmgren, R., 214
Malone, E., 484
Malouf, J. L., 102
Mamelle, N., 283
Mamish, M. E., 291
Mandel, F. S., 6
Manderscheid, R., 364
Manderscheidt, R. W., 86
Mangelsdorff, A. D., 5, 85
Manis, M., 28
Mann, B. D., 444
Mann, C. A., 349
Manning, W. G., 51
Manson, J. E., 283
Manuel y Keenoy, B., 341, 342
Marbach, J. J., 227
Marchand, S., 75
Marcille, P. J., 74
Marcus, B. H., 51
Marcus, S., 304
Margolin, A., 184
Margolis, R. B., 225
Margulies, I., 75
Marks, I., 340
Marks, J., 254
Marlowe, D., 21
Marmot, M., 254
Marrero, D., 283, 287
Marsh, G. R., 396
Martens, H., 399
Martin, J. L., 283
Martina, R., 226
Martinoff, J. T., 225
Martus, P., 241
Marucha, P. T., 11
Marxer, F., 254
Mas, F. G., 127
Maseri, A., 252
Masi, A. T., 324, 408
Mason, J. W., 46
Mass, R., 242, 243
Massimini, F., 24
Mathew, N. T., 208, 209

Mathews, H. L., 450
Mathews, M., 252
Mathews-Simonton, S., 452
Matousek, M., 123, 127
Matsuura, M., 127
Mattiasson, I., 282
Mattos, C., 228
Maxton, D. G., 153
May, A., 207
May, W. F., 100
Mayer, D. J., 154
Mayman, M., 28
Mayne, T., 241, 242
McCabe, M. P., 154
McCahill, M. E., 85
McCain, C., 153
McCain, G., 341, 342
McCane, L. M., 128
McCann, G., 155
McCarney, S. B., 350
McCarty, D. J., 275
McCarty, R. C., 341
McCaskill, C. C., 288
McCauley, J., 20, 49
McClelland, D., 253
McClelland, D. C., 50
McClish, D. K., 318
McCloskey, J., 452
McConkey, M., 154
McCoy, G. C., 290, 291
McCrae, R. R., 75
McCraty, R., 254, 370
McCrory, D. C., 213
McCullough, M. E., 50, 192, 195, 196, 197, 484
McDaniel, L. K., 413
McDaniel, R. J., 230
McDaniel, S. H., 12
McDermott, J., 424
McDermott, M. A., 483
McDonald, R. D., 23, 72, 76, 154
McDonald, R. V., 73, 76
McEwen, B. S., 45, 49
McFarland, D. J., 128
McFarlane, A., 6
McGlynn, F. D., 231
McGonagle, K. A., 359
McGrady, A., 43, 44, 116, 117, 153, 155,
    212, 289, 290, 291
McGrath, P., 22, 153, 155
McGregor, N., 341
McGuigan, F. J., 110, 139
McKinney, M. W., 229
McLaughlin, D. M., 154
McLellan, A. T., 7
McLeod, C., 153
McLeod, K., 483
McMurry, J. F., 282, 283
McNamara, J. A., 226
McNeely, E., 14

McShane, D. J., 409, 410
Meaden, P. M., 389
Meara, N. M., 93
Medical Economics Company, 459, 462
Medina, J. L., 214
Meenan, R. F., 413
Meinders, A. E., 287
Mellgren, S. I., 408
Melzack, R., 262, 325
Memel, D. S., 313
Mendelson, M., 382
Mendlein, J. M., 291
Menezes, J., 228
Menitsky, D. N., 243
Mercier, L., 71, 76
Mercier, M. A. S., 387
Merendino, R. A., 70, 76
Merikangas, K. R., 211
Merkin, M., 127
Merrill, J. M., 444
Mersky, H., 325
Merton, T., 483
Meyer, K., 307
Mezzasalma, M. A., 362
Miaskowski, C., 22, 26, 35, 153
Michalek, J., 324
Michalek, J. E., 338
Michel, P., 210
Michelotti, A., 226
Middaugh, S. J., 118
Mieczkowski, T. A., 422
Miettinen, A., 276
Migliori, G. B., 244
Mikami, A., 485
Millar, A. P., 86
Millar, D. R., 318
Miller, B. A., 349
Miller, D. K., 348
Miller, G. E., 46, 51
Miller, J. F., 431, 432, 436
Miller, M. A., 47
Miller, N. E., 110
Miller, T. I., 151, 155, 156
Miller, V., 305, 307
Miller, W. R., 194
Milman, H., 253
Milsom, I., 317, 319
Mineka, S. L., 24
Miner, L. A., 128
Mishel, M. H., 436, 438
Mitchell, E. S., 420, 422, 423
Mitchell, J. H., 139
Mitchell, T. F., 59
Miya, P. A., 102
Miyaoka, H., 282
Miyaoka, Y., 282
Mochs, J., 127
Mock, J., 382
Modell, J. G., 339, 340

Mohn, U., 116
Mokdad, A. H., 291
Moldofsky, H., 324, 409
Monastra, V. J., 127, 349
Monga, T. N., 265
Monjaud, I., 283
Monroe, S. M., 386
Montanari, E., 317, 318
Montgomery, A., 348
Montgomery, G., 151, 152, 156
Montjoy, C. Q., 378
Mooney, R., 317
Moore, J. E., 51
Moore, N. C., 131, 370
Moore, P. J., 207, 212
Moore, R. J., 59
Moore, T., 477
Moorkens, G., 341, 342
Moos, R., 420, 425
Moos, R. H., 30
Mooy, J. M., 281, 282
Morabia, A., 280
Moran, G., 253
Morgan, A. H., 155
Morgan, M., 423
Morin, C., 396
Morin, C. M., 22, 23
Morley, S., 168
Morse, C. A., 425, 426
Morse, G., 425, 426
Mortola, J. F., 420
Morton, S., 432
Moscovitch, M., 28
Moss, D., 4, 9, 10, 11, 84, 113, 116,
    364, 467, 477, 481, 486
Mossey, C., 323
Moss-Morris, R., 167
Motomiya, T., 282
Moulton, A. W., 444
Mountz, J. M., 339, 340
Mubbashar, M., 88
Mubbashar, S., 88
Mueller, H., 323, 324, 325, 327, 329, 330
Mueller-Oberlinghausen, B., 383
Muenchen, R. A., 349
Mulder, P., 254
Mulholland, T., 110
Muller-Lisner, S., 300, 303, 304
Munoz, P., 205
Muñoz, R. F., 173, 174
Murphy, A. I., 155
Murphy, D., 156
Murphy, G. E., 387
Murray, T. J., 205
Murthy, K. C., 243
Musselman, D. L., 50
Musso, A., 290, 291
Myer, A., 377
Myers, M. A., 50

Myers, T. C., 210
Mykkanen, L., 276
Myllykangas-Luosujarvi, I., 408
Myran, D., 176, 305, 307

Nace, E, P., 154
Nadeau, M., 11
Nadon, R., 29, 154
Nadsady, P. A., 291
Naeser, M. A., 184
Nagano, Y., 485
Nagaraja, H. N., 338
Nagel, R., 43, 44, 153, 155
Nahmias, C., 151
Nakagawa-Kogan, H., 4
Nakao, M., 290
Naliboff, B. D., 289
Nam, C., 484
Napoli, L., 211
Nappi, G., 211
Nardi, A. E., 362
Narrow, W. E., 86, 359, 361, 364
Nascimento, I., 362
Nash, J., 154
Nash, M. R., 157
Natelson, B. H., 341
National Academy of Sciences,
    Institute of Medicine, 29
National Association of Cognitive-Behavioral
    Therapists, 453
National Center for Complementary and
    Alternative Medicine (NCCAM), 58, 62,
    64, 66, 437, 445, 454
National Certification Board for Therapeutic
    Massage and Bodywork, 454
National Commission on Sleep Disorders
    Research, 393
National Heart, Lung, and Blood Institute,
    236, 238, 245, 253, 329
National Institute of Dental and Craniofacial
    Research, 231
National Institutes of Health (NIH), 57, 58, 64, 65,
    181, 184, 187, 198, 315, 339, 351, 413, 437,
    445, 452, 474
National Institutes of Health Technology
    Assessment Panel, 30
National Sleep Foundation, 394
Nawrocki, T., 378
Neblett, J., 230
Needham, J., 187
Neel, J. V., 277, 280, 281
Neely, R. D., 287
Nehra, V., 300
Neimeyer, R., 172
Nelesen, R. A., 46
Nelson, C. B., 359
Nelson, D., 325, 327, 330
Nelson, D. V., 262
Nelson, R. F., 205

Nemeroff, C., 50
Nemiah, J. C., 25
Neri, M., 244
Nesse, R. M., 362
Neufeld, J. D., 207, 212
Neumann, L., 323
Nevitt, M., 413
Newberg, A., 481
Newell, R., 305
Newman, L. C., 209
New York College of Health Professions, 451
Nezu, A. M., 168
Ng, N. K. Y., 187
Niaura, R., 44
Nicassio, P. M., 396, 411
Nicholson, J. A., 118
Nicolaisen, T., 265
Nielan, B. A., 444
Nieman, L. Z., 444
Nilsson, A., 276
Nisenbaum, R., 339
Nixon, P., 250, 251, 252, 255
Nixon, P. G. F., 361
Nobel, E., 348
Nochasjski, T., 318
Nohr, S. B., 318
Nolen-Hoeksema, S., 170, 172
Nollet-Clemencon, C., 364
Nomura, S., 290
Norcross, J. C., 50, 434, 435, 436
Nordahl, T., 348
Norell, J. S., 5
Norlock, F. E., 58, 60
Norrie, J., 287
Norris, P. A., 144
Northen, A., 319
Northridge, M. E., 280
Northrup, C., 437
Norton, N. J., 301, 302, 304
Norton, P., 317
Nouwen, A., 265
Nouwen, H. J. M., 483
Nunez, P. L., 126
Nussbaum, G., 46
Nutt, D. J., 359, 404
Nyhlin, K. T., 431

Oakland University, 461
Oakman, J. M., 155
O'Banion, K., 237
O'Brien, C. P., 7
O'Brien, P. M., 423
Ochs, L., 328, 329
O'Connell, P., 211
O'Connor, P. D., 265
O'Connor, R., 378, 383
O'Donnell, F., 205, 211
O'Donnell, P., 352
Ogata, M., 485

Okabe, S., 237
O'Keane, V., 339, 340
Okubo, Y., 127
Olander, R. T., 184
Oldenburg, B., 51
Older, S., 323, 324
O'Leary, A., 413
O'Leary, T. A., 369
Olesen, J., 207, 212
Olfson, M., xv
Olik, D., 187
Olmsted, M., 171
Olness, K., 30, 72, 77
Olsen, C. G., 435, 436
Olson, A., 304
Olson, J. K., 483
Orchard, T. J., 281
Orebaugh, C., 117, 290
Orgill, A. A., 127, 353
Orleans, C., xv
Orne, E. C., 21, 154
Ornish, D., 196, 255
Oros, M. T., 450, 451
Orr, M., 324
Orth-Gomer, K., 280
Oschman, J. L., 62
Ostbye, T., 323, 324, 326
Ostensen, M., 408
Osterhaus, J. T., 205
Ottenweller, J. E., 341
Otto, M. W., 387
Ouslander, J. G., 313
Owaid, I., 252
Owens, J. E., 452
Oxman, T. E., 47

Packard, R. C., 211
Packer, M., 250
Padesky, C. A., 174, 175, 176
Padgett, L., 432
Padus, E., 385
Page, A., 244
Page, G. G., 11
Pagliaro, A. M., 351
Pagliaro, L. A., 351
Palenque, M., 241
Pallmeyer, T. P., 290, 291
Palsson, O. S., 28, 90, 300, 307, 444, 445
Palta, M., 404
Panagiotides, H., 378
Panayi, G. S., 408
Paneral, A. A., 153
Paoletti, C., 184
Papp, L. A., 361
Para, V., 44
Pareja, J., 341
Pargament, K. I., 484
Park, S. J., 244
Parker, J., 343

Parker, J. C., 411, 413
Parks, P., 244
Parry, B., 422
Partanen, J., 265
Partinen, M., 404
Parton, E., 288, 289
Pascual, J., 205
Paskewitz, D. A., 153
Pasquale, R., 127
Pasquali, R., 282
Passatore, M., 139
Patanar, S. K., 306
Paterson, B. L., 431, 432
Patterson, D. R., 151, 156
Payne, A., 168, 307
Payne, L. C., 408
Pearce, K. L., 318
Pearce, S., 409
Pearlstein, T., 419, 420, 421,
    422, 423, 424
Pearson, S. D., 51
Peck, C. L., 72, 76
Peckham, P. H., 128
Pelcovitz, D., 6
Pellegrino, E. D., ix
Pemberton, J. H., 300, 304
Peniston, E. G., 353, 481
Pennington, D., 156
Penttila, I., 276
Penzien, D. B., 74, 116, 213, 215
Peper, E., 242, 243, 244
Perelmouter, J., 128
Perlis, M. L., 396
Perlstrom, J. R., 22, 23, 153
Perozo, S. E., 306
Perry, C., 153, 154
Perry, J., 9
Perry, J. D., 116
Persons, J. B., 170
Persson, J., 314
Pert, C., 196
Petersen, I., 123, 127
Peterson, A. L., 230
Peterson, D. L., 333, 334, 335, 336
Peterson, P. K., 341
Peterson, Z. L., 211
Petrash, V. V., 243
Petrie, K. J., 167
Petroni, M. L., 282
Pettei, M. J., 304
Pettinati, H. M., 22, 153, 154
Peyrot, M., 282, 283
Pfeifer, J., 304
Pfurtscheller, G., 128
Phaneuf, D., 335, 339
Pheley, A. M., 341
Phillips, A., 349
Piccione, C., 155
Pichert, J. W., 284, 291

Pichugin, V. I., 243
Pickens, J., 378
Pickering, T. G., 254
Pieper, C., 254
Pierei, A., 210
Pikoff, H., 207, 212
Pilkonis, P. A., 169
Pincus, T., 409, 410, 411
Pingel, J. D., 215
Pinto, B. M., 51
Pi-Sunyer, F. X., 275
Pittler, M. H., 8, 12
Plante, T. G., 195
Plioplys, A. V., 335
Poehlmann, K. M., 45
Pollak, C. P., 338
Pollet, S. M., 156
Pomerantz, B., 26
Pomeranz, B., 184, 187
Pope, A. T., 23, 24, 25, 26, 28, 153
Pope, M., 261
Popkin, M. K., 27
Porges, S., 243, 244
Porges, S. W., 26, 46, 366, 370
Portenoy, R. K., 338
Posner, M. I., 348
Posner, S. F., 313
Post, S. G., 486
Potapova, T., 243
Pothmann, R., 116
Potter VanLoon, B. J. P., 287
Potts, J. T., 139
Potvin, L., 254
Powell, B. T., 196
Powell-Griner, E. E., 434
Power, M. J., 341
Pranikoff, K., 318
Prescott, C. A., 49
Pribram, K., 127, 154
Price, B., 433
Price, D., 22, 25, 26, 153, 155
Price, J. H., 459
Price, J. R., 168, 340, 341
Prichep, L. S., 65, 123, 127, 353
Priestley, D., 412
Prince, S. E., 171
Prior, A., 151, 156, 300, 304, 305, 307
Prochaska, J. O., 434, 435, 436
Prohaska, T. R., 167
Proietti Cecchini, A., 211
Pruitt, S. D., 51, 90
Pryse-Phillips, W., 205
Puchalski, C., 486
Pulos, S. M., 384
Pumpria, J., 292
Purcell, M., 131
Putignano, P., 282
Putnam, F. W., 153
Pyorala, K., 276

Qualls, P. J., 75, 158
Quigly, M. A., 253
Quill, T. E., 5, 21
Quiller-Couch, A., 480
Quillian, R. E., 396
Quinn, A. A., 450
Quinn, J. A., 451

Rabin, B. S., 46
Rachman, S. J., 359, 363
Raczynski, J. M., 265
Radder, J. K., 287
Rademaker, A. W., 335
Radil, T., 153, 155
Radnitz, C. L., 208, 214
Radojevic, V., 352, 411
Radtke, R. A., 396
Rae, D. S., 86, 359, 361, 364
Raezer, L. B., 411
Rahe, R. H., 47
Rai, L., 243
Raichle, M. E., 348
Rainford, G. L., xiii
Rainforth, M., 289
Rains, J. C., 213
Ram, K., 243
Ramadan, N. M., 206
Ramey, D., 413
Ramm, M., 242
Rammohan, K. W., 338
Ramsey, S. D., 8
Randles, J., 305, 307
Ranganath, C., 382, 383
Rao, M., 383
Rao, S. S., 300, 304, 305, 306
Raphael, K. G., 227
Rapkin, A. J., 423
Rapoport, A. M., 209, 213
Rasey, H., 124
Rasker, J. J., 411, 412
Rasmussen, B. K., 207, 212
Ratcliffe, M. A., 156
Ratey, J. J., 351
Rath-Harvey, D. M., 300
Rause, V., 481
Ravussin, E., 276
Ray, W. J., 153
Rea, M. R., 284, 291
Read, J., 343
Read, L., 318
Reed, M. L., 205
Rees, A., 386, 387
Reeves, W. C., 339
Regier, D. A., 86, 359, 361, 364
Register, P. A., 29, 154
Regland, B., 342
Rehm, L. P., 168
Reid, R., 421, 422
Reid, S. A., 444

Reinecke, M., 453
Remler, H., 22
Ren, C., 154
Rendina, V., 282
Rescorla, R. A., 23
Resnick, R. J., 351, 352
Reston, J., 182
Reyes, M., 339
Reynolds, C. F., III, 401
Reynolds, R. V., 4
Reynolds, R. V. C., 244
Reynolds, S., 386, 387
Rezende, R., 228
Rhodes, J., 305
Rhodes, L., 434
Riccio, C. A., 349
Rice, B. I., 289
Rice, D., 430, 443
Rice, K. M., 131
Rich, S., 24, 155
Richards, J. M., 50
Richards, P. S., 195
Richardson, G. S., 399
Richardson, M. T., 341, 343
Richardson, P. H., 187
Richardson, W. S., 7
Rich-Edwards, J. W., 283
Richman, J. A., 335, 340
Richter, H. E., 319
Richter, R., 242, 243, 244
Rieder, C. E., 225
Riemsma, R. P., 411, 412
Rigden, S., 342
Riley, D., 66
Ritcher, C., 254
Ritchie, T., 348
Ritter, P., 430, 431, 432
Ritz, T., 242
Rivera-Tovar, A., 422
Roatta, S., 139
Robbins, J. M., 44
Robert, J. J., 364
Roberts, A. H., 71, 76
Roberts, L., xiii
Roberts, S. J., 20
Robertson, L. S., 20
Robinson, E., 411, 412
Robinson, F. P., 450
Robinson, H., 146, 147
Robinson, J. C., 318
Robinson, M. E., 265
Roche, S. M., 154
Rockland, C., 384
Rodin, J., 156
Rodriguez, M. S., 48
Roeykens, J., 341
Rogers, L., 116
Rogers, M. E., 449
Rogers, R., 484

Rohan, K. J., 421, 422
Rokicki, L. A., 114
Rokke, P. D., 168
Rolls, E. T., 383
Romano, J., 43, 48
Romeo, R., 226
Romunde, L. K. J., 156
Rosa, R. R., 401
Rose, R., 152
Rosenberg, J. H., 338
Rosenberg, R. S., 400
Rosenberg, W., 7
Rosenfeld, J. P., 127, 131, 382, 383, 384, 388
Rosenfeld, P. J., 270
Rosenman, R. H., 252
Rosenthal, M. J., 289
Rosenthal, N. E., 400
Ross, K., 323, 324
Ross, S. L., 288
Rossiter, T., 117
Rossiter, T. R., 129, 130, 352
Rossner, S., 25
Rost, K., 6
Rostel, G., 156
Roth, M., 378
Roth, S., 6
Roth, W. T., 8, 362
Rouan, G. W., 6
Rovito, M. A., 444
Rowan, A. B., 51
Rowe, P. C., 335, 339
Rowley, M. J., 276
Roy, A. J., 307
Roy, S. H., 265
Rozanski, A., 250, 254
Rudell, A., 127
Ruff, M., 196
Rugh, J. D., 74, 225, 226
Rumsey, J., 348
Rusanovskii, V. V., 243
Rush, A. J., 176
Russe, C., 265
Russell, H. W., 319
Russell, I., 323, 324
Russell, I. J., 338
Russo, A., 276
Russo, M., 226
Ruth, T. J., 70
Rutherford, C., 336
Rutledge, C., 28
Ruzyla-Smith, P., 153, 154
Ryan, M., 473
Rybarczyk, B., 51
Ryden, J., 20
Rydhstroem, H., 314

Sachdeva, A. K., 444
Sachs, R. G., 153
Sack, R. L., 400

Sackett, D. L., 7
Sadlier, M., 305
Sadock, B. J., 378, 379, 381, 382, 384, 386
Sainard-Gainko, J., 207, 212, 212
Saito, Y., 485
Sakai, S., 226
Salen, P., 283
Salfield, S. A., 214
Salis, J. F., 51
Salit, I. E., 335, 336
Salkovskis, P., 425
Salkovskis, P. M., 176, 363
Salladay, S. A., 102
Salley, A., 411, 412
Sand, P. K., 319
Sanders, E., 319
Sandler, H. M., 484
Sandner, D., 193
Sandrini, G., 211
Saper, J. R., 209
Sapirstein, G., 151, 152, 156
Sarason, B. R., 30
Sarason, I. G., 30
Sarelin, L., 276
Sargunaraj, D., 241
Sasaki, Y., 485
Saskin, P., 396
Sattar, N., 287
Sattlberger, E., 362, 370
Sattlberger, M. A., 362, 370
Saunders, K., 226
Saunders, K. W., 51
Saunders, M. J., 226
Savino, M., 382
Sawyer, S. M., 244
Saxon, J., 22, 23, 24, 26, 27, 73, 153, 155
Sayegh, R., 424
Scafidi, F. A., 453
Scarisbrick, P., 324
Schabmann, A., 292
Schalk, G., 128
Schamberg, W., 51
Schamberger, W., 290
Scharff, L., 305, 306
Schatzberg, A. F., 359, 386
Schayck, R. V., 207
Schenck, C. H., 341
Scherger, C., 155
Schiff, I., 424
Schiffman, E. L., 225
Schindler, J. V., 289
Schlundt, D. G., 284, 291
Schlusche, C., 292
Schmid, C., 323
Schneck, J. M., 401
Schneider, C., 115
Schneider, D., 128
Schneider, M. S., 282
Schneider, P., 115

Schneider, R. H., 289
Schnyer, R., 65
Schoenen, J., 207, 212, 212
Schonberger, L. B., 336
Schondorf, R., 335, 339
School, P. J., 115
Schore, A. N., 362
Schroeder, A. F., 20, 49
Schroevers, M., 211
Schultz, J. H., 137, 139, 144, 145, 148
Schultz, J., 110
Schultz, L. R., 211
Schulz, L. O., 276
Schulzer, M., 70
Schuman, S. H., xiii
Schumann-Brzezinski, C., 291
Schuster, M. M., 304, 305, 307
Schuyler, D., 88
Schwartz, B. S., 205
Schwartz, G. E., 27, 138
Schwartz, M. S., 102
Schwartz, M., 9, 113, 115, 117, 120, 205,
    215, 467, 474
Schwartz, R. B., 335, 336
Schwarz, S. P., 305, 306
Schwarz-McMorris, S. P., 305
Schwitzgebel, R., 75
Seaward, B. L., 192
Seely, E. W., 399
Segal, D., 207, 209, 212
Segal, N. L., 155
Segal, Z. V., 169, 170, 172, 175, 176, 305, 307
Segreto, J., 242
Seidel, H., 265
Seleshi, E., 207, 212
Sella, G., 266, 323, 324, 325, 326, 327, 329
Selmi, P. M., 387
Selye, H., 113
Selzer, S., 214
Semple, W. E., 348
Senthilselvan, A., 364
Serdula, M. K., 291
Serfontein, G., 127, 353
Seveso, M., 317, 318
Seydel, E. R., 412
Shaffer, F., 484
Shafranske, E. P., 191
Shah, N., 355
Shanker, J., 229
Shannon, S., 61
Shapiro, A., 70, 71
Shapiro, D. A., 386, 387
Sharma, A. M., 281
Sharpe, M., 44, 340
Sharpe, M. C., 336, 337
Sharpe, N., 167
Shaughn O'Brien, P. M., 424
Shaver, J., 420, 422, 423
Shaver, J. R., 403

Shaw, B. F., 170, 171, 176
Shaw, G., 305
Shea, S., 280
Shear, M. K., 8
Shedler, J., 28
Sheehan, D. V., 155
Sheehan, M., 291
Sheehan, P. W., 75, 158
Sheftell, F. D., 213
Shellenberger, R., 115, 117
Shelton, R. C., 386
Shen, Y., 127
Shepherd, J., 286
Sheppard, W., 289
Sheridan, P., 348
Sherman, A. C., 195
Sherman, M., 253
Shertzer, C. I., 22, 153, 155
Sherwood, A., 254, 289
Shevrin, H., 28
Shidara, T., 124
Shimosawa, T., 290
Shipley, M. J., 280
Shirato, K., 237
Shoor, S., 413
Shor, R. E., 21, 154
Shouse, M. N., 117, 128, 352
Shum, K., 154
Sibbald, B., 88
Siegel, S., 72, 73, 76
Siegfried, W., 241
Sierpina, V., 462, 463
Sierpina, V. S., 88
Siever, D., 389
Sifneos, P. E., 25
Sigal, R. J., 283
Sigmon, S. T., 421, 422
Sihvonen, T., 265
Silberstein, R. B., 126
Silberstein, S. D., 206, 208, 211, 213
Silman, A. J., 407
Silver, R. C., 44, 50
Silverglade, L., 241
Simkin, P., 453
Simkin, S., 340
Simmons, J., 195
Simon, D., 205
Simon, G. E., 51
Simone, D., 423
Simons, A. D., 386, 387
Simons, D., 261
Simonton, O. C., 452
Sindrup, S., 210
Singer, D., 370
Singh, G., 413
Sirr, S. A., 341
Sisson, R., 450
Sisto, S. A., 341
Skatrud, J., 404

Skinner, J. E., 46
Skoner, D. P., 46
Skriver, C., 153
Sletten, I., 154
Sliwinski, M., 208
Sloan, R., 253
Sloan, R. P., 196, 484
Smarr, K. L., 411, 413
Smetankine, A., 243, 244
Smilgin-Humphreys, S., 300
Smith, G. R., 20
Smith, G. R., Jr., 6
Smith, J., 6
Smith, J. C., 139
Smith, J. F., 341, 343
Smith, J. P., 438
Smith, M. L., 151, 155, 156
Smith, S., 5
Smolensky, M., 400
Smyth, J. M., 241
Smythe, H. A., 323, 324, 329, 409
Snelling, L. S., 327
Sobel, D. S., 3, 4
Soefer, M. H., 241
Solari-Twadell, P. A., 483
Solberg, W. K., 225
Solomon, C. G., 283
Solomon, S., 209
Sommaruga, M., 244
Sommer, S., 317
Sontag, S., 429
Sorbi, M., 211
Sorrell, S. P., 387
Sossi, V., 70
Sotsky, S. M., 169
Soufer, R., 253
South-Paul, J., 419, 420
Southwick, S. M., 46
Sovak, M., 116
Sowers, J. R., 282
Sox, H. C., Jr., 75
Spalton, A. P., 214
Spanevello, A., 244
Spangler, D. L., 386
Spangler, J. G., 281
Spanos, N. P., 70
Sparrow, D., 254
Speckman, E.-F., 124
Spector, S., 237
Speechley, M., 323, 324, 326
Speizer, F. E., 283
Spencer, J. W., 59
Sperry, R., 24, 25
Spiegel, D., 22, 59, 151, 153, 154, 155, 156, 157, 197
Spiegel, H., 154
Spiegel, K., 50
Spieker, S., 378
Spielman, A. J., 396
Spierings, E. L., 211
Spiers, P., 424

Spinter, D., 155
Spire, J. P., 400
Spitzer, L. R., xv
Spitzer, R. L., 43
Srinivasan, R., 126
Srivastava, E. D., 305
Sroka, L., 127
Srour, J. W., 304, 305, 307
Staats, J. M., 22, 153, 154
Staggers, F., 289
Stam, H. J., 22, 24, 73, 153, 155
Stamler, J., 276
Stamler, R., 276
Stanton, H. E.
Stanton, R., 305
Stanton, S. L., 315
Starfield, B., x
Starkey, P., 424
Staropoli, C. A., 444
Starr, K., 411
Starr, N. J., 244
Startup, M., 386, 387
Staten, M. A., 276
Staubach, L. B., 86
Steege, J. F., 425
Stefanick, M. L., 291
Stein, J., 361
Steiner, M., 419, 420, 421, 422, 423, 424, 426
Stennett, J., 450
Stensland, M., 205, 211
Stenstrom, R. J., 70
Stepanski, E. J., 396
Stephenson, J., 283
Sterman, M. B., 114, 128, 129, 130
Stern, J. A., 154
Stern, K., 378
Sternbach, R., 5, 6
Sternbach, R. A., 116
Sternberg, E., 152
Sternberg, E. M., 46
Stevens, D. E., 211
Stevenson, J., 400
Stevinson, C., 8, 12
Stewart, A. L., 430, 431, 432
Stewart, D. E., 151, 155
Stewart, J. W., 387
Stewart, R., 214
Stewart, W. F., 205
Stickney, S. K., 27
Stiles, T. C., 341
Still, G. F., 348
Stockley, H., 131
Stoessl, A. J., 70
Stolberg, S., 463
Stolze, H., 210
Stone, A. A., 241
Stone, A. B., 419, 420, 421, 422
Storrie, J. B., 307
Stoudemire, A., 195
Strain, L. A., 432

Strang, P. E., 205
Strasser, M. R., 408
Straus, S. E., 7, 334, 335, 336, 337, 339, 340
Strebel, B., 378
Streeten, D., 335
Strehl, U., 128, 129
Strelakov, S. A., 243
Striefel, S., 94, 95, 98, 99, 102, 128, 129, 212
Strong, S. R., 22, 23
Strong, W. B., 51, 289
Strube, M. J., 154
Stuart, E. M., 291
Stuart, M., 462, 463
Stucky-Ropp, R. C., 411, 413
Stutman, R. K., 22, 153
Stux, G., 187
Suarez, L., 276, 278
Suchowersky, O., 210
Sudderth, D. B., 351
Suematsu, H., 124
Sulkhanova, A., 408
Sullivan, E. M., 463
Sullivan, M. D., 43, 48
Summerson, J. H., 281
Sung, H., 430
Sung, H.-Y., 443
Superio-Cabuslay, E., 413
Superko, R., 255
Surawy, C., 340
Surwit, R. S., 282, 288
Susset, J. G., 318
Svedlund, J., 305
Swallow, S. R., 172
Swan, R., 197
Swann, P., 305
Swartwood, D. I., 128
Swartwood, J. N., 352
Swartwood, M. O., 128, 352
Swartzman, L., 155
Swindle, R., 51
Syme, S. L., 254
Szechtman, H., 151
Szold, A., 26

Taal, E., 411, 412
Tabacchi, K. N., 229
Tafti, M., 409
Tait, R. C., 225
Taitel, M. A., 244
Talcott, G. W., 230
Talley, N. J., 299, 300, 301, 303
Talukdar, B., 289
Tamura, G., 237
Tan, S. Y., 290
Tang, T. Z., 168
Tansey, M., 352
Tarakeshwar, N., 485
Tart, C., 110
Tatman, S. M., 153
Taub, E., 115

Taylor, A., 211
Taylor, A. E., 116, 305, 306
Taylor, A. G., 452
Taylor, A. W., 313, 314
Taylor, C. B., 253
Taylor, D., 425, 426
Taylor, E. E., 153
Taylor, R., 340
Taylor, R. R., 335
Taylor-Vaisey, A., 47
Teasdale, J. D., 175
Teders, S. J., 4
Tellegen, A., 21, 24, 29, 75, 152, 154, 155
Temple, R., 129
Temple, R. D., 299
Tennen, H., 409
Tennessee State University, 451
Tepley, N., 206
Ter Riet, G., 184
Terry, R., 413
Terwiel, J. P., 156
Test of Variables of Attention (TOVA), 350
Thase, M. E., 386, 387
Thatcher, R. W., 65, 126, 127
Theofanous, A. G., 215
Theorell, T., 254
Thoft, J. S., 422
Thomas, G. I., 70, 76
Thomas, J. E., 362, 370
Thomasma, D. C., ix
Thompson, L., 130, 352
Thompson, M., 130, 352
Thompson, W. G., 299, 300, 301, 303, 304
Thong, D., 198
Thoresen, C., 50
Thorn, B. E., 44
Thornby, J. I., 444
Thorne, S. E., 430, 431, 432, 433
Thornton, K., 128
Thorogood, M., 284
Thorpy, M. J., 396
Thuras, P., 131
Thys-Jacobs, S., 424
Tian, J., 424
Tibbetts, V., 242
Tice, H. M., 335, 336
Tiemens, B., 434
Tiller, W., 370
Tiller, W. A., 254
Timmermann, D. L., 128
Timmons, B., 361
Tkach, W., 182
Tobin, D. L., 116
Tobin, L. R., 74
Tomenson, B., 305
Toner, B. B., 22, 28, 176, 300, 305, 307
Topper, M. D., 198
Toro, M., 127
Torrey, E. F., 198
Tosi, D. J., 241

Totka, J., 288, 289
Touboul, P., 283
Tougas, G., 184
Townsend, D., 230
Trabert, W., 362
Tranel, D., 383, 384
Traugott, M., 75
Travell, J., 261
Treiber, F. A., 51, 289
Trepetin, M., 127
Triana-Alexander, M., 339, 340
Tries, J., 315, 318
Trill, K., 241
Trimarco, B., 282
Trotter, R. T., III, 193
Truax, P. A., 171
Trudeau, D. L., 131
Truong, X. T., 70, 73
Tuason, V. B., 169
Tucker, D. M., 126
Tuftin, M., 300
Tugwell, P., 205
Tunis, M. M., 206
Tuomi, T., 276
Turek, F. W., 399
Turk, D., 325
Turk, D. C., 168, 212
Turner, D. C., 432
Turner, I. C., 307
Turner, J., 115
Turner, J. A., 43, 48, 70, 71
Turner, J. R., 289
Turner, L., 51, 290
Turner, M. J., 307
Turner, R., 51, 192
Turner, R. A., 413
Turner, S. L., 214
Turner, T., 50
Türp, J. C., 226

U.S. Department of Health and Human Services, 4
Uematsu, S., 75
Uleman, J. S., 28
Ulett, A., 154
Ullman, L. P., 154
Ulmsten, U., 317, 318, 319
Umberson, D., 30
Unitzer, J., 46, 49
University of California at San Francisco, 451
University of Virginia Health System, 452
Uppal, A., 289
Urrows, S., 409
Utz, S. W., 291, 432

Vaccarino, A., 325
va der Wal, R., 51
Vaes, J., 49
Vaisberg, G., 323
Valdeon, C., 453

Valdez, P., 127
Valecha, A., 243
Valenca, A. M., 362
Valencia, M. E., 276
Vallis, M., 171
VanAkkerveeken, P. F., 265
Vanast, W. J., 208
Van Cauter, E., 50
van der Kolk, B. A., 6
Vanderpool, H. Y., 484
van der Wal, R., 290
Van Deusen, P., 127, 349
Van Dulmen, A. M., 307
Van Horn, Y., 412
Van Rompay, M., 13, 14, 58, 60, 87, 430, 431, 437, 459, 462
Vanselow, N. A., xi, xv
Van Sweden, B., 327
van Weel, C., 319
Varady, A. N., 280
Varhos, G., 317, 318, 319
Varnavides, K., 425, 426
Varner, R. E., 313, 319
Vaschillo, B., 243
Vaschillo, E., 243, 244
Vaughan, F., 199
Vaughan, S. C., 28
Vaughan, T. M., 128
Vazquez, M. I., 241, 242
Vedanthan, P. K., 243
Velten, E., 24, 153
Vera, M., 364
Verge, M., 409
Verleger, R., 127
Verri, A. P., 211
Versloot, J. M., 265
Vertommen, J., 341, 342
Vicennati, V., 282
Viera, A. J., 317
Vila, G., 364
Villamirqa, M. A., 153
Vincent, C. A., 187
Vincenz, L. M., 26
Viol, G. W., 117, 290
Vipaio, G., 324
Vipraio, G. A., 338
Vogel, P. A., 341
Vokonas, P. S., 254
Volpe, M., 282
Von Bertalanffy, L., xii
Von Korff, M., xviii, 51, 70, 71, 434
Von Korff, M. R., 226
Von Scheele, B. H. C., 361, 370
von Scheele, I. A. M., 361
Voss, R. W., 198
Voudouris, N. J., 72, 76

Wadden, T. A., 153, 155, 156
Wade, J. H., 22, 153, 154

Wagaman, M. J., 22, 28
Wagener, D. K., 364
Wagner, C., 242
Wagner, E. H., xviii
Wagner, L., 340
Wagner, T. H., 313
Wagner-Nosiska, D., 292
Wahl, E., 43
Wahlby, V., 46
Wais, R., 242
Waitzkin, H., 44, 50
Walach, H., 7, 8, 66
Walczyk, J., 335
Wald, A., 300, 301, 302, 304
Waldforgel, S., 90
Walker, E. A., 46, 49, 300
Walker, L. G., 156
Walker, R. A., 127
Wall, J., 283
Wall, K., 324
Wall, P. D., 262
Wall, V. J., 156
Walter, S., 318
Walter, W. G., 123
Walters, E. D., 10, 109, 110
Wamala, S. P., 280
Wang, M., 341, 343
Ward, C., 382
Ward, J., 323, 324
Ward, M. M., 413
Ward, P., 431, 432
Wardley, B. L., 214
Ware, C., 22, 23, 153
Ware, J. C., 22, 23
Warner, D., 153, 154
Warwick, A. M., 154
Warwick, H. M. C., 176
Watier, A., 300
Watkin, L., 254
Watkins, J. T., 169
Watkins, L. R., 46
Watson, D., 21, 30, 152
Watson, J., 449, 449
Watson, S., 453
Waugh, R., 289
Weaver, M. T., 291
Webb, R. A., 23, 72, 76, 154
Weber, R., 196
Weber, S., 404
Weder, A. B., 277, 280, 281
Weeks, C., 369
Weg, J. G., 362
Weil, A., 89
Weiler, C., 207
Wein, T., 335, 339
Weinberger, D. A., 27, 28
Weinberger, M. W., 319
Weinman, J., 167
Weinstein, T. A., 304

Weise-Kelly, L., 73, 76
Weisman, M. H., 411
Weiss, R. L., 154
Weiss, S. T., 254
Welch, K. M. A., 206
Welch, P., 191, 192
Wells, A., 363
Wells, G., 411
Wendorf, M., 281
Wenig, P., 116
Werbach, M. R., 88
Werner, K. E., 450
Wessel, M., 243
Wessley, S., 340
Westdorp, A. F., 126
Wester, F., 432
Westgate, C. E., 195
Westley, C. J., 430, 437
Westmorland, B., 327
Wetzel, M. S., 457, 459, 460
Wetzel, R. D., 387
Wexner, S. D., 300, 301, 304
Weyand, C. M., 408
Whalen, C. K., 347
Wheeden, A., 453
Whelan, V., 305, 307
Whelton, P., 277
Whelton, P. K., 289
White House Commission on Complementary and
    Alternative Medicine Policy, 454
White, A., 8, 12
White, C. A., 168, 170, 172, 176
White, K., 323, 324, 326
Whitehead, E. W., 299, 300, 301, 303
Whitehead, W. E., 300, 301, 302, 304,
    305, 307, 318
Whitworth, P., 387
Whorton, J. C., 13
Whorwell, P. J., 151, 153, 156, 300, 304, 305, 307
Wickless, C., 154
Wickramasekera, I., v, 6, 9, 10, 11, 19, 21, 22, 23,
    24, 25, 26, 27, 28, 29, 30, 31, 33, 48, 70, 72,
    73, 74, 75, 76, 77, 90, 114, 151, 152, 153,
    154, 155, 156, 157, 158, 212, 365, 446, 473
Wickramasekera, I., II, 156
Widen, E., 276
Widmark, G., 226
Wiederhold, B., 474
Wiederhold, M., 474
Wiegman, O., 411, 412
Wigal, J. K., 4, 244
Wigers, S. H., 341
Wilber, K., 60, 61, 63
Wilcox, K. J., 24, 155
Wilcox, S. A., 225
Wilcoxon, L. A., 70
Wilder, R. L., 46
Wilhelm, F. H., 8, 362
Wilke, W. S., 335

Wilkey, S., 13, 14, 58, 60, 87, 430, 431, 437, 459, 462
Wilkinson, M., 209
Willett, W. C., 283
Williams, A., 168
Williams, B., 317
Williams, D. A., 168
Williams, J. B., xv, 43
Williams, J. M. G., 172, 173, 175
Williams, K. M., 225
Williams, R. B., 253
Williams, W. J., 28
Williamson, D., 254
Williamson, D. F., 291
Williamson, P. R., 306
Wilson, D., 313, 314
Wilson, G. T., 44, 281, 291
Wilson, J., 432
Wilson, K., 409
Wilson, S. R., 244
Wing, W., 127, 349
Wingard, D. L., 276, 278
Winkelman, M. J., 192
Winkleby, M. A., 280
Wise, C. G., 304
Wise, P. S., 241
Wisen, O., 25
Witek-Janusek, L., 450
Wittert, G. A., 276
Witty, T. E., 343
Woerner, M., 290, 291
Wohlgenmuth, W. K., 396
Wolf, S., 254
Wolf, S. L., 14, 265
Wolf, S. M., 126
Wolfe, F., 323, 324, 329, 409, 410
Wolff, H. G., 206
Wolfson, S. K., 281
Wolk, A., 280
Wolner-Hanssen, P., 314
Wolpaw, J. R., 128
Womack, W., 156
Wong, M., 225
Wood, L. M., 127
Wood, L. W., 146, 147
Wood, P. D., 291
Woods, N. F., 403, 420, 422, 423
Woods, S. W., 8
Woodward, S., 403
Woody, E., 151
Woolfolk, R. L., 137, 138, 140
World Health Organization, 88, 184, 420, 422, 423
Wormsley, S. B., 333, 334, 335, 336
Wouters, J. M., 411
Wright, E. W., 230
Wright, G. E., 411
Wright, L., 308
Wulff, D. N., 196
Wulsin, L. R., 6
Wurtman, J., 424

Wurtman, R., 424
Wyatt, K. M., 423, 424
Wyman, J. F., 318
Wynne, E., 243

Xiangcai, X., 14, 361, 481
Xu, T., 14

Yaffe, M. J., 44
Yamaguchi, J., 171
Yanovski, S. Z., 44, 281, 291
Yasushi, M., 124
Yeager, R. J., 196
Yeap, B. B., 276, 342
Yehuda, R., 46
Yelin, E., 413
Yen, S. S., 420
Yingling, K. W., 6
Yokode, M., 485
Yonker, R., 290
Yordy, K. D., xi, xv
Young, G. A., 242
Young, L. D., 413
Young, M. A., 389
Young, T., 404
Youngren, M. A., 173, 174
Yudkin, P., 284
Yuen, E. J., 90
Yunus, M. B., 323, 324, 329

Zachariae, R., 151, 152, 153, 154
Zakharevich, A. S., 243
Zamble, E., v
Zametkin, A. J., 348
Zanelli, E., 407
Zanetti, G., 317, 318
Zang, T. Z., 171
Zarcone, V., 397
Zarski, J. J., 30
Zborowski, M. J., 70
Zee, P. C., 399
Zeigler, D. K., 214
Zeiss, A. M., 173, 174
Zhang, M., 6
Zhao, S., 359
Ziebland, S., 284
Zimbardo, P. G., 155
Zimmer, P. A., 276
Zimmer, P. Z., 275
Zimmerman, A. W., 349
Zimmerman, G. L., 435, 436
Zimmerman, M., 382
Zin, W. A., 362
Zingerman, A. M., 243
Zinn, M., 153
Zocco, L., 30
Zsembik, C., 44, 153
Zuckerman, E. L., 97
Zwinderman, A. H., 287

# Subject Index

Abdominal bloating, functional, 299
    diagnostic requirements, 302
Abdominal pain syndrome, functional, 299, 300
    conventional medical treatment and, 303
    diagnostic requirements, 302
Absorption, hypnotic, 24, 25, 75, 155
    genetic predisposition, 155
    stress-related disorders and, 155
Absorption test, 154-155, 159
Abuse victims:
    disengagement by, 50
    physical illness and, 49
Academy for Guided Imagery (AGI), 452-453
Accreditation Review Commission on Education for
    the Physician Assistant (ARC-PA), 458
Acupressure, 451
Acupuncture, 12, 13, 14, 59, 60, 62,
    181-187, 430, 445, 463
    applications, 184
    back pain and, 266
    case studies, 185-186
    chronic fatigue syndrome and, 339
    chronic illness and, 437
    emergence in United States, 182
    fibromyalgia and, 339
    myofascial pain and, 339
    origins, 181-182
    practice issues, 184-185
    traditional pain syndromes and, 339
    training/certification, 186-187
    Western acceptance, 181
    *See also* Traditional Chinese Medicine
Acupuncture anesthesia, 182
Acute care medical model, 4
Addictive disorders:
    biofeedback and, 10
    neurotherapy and, 123, 131
Adjustment disorder with anxious features, 364
Affective disorders, physical illness and, 48
African American churches, 195, 199
Agency for Healthcare Research and Quality, 438
Agoraphobia, PMS and, 422
AIDS patients, spiritual experiences and, 197

Alcoholism treatment:
    biofeedback, 10
    neurofeedback, 66
Allopathic healing, 193
Allopathic practitioners, 191, 195, 199
Allostasis, 45
Allostatic load, 45, 49, 50
Altered states of consciousness, 481
Alternative medicine, 445
    legitimizing, 57-58
Alternative treatments:
    versus complementary treatments, 59
American Academy of Allergy, Asthma, and
    Immunology, 244
American Academy of Medical Acupuncture, 187
American Academy of Neurology-U.S.
    Consortium, 213
American Association of Colleges of Nursing
    (AACN), 450, 454
American Board of Psychological Hypnosis, 152
American Boards of Hypnosis, 158
American College of Allergy, Asthma, and
    Immunology, 244
American College of Physicians, 458
American College of Rheumatology (ACR), 409
    fibromyalgia diagnostic criteria, 323, 329, 330
American Council of Hypnotist Examiners, 453
American Lung Association, 244
American Medical Association, 458
    Current Procedural Terminology (CPT) codes, 12
American Society of Internal Medicine, 458
Anemia, menstrual cycle and, 421
Anger control, biofeedback-assisted, 153
Anger research, 252-254
    hostility and Type A behavior, 253
    real-time effects on heart, 253
    Type A behavior, 252-253
Anorectal pain, functional, 299
    conventional medical treatment and, 303
    diagnostic requirements, 302
Anxiety, 7
    as CAD risk, 254
    back pain and, 270

biofeedback and, 10
cognitive-behavior therapy and, 168
diabetes-related, 288
fibromyalgia and, 328
functional bowel/anorectal disorders and, 300
in primary care sector, 43
metabolic syndrome and, 282
*See also* Anxiety disorders
Anxiety disorders, 6, 359
age and, 359
age of onset, 359
AP/B applications, 473
demographic profile, 359
gender and, 359
generalized, 361, 362, 364, 370
hyperventilation and, 361, 365
hypocapnia and, 361
identifying, 371
in primary care sector, 43, 47
medical illness and, 364
medical illnesses mimicking, 365
physical symptoms, 361
PMS and, 422
prevalence, 359
psychological profile, 359
sleep disorders and, 401
symptoms, 363
*See also* Anxiety disorders, assessment of; Anxiety
    disorders, comprehensive model of; Anxiety
    disorders, treatment/interventions for; Panic
    disorder; Phobias
Anxiety disorders, assessment of:
behavioral, 368
capnometric, 367
cognitive, 367-368
neurometric, 367, 370
QEEG, 370
Anxiety disorders, comprehensive model of, 359-364
avoidance behavior/stimulus
    generalization, 363-364
biochemical vulnerability, 360
neurocortical activation patterns, 362
neurophysiological activation, 361
physiology and cognition, 363
respiratory psychophysiology, 361-362
Anxiety disorders, screening for, 364-368
conceptualizing patient's anxiety disorder, 368
diagnostic categories, 364-365
HMO's and, 364
in medical settings, 364
medical, 365
psychophysiological, 365-368
*See also* Anxiety disorders, assessment of
Anxiety disorders, treatment/interventions for:
antidepressants, 359, 369
anxiolytic medications, 359, 360, 369
autogenic training, 370
biofeedback, 65, 116, 117, 359, 366, 370, 371
breathing retraining, 359, 371

clinically standardized meditation, 370
cognitive-behavioral, 359, 363, 369, 371, 372
combination, 371
conventional, 359
EMG biofeedback, 370
heart rate variability biofeedback, 370
integrating, 371
mind-body, 359
neurofeedback, 359, 370, 371
neurotherapy and, 123, 131
patient education, 371-372
pharmacotherapy, 369, 371, 372
progressive muscle relaxation, 370
relaxation therapy, 359, 366, 371
relaxation training, 370
systematic desensitization, 364
thermal biofeedback, 370
Anxiety management skills, 372
Apache disease, 193
Apache shamanism, 195
Applied kinesiology, 64
Applied psychophysiology, 90, 467
in primary care, 473
Applied psychophysiology and biofeedback (AP/B),
    behavioral health practitioners and, 467-470,
    472-473
Applied psychophysiology and biofeedback (AP/B),
    innovative uses of, 472-474
Aromatherapy, 13, 449, 451, 453
chronic illness and, 437
Arthritis, 7, 430. *See also* Rheumatoid arthritis
Arthritis Self-Management Program (ASMP), 412-413
Art therapy, 58
Asthma, 235-237
biofeedback and, 117
clinical efficacy/cost-effectiveness, 244
defining characteristics, 235
ethnicity and, 237
exacerbations, 235
flare, 237, 238
in African Americans, 237
information sources, 244
in Hispanics, 237
menstrual cycle and, 421
morbidity and, 237
physiology of, 238
prevalence, 235
sample action plan, 240-241
severity classification, 236
symptoms, 235, 236-237
treatment protocols, 244
triggers, 235, 236, 237
*See also* Asthma, behavioral intervention research
    and; Asthma, pathophysiology of
Asthma, behavioral intervention research
    and, 238-241
asthma education, 235, 238-239
psychosocial interventions, 241
stress management, 241

written emotional expression exercises, 239-241
Asthma, pathophysiology of:
    psychological treatments and, 241-245
    *See also specific types of biofeedback;*
        Relaxation training
Asthma and Allergy Foundation of America, 244
Asthma diagnosis, 235, 237-238
Asthma screening questions, 237
Asthma treatment, selection of alternative, 244-245
Atopic eczema, high hypnotic ability and, 153
Attention Deficit Disorders Evaluation Scale
    (ADDES), 350
Attention deficit hyperactivity disorder
    (ADHD), 347-349
    behavioral profile, 348-349
    biofeedback and, 10, 117
    combined form, 347
    comorbidities, 349
    EEG biofeedback and, 347
    genetic basis for, 347, 348
    hyperactive-impulsive form, 347, 348
    inattentive form, 347
    neurofeedback and, 66, 347
    neurotherapy and, 123, 124, 127, 128, 130
    screening for, 349
    symptom profile/assessment, 349-350
    *See also* Attention deficit hyperactivity disorder
        (ADHD), treatment/inventions for
Attention deficit hyperactivity disorder (ADHD),
    treatment/inventions for:
    alternative, 352
    conventional, 351
    EEG biofeedback, 352-353, 354
    effective, 353-354
    future of, 354-355
    longterm outcome studies on, 354
    neurofeedback, 352-353, 354-355
    patient and family education, 353
    patient compliance and, 351
    stimulant medications, 351
Audiovisual stimulation (AVS), 124
Australasian College of Herbal Studies, 453
Autogenic training, 110, 137, 139, 148
    anxiety disorders and, 370
    biofeedback and, 14
    fibromyalgia and, 329
    handwarming and, 144
    specific effects, 138
    standard exercises, 145
    stress management and, 138, 305
    treatment protocol, 144-146
Ayurvedic medicine, 14, 58, 59, 64

Back pain:
    anatomy/physiology/pathology of, 264-265
    behavior intervention research on, 265-266
    behavioral profile, 262
    diagnostic assessment, 262-264
    gate theory and, 262

    lower, 22
    medical profile, 259
    medical testing in assessment of, 264
    neuromatrix theory and, 262
    pathophysiological profile, 259-261
    psychophysiological/psychological
        profiles, 261-262
    reasons for psychological testing in
        assessment of, 264
    symptom profile, 262
Back pain, outcome studies on, 270-271
    clinical efficacy, 270-271
Back pain treatment protocols:
    alternative medical, 266, 271
    behavioral, 266, 270
    classical medical, 266, 271
    cost effectiveness, 271
    neurofeedback, 270
Beck Anxiety Inventory, 367
Beck Depression Inventory, 32, 288, 382,
    386, 387, 388
Behavioral headache interview, 205
Behavioral health practitioners, 467, 474
    certification/credentialing, 474
    necessity for, 467-468
    professional roles, 472
Behavioral health practitioners, education/training
    for, 468-470
    doctoral level, 468, 470, 472
    documented competencies, 471-472
    master's level, 468, 469-470, 472
    required knowledge/skills, 470-472
    unlicensed, 468, 472
Belief/placebo effects, physician assistants
    and, 457, 461, 464
Bell's palsy, acupuncture and, 182, 185-186
Bioelectromagnetism, chronic illness and, 437
Bioenergetics, 13
Biofeedback, 3, 6, 9-11, 12, 13, 30, 51, 58, 64, 66,
    90, 109, 119, 159, 444, 463, 467-468, 481
    anatomy/physiology and, 113-114
    and "letting go," 478, 480
    anxiety disorders and, 359, 366, 370, 371
    autonomic nervous tension and, 10
    back pain and, 266, 270
    biomedical instruments and, 75
    brain blood flow and, 10
    chronic fatigue syndrome and, 339
    controlled breathing, 111
    creation of different state of consciousness, 111
    depression and, 377
    efficacy of, 74-76
    electric wave brain activity and, 10
    for fecal incontinence, 306
    for pelvic floor dyssynergia, 306
    functional bowel/anorectal disorders and, 305
    goal, 109
    headache treatment and, 213, 215-216
    heart rate and, 10

hypertension and, 290
imagery, 111
mental health applications, 10
muscle relaxation, 111
openness to change and, 75
origins, 109
placebo effect and, 69-77, 116
repetition of words, 111
respiration and, 10
selective remembering, 111
skin temperature and, 10
stress management and, 138, 305
understanding mind-body link, 10
urinary incontinence and, 9, 117, 318, 319
*See also* specific types of biofeedback;
    Biofeedback, applications of; QEEG
    assessment; Trait hypnotic ability
Biofeedback, applications of, 115-118
anxiety disorders, 65, 116, 117
asthma, 117
attention deficit disorder, 117
bruxism, 117
chronic pain, 117
dermatological disorders, 117
epileptic seizures, 117
essential hypertension, 116-117
fecal incontinence, 117
global effects, 115-116
headaches, 115, 116, 117
hypertension, 115-116, 117
irritable bowel syndrome and, 9, 117
motion sickness, 117
muscles disorders, 117
muscle tension and, 10, 115
nausea/vomiting, 117
nocturnal enuresis, 117
phantom-limb pain, 117
Raynaud's disease, 116, 117
Temporomandibular joint dysfunction, 117
tinnitus, 117
urinary incontinence and, 9, 117
Biofeedback-assisted relaxation therapy,
    diabetes and, 289
Biofeedback Certification Institute of America
    (BCIA), 468, 474
Biofeedback learning principles, 114-115
    shaping, 115
Biofeedback outcome research,
    methodological problems in, 117-118
Biofeedback practitioners, 4
    personality of, 115
Biofeedback Research Society, 110
Biofeedback Society of American, 474
Biofeedback system, basic, 10
Biofeedback training:
    in diaphragmatic breathing, 8
Biomedical instruments/procedures, 109, 111-113
electrocardiogram, 113
electroencephalograph, 112

electromyograph, 111
photoplethysmograph 113
placebo effects and, 75-76
respiration feedback, 113
skin conductance, 112
skin temperature, 111-112
*See also* EEG biofeedback; EMG biofeedback;
    Heart rate variability (HRV) biofeedback;
    Respiratory sinus arrhythmia (RSA)
    biofeedback; Temperature biofeedback
    (TEMP)
Biomedical model, 195
Biomedicine, 57
historical roots, 59-60
Biopsychosocial model, xii, xiii, 11, 83, 86, 443, 448
Bipolar disorder I, 379, 380, 382
with rapid cycling, 382
*See also* Bipolar disorders
Bipolar disorder II, 379, 380, 382
with rapid cycling, 382
*See also* Bipolar disorders
Bipolar disorders, 382
criteria, 381
hypomanic episode, 381
manic episode, 381
Body sensations, shifts in, 193
Bowel and anorectal disorders, functional, 299
diagnostic requirements, 302
prevalence, 299
primary care clinicians and treatment of, 308
psychological distress and, 300-301
psychological functioning and, 301
social functioning and, 301
symptom profile/assessment, 301-303
*See also* specific functional bowel and anorectal
    disorders; Bowel and anorectal disorders,
    treatment/interventions for functional
Bowel and anorectal disorders,
    treatment/interventions for functional, 306-307
antidepressant medications, 303
conventional medical treatment, 303-305
fiber supplementation, 303
laxatives, 303-304
long-term outcome studies, 307
stress management training, 305
*See also* specific interventions and bowel and
    anorectal disorders
Breast cancer, spiritual experiences and, 197
Breathing retraining, anxiety disorders and, 359, 371
Bruxism, biofeedback and, 117
Bulimia, 22
high hypnotic ability and, 153

Calendar of Premenstrual Experiences (COPE), 420
California Board of Registered Nursing, 453
Cancer, psychological effects of:
cognitive-behavior therapy and, 168
Capitation, shared-risk model of, 90
Cardiac behavioral intervention research, 252-254

anger, 252-254
anxiety, 254
depression, 254
social isolation, 254
Cardiac disease, low hypnotic ability and, 153
Cardiac disorder, functional:
    AP/B applications, 473
Cardiac dynamics, anatomy/physiology of, 250
Cardiac psychology, 473
Cardiac rehabilitation, AP/B applications, 473
Cardiac surgery response, low hypnotic ability
    and, 153
Cartesian mind-body dualism, 83-84
Center for Studying Health System Change, 87
Center for the Study of Complementary and
    Alternative Therapies, University of
    Virginia, 452
Center for the Study of Ethics in Professions, 99
Centers of Alternative Medicine,
    NIH-sponsored, 64
Chantilly Report, 57-58
Chemotherapy, anticipatory nausea and
    vomiting and:
    absorption and, 155
Chest pain:
    absorption and, 155
    low hypnotic ability and, 153
    nonorganic, 22
Child bearing, urinary incontinence and, 314
Chiropractic therapies, 12, 13
Chiropractors, 4
Christian mystics, 480-481
Chronic/illness, 7, 429, 478
    children with, 430
    definition, 430
    doctor visits for, 48
    management principles, xviii
    most prevalent, 430
    perception of threat in, 479
    prevalence, 429, 430
    reaction to diagnosis, 44
    symptoms, 4
    through life cycle, 479
    *See also specific chronic diseases and conditions*
Chronically ill people:
    caring for, 429-438
    enhancing health behaviors/self-care, 434-437
    medical management principles, 433-434
    *See also* Stages of change; Stepped care,
        individualized
Chronically ill people, assessment of, 431-433
    cultural understanding, 432
    personal perspectives, 432
    therapeutic partnership, 431-432
    trusting relationship, 431
Chronically ill people, task lists for, 432, 438
Chronic benign pain:
    definition, 325
    fibromyalgia and, 324-325

Chronic fatigue:
    differentiating from chronic fatigue syndrome, 333
    prevalence, 333
Chronic fatigue syndrome (CFS), 47, 89, 263,
    327, 333
    AP/B applications, 473
    behavioral/neuropsychiatric aspects, 338-339
    cognitive-behavior therapy and, 168
    defining, 336
    defining characteristics, 333
    depression and, 339
    differentiating from chronic fatigue, 333
    dysautonomia and, 335
    epidemiology, 334-335
    etiology, 333, 334
    fibromyalgia and, 333
    gender and, 334
    laboratory findings and, 336
    most common concerns in, 338
    neurofeedback and, 66
    overlap syndromes, 333
    pathophysiology, 335
    physical examination findings and, 335-336
    radiological findings and, 336
    signs and diagnostic criteria, 335-336
    stress and, 339
    symptoms, 333, 334
    versus major depression, 340
Chronic fatigue syndrome (CFS),
    management/interventions for:
    activity, 337
    acupuncture, 339
    aerobic activity, 341
    alternative and traditional combination, 343
    alternative therapies, 339
    amphetamine-like drugs, 338
    antidepressant medications, 338
    behavioral, 339-340
    biofeedback, 339
    cognitive-behavioral, 340-341
    dietary changes, 339
    exercise, 339
    herbal remedies, 339, 342
    homeopathy, 339
    hypnosis, 339
    long-term, 342-343
    meditation, 339
    neurofeedback, 339
    physical therapies, 341-342
    sleep medications, 338
    nutrition, 337-338, 342
    pain medications, 338
    reassurance/education, 336-337
    relaxation training, 339
    traditional management of, 336-338
    unusual/extreme, 342
    vitamins, 339, 342
Chronic obstructive pulmonary disease, 430
Chronic pain, 22

CBT treatment protocol, 176
cognitive-behavior therapy and, 168
in primary care sector, 43
low hypnotic ability and, 153
Chronic pain care:
  AP/B applications, 473
Chronic urticaria intensity, high hypnotic
  ability and, 153
Clinical/dental phobia severity, high hypnotic ability
  and, 153
Clinically standardized meditation (CSM), 137
  treatment protocol, 146-147
Clinical psychophysiology, 3, 6, 11
Cognition, levels of:
  automatic thoughts, 169, 174-175
  core beliefs, 169, 170, 174, 176
  underlying assumptions, 169-170, 174, 175
Cognitive-behavioral therapy (CBT), 8, 30,
  138, 449, 453
  anxiety disorders and, 359, 363, 369, 371, 372
  asthmatic children and, 244-245
  chronic fatigue syndrome and, 340-341
  computer-administered, 387
  functional bowel/anorectal disorders and, 305
  goals, 217
  headaches and, 217-218
  hypnosis and, 156
  irritable bowel syndrome and, 9, 307
  migraines and, 213
  mood disorders and, 387, 388
  problems, 341
  purpose, 411
  rheumatoid arthritis and, 407, 411-414
  self-statements, 217
  sleep disorders and, 393, 396
  tension headaches, 213
Cognitive-behavior therapy (CBT) applications:
  activity scheduling, 172, 173
  behavioral experiments, 174
  behavioral intervention strategies, 172-174, 177
  cognitive continuum to modify beliefs, 174
  cognitive strategies, 172, 174-176, 177
  core belief log, 174
  cost-benefits analysis of beliefs, 174
  distraction, 172
  downward arrow technique, 174
  exercise, 172
  exposure, 172, 174
  graded task assignment, 172, 173
  historical test of core belief, 174
  identifying cognitive distortions, 174
  "pie" technique, 174
  reinforcement, 172, 173-174
  relaxation, 172
  rational-emotional role play, 174
  role play, 172
  social skills training, 172
  targeting automatic thoughts, 174-175
  targeting core beliefs, 176

  targeting intermediate beliefs, 175
  thought records, 174
Cognitive beliefs:
  catastrophizing, 411
  helplessness, 411
  rheumatoid arthritis and, 410-411
  self-efficacy, 411
  Cognitive therapy, 168, 176, 218
  asthma and, 241
  back pain and, 270
  functional bowel/anorectal disorders and, 305
  irritable bowel syndrome and, 306
  PMDD and, 419, 424, 427
  PMS and, 419, 425, 426, 427
  reframing, 426
  stress management training and, 305
  *See also* Cognitive behavioral therapy (CBT)
Collaborative Curriculum Survey, 450
Colorado Center for Healing Touch, 453
Complementary and alternative medicine (CAM),
  12-14, 57, 63, 64, 87, 450
  chronic illness and, 430, 437
  encouraging disclosure/evaluation of, 437
  favors factoring, 60
  favors limiting, 60
  fundamental assumptions, 168
  goal, 176
  in medical school curricula, 445
  medical disorders and, 168
  origins for medical disorders, 167-168
  paradigm, 13
  prevalence of use, 14
  principles of, 168-172
  providers, 83
  psychological disorders and, 168
  structuring treatment, 176-177
  Western medical paradigm and, 58-59
  *See also specific CAM interventions;*
    Complementary treatments
Complementary treatments, 59
  emerging, 63-66
  versus alternative treatments, 59
  *See also specific CAM interventions;*
    Complementary and alternative
    medicine (CAM)
Conditioned placebo hope response,
  biofeedback and, 75-76
Conditioned response model, 76-77
  origins, 73-74
Conditioned responses, personality factors and, 72-73
Congestive heart failure (CHF), 249-250, 251
  management, 250
  prevalence, 249
Constipation, functional, 299
  diagnostic requirements, 302
Coronary artery disease (CAD), 249, 250
  clinical manifestations, 249
  conventional medical treatment for, 251
  diagnosis, 251

outcome studies, 256
prevalence, 249, 250
psychophysiological protocol, 255-256
risk factors, 250
symptoms, 251
Cranial sacral therapy, fibromyalgia and, 329
Cults, fanatical, 196
Culture-bound syndromes, 197
*Curanderas,* 193
*Curanderismo,* 195
*Curanderos,* 193
Cushing's syndrome, 281
Cybernetics, 110
Cyclothymic disorder, 379

Dance therapy, 58
Depression, 6, 7
  as CAD risk, 254
  back pain and, 270
  biofeedback and, 10
  chronic fatigue syndrome and, 339
  cognitive-behavior therapy and, 168
  definition, 377
  epidemiology, 382-383
  etiology, 377
  fibromyalgia and, 328
  functional bowel/anorectal disorders and, 300
  Hopi Indians and, 197
  in children, 383
  in primary care sector, 43
  metabolic syndrome and, 282
  neurobiology, 377, 383-384
  neurotherapy and, 123
  prevalence, 382
  Traditional Chinese Medicine (TCM) and, 64-65
  versus PMDD, 423
  *See also* Depression, major; Depression, symptoms of; Depressive disorders; Depressive disorder, major
Depression, major, 379
  criteria, 380
  high hypnotic ability and, 153
  PMDD and, 422
  sleep disorders and, 401
  versus chronic fatigue syndrome, 340
  *See also* Depressive disorder, major
Depression, symptoms of, 381
  cognitive, 381, 382
  emotional, 381, 382
  vegetative, 381, 382
Depression screening/diagnostic evaluation, 379-382
Depressive disorder, major:
  sleep disorders and, 403
  *See also* Depression, major
Depressive disorder not otherwise specified, 379
Depressive disorders, 6, 197
  diagnosis, 377
  obesity and, 49
  physiological hypoarousal and, 47

stressful life events and, 49
  *See also* Depression; Depression, major; Depressive disorder, major
Dermatological disorders, biofeedback and, 117
"Desert fathers," 483
Diabetes, 430
  menstrual cycle and, 421
  *See also* Diabetes, Type 2; Diabetes mellitus
Diabetes, Type 2, 275, 278, 280, 281, 282, 283
  behavioral therapies, 287-289
  care flow sheet, 287
  circulation-related problems, 289
  definition, 276
  diagnosis, 276, 277
  in Pima Indian population, 276
  laboratory evaluation components for, 286
  medical history components for, 285
  physical examination components for, 286
  prevalence, 276
  screening, 279
  stress management and, 289
  treatment response prediction, 291-292
Diabetes management plan:
  evaluation, 288
Diabetes mellitus, 7
  obesity and, 49
  urinary incontinence and, 314
Diabetics, standards of care for, 284-287
*Diagnostic and Statistical Manual of Mental Disorders:*
  cross-cultural limitations, 197
  IV, 20, 29, 32, 158, 197, 198, 347, 364, 372, 377, 378, 379, 380, 382, 420
  IV-TR, 377
  mental diagnosis, xvi
  I, 377
  III, 377, 378
  III-R, 420
  II, 377
Diarrhea, functional, 299
  antidiarrheal medications and, 304
  diagnostic requirements, 302
Direct blood pressure feedback, hypertension and, 290
Disease:
  versus illness, 195
Dissociation, 6
Dissociative disorders, high hypnotic ability and, 153
Dissociative identity disorder, 197
Dissociative trance disorder, 197
Donaldson Protocol, 328
Dysmenorrhea, primary, 22
Dyssomnias, 395-400
  alcohol-dependent sleep disorder, 395, 399
  altitude insomnia, 398, 399
  circadian rhythm sleep disorders, 395, 399-400
  environmental sleep disorder, 398
  extrinsic sleep disorders, 395, 398-399
  inadequate sleep hygiene, 398

intrinsic sleep disorders, 395-398
narcolepsy, 397
obstructive sleep apnea, 397-398, 404
periodic limb movement disorder, 396
psychophysiological insomnia, 395-396
restless legs syndrome, 396-397
stimulant-dependent sleep disorder, 398-399
See also Sleep disorders
Dysthmymia, 378. See also Depression
Dysthmymic disorder, 379
criteria, 380
diagnosis, 380-381

Education. See Behavioral health practitioners,
education/training for; Mind-body medicine,
medical education for; Mind-body medicine,
education of physician assistants in; Mind-body
nursing, nursing education for
EEG biofeedback, 57, 59, 64, 65, 66, 71, 74, 75, 110,
112, 118, 123, 124, 127, 157, 158
ADHD and, 347, 352-353, 354
back pain and, 270
chronic fatigue syndrome and, 339-340
fibromyalgia and, 325, 329
mood disorders and, 384, 388
muscle tension headaches and, 118-119
terminology, 124-127
See also Neurofeedback
EMG biofeedback, 71, 75, 111, 118, 158, 288, 305
anxiety disorders and, 370
asthma and, 242-243
as TMD treatment, 229-230
fibromyalgia and, 329
headaches and, 73-74, 116
hypertension and, 117, 290
migraines and, 213
sleep disorders and, 396
tension headaches and, 213, 216
Emotional illness:
in primary care sector, 43
Endometriosis, menstrual cycle and, 421
Energy medicine, 57, 60, 62, 64, 65
Energy therapy, 454
Epileptic seizures, biofeedback and, 117
Ethical decision-making models, 102
Ethical functioning, 105
aspirational, 95
aspirational versus mandatory, 95
continuing education and, 105
discussion and, 105
mandatory, 95
reflection and, 105
Ethical principles, core, 94, 95-98
accepting accountability, 98
according dignity, 97
being just, 96
beneficence, 96
fidelity, 97
nonmaleficence, 96

pursuing excellence, 97-98
respecting autonomy, 96
treating others with care and compassion, 97
Ethical professional, 94
Ethics, 95
mandatory, 95
principle, 100
Ethics, code of, 99
American Chiropractic Association, 99
American Occupational Therapy Association, 99
compliance, 95
role, 94
values listed in, 99
See also Ethical functioning; Ethical principles,
core; Ethical professional; Ethics,
professional; Practice standards;
Virtue ethics
Ethics, problematic situations and, 102-105
advanced planning, 102-103
appropriate, 103-104
boundary issues, 103
conflict of interest, 104-105
Ethics, professional, 93-94. See also Ethical
functioning; Ethical principles, core; Ethical
professional; Ethics, code of; Practice standards;
Virtue ethics
Evidence-based medicine, 3, 7-9
challenges, 8-9
faith and, 9
paradigm shifting and, 9
placebo and, 9
reaching decisions, 8
Evolution, primary care in, 87-88
Exercise therapies, 13
Exorcism, 194
Experimental pain intensity, high hypnotic ability
and, 153

Facial pain intensity, high hypnotic ability and, 153
Faith:
role in healing, 9
Family medicine, 84-85
as medical specialty, 84
FDA testing, 463
Feldenkreis physical therapy, 13
fibromyalgia and, 329
Fibromyalgia, 47, 263, 323-324, 330
aerobic activity and, 341
AP/B applications, 473
biological theory of, 324
chronic benign pain and, 324-325
chronic fatigue syndrome and, 333
cognitive deficits, 323
diagnosis, 323, 325-327
etiological theories, 324
fatigue and, 338
neural plasticity model of, 325
onset, 323
patient age, 323

patient gender, 323
prevalence, 324
psychological theory of, 324
reduced energy, 323
screening questions, 324
sleep disturbance, 323
sleep-related theory of, 324
stress and, 339
tender points, 323, 327, 330
trigger points, 327
versus myofascial pain syndrome, 325
*See also* EEG biofeedback; Fibromyalgia,
    treatment/interventions for; SEMG testing
Fibromyalgia, treatment/interventions
    for, 327-329
    alternative, 329
    behavioral, 328
    medication, 327-328
    multidisciplinary, 329
    outcome studies on, 329-330
    *See also specific treatments and interventions*
Fibromyalgia Impact Questionnaire, 330
Functional improvement, 89
Functional syndromes, managing, 51

Gastroenterology, acupuncture and, 184
Gastrointestinal (GI) disorders, 299, 308
    treatment of in children, 308
    *See also* Rome criteria; Rome II criteria
Geriatrics, 89
Guided imagery, 58, 449, 451, 452-453, 463
    asthma management and, 241

Hamilton Anxiety Scale, 367
Hamilton Depression Scale, 382, 389
    Structured Interview Guide (SAD version), 389
Harvard scale, 32
Headache diary, 205, 213, 214, 218
Headache disorders, primary:
    prevalence, 205
    profile, 205-208
        *See also* Migraine headaches; Tension-type
        headaches
Headache disorders, secondary, 205
Headache management, biobehavioral approach to,
    209-218
    assessment, 209-212
    clinical interview, 209-212, 218
    education, 213
    patient education and, 209
    psychophysiological evaluation, 212
    skills acquisition, 213-218
    treatment, 212-213
Headaches, 30
    biofeedback and, 115, 116, 117
    chronic daily, 205, 207, 208
    functional muscular, 22
    vascular, 22
    *See also specific types of headaches*

Headache triggers, 213
    dietary, 213-214
Head injuries, closed:
    neurotherapy and, 123
Healing ceremonies, Navajo, 192
    chanting and, 192
    sand painting and, 192
Healing touch, 454
Health risk factors, 7
    inactivity, 7
    obesity, 7
    stress level, 7
Heart disease, 7, 430
    dynamic factors in, 251-252
    mind-body interventions and, 254-256
    psychosocial factors and, 196
Heart rate variability (HRV) biofeedback,
    113, 157, 158
    anxiety disorders and, 370
    hypertension and, 290
Herbal medicine/supplements, 12, 13, 59, 64, 66
Herbal remedies, 430, 445
    back pain and, 266
Hidden information:
    prevalence/psychophysiology, 28-29
High hypnotic ability:
    psychological disorders and, 153
    psychophysiological disorders and, 153
    *See also specific psychological and
        psychophysiological disorders*
High hypnotizables, 22-23, 35
    cognitive style, 23-24
    physiology and psychology and, 154
High risk model of threat perception, 5, 19, 30, 31,
    48, 152-153
    empirical tests of, 35
    predictions from, 35
Holistic cardiology, 249
Holistic care, 431, 438
    client and, 433
    health care professional and, 433
Homeopathic medicine, 58
Homeopathy, 9, 60, 62, 64, 445
    chronic illness and, 437
Hopi Indians, depression and, 197
Hormone replacement therapy (HRT),
    sleep disorders and, 404
Hyperhydrosis, 22
Hyperinsulinemia, 282
Hyperlipidemia, 275, 277-278, 280, 281
    definition, 277
    diagnosis, 277-278
    prevalence, 278
    therapy, 278, 291
Hypertension, 7, 275, 276-277, 278, 280, 281, 430
    biofeedback and, 115, 116-117
    definition, 276
    diagnosis, 276-277
    in African American population, 277

obesity and, 49
prevalence, 277
preventing, 283
primary, 22, 27
stress management education for, 52, 289-291
"white coat," 290
Hyperventilation, anxiety disorders and, 361, 365
Hypnosis, 30, 58, 151, 159, 444, 453, 463
as information processing, 152
asthma and, 243
back pain and, 266, 270
chronic fatigue syndrome and, 339
contraindications, 157-158, 159
fibromyalgia and, 329
irritable bowel syndrome and, 9
placebo effect, 151, 156
stress management training and, 305
See also High risk model of threat perception;
Hypnotherapy
Hypnotherapy, 13, 151-152, 155, 159, 449
contraindications, 157-158, 159
definition, 151
irritable bowel syndrome and, 305, 306-307
professional organizations, 158
psychological techniques, 155
Hypnotizability, 151, 153-155
empirical efficacy of nonspecific hypnotherapy
and, 155-157
empirical efficacy of specific hypnotherapy
and, 155
genetic predisposition, 155
See also High hypnotizables; Hypnotizability, tests
of; Low hypnotizables
Hypnotizability, tests of, 154
clinical applications, 158
Harvard Group Scale of Hypnotic Susceptibility
Form A, 154
Hypnotic Induction Profile, 154
Stanford Hypnotic Susceptibility Scale
Form C, 154
See also Absorption test
Hypocapnia, anxiety disorders and, 361
Hypochondriasis, 44

Idiopathic flushing, 22
Illness:
phenomenology of, 478-479
psychology of, 477
spirituality and, 479-480
versus disease, 195
Illness conviction, 48
Immune function, high hypnotic ability and, 153
Incontinence, functional fecal, 299, 301
behavioral/psychophysiological interventions, 305
biofeedback and, 117, 306
management of childhood, 304
diagnostic requirements, 302
Incontinence, urinary, 313-319
AP/B applications, 473

assessment/diagnosis, 315
determining severity of, 316
functional incontinence, 315
mixed, 315
overflow incontinence, 314-315, 316
reasons for, 313
risk factors, 314
stress incontinence, 315, 316, 317, 318, 319
symptom profiles, 314-315
types, 216
urge incontinence, 314, 316, 317, 318
Incontinence, treatments/interventions for
urinary, 313, 318
behavioral/psychophysiological, 313, 317-318
biofeedback, 9, 117, 318, 319
bladder training, 313, 317-318, 319
conventional medical, 315-317
electrical stimulation of pelvic floor, 317
future of, 319
long-term outcome studies on, 319
medication, 313, 316-317
patient education, 318
pelvic floor exercises, 313, 317, 318, 319
pessaries, 317
positive reinforcement, 318
surgery, 313, 317, 318, 319
vaginal weights, 317
Indigenous healers, 192
instrumentation/procedures, 192-195
Indigenous healing models, 191, 193
Insomnia, 27, 30
primary, 22
Insomnia, chronic:
low hypnotic ability and, 153
Insomnia, EEG-defined:
high hypnotic ability and, 153
Institute of Integrative Aromatherapy, 453
Integrated care, 3, 11-12
barriers, 12
definition, 12
Integrative medicine, 3, 12-14, 59, 62-63, 66-67
opponents, 62
proponents, 63
Intentional healing at distance, 58
International Association for the Study of Pain, 325
International Case Definition Criteria for
CFS, 336, 337
International Headache Society (IHS), 205, 207
International Society of Hypnosis, 158
Interventions, short-term, 51
Inventory to Diagnose Depression, 382
Irritable bowel syndrome (IBS), 22, 30, 299, 300, 301
antidiarrheal medications and, 304
AP/B applications, 473
behavioral/psychophysiological interventions, 305
biofeedback and, 9, 117
CBT treatment protocol, 176
cognitive behavioral therapy and, 9, 168, 307
cognitive therapy and, 305

combined treatment, 305-306
conventional medical treatment and, 303
diagnostic requirements, 302
education and, 306
hypnosis and, 9
hypnotherapy and, 305, 306-307
interpersonal therapy and, 305
menstrual cycle and, 421
prevalence, 301
psychodynamic therapy and, 305
research on, 307-308
stress management training and, 305
work absenteeism and, 301

Joint Commission on Hospital Accreditation, 450

"Kingdom of the sick," 429, 478-479

Lakota Sioux:
  shaman, 198
  tribalism, 198
Learning under anesthesia, 28
Levator ani syndrome:
  diagnostic requirements, 302
Liebowitz Social Anxiety Scale, 367
Life Events Scale, 47, 48
Light therapy:
  depression and, 377, 389
  PMDD and, 424
  sleep disorders and, 403
Low hypnotic ability:
  psychological disorders and, 153
  psychophysiological disorders and, 153
  *See also specific psychological and
    psychophysiological disorders*
Low hypnotizables, 23, 35
  cognitive style, 24-27

Magnetic devices, 62
Managed care, xiii-xiv, 12, 473
  gatekeeper, 87
  limitations presented by, 63
  "mental health carve-out," 12, 90
  neurofeedback and, 355
Manual therapies, 13
Marlowe-Crowne high scoring people, 23, 35
  cognitive style, 27-28
  with IBS, 28
  with severe asthma, 28
Marlowe-Crowne test, 32
Massage therapy, 13, 59, 64, 430, 449, 451,
    453-454, 463
  chronic illness and, 437
  fibromyalgia and, 329
McGill Pain Questionnaire, 329
Medical practice, redefining purpose of, 89
"Medical world," 479
Medication management, 63
Medicine, evolution of:

Dossey's three-era medicine model,
    57, 61, 62, 254
  redefining, 61
Meditation, 50, 51, 58, 137, 139-140, 148,
    451, 478, 485
  and "letting go," 478, 480
  anxiety disorders and, 370
  Buddhist mindfulness, 483
  chronic fatigue syndrome and, 339
  medical benefits, 137
  modifying brain states, 481
  sleep disorders and, 396
  specific effects, 138
  stress management and, 138
  *See also* Clinically standardized meditation (CSM)
Meditative traditions, 480
Med-Plus, 90
Menopause:
  HRT and, 404
  sleep disorders and, 403-404
Menstrual cycle:
  exacerbation of medical conditions, 421
  sleep disorders and, 402-403
  *See also specific medical conditions*
Menstrual Distress Questionnaire, 420, 425
Menstrual Symptom Severity List, 425
Mental health:
  primary care and, xi
  problems, xv-xviii
Mental health care, integrated, 90
Mental illness:
  in primary care sector, 43
Mental imagery, unusual, 193
Mental relaxation, 74
Metabolic syndrome, 275-276, 282
  African Americans and, 280
  and cardiovascular disease risk, 275
  and cerebrovascular disease risk, 275
  components, 280
  long-term complications, 278
  overt symptoms, 275
  stressful life events and, 281
  thrifty-gene hypothesis and, 281
  underlying psychophysiological mechanisms, 280
Metabolic syndrome, treatment/interventions for,
    282-284
  diet modification barriers and, 284
  goals, 284
  patient compliance and, 275
Migraine headaches, 205-207
  AP/B applications, 473
  chronic, 207, 208
  diagnostic criteria, 206, 207
  episodic, 209
  high hypnotic ability and pain intensity, 153
  hyperexcitable brain and, 206
  menstrual cycle and, 421
  transformational, 208
  treatment options, 213

Mind-body interventions, 58, 445. *See also specific mind-body interventions*; Mind-body therapy
Mind-body medicine, 3-4, 445
  definition, 58
  functional integration of primary care and, 89-90
Mind-body medicine, competencies for physician assistants practicing, 461-463
Mind-body medicine, medical education for, 443-448
  Eastern Virginia Medical School and, 446-448
  establishing mind's physical/medical relevance, 444-445
  gap, 443-444
  obstacles, 444
  practical mind-body skills, 445-446
Mind-body medicine, physician assistant education in, 457-464
  appropriate, 457-458
  conceptual model, 461
  interviewing/communication skills, 457
  optimal models, 460
  potential safety problems, 459
  primary care emphasis, 457
  problems with present, 460
  psychoneuroimmunology model, 457, 461
Mind-body models, primary care and, 47-52
  brief interventions, 51
  chronic illness visits, 48
  managing functional syndromes, 51
  mind-body therapy models, 48-50
  motivation for change, 50
  spiritual factors, 50
  therapist-intensive interventions, 51-52
  treating stress/mood disorders, 50-51
  wellness checkups, 47-48
Mind-body nursing, nursing education for, 449-454
Mind-body specialists, 4. *See also specific types of mind-boy specialists*
Mind-body therapies, models for, 48-50. *See also* High risk model of threat perception
Mind-body therapy, criteria for empirically valid, 306-307
Minnesota Multiphasic Personality Inventory (MMPI), 32, 388
Mood:
  definition, 379
  depressed, 379
  manic, 379
Mood disorder, substance-induced, 379
Mood disorder due to general medical condition, 379
Mood disorders, 377, 378-379
  as mental illnesses, 379
  chronic, 382
  etiology, 378
  in primary care sector, 43, 47
  major subtypes, 379
  physical illness and, 49
  sleep disorders and, 401, 403
  *See also specific mood disorders*; Depression

Mood disorders, treatments/interventions for, 50-51, 384-388
  aerobic exercise, 385
  alternative nonprescription medications, 386
  asymmetry training, 388
  bibliotherapy, 387
  cognitive, 384, 385
  cognitive-behavioral therapy, 387, 388
  computer-administered cognitive-behavioral therapy, 387
  conventional, 384
  EEG biofeedback, 384, 388
  future of mind-body, 388-389
  hospitalization, 384
  interpersonal, 384, 385, 387
  light therapy, 377, 389
  MAOIs, 385, 386
  medication, 384
  neurofeedback, 388
  outcome studies on, 386-387
  psychodynamic, 384, 385, 387
  psychopharmacology, 385-386, 387
  relaxation therapy, 387
  shock therapy, 384
  SSRIs, 385, 386
  stimulants, 385
  transcranial magnetic stimulation, 384
  *See also* Psychotherapy
Morals, 95
Moral values, 98-99
  mind-body services and, 98-99
Morning sickness, high hypnotic ability and, 153
Mother Teresa effect, 253
Motion sickness, biofeedback and, 117
Moxibustion, back pain and, 266
MULTIFIT program, Kaiser Permanente, 256
Muscle disorders, biofeedback and, 117
Muscle tension, biofeedback and, 10, 115
Musical performance anxiety, high hypnotic ability and, 153
Music therapy, 58
Myofascial pain syndrome (MPS), 263, 266, 270
  AP/B applications, 473
  versus fibromyalgia, 325
Mystical experiences, 194

National Allergy and Asthma Network/Mothers of Asthmatics, 244
National Association of Cognitive-Behavioral Therapists, 453
National Certification Commission for Acupuncture and Oriental Medicine, 186, 451
National Guideline Clearinghouse, 438
National Jewish Medical and Research Center Information Service, 244
National League for Nursing, 450, 451
National Organization of Nurse Practitioner Faculty (NONPF), 450
Native healers, 192

Naturopathic medicine, 58
Nausea/vomiting, biofeedback and, 117
Navajo practitioners, 198
Navajo shamans, 198
Negative moods, high hypnotic ability and, 153
Neurofeedback, 65, 66, 112, 123, 124, 159, 478
    ADHD and, 66, 347, 352-353, 354-355
    alcoholism and, 66
    anxiety disorders and, 359, 370, 371
    chronic fatigue syndrome and, 66, 339-340
    fibromyalgia and, 328
    mood disorders and, 388
    Peniston protocol, 481-482
    PMDD and, 424
    post-stroke treatment and, 66
    *See also* EEG biofeedback; Neurotherapy
Neurology, acupuncture and, 184
Neurotheology, 481
    modifying brain states, 481
Neurotherapy, 65, 123
    learning principles, 127-128
    origins, 123-124
    *See also* EEG biofeedback; Neurofeedback
Neurotherapy applications, 128-131
    addictive disorders, 123, 131
    affective disorders, 131
    anxiety disorders, 123, 131
    attention deficit hyperactivity disorder, 123, 124,
        127, 128, 130
    depression, 123, 131
    head injuries (closed), 123
    schizophrenia, 131
    seizure disorder, 123, 127-128, 129-130
    stroke, 131
Neuroticism, functional bowel/anorectal disorders
    and, 300
Nightingale, F., 449, 451
Nightmares, 22, 401
Nightmares, predisposition to:
    absorption and, 155
    high hypnotic ability and, 153
Nocturnal enuresis, biofeedback and, 117
Nursing, mind-body approaches:
    history, 449-450
Nursing education, mind-body principles
    in, 450, 454
    curricula/programs, 451-454
    examples, 452-454
    required knowledge/skills, 450-451
Nursing science:
    traditional holistic view, 449
Nutritional therapies, 12, 13

Obesity, 275, 280, 281
    depression and, 49
    diabetes and, 49
    hypertension and, 49
    stress and, 45, 49
    urinary incontinence and, 314

Western society and, 281
    *See also* Obesity (moderate); Obesity (Morbid)
Obesity (moderate), 22
    high hypnotic ability and, 153
Obesity (morbid), 22
    absorption and, 155
    low hypnotic ability and, 153
Obesity management:
    depressive symptoms and, 44
    emotional factors, 44
    social factors, 44
Obsessive-compulsive disorder, 364, 370
    cognitive-behavioral interventions and, 364
    SSRIs and, 364, 369
Office of Alternative Medicine (OAM), 14, 57-58. *See
    also* National Center for Complementary and
    Alternative Medicine (NCCAM)
Ontogeny recapitulating phylogeny, 84
Oxford Brooks University, 453

Pain:
    acupuncture and, 184
    acute, 70
    biofeedback and chronic, 117
    clinical, 70
    experimental, 70
    *See also* Chronic pain; Chronic benign pain;
        Chronic pain care
Pain experience:
    reactive component, 215, 216-218
    sensory component, 215-216
Pain tolerance, perception and, 215
Panic attacks, 362
    PMS and, 422
    *See also* Panic disorder
Panic disorder, 6, 8, 361, 362, 363, 364
    adult asthmatics with, 245
    catastrophic fears and, 363
    CBT treatment and, 176, 245
    exertion-triggered, 366
    hyperventilation and, 361
    sleep disorders and, 401
    *See also* Panic attacks
Papago Indians, 198
Parasomnias, 395, 400-401
    arousal disorders, 395, 400
    night terrors, 400
    primary snoring, 401
    REM sleep-associated, 395, 400-401
    SIDS, 401
    sleep bruxism, 401
    sleep enuresis, 401
    sleep-wake transition disorders, 395, 400
    sleepwalking, 400
    *See also* Sleep disorders
Parasympathetic dysregulation hypothesis, 25
Parish nurses, 483
Pastoral care, 483
Pastoral counseling, 483

Patient education, 4, 6
Patient empowerment, physician assistants and, 457
  counseling patients, 461
  facilitating health-promoting behavior, 461
Patient self-management, 4, 6
"Patient's world," changes in:
  changes in body and, 479
Pediatrics, AP/B applications, 474
Pelvic floor dyssynergia, 299, 300
  behavioral/psychophysiological interventions, 305
  biofeedback for, 306
  diagnostic requirements, 302
Perception:
  implicit, 28
  subliminal, 28
Personal Health Improvement Program, Harvard
    Pilgrim Health Care, 86
Phantom-limb pain, biofeedback and, 117
Phobias, 27, 361, 363, 364, 370. See also
    Social phobias
PHQ, xvii
Physical symptoms, emotionally derived, 19
Physical therapy:
  active, 266
  fibromyalgia and, 329, 330
  passive, 266
Physician assistant education programs:
  accredited, 458
  general philosophy, 458
  hallmarks, 458
  versus physician education programs, 458-459
Physician assistant services, 459
Physician assistants (PAs), 457
  as patient education resource, 460
  own experiences with mind-body therapies, 463
  professional roles, 463-464
  required knowledge/skills, 458-459
  use of mind-body approaches, 457
Physician education, 4
Physiotherapy, fibromyalgia and, 329
Placebo effect, 457, 461, 464
  chemical treatments, 70, 71
  conditioned response model, 72
  definition, 69-70
  empirical efficacy of, 70-72
  in biofeedback therapy, 69-77
  maximizing, 76-77
  Prozac and, 69-70
  psychological therapy, 70, 71
  surgical treatment, 70
  theories, 72
  See also Conditioned response model; Conditioned
    responses; Placebos
Placebo learning, 73, 76-77
Placebos:
  ethical issues, 117
  in healing, 9
  uses, 70
  See also Placebo effects

Polarity therapy, 62, 64
Polypharmacy, adverse effects of, 7
Possession, 197
Possession trance, 197
Posttraumatic conditions, 4, 6
Posttraumatic stress disorder (PTSD), 6, 47, 364, 370
  high hypnotic ability and, 153
  symptom intensity, 22
Practice standards, 93-94
  role, 94
Prayer, 12, 13, 50, 58, 483, 484
  wellness and, 478
  See also Religiosity
Pregnancy, sleep disorders and, 403
Premenstrual dysphoric disorder (PMDD), 419, 427
  anatomy/physiology and, 423, 427
  cultural influences, 420, 427
  major depression and, 422
  patterns of symptom activity, 419-420
  physiological influences, 420, 427
  prevalence, 419, 427
  psychological influences, 420, 427
  screening/diagnostic assessment, 420-423
  social influences, 420, 427
  versus depression, 423
Premenstrual dysphoric disorder (PMDD),
    treatments/interventions for:
  alternative, 424-426
  asymmetry training, 424
  audiovisual stimulation, 424
  cognitive therapy, 419, 424, 427
  dietary changes, 419
  electromagnetic stimulation, 424
  lifestyle/behavioral, 424, 427
  light therapy, 424
  neurofeedback training, 424
  nutritional supplements, 419, 424
  pharmacological, 423, 427
  SSRIs and, 423, 427
  stress management training, 419
  vitamins, 424
Premenstrual syndrome (PMS), 419, 427
  anatomy/physiology and, 423, 427
  cultural influences, 420, 427
  physiological influences, 420, 427
  prevalence, 419, 427
  psychological influences, 420, 427
  screening/diagnostic assessment, 420-422
  social influences, 420, 427
  symptoms, 419
Premenstrual syndrome (PMS),
    treatment/interventions for:
  cognitive therapy, 419, 425, 426, 427
  dietary changes, 419, 426
  effective nonpharmacological, 426
  lifestyle/behavioral, 425-426, 427
  nutritional supplements, 419
  pharmacological, 423, 427
  stress management training, 419

Premenstrual Tension Scales, 420
Primary care:
  as academic discipline, 84
  challenging problems, 4-7
  core attributes, xi, xv
  definition, xi
  evolution of, 87-88
  functional integration of mind-body
    medicine and, 89-90
  future, 88-89
  mental health and, xi, 83
  psychiatry and, 86-87
  scientific/intellectual basis, xi-xiii
  society's obligation, ix
  visits for mind-body disorders, 467, 472
  *See also* Primary care practice
Primary care physicians, mental health
    education of, 90
Primary care practice, exactitude versus
    ambiguity in, 85-86
PRIME-MD, xvii, 43, 47, 48
Problem-solving therapy, 168
Proctalgia fugax:
  diagnostic requirements, 302
Professional culture:
  physician versus psychologists, 12
Progressive muscle relaxation, 110, 137,
    139, 145, 148
  anxiety disorders and, 370
  fibromyalgia and, 329
  irritable bowel syndrome and, 306
  sleep disorders and, 396
  specific effects, 138
  stress management and, 138, 305
  treatment protocol, 140-144
Prospective Record of the Impact and Severity of
    Menstruation (PRISM), 420
  symptoms listed, 422
Psychiatric disorders, menstrual cycle and, 421
Psychiatry:
  lack of unifying theory, 60-61
  primary care and, 86-87
Psychoneuroimmunological (PNI) paradigm, 196, 450
Psychophysiological disorders, 4, 5-6, 19
  risk factors, 19
  *See also specific types of psychophysiological
    disorders*
Psychophysiological Stress Profile (PSP), 365, 367
  format, 366
Psychosocial stress, 4
Psychosomatic illness:
  CBT treatment protocol, 176
Psychotherapy, 58, 61
  back pain and, 266, 270
  biofeedback and, 10
  choosing right, 387-388
  hypnosis and, 156, 157-158
  mood disorders and, 384
Pulmonary disease, 430

QEEG assessment, 65, 66, 123, 124, 128
  normative databases, 127
Qigong, 13, 14, 62, 64, 65

Rational emotive behavior therapy, 168
Raynaud's disease, biofeedback and, 116, 117
Reflexology, chronic illness and, 437
Reiki, 59, 64, 65
Relaxation exercises, 481
  and "letting go," 478, 480
Relaxation techniques, 51, 37-138, 140, 147-148
  teaching, 139
  *See also specific relaxation techniques*
Relaxation therapy:
  anxiety disorders and, 359, 366, 371
  mood disorders and, 387
  *See also* Relaxation training
Relaxation training, 444
  anxiety disorders and, 370
  asthma and, 235, 241-242
  by physician assistants, 457, 461
  chronic fatigue syndrome and, 339
  fibromyalgia and, 329
  headaches and, 213, 215
  migraines and, 213
  procedures, 215
  progressive, 288-289
  rheumatoid arthritis and, 407, 413, 414
  sleep disorders and, 393, 396
  tension headaches and, 213
Religiosity:
  as coping mechanism, 482
  negative aspects, 485
  wellness and, 196, 477, 478, 483-485, 486
  *See also* African American churches; Prayer
Religious experiences, dramatic, 193-194
Religious signs/symbols, 193
Respiratory resistance biofeedback, asthma and, 243
Respiratory sinus arrhythmia (RSA) biofeedback, 113
  asthma and, 243
  hypertension and, 291
Rheumatoid arthritis, 407, 414
  cardiovascular complications, 408
  characteristics, 407, 414
  cognitive beliefs/psychological processes
    and, 410-411
  Epstein-Barr virus and, 407
  fatigue and, 409, 414
  gender and, 407, 408
  genetic factors, 407
  menstrual cycle and, 421
  parvovirus and, 407
  pathophysiology, 407-408
  prevalence, 407, 414
  sleep disturbances and, 409
  work-related disability and, 413
Rheumatoid arthritis, diagnosing, 409
  classification criteria, 410
  functional status classification, 410

laboratory tests, 409
pattern of joint involvement, 409
symptoms, 409
x-rays, 409
Rheumatoid arthritis, treatments/interventions for, 407, 414
cognitive-behavioral therapy, 407, 411-414
economic outcomes, 413-414
NSAIDs, 413-414
patient education, 407, 412, 413, 414
relaxation training, 407, 413, 414
treatment outcomes, 413
Rolfing, 64
Rome criteria, 301
Rome II criteria, 301

SABRES model, 255
Sahrmann muscle work, fibromyalgia and, 329
Scanning, 65
Science of Unitary Human Beings, 449
Seasonal affective disorder (SAD), 389
audiovisual entrainment and, 389
light therapy and, 403
sleep disorders and, 403
Seizure disorders,neurotherapy and, 123, 127-128, 129-130
Seizures, menstrual cycle and, 421
Self-efficacy, 10
Self-hypnosis:
fibromyalgia and, 329
sleep disorders and, 396
Self-management therapy, 168
SEMG biofeedback, 270, 271
fibromyalgia and, 329
SEMG testing, 265, 267, 268-269, 271
fibromyalgia and, 325, 326, 328
studies, 265
See also SEMG biofeedback
Sensory restriction, 74
Sick role, 45
Sleep:
neurophysiology, 393-394
non-REM, 393-394
REM, 393, 394
Sleep deprivation, impact of, 394
Sleep disorders, 393
advanced sleep phase syndrome, 399
cataplexy, 397
delayed sleep phase syndrome, 399
diagnosis of, 404
gender and, 393
hormone replacement therapy and, 393
hypnogogic hallucination, 397
nightmares, 401
night terrors, 400
nocturnal leg cramps, 400
non-24-hour sleep-wake disorder, 399
prevalence, 393
REM sleep behavior disorder, 401

rhythmic movement disorder, 400
sleep paralysis, 397, 401
sleep starts, 400
sleep talking, 400
sleep walking, 400
See also Dyssomnias; Parasomnias; Sleep disorders, classification of
Sleep disorders, classification of, 395
mental/neurological/medical-related, 395, 401-404
See also Dyssomnias; Parasomnias
Sleep disorders, treatments/interventions for, 393
behavioral, 401
behavioral sleep hygiene, 393
chronotherapies, 399-400
cognitive behavioral therapy, 393, 396
CPAP, 397-398
deep breathing, 396
EMG biofeedback, 396
HRT, 404
light therapy, 403
medication, 397
meditation, 396
melatonin, 400
progressive muscle relaxation, 396
relaxation training, 393, 396
self-hypnosis, 396
sleep restriction therapy, 393, 396
stimulus control therapy, 393, 396
Sleep learning, 28
Smoking cessation, acupuncture and, 184
cognitive-behavior therapy and, 168
Social information processing, 28
Social isolation:
as CAD risk, 154
Social phobias, 361, 362
PMS and, 422
Society for Clinical and Experimental Hypnosis, 158
Society for Neuronal Regulation (SNR), 66
Society of Clinical Psychology Task Force on Promotion and Dissemination of Psychological Procedures, 128
Somatic complaints, absorption and, 155
Somatic disorders, risk factors and, 19, 22
blocking consciousness, 22-28
high hypnotic ability, 21, 22, 29
low hypnotic ability, 21, 22, 29
Marlowe-Crowne scale score, 21, 22, 29
See also specific somatic disorders; High hypnotizables; Low hypnotizables; Marlowe-Crowne high scoring people; Somatoform patients
Somatic symptoms, chronic:
high hypnotic ability and, 153
Somatic symptoms, psychiatric disorder, 4, 6-7. See also Anxiety disorders; Depressive disorders
Somatization, xv-xvi, 6, 19, 21, 85
functional bowel/anorectal disorders and, 300
Somatization disorder, 4, 5
Somatization symptoms, 6

Somatizing patients, 85
   challenge of treating, 19-21
   *See also* Somatoform patients
Somatoform disorders, 19. *See also* Somatic disorders,
    risk factors and; Somatizing patients;
    Somatoform patients
Somatoform patients, 20, 21. *See also* Somatizing
    patients; Somatoform patients, risk factors and
Somatoform patients, risk factors and:
   high hypnotic ability, 21
   low hypnotic ability, 21
   Marlowe-Crowne scale score, 21
   testing for, 29-30
   *See also* High risk model of threat perception;
     Somatic disorders, risk factors and;
     Somatoform patients
Somatoform patients, treating, 30, 32
   Trojan horse role induction and, 30
Spielberger State-Trait Anger Expression
    Inventory, 253
Spielberger State-Trait Anxiety Inventory, 367
Spindrift Institute, 484
Spirit communication, 193
Spiritual addiction, 199
Spiritual ambition, 199
Spiritual concepts, 478, 482
Spiritual counselors, 4
Spiritual crises, 194
Spiritual disciplines, 483
Spiritual Emergence Network, 193
Spiritual experiences, 478, 485
   versus psychotic experiences, 194
Spirituality, 191, 199
   African Americans and, 192
   life wisdom and, 482-483
   versus religion, 191-192
   wellness and, 477, 486
   *See also* Spirituality, healing and
Spirituality, healing and, 12, 13, 191-199
   classification/diagnostic issues, 197-199
   documented applications, 195-197
Spiritual liturgies, 478, 482
Spiritually well person, 195
Spiritual music, 482, 483
Spiritual psychotherapy, 195
Spiritual symbols, 192, 478, 482
Spiritual texts, 478, 482, 483
   Judaic-Christian, 481
Spiritual traditions, 478
Stages of change, 434-437
   action, 435, 436
   contemplation, 435
   maintenance, 435, 436
   precontemplation, 435
   preparation, 435, 436
   strategies/techniques, 435-437
Standard of care, minimum, 99
Stanford Hypnotic Susceptibility Scale Form, 32
State hypnotic ability, 75

State-Trait Anxiety Inventory, 484
Stepped care, individualized, 433-434, 437, 438
Stress:
   cancer and, 137
   cortisol levels and, 46-47
   development/maintenance of physical disorders
    and, 45-47
   heart disease and, 137
   high blood pressure and, 46, 137
   illness and, 137
   immune system response to, 46
   low blood pressure and, 46
   outpatient physician visits and, 137
Stress-diathesis model, 5
Stress disorders, acute, 364
Stress management, 52
   diabetes and, 289
   PMS and, 419
Stress management education, 6, 372
Stress management training, 305
   biofeedback and, 305
   cognitive therapy and, 305
   hypnosis and, 305
   *See also* Autogenic training; Progressive muscle
    relaxation
Stress-related illness, treating, 50-51
Strokes, neurotherapy and, 66, 131
Substance abuse, 22
   high hypnotic ability and, 153
Substance abuse cessation, acupuncture and, 184
Symptom Check List, 32
Symptom Check List-90-R, 330
Systemic lupus erythematosus, menstrual
    cycle and, 421

Tai chi, 13, 14
Talk therapists, 63
Tart, C., 481
Temperature biofeedback (TEMP), 111-112
   headaches and, 116
   hypertension and, 117
   Raynaud's disease and, 116
Temporomandibular disorders (TMD), 223
   age effects, 225
   assessment/differential diagnosis standards,
    227-229, 231
   clinical signs/symptoms, 223
   gender effects, 225
   initiation factors, 225
   insurance coverage and, 227
   patient education information for, 230
   prevalence, 225
   progression factors, 225
   *Research Diagnostic Criteria (RDC)* for,
    224-225, 227, 228, 229
   tests, 229
   typical symptom profile, 226-227
   *See also* TMD patients, psychological/behavioral
    profile of

Temporomandibular disorders (TMD),
    behavioral/psychosocial intervention literature
    on, 229-231
Temporomandibular joint (TMJ), 223, 226
    biofeedback and dysfunction of, 117
    dysfunction, 22
    imaging, 229
    medical profile, 223-225
Tension-type headaches, 205
    chronic, 207
    diagnostic criteria, 208
    episodic, 207, 209
    pathophysiology of, 207-208
Therapeutic touch, 57, 62, 449, 454
    for stress-related diseases, 65
Therapist-intensive interventions, 51-52
Thermal biofeedback, 305
    anxiety disorders and, 370
    hypertension and, 290, 291
    irritable bowel syndrome and, 306
Thermal biofeedback-assisted relaxation:
    diabetes and, 289
    headaches and, 216
    migraines and, 213
Thought:
    unattended, 28
    unintended, 28
Threat perception. See High risk model of threat
    perception
Tinnitus, biofeedback and, 117
TMD patients, psychological/behavioral profile of,
    225-226
Traditional Chinese Medicine (TCM), 14, 57,
    58, 59, 64, 66
    depression and, 64-65
    meridians, 181, 182-184
    qi, 181, 182
Traditional Chinese philosophy, 481
Traditional healers, 192

Trait hypnotic ability, 72-73, 75, 151
    biofeedback and, 75
Trance, 197
Treatment compliance, 7
Trojan horse role induction, 19, 30, 35, 341
    case study, 32-35
    treating somatoform patients, 30, 32
Type D personality, 49

U.S. Food and Drug Administration, 181
Undifferentiated complaints, 4, 5
United Health Foundation, 85
Universal health care:
    coverage, 89
    dispute, ix
Urticaria, chronic, 22

Vasovagal syncope, 22, 30
Virtue ethics, 94, 99. See also Virtues
Virtues, 99-102
    compassion and caring, 101
    integrity, 100
    prudence, 100
    respectfulness, 100-101
    trustworthiness, 101-102
Visual imaging, 139
Visualization, fibromyalgia and, 329

Wellness checkups, 47-48
World Medical Association:
    Declaration of Helsinki, 117

Yale-Brown Obsessive-Compulsive Scale, 367
Yoga, 12, 13, 51, 58
    asthma and, 243
    diabetes and, 289
Yoga teachers, 4

Zen monks, 485

# About the Editors

**Donald Moss,** Ph.D., is a partner in West Michigan Behavioral Health Services, adjunct graduate faculty for Saybrook Graduate School, San Francisco, and mental health director for the humanitarian Trelawny Outreach Project in Western Jamaica. He is president of the Association for Applied Psychophysiology and Biofeedback, editor of *Biofeedback,* and consulting editor for the *Journal of Neurotherapy.* He serves on advisory boards for the Advanced Learning Foundation in Colorado, BioCom Technologies of Seattle, Washington, and the Behavioral Medicine Research and Training Foundation of Suquamish, Washington. Dr. Moss's third book, *Humanistic and Transpersonal Psychology,* was released in 1998, and he has published numerous book chapters and journal articles on humanistic psychology, philosophy of medicine, anxiety disorders, and behavioral medicine.

**Angele McGrady,** Ph.D., is professor of psychiatry and adjunct professor of physiology and molecular medicine at the Medical College of Ohio in Toledo. Dr. McGrady is the past president of the Association for Applied Psychophysiology and Biofeedback and is an editor of the journal *Applied Psychophysiology and Biofeedback.* In addition, she is a reviewer for *Physiology and Behavior* and *Diabetes Care* and the author of numerous journal articles applying physiological research methodology to chronic medical conditions, such as diabetes and hypertension.

**Terence C. Davies,** MD, is professor and chair of family and community medicine at Eastern Virginia Medical School, and a practicing family physician. He is the Glennan Endowed Chair of Generalist Medicine at EVMS. Dr. Davies has a special interest in behavioral medicine interventions in primary care settings and established a division of behavioral medicine in his department three years ago.

**Ian Wickramasekera,** Ph.D., ABPP, ABPH, is past president of the Association for Applied Psychophysiology and Biofeedback and was cofounder of AAPB's primary care section. Dr. Wickramasekera developed the high risk model of threat perception, an empirical approach to the diagnosis and treatment of psychophysiological disorders. He is the author of *Clinical Behavioral Medicine* as well as more than 80 articles and book chapters on topics ranging from hypnosis to psychophysiological psychotherapy and somatization disorder.

# About the Contributors

**Elsa Baehr**, Ph.D., is a clinical associate in the Department of Psychiatry and Behavioral Science at Northwestern University Medical School. She is also a consultant to the outpatient Mental Health Clinic at the Lakeside Veterans Administration. She is the director of the NeuroQuest Clinic in Evanston, Illinois, where she shares a private practice with her husband, Dr. Rufus Baehr. She published research on brain-wave asymmetry and depression, and coauthored two chapters on depression. She has presented at professional meetings sponsored by the Association for Applied Psychophysiology and Biofeedback, the Society for Neuronal Regulation, and Future Health.

**Barbara Bailey**, RN, MSN, CDE, earned her BSN in 1979 from the University of Toledo and her MSN in 1984 from the Medical College of Ohio in Toledo. She is a diabetes nurse educator for St. Vincent Mercy Medical Center in Toledo and serves as coinvestigator in several research studies about biofeedback, stress, and diabetes mellitus.

**Steven M. Baskin**, Ph.D., is the director of the New England Institute for Behavioral Medicine in Stamford, Connecticut, and an attending psychologist in neurology and psychiatry at Greenwich Hospital of Yale-New Haven Health. He is currently the treasurer of the Association of Applied Psychophysiology and Biofeedback and is a former board member at large of the American Headache Society. He has authored numerous scientific papers and chapters on primary headache disorders.

**Kusum Bhat**, Ph.D., is the clinical director of Cybernetix Medical Institute in Concord, California. Her doctoral thesis at the American School of Professional Psychology was titled *The Role of Biofeedback Assisted Anger Control in Reversing Heart Disease*. She treats coronary heart patients using cognitive behavioral methods, including biofeedback, and works as a mental health clinical specialist at Contra Costa County Hospital. She is also a certified physician assistant from the University of California at San Diego.

**Naras Bhat**, MD, is a board-certified specialist in internal medicine and a certified specialist in stress management education. He is a professor of behavioral medicine at Rosebridge College of Integrative Psychology and teaches at the University of California at Berkeley. Dr. Bhat is the author of the book *How to Reverse and Prevent Heart Disease and Cancer* and has produced two popular videos, *Uprooting Anger* and *Meditation Prescription*.

**Raymond Bourey**, MD, is a clinical assistant professor of medicine at The Medical College of Ohio. He has a background in cell biology research as well as subspecialty training in applied physiology, endocrinology, diabetes, metabolism, and sleep medicine. He has studied the basis of the metabolic syndrome and insulin resistance at the molecular level as well as in human studies. Most recently, Dr. Bourey has turned his efforts toward clarification of the impact of sleep apnea and sleep deprivation on the metabolic syndrome. He currently applies his research as an internal medicine physician in primary care.

**Cheryl Bourguignon**, Ph.D., RN, is an assistant professor and a research fellow in complementary and alternative medicine at the Center for the Study of Complementary and Alternative Therapies at the University of Virginia School of Nursing. Her current studies investigate the effects of sex hormones on symptoms (pain, fatigue, sleep disturbance, mood), stress reactivity, functional status, and inflammation in pre- and postmenopausal women with rheumatoid arthritis. Dr. Bourguignon is currently expanding her research to investigating the effectiveness of relaxation, imagery, and other complementary practices and products in improving the symptoms, stress, inflammation, and functional status in women with rheumatoid arthritis.

**Patricia Carrington**, Ph.D., is a clinical professor of psychiatry at the University of Medicine and Dentistry of New Jersey, Robert Wood Johnson Medical School. She has authored more than 35 research and theoretical papers in psychological and psychiatric journals on the topics of sleep and dream research, modern meditation techniques, and the new meridian-based desensitization methods. She is the author of five books: *Freedom in Meditation*, *Releasing*, *The Clinically Standardized Meditation Instructors Course*, *The Power of Letting Go*, and *The Book of Meditation*.

**Robert W. Collins**, Ph.D., has published scientific and review articles on enuresis and encopresis. He recently published *The Dry Bed Manual* for bed wetters and *The Clean Kid Manual* for soiling children, which are available from his website at www.soilingsolutions.com. He has recently retired from office practice. Dr. Collins has been president of the Michigan Psychological Association and the Michigan Society of Behavioral Medicine and Biofeedback.

**Margaret Davies**, MD, is a professor of family and community medicine at Eastern Virginia Medical School. She is assistant dean of student affairs at EVMS and pioneered an innovative student wellness program that has received national attention. Dr. Davies is a practicing family physician and has special interests in family issues and in training medical students, medical residents, and physicians to address psychosocial problems that affect the health and well-being of primary care patients.

**Frank V. deGruy, III,** MD, is the Woodward-Chisholm Professor and chair of the Department of Family Medicine at the University of Colorado School of Medicine. He has been researching and writing about mind-body problems, particularly mental health problems in the primary care setting, for 20 years. Dr. deGruy has been funded by the National Institute of Mental Health to study somatization in primary care and has served as a grant reviewer for the NIMH's Services Research Grant Review Group. Currently, he is chair of the National Advisory Committee of the Robert Wood Johnson Depression in Primary Care Program.

**C. C. Stuart Donaldson,** Ph.D., is a psychologist in private practice in Calgary, Alberta, Canada. He is the director of a multidisciplinary pain treatment and rehabilitation center and a pioneer in the field of surface EMG and chronic pain. His recent work has involved the integration of SEMG, quantitative EEG, and chronic pain. Dr. Donaldson has published extensively on biofeedback and chronic pain.

**Jonathan M. Feldman,** MS, is currently pursuing his Ph.D. in clinical psychology at Rutgers University and completing a predoctoral internship in the Department of Psychiatry and Behavioral Sciences at the University of Washington School of Medicine. Mr. Feldman has been conducting research on comorbidity between psychiatric disease and asthma as well as identifying behavioral factors that can complicate asthma self-management. He is the principal investigator on a National Institute of Mental Health predoctoral fellowship examining the impact of panic disorder on asthma. His clinical expertise is in cognitive-behavioral treatment for anxiety and mood disorders.

**Annabaker Garber,** Ph.D., R.N., is currently an associate editor with *Milliman Care Guidelines,* a division of Milliman USA. Her background includes a Ph.D. in physiological psychology and a master's in psychosocial nursing. Her career includes research faculty experience working on three grants, including one as a coprincipal investigator at the University of Washington School of Nursing. Dr. Garber has developed and taught professional training programs in psychophysiology, had a private practice, and, as the clinical director for a medical device manufacturer, designed and published psychophysiology treatment protocols. Her areas of expertise are behavioral treatment for stress-related disorders and psychophysiology.

**Richard Gevirtz,** Ph.D., is a professor in the health psychology program at the California School of Professional Psychology, Alliant International University,

San Diego. He has been involved in research and clinical work in applied psychophysiology for the last 25 years, with primary interests in understanding the physiological and psychological mediators involved in disorders such as chronic muscle pain, gastrointestinal pain, fibromyalgia, chronic fatigue syndrome, panic disorder, and functional cardiac disorder. Dr. Gevirtz is the author of many journal articles and chapters on these topics.

**Nicholas Giardino, Ph.D.**, is a postdoctoral fellow in the Department of Rehabilitation Medicine at the University of Washington School of Medicine. His research focuses on respiratory psychophysiology in chronic respiratory diseases, such as asthma and chronic obstructive pulmonary disease, and functional somatic syndromes, such as chronic fatigue syndrome and chemical intolerance. Dr. Giardino also performs clinical and epidemiological research in the area of comorbid psychological and chronic respiratory disorders. His clinical work focuses on behavioral and psychophysiological interventions for chronic respiratory disease and pain.

**Christopher D. Gilbert, Ph.D.**, is a licensed psychologist who since 1974 has used biofeedback as an aid in treating psychophysiological and anxiety disorders. He received his doctorate in psychology from Michigan State University and until recently taught psychology at Ramapo College of New Jersey. He is coauthor of *Multidisciplinary Approaches to Breathing Pattern Disorders*, is on the international advisory board of the *Journal of Bodywork and Movement Therapies*, has written several articles on hyperventilation, and edits the newsletter of the International Society for the Advancement of Respiratory Psychophysiology. Dr. Gilbert is now associated with the chronic pain management program of the Kaiser Permanente Medical Center in San Francisco.

**Alan G. Glaros, Ph.D.**, is the Beulah McCollum Professor of Dentistry at the University of Missouri-Kansas City in the Department of Dental Public Health and Behavioral Science. He has held positions in the Department of Psychology at Wayne State University and the Department of Clinical and Health Psychology at the University of Florida. Dr. Glaros maintains an active clinical and research program in temporomandibular disorders.

**Robert W. Jarski, Ph.D., PA-C**, is the founder and director of the complementary medicine and wellness program at Oakland University in Rochester, Michigan. Dr. Jarski completed specialized training in behavioral medicine at the Harvard Medical School and is formally trained in interactive guided imagery and mindfulness meditation. He received a major research grant from the Michigan Department of Public Health to study stress management and has served as a grant project reviewer for the National Institutes of Health National Center for Complementary and Alternative Medicine. Dr. Jarski is a referee and editorial board member of several professional journals, has published numerous articles in scientific journals and books, and is a hospice volunteer. His expertise lies in education for health and healing from the curricular level, where students consciously learn, to the cellular level, where the body learns to heal itself.

**Stanley Krippner, Ph.D.,** is professor of psychology at Saybrook Graduate School, San Francisco. He is a fellow of the American Psychological Association, the American Psychological Society, the American Society of Clinical Hypnosis, and the International Society for Clinical and Experimental Hypnosis, and past president of two divisions of the American Psychological Association. Dr. Krippner is coauthor of *The Mythic Path*, editor of *Dreamtime and Dreamwork*, and coeditor of *Varieties of Anomalous Experience*, recently published by the American Psychological Association.

**James Lake, MD,** is a board-certified psychiatrist with long-standing interests in the interface between mental health and culture and in the philosophical and scientific perspectives of different systems of medicine as they pertain to diagnosis and treatment of psychiatric disorders. Presently, he is in private practice in Pacific Grove, California, where he integrates conventional biomedical therapies and evidence-based alternative therapies for adult psychiatric disorders. Dr. Lake was recently selected to create and chair a committee on complementary and integrative medicine at a private hospital in Monterey with the goal of introducing complementary and integrative treatments into the hospital setting and affiliated clinics. From 1999 through 2000, he was an attending physician at Stanford University Hospital, where he consulted on psychiatric cases in the Complementary Medicine Clinic.

**Charles W. Lapp, MD,** is director of the Hunter-Hopkins Center and assistant consulting professor in community and family medicine at Duke University. He is a diplomate of the American Boards of Internal Medicine, Pediatrics, and Independent Medical Examiners, and is a fellow of the American Academies of Pediatrics, Family Physicians, and Disability Evaluating Physicians. Dr. Lapp has published extensively on the neurobiology, assessment, and treatment of chronic fatigue syndrome.

**Mark A. Lau, Ph.D.,** is a psychologist at the Cognitive Behaviour Therapy Unit at the Centre for Addiction and Mental Health in Toronto and is an assistant professor in the Department of Psychiatry at the University of Toronto. He has an active interest in cognitive-behavioral therapy training and supervision and a nationally funded program of research interests investigating the role played by inhibitory deficits in depressive thinking styles. Dr. Lau is a founding fellow of the Academy of Cognitive therapy.

**Leonard Lausten, DDS,** is an associate professor in the Department of Dental Public Health and Behavioral Science and director of the Special Patient Care Center at the University of Missouri–Kansas City School of Dentistry. He has served on the faculty at Marquette University, where he also directed the advanced education program in general dentistry and taught in the oral medicine program. Dr. Lausten maintains a clinical practice serving patients with temporomandibular disorders and those who are medically compromised or have dental fears.

**Theodore J. La Vaque**, Ph.D., has graduate and postgraduate education in both physiological psychology and clinical psychology. He was a research associate in behavioral neuroendocrinology at the West Side Veterans Administration Hospital in Chicago and assistant professor in the Department of Psychiatry at Abraham Lincoln School of Medicine, University of Illinois. Dr. La Vaque has been in private practice since 1975 and is currently the director of the Clinical Psychophysiology Center, Rogers Memorial Hospital, Milwaukee, Wisconsin. He is also an associate editor of *Biofeedback,* the newsmagazine of the Association of Applied Psychophysiology and Biofeedback.

**Debra E. Lyon**, RN, Ph.D., is an assistant professor in the School of Nursing and a postdoctoral fellow in the CAM Research Training Program in the Center for the Study of Complementary and Alternative Therapies at the University of Virginia. Her scholarly articles have appeared in several journals, including *Journal of the Association of Nurses in AIDS Care, Journal of School Nursing, Issues in Mental Health, Applied Nursing Research,* and *Journal of Nursing Scholarship.* Dr. Lyon has also written book chapters, including one on women as individuals in *Women's Health: A Relational Perspective Across the Lifespan.*

**Paul Lehrer**, Ph.D., is a clinical psychologist and professor of psychiatry, at the University of Medicine and Dentistry of New Jersey, Robert Wood Johnson Medical School, where he directs the Center for Stress Management and Behavioral Medicine. He also is professor of psychology at Rutgers University, where he teaches in the graduate clinical psychology program. His research interests are in respiratory psychophysiology, cardiovascular variability, and the interrelationships among anxiety disorders, disordered breathing, and somatization disorder. He has published more than a hundred scientific papers on these topics and is senior editor of the book *Principles and Practice of Stress Management*, which is now in its second edition. He is president-elect of the Association for Applied Psychophysiology and Feedback.

**Joel F. Lubar**, Ph.D., is professor of psychology at the University of Tennessee. He has published more than a hundred papers, many book chapters, and eight books in the areas of neuroscience and applied psychophysiology. He is president of the EEG division of the Association for Applied Psychophysiology and Biofeedback and was the president of AAPB in 1995–1996. He was responsible for developing the use of EEG biofeedback (neurofeedback) as a treatment modality for children, adolescents, and adults with attention deficit hyperactivity disorder, starting with controlled studies in the mid-1970s. Dr. Lubar is currently developing databases for the assessment of individuals with ADD/HD and is the scientific advisor and developer for several controlled multicenter studies evaluating the effectiveness of neurofeedback.

**Olafur S. Palsson,** Psy.D., is a licensed clinical psychologist. He completed a two-year postdoctoral fellowship in behavioral medicine at the University of North Carolina at Chapel Hill. From 1996 to 2000, Dr. Palsson was director of behavioral medicine and assistant professor of psychiatry and family medicine at Eastern Virginia Medical School, where he conducted clinical work and research in mind-body medicine and taught medical students and family medicine residents. He is currently a research associate in the division of digestive diseases and nutrition at UNC-Chapel Hill, treats patients with psychophysiological disorders, and conducts research on functional gastrointestinal disorders.

**J. Peter Rosenfeld,** Ph.D., is a professor of psychology, neurobiology, and physiology at Northwestern University and is past president of the Association for Applied Psychophysiology and Biofeedback. He serves on the editorial board for the journals *Applied Psychophysiology and Biofeedback* and *International Journal of Rehabilitation and Health* and has served as consulting editor for numerous scientific journals. His research has recently focused on the detection of brain signatures for false memories, the detection of deception and malingering through patterns in event-related brain-wave amplitudes, and the asymmetry protocol for the neurofeedback treatment of depression.

**Zindel V. Segal,** Ph.D., is head of the Cognitive Behaviour Therapy Unit at the Centre for Addiction and Mental Health in Toronto. At the University of Toronto, he is a professor in the Departments of Psychiatry and Psychology and head of psychotherapy research for the psychotherapy program in the Department of Psychiatry. He holds the Morgan Firestone Chair in Psychotherapy. Dr. Segal is a founding fellow of the Academy of Cognitive Therapy and is an associate editor for *Cognitive Therapy and Research.*

**Gabriel E. Sella,** MD, is a physician specializing in family and preventive medicine as well as occupational disability and pain management. His research and teaching focus on muscle physiology, electromyographic assessment, and biofeedback. He has published 10 textbooks and more than 80 articles and has given over 250 professional presentations and seminars nationally and internationally. Dr. Sella is a board member of the SEMG Society of North America and the American Academy of Pain Management and has seven fellowships and three board certifications. He is particularly interested in the subject of myofascial pain and its treatment, with special emphasis on EMG assessment and neuromuscular reeducation.

**Mahmood Siddique,** DO, FACP, FCCP, is a clinical assistant professor of medicine in the division of pulmonary and critical care medicine at University of Medicine and Dentistry of New Jersey, Robert Wood Johnson Medical School. He is in private practice in Hamilton, New Jersey. Dr. Siddique completed residency in internal medicine at the Robert Wood Johnson Medical School and a fellowship in pulmonary and critical care medicine at Case Western Reserve University. He is board certified in internal medicine, and pulmonary and critical care medicine and specializes in sleep medicine. He is currently an advisory committee member of the Global Initiative for Asthma.

**Emanuel Stein**, MD, is professor of family and community medicine and internal medicine at Eastern Virginia Medical School. He is a diplomate of the American Board of Internal Medicine, a diplomate of the subspecialty Board of Cardiovascular Disease, and a fellow of the American College of Physicians, the American College of Chest Physicians, and the American College of Cardiology. Dr. Stein also holds a master's degree in public health from Columbia University and has served as clinical cardiologist, educator, researcher, and administrator. His books have been translated into French, German, Indonesian, Italian, Japanese, and Spanish. Dr. Stein is licensed to practice acupuncture in Virginia.

**Sebastian Striefel**, Ph.D., became a professor emeritus in the Department of Psychology at Utah State University in September 2000. For 26 years, he taught graduate-level courses in ethics and professional conduct, clinical applications of biofeedback, clinical applications of relaxation training, and behavior therapy. As the director of the division of services at the Center for Persons with Disabilities at Utah State University, Dr. Striefel managed a variety of programs, including an outpatient clinic, a biofeedback lab, and an early intervention program. He is past president of the Association of Applied Psychophysiology and Biofeedback, current president of the neurofeedback division of AAPB, and secretary/treasurer of the international section of AAPB. In addition, he writes an ongoing ethics column and conducts workshops on ethics, standards, and professional conduct.

**Diana Taibi**, MSN, RN, is a doctoral student in nursing at the University of Virginia. As a research assistant, she works closely with Dr. Cheryl Bourguignon on research investigating changes in pain, sleep, mood, and fatigue over the menstrual cycle in women with rheumatoid arthritis. Ms. Taibi will continue to focus on pain and symptom management in rheumatoid arthritis as a doctoral student and predoctoral trainee at the Center for the Study of Complementary and Alternative Therapies at the University of Virginia School of Nursing.

**Ann Gill Taylor**, MS, Ed.D., FAAN, is the Betty Norman Norris Professor of Nursing and director of the Center for the Study of Complementary and Alternative Therapies at the University of Virginia. As part of her 30-year focus on academic nursing, she developed the critical care master's program in nursing at the University of Virginia. Dr. Taylor has published numerous journal articles and book chapters on complementary and alternative therapies, therapeutic touch, and pain management. Her current research is investigating links among the musculoskeletal, vascular, neuroendocrine, and central nervous systems in fibromyalgia.

**Sharon Williams Utz,** Ph.D., RN, is associate professor and chair of the division of acute and speciality care of adults at the University of Virginia School of Nursing. Educated and experienced in the care of adults with cardiovascular conditions, she has held positions in hospitals, rehabilitation centers, and university schools of nursing. Her current research and teaching focus is on care of chronically ill adults, with a focus on self-care and cultural competence among health care providers. Awards include appointment as a University of Virginia Shannon Scholar, a scholar of the American Nurses Foundation, and two citations for papers presented at annual conferences of the Association for Applied Psychophysiology and Biofeedback. Relevant publications include articles and book chapters on care of patients with hypertension and heart attack, use of biofeedback, the self-care model, and the case-management model of care.

**Randall E. Weeks,** Ph.D., is a clinical psychologist specializing in behavioral medicine and neuropsychology. He is director of the New England Institute for Behavioral Medicine and clinical program director of the New England Heachache Treatment Program. Dr. Weeks has numerous publications in headache classification and treatment with an emphasis on the role of analgesic overuse in headache maintenance.

**Suzanne Woodward,** Ph.D., is an assistant professor of psychiatry at Wayne State University School of Medicine in Detroit. Her research interests have concentrated on sleep in women during menopause, and she is a nationally recognized expert and invited speaker in this area. She has published numerous articles and chapters on sleep in women. Dr. Woodward is a charter member of the North American Menopause Society as well as a member of the Association of Professional Sleep Societies. She has been a member of the Association for Applied Psychophysiology and Biofeedback since 1980 and has served on the board of AAPB. She is a concerned proponent of the integration of behavioral medicine into traditional medical education programs.

**Ari E. Zaretsky,** MD, received his medical degree from the University of Toronto and then completed a psychiatry residency there. He pursued a fellowship in cognitive therapy both at the Centre for Addiction and Mental Health in Toronto and Massachusetts General Hospital in Boston. Dr. Zaretsky is Head of the Cognitive Behaviour Therapy Clinic at Sunnybrook & Women's College Health Sciences Centre, and an assistant professor in the Department of Psychiatry, University of Toronto. He is a Founding Fellow of the Academy of Cognitive Therapy and has a national reputation as a teacher of cognitive therapy. He has published on supervision in cognitive therapy and on cognitive therapy for bipolar disorder and has received peer-reviewed funding from CIHR and NARSAD. His current research activities include CBT for bipolar disorder, prophylactic CBT for women at risk for postpartum depression, and CBT for HIV+ individuals.